OPHTHALMOLOGICAL IMAGING AND APPLICATIONS

Edited by

E. Y. K. Ng

U. Rajendra Acharya

Rangaraj M. Rangayyan

Jasjit S. Suri

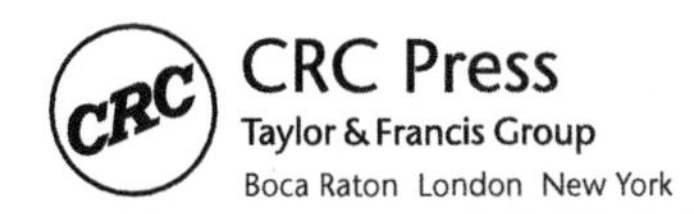

CRC Press is an imprint of the
Taylor & Francis Group, an **informa** business

CRC Press
Taylor & Francis Group
6000 Broken Sound Parkway NW, Suite 300
Boca Raton, FL 33487-2742

First issued in paperback 2017

ISBN-13: 978-1-4665-5913-4 (hbk)
ISBN-13: 978-1-138-07479-8 (pbk)

Visit the Taylor & Francis Web site at
http://www.taylorandfrancis.com

and the CRC Press Web site at
http://www.crcpress.com

Contents

Preface

The human eye is one of the most important organs and works like a camera. It is tedious and time consuming to decipher minute changes in the anatomy of the eye caused by the progression of abnormalities. The growth in image processing, artificial intelligence, high-performance computing, and modeling techniques has had a significant impact on the detection and treatment of eye diseases. Optical, digital fundus, infrared, optical coherence tomography (OCT), and Heidelberg retina tomograph images have been widely used to diagnose eye abnormalities.

This book covers wide-ranging topics such as computer-aided diagnosis of diabetic retinopathy (DR), maculopathy, glaucoma, dry eyes, cysts, imaging of the eye after glaucoma surgery, optic nerve analysis, anterior segment imaging of the eye, infrared imaging of the eye, confocal microscopy of the cornea, OCT, scanning laser ophthalmoscopy (SLO), fundus perimetry, fundus autofluorescence (FAF) imaging, in vivo confocal microscopy, hybrid finite element simulation of bioheat transfer in the human eye, and effects of electromagnetic (EM) fields on specific absorption rates. FAF is a relatively new, noninvasive imaging modality that has been developed over the past decade.

The retina provides an ideal opportunity to explore the role of microvascular pathology in the pathophysiology of cardiovascular diseases. Over the last decade, advances in retinal vascular imaging allowed the development of accurate and reliable quantitative parameters such as retinal vascular calibers. Using these parameters, several large population-based studies have shown that retinal vascular calibers are related to cardiovascular diseases.

Chapter 1 presents the clinical application of retinal vascular imaging and its limitation. Changes in the vascular structure of the retina can indicate the presence of several types of pathology, such as hypertension, arteriosclerosis, proliferative diabetic retinopathy, myopia, and retinopathy of prematurity.

Chapter 2 proposes parabolic modeling methods using the generalized Hough transform to detect, measure, and parameterize the architecture of the major temporal arcade in retinal fundus images.

An automated diagnosis system to diagnose DR using higher order spectra (HOS) cumulants with digital fundus images is proposed in Chapter 3. HOS cumulants coupled with a support vector machine yielded an accuracy rate of 97.06% in classifying normal and DR images.

Chapter 4 presents new wavelet weighted distortion measures to quantify information loss in retinal features. These measures are defined after carrying out analysis of retinal image information in different wavelet subbands. It was shown that significant information of a retinal feature was captured only in a few subbands. The analysis of retinal fundus images is an important noninvasive procedure that allows early diagnosis and effective monitoring of the response to retinopathy therapy. In order to derive a quantitative evaluation of clinical features, an accurate identification of the vessel network has to be provided.

A system for automatic extraction of the retinal vasculature based on a multidirectional graph search approach is proposed and discussed in Chapter 5.

Chapter 6 presents the usefulness of FAF in understanding the pathophysiological mechanisms, diagnostics, and identification of predictive markers for disease progression and for monitoring novel therapies. At present, DR screening in India is undertaken in various ways such as in eye camps, evaluation of the fundus of all diabetics attending eye care facilities for any ocular problem, and through telemedicine, where digital retinal images are analyzed by remotely placed experts.

Chapter 7 proposes an efficient imaging system that can be installed not only at a national-level hospital but at the grass-root level as well, such as at primary health-care units, so as to be able to image a layperson unaware of the problems related to diabetes and DR. The fundus of the eye is situated at the back of the interior of the eyeball, which can be viewed through the pupil using an ophthalmoscope.

Chapter 8 presents imaging of the ocular fundus with color photography, photography with filters, and fluorescence angiography. The diagnosis of glaucoma and monitoring its progression are challenging and difficult to the general ophthalmologist. In a setting where there is lack of glaucoma expertise, instruments that quantify reproducible parameters and are easy to interpret could improve diagnostic accuracy.

Chapter 9 presents a discussion on the strengths and weaknesses of each imaging modality which resulted in accelerated modifications to improve its efficacy. The advent of newer imaging technologies has enabled more detailed and comprehensive imaging than previously possible.

Chapter 10 provides an analysis on how morphological data provided by bleb imaging may assist in the clinical management of glaucoma patients after filtration surgery. In addition, bleb imaging may have a role in investigating novel surgical approaches. The confocal microscope is one of the wonderful innovations in recent times; it is becoming more popular every day and its indications are expanding.

Chapter 11 describes the usefulness of the confocal microscope for clinical diagnosis, follow-up, and analysis of corneal lesions. Corneal analysis has evolved with recent software technologies since the advent of the Placido's disk.

Chapter 12 describes how advancing technologies have evolved patient care to its current stage where analysis of corneal topography is part of the standard care in the present-day practice of the cornea and refractive surgeon. Retinal microcirculation can vary in the presence of retinopathies. One of the most widely used techniques for analyzing these variations is fluorescein angiography. SLO sequences are obtained of a patient in whom a fluorescent dye is injected. SLO techniques are useful for measuring biomedical metrics such as the arteriovenous passage time.

Chapter 13 deals with the application and validation of the registration approach by automatically estimating the dye dilution curves and computing arteriovenous passage time in fundus images.

OCT is widely used in imaging biological tissues such as eye, skin, and most recently blood vessels. Chapter 14 provides a brief history of OCT and its development, especially in recent years. It focuses on the applications of OCT in the ophthalmological field, newer developments in OCT technologies with a focus on research topics, and future directions of use in ocular diseases.

Chapter 15 introduces clinical and research applications of OCT to understand the anatomical structures and functions of the anterior segment of the eye. It covers the usage of anterior segment OCT (AS-OCT) in corneal and glaucoma imaging by explaining the pathophysiology of the diseases or conditions and the usefulness of AS-OCT in these conditions. AS-OCT is applicable to assess a wide variety of anterior segment conditions. As a noncontact method, AS-OCT is likely to become an essential tool for screening eye diseases like primary angle closure, corneal lesions, and lens opacity.

Information obtained via OCT could be used in the assessment of the guidelines for medical or surgical treatment and are discussed in Chapter 16. One of the retinal alterations that is present in a wide number of pathologies is cystoid macular edema. It can be easily detected using OCT, and its presence significantly affects visual function and guides the therapeutic approach to follow in the case of pathologies with intraretinal cysts.

Chapter 17 deals with the detection of cysts and their monitoring using OCT. SLO-automated fundus perimetry, also known as microperimetry, is a relatively new imaging modality bound to the study of the macular function. SLO fundus perimetry provides a quantitative assessment of the retina's sensitivity to light within the central posterior pole.

Chapter 18 focuses on the evolution of fundus perimetry technology. It also describes the features of different SLO fundus perimeters and their limitations and applicability to specific diseases. A major advantage of confocal images is providing histological information without prior staining and excising of the tissue, giving clinicians more control over diagnosis. The slit scanning in vivo confocal microscope (IVCM) is used in ophthalmology for obtaining useful information about the structure and function of the cornea and other ocular surface structures, along with quantitative diagnosis of cell morphology, cell count, and infections.

Chapter 19 provides a discussion on applications of IVCM in both the clinical setting and research. There are many tortuosity estimates that can be correlated with blood pressure. Their behavior in simplified conditions is worthy of investigation.

The finite element method was used to model blood vessels and validated experimentally in the work presented in Chapter 20. Numerical simulation of bioheat transfer in a two-dimensional human eye model including multiple material domains is performed using the newly developed fundamental solution-based hybrid finite element formulation.

In the absence of blood perfusion in the eyeball, Chapter 21 presents a method that is verified by comparing with the results of numerical methods. Consequently, the effect of the blood perfusion rate in the sclera on temperature change is investigated to study bioheat transfer behavior caused by interior heat energy exchange from the blood vessels in the sclera region into the eyeball. A two-dimensional eye model is used to simulate tissue-specific absorption rate and temperature distributions. EM wave propagation in the eye is investigated using Maxwell's equations.

An analysis of heat transfer in the eye exposed to a transverse magnetic mode of EM fields is investigated using a heat transfer model in Chapter 22. Dry eye diagnosis is difficult to perform, especially because of its multifactorial nature. Thus, there are several clinical tests to measure tear quality and quantity. Some tests assess the tear film by evaluating the interference lipid pattern.

Chapter 23 describes an automatic image-processing methodology to perform the analysis of the interference lipid pattern using Tearscope plus and Doane's interferometer as instruments to acquire tear film images. Infrared cameras are nowadays increasingly applied in medical settings, with high sensitivity and reliability, the results of which can be appreciated in a color-coded display.

Chapter 24 presents the application of infrared images to detect OST and the ocular factors influencing OST, as well as the limitations and possibilities of ocular thermography.

Many esteemed authors have contributed generously and made this book possible by their diligent hard work and valuable time. We thank them wholeheartedly for their significant contributions. The authors and their affiliations are listed in the following Contributors section.

This book covers several aspects of multimodality imaging in ophthalmology and applications. It focuses on methods and techniques for imaging and their applications in eye care. The chapters in the book cover theories and principles of imaging and present results of practical applications. They are written in simple language for easy readability and understanding.

The main purpose of this book is to present a unified work on eye imaging and modeling techniques that have been proposed and applied to ophthalmologic problems. It represents a novel and well-timed effort and is a substantial addition to literature in the field. The book also represents various applications in this area. It is unique in its focus and is of interest to researchers, students, and practitioners.

This book is intended for individuals engaged in research or in industry who are developing software incorporating elements of image processing and machine vision. It is also suitable for a graduate course on image processing and machine vision, including elements of algorithm design and performance evaluation.

E.Y.K. Ng
U. Rajendra Acharya
Rangaraj M. Rangayyan
Jasjit S. Suri

MATLAB® is a registered trademark of The MathWorks, Inc. For product information, please contact:

The MathWorks, Inc.
3 Apple Hill Drive
Natick, MA 01760-2098 USA
Tel: 508-647-7000
Fax: 508-647-7001
E-mail: info@mathworks.com
Web: www.mathworks.com

Editors

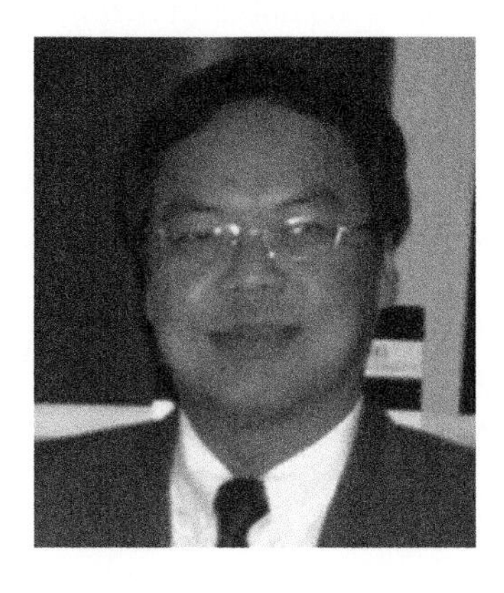

E.Y.K. Ng, PhD, earned his PhD from Cambridge University with a Cambridge Commonwealth Scholarship. His main areas of research are in thermal imaging, biomedical engineering, and computational fluid dynamics and heat transfer. He is currently an associate professor at the Nanyang Technological University in the School of Mechanical and Aerospace Engineering. Ng is a member of the Singapore Biomedical Standards Committee and an adjunct scientist at the National University Hospital. He has published more than 370 papers, including articles in refereed international Science Citation Index (SCI) journals (195) and international conference proceedings (71) as well as textbook chapters (82) and other publications (22). Dr. Ng is editor-in-chief of the *Journal of Mechanics in Medicine and Biology* and the *Journal of Medicinal Imaging and Health Informatics*. He is also the strategy associate editor-in-chief of the *World Journal of Clinical Oncology* and the associate editor of the *International Journal of Rotating Machinery; Computational Fluid Dynamics Journal; International Journal of Breast Cancer; The Journal of Chinese Medicine; Open Medical Informatics Journal; Open Numerical Methods Journal*; and the *Journal of Healthcare Engineering*. He also serves as guest editor of various other journals. Dr. Ng is an invited keynote speaker for many international scientific conferences and workshops. He has coedited nine books, which include the following: *Cardiac Perfusion and Pumping Engineering* (WSPC Press, 2007); *Human Eye Imaging and Modeling* (Artech House, 2008); *Distributed Diagnosis and Home Healthcare, D_2H_2*, vols. 1 and 3 (ASP, 2010, 2012); *Performance Evaluation in Breast Imaging, Tumor Detection & Analysis* (ASP, 2010); *Computational Analysis of the Human Eye with Applications* (WSPC Press, 2011); *Multimodality Breast Imaging* (SPIE, 2013); and *Human Eye Imaging and Modeling* and *Image Analysis and Modeling in Ophthalmology* (CRC Press, 2012, 2013). He has also coauthored a textbook entitled *Compressor Instability with Integral Methods* (Springer, 2007). More details are available upon request and at http://www.researcherid.com/rid/A-1375-2011.

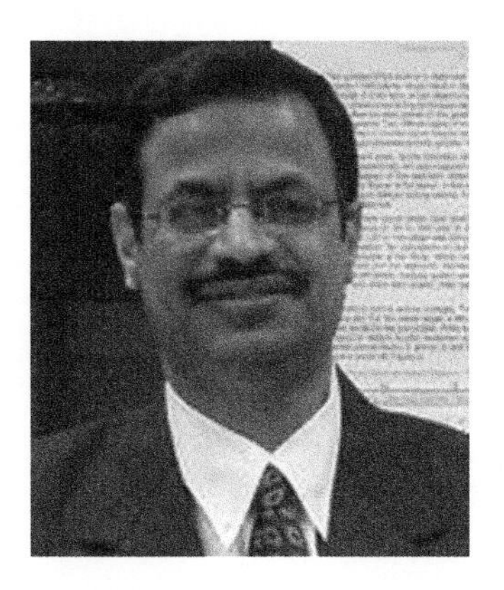

U. Rajendra Acharya, PhD, DEng, is a visiting faculty at the Ngee Ann Polytechnic, Singapore. He is also an adjunct professor at the University of Malaya, Malaysia; an adjunct faculty at the Singapore Institute of Technology–University of Glasgow, Singapore; an associate faculty at the SIM University, Singapore; and an adjunct faculty at the Manipal Institute of Technology, Manipal, India. He earned his PhD from the National Institute of Technology Karnataka, Surathkal, India, and DEngg from Chiba University, Japan. He has published more than 270 papers, including articles in refereed international SCI-IF journals (229) and international conference proceedings (42) and books (16, including those in press) with an h-index of 28 in SCOPUS without self-citations. He has also worked on various funded projects with grants worth more than two million SGD. Dr. Acharya serves on the editorial boards of many journals and has previously served as a guest editor for several journals. His major interests are in biomedical signal processing, bioimaging, data mining, visualization, and biophysics for better health-care design, delivery, and therapy. More information is available in http://urajendraacharya.webs.com/.

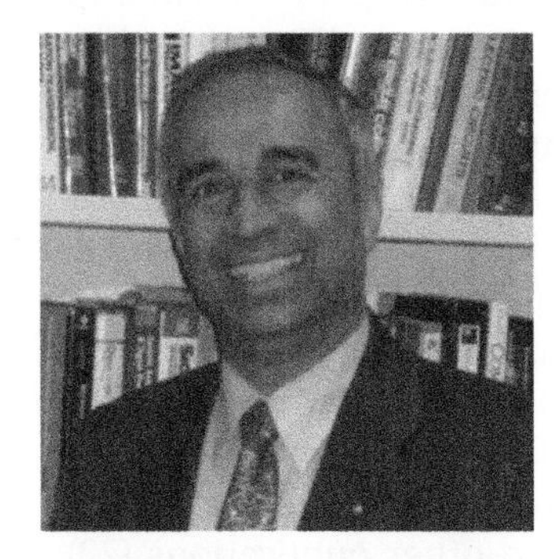

Rangaraj M. Rangayyan is a professor at the University of Calgary, Calgary, Alberta, Canada. He is a pioneer in the field of computer-aided diagnosis and is a fellow of the IEEE, AIMBE, SPIE, EIC, SIIM, CMBES, and CAE. His research interests are in the areas of digital signal and image processing, biomedical signal and image analysis, and medical imaging. He was awarded the 2013 outstanding engineer medal of IEEE Canada.

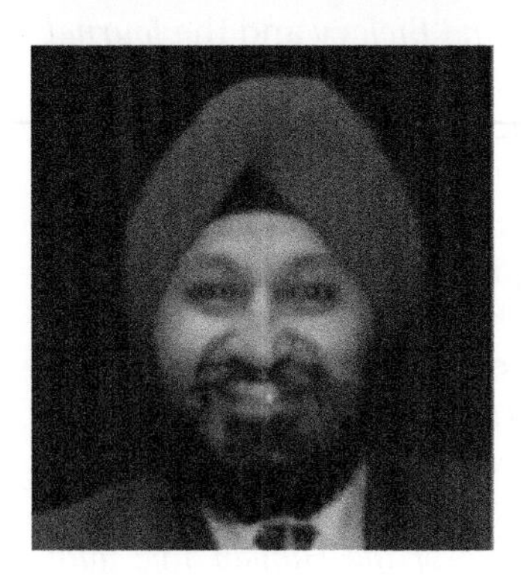

Jasjit S. Suri, MS, PhD, MBA, fellow AIMBE, is an innovator, visionary, scientist, and an internationally known world leader in biomedical devices and biomedical imaging sciences and its applications. He has spent over 25 years in the field of biomedical engineering/sciences and its management. He earned his master's degree from the University of Illinois, Chicago; his doctorate from the University of Washington, Seattle; and his MBA from the Weatherhead School of Management, CWRU, Cleveland. Dr. Suri is a committee member of several journals and companies. He was awarded the Director General's Gold Medal in 1980. He was also named a fellow of the American Institute of Medical and Biological Engineering (AIMBE) and was honored by the National Academy of Sciences, Washington, DC, in 2004. Dr. Suri has been the chairman of the IEEE Denver section and has won over 50 awards during his career.

Contributors

U. Rajendra Acharya
Department of Electronic & Computer Engineering
Ngee Ann Polytechnic
Singapore

and

Faculty of Engineering
Department of Biomedical Engineering
University of Malaya
Kuala Lumpur, Malaysia

Abeer Akhtar
Ocular Imaging Research and Reading Center
Stanley M. Truhlsen Eye Institute
University of Nebraska Medical Center
Omaha, Nebraska

and

Harvard Medical School
Cambridge, Massachusetts

Maria Cecilia D. Aquino
Department of Ophthalmology
National University Hospital
National University Health System
Singapore

Reema Bansal
Advanced Eye Centre
Post Graduate Institute of Medical Education and Research
Chandigarh, India

Millena G. Bittencourt
Retinal Imaging Research and Reading Center
Wilmer Eye Institute
School of Medicine
Johns Hopkins University
Baltimore, Maryland

P.K. Bora
Department of Electronics and Electrical Engineering
Indian Institute of Technology Guwahati
Guwahati, India

Zheng Ce
Department of Ophthalmology
National University Health System
Singapore

Pablo Charlón
Institute of Ophthalmology Gómez-Ulla
Santiago de Compostela, Spain

Caroline Ka Lin Chee
Department of Ophthalmology
National University Hospital
and
Yong Loo Lin School of Medicine
National University of Singapore
National University Health System
Singapore

Carol Y. Cheung
Department of Ophthalmology
Yong Loo Lin School of Medicine
National University of Singapore
and
Singapore Eye Research Institute
Singapore National Eye Centre
and
Centre for Quantitative Medicine
Duke-NUS Graduate Medical School
Singapore

Paul Tec Kuan Chew
Department of Ophthalmology
National University Hospital
National University Health System
Singapore

Chua Kuang Chua
Department of Electrical Communication Engineering
Ngee Ann Polytechnic
Singapore

S. Dandapat
Department of Electronics and Electrical Engineering
Indian Institute of Technology Guwahati
Guwahati, India

Diana J. Dean
Creighton School of Medicine
and
Ocular Imaging Research and Reading Center
Stanley M. Truhlsen Eye Institute
University of Nebraska Medical Center
Omaha, Nebraska

Diana V. Do
Ocular Imaging Research and Reading Center
Stanley M. Truhlsen Eye Institute
University of Nebraska Medical Center
Omaha, Nebraska

Anna L. Ells
Division of Ophthalmology
Department of Surgery
Alberta Children's Hospital
Calgary, Alberta, Canada

Alba Fernandez
Computer Vision and Pattern Recognition Group
University of A Coruña
A Coruña, Spain

Daniel Araújo Ferraz
Ocular Imaging Research and Reading Center
Stanley M. Truhlsen Eye Institute
University of Nebraska Medical Center
Omaha, Nebraska
and
Department of Ophthalmology
University of São Paulo
São Paulo, Brazil

Karthikeyan Ganesan
Department of Electronic & Computer Engineering
Ngee Ann Polytechnic
Singapore

Carlos García-Resúa
Optometry Group
University of Santiago de Compostela
Santiago de Compostela, Spain

F. Gomez-Ulla
Ophthalmologic Technological Institute
Santiago de Compostela, Spain

Ana González
Computer Vision and Pattern Recognition Group
University of A Coruña
A Coruña, Spain

Amod Gupta
Advanced Eye Centre
Post Graduate Institute of Medical Education and Research
Chandigarh, India

Yamama Hafeez
Kansas City University of Medicine and Biosciences
Kansas City, Missouri
and
Ocular Imaging Research and Reading Center
Stanley M. Truhlsen Eye Institute
University of Nebraska Medical Center
Omaha, Nebraska

Ming-Yue Han
Department of Mechanics
Henan University of Technology
Zhengzhou, Henan, People's Republic of China

Mostafa Hanout
Ocular Imaging Research and Reading Center
Stanley M. Truhlsen Eye Institute
University of Nebraska Medical Center
Omaha, Nebraska

Mohamed A. Ibrahim
Ocular Imaging Research and Reading Center
Stanley M. Truhlsen Eye Institute
University of Nebraska Medical Center
Omaha, Nebraska

Mohammad Kamran Ikram
Department of Ophthalmology
Yong Loo Lin School of Medicine
and
Singapore Eye Research Institute
Singapore National Eye Centre
and
Centre for Quantitative Medicine
Duke-NUS Graduate Medical School
and
Memory, Aging & Cognition Centre
National University Health System
Singapore

Darius Jegelevičius
Department of Electronics Engineering
Biomedical Engineering Institute
Kaunas University of Technology
Kaunas, Lithuania

Victor Koh
Department of Ophthalmology
National University Health Systems
Singapore

Audris Kopustinskas
Department of Electronics Engineering
Biomedical Engineering Institute
Kaunas University of Technology
Kaunas, Lithuania

Irmantas Kupčiūnas
Department of Electronics Engineering
Biomedical Engineering Institute
Kaunas University of Technology
Kaunas, Lithuania

Augustinus Laude
National Healthcare Group Eye Institute
Tan Tock Seng Hospital
Singapore

Sze-Yee Lee
Ocular Surface Research Group
Singapore Eye Research Institute
Singapore

Dawn K.A. Lim
Department of Ophthalmology
National University Hospital
National University Health System
Singapore

Gopal Lingam
Department of Ophthalmology
National University Hospital
and
Yong Loo Lin School of Medicine
National University of Singapore
National University Health System
Singapore

Hongting Liu
Retinal Imaging Research and Reading Center
Wilmer Eye Institute
School of Medicine
Johns Hopkins University
Baltimore, Maryland

Seng Chee Loon
Department of Ophthalmology
National University Health Systems
Singapore

Arūnas Lukoševičius
Department of Electronics Engineering
Biomedical Engineering Institute
Kaunas University of Technology
Kaunas, Lithuania

Aria E. Mangunkusumo
Department of Ophthalmology
National University Hospital
National University Health System
Singapore

C. Marino
Computer Vision and Pattern Recognition Group
University of A Coruña
A Coruña, Spain

Vaidotas Marozas
Department of Electronics Engineering
Biomedical Engineering Institute
Kaunas University of Technology
Kaunas, Lithuania

Roshan Joy Martis
Department of Electronic & Computer Engineering
Ngee Ann Polytechnic
Singapore

Narissa Mawji
Ocular Imaging Research and Reading Center
Stanley M. Truhlsen Eye Institute
University of Nebraska Medical Center
Omaha, Nebraska

and

University of British Columbia
Vancouver, British Columbia, Canada

Lim Choo Min
Department of Electronic & Computer Engineering
Ngee Ann Polytechnic
Singapore

Antonio Mosquera
Computer Vision Group
University of Santiago de Compostela
Santiago de Compostela, Spain

Sudipta Mukhopadhyay
Department of Electronics and Electrical Communication Engineering
Indian Institute of Technology Kharagpur
Kharagpur, India

Thet Naing
Department of Ophthalmology
National University Hospital
National University Health System
Singapore

Mohamed Naeem Naser
Department of Ophthalmology
National University Hospital
National University Health System
Singapore

Humzah Nasir
Retinal Imaging Research and Reading Center
Wilmer Eye Institute
Johns Hopkins University
Baltimore, Maryland

E.Y.K. Ng
School of Mechanical and Aerospace Engineering
Nanyang Technological University
Singapore

Rachel Nge
Singapore Eye Research Institute
Singapore

Quan Dong Nguyen
Ocular Imaging Research and Reading Center
Stanley M. Truhlsen Eye Institute
University of Nebraska Medical Center
Omaha, Nebraska

S.R. Nirmala
Department of Electronics and Communication Engineering
Guwahati University
Guwahati, India

J. Novo
Computer Vision and Pattern Recognition Group
University of A Coruña
A Coruña, Spain

Faraz Oloumi
Department of Electrical and Computer Engineering
Schulich School of Engineering
University of Calgary
Calgary, Alberta, Canada

Yi Ting Ong
Singapore Eye Research Institute
Singapore National Eye Centre
Singapore

Marcos Ortega
Computer Vision and Pattern Recognition Group
University of A Coruña
A Coruña, Spain

Martynas Patašius
Department of Applied Informatics
Biomedical Engineering Institute
Kaunas University of Technology
Kaunas, Lithuania

Manuel G. Penedo
Computer Vision and Pattern Recognition Group
University of A Coruña
A Coruña, Spain

Brian Perez
Ocular Imaging Research and Reading Center
Stanley M. Truhlsen Eye Institute
University of Nebraska Medical Center
Omaha, Nebraska

and

School of Medicine
El Bosque University
Bogota, Colombia

Enea Poletti
Department of Information Engineering
University of Padua
Padua, Italy

Qing-Hua Qin
Research School of Engineering
Australia National University
Canberra, Australian Capital Territory, Australia

Rangaraj M. Rangayyan
Department of Electrical and Computer Engineering
Schulich School of Engineering
University of Calgary
Calgary, Alberta, Canada

Phadungsak Rattanadecho
Department of Mechanical Engineering
Center of Excellence in Electromagnetic Energy Utilization in Engineering
Thammasat University
Pathumthani, Thailand

Manotosh Ray
Department of Ophthalmology
National University Hospital
and
Yong Loo Lin School of Medicine
National University of Singapore
Singapore

Shakil Rehman
Singapore-MIT Alliance for Research and Technology Centre
Singapore

Beatriz Remeseiro
Computer Vision and Pattern Recognition Group
University of A Coruña
A Coruña, Spain

Alfredo Ruggeri
Department of Information Engineering
University of Padua
Padua, Italy

Mohammad Ali Sadiq
Ocular Imaging Research and Reading Center
Stanley M. Truhlsen Eye Institute
University of Nebraska Medical Center
Omaha, Nebraska

Patrick A. Santiago
Department of Ophthalmology
National University Hospital
National University Health System
Singapore

and

Department of Ophthalmology
Far Eastern University
Manila, Philippines

Yasir J. Sepah
Ocular Imaging Research and Reading Center
Stanley M. Truhlsen Eye Institute
University of Nebraska Medical Center
Omaha, Nebraska

Rosalynn Grace Siantar
Department of Ophthalmology
National University Health Systems
Singapore

Shaun Sim
Department of Ophthalmology
Yong Loo Lin School of Medicine
National University of Singapore
Singapore

Mandeep S. Singh
Department of Ophthalmology
National University Hospital
National University Health System
Singapore

Jasjit S. Suri
Global Biomedical Technologies, Inc.
Roseville, California

and

Department of Biomedical Engineering
Idaho State University
Pocatello, Idaho

Anna W.T. Tan
Department of Ophthalmology
National University Hospital
National University Health System
Singapore

Louis Tong
Cornea and External Eye Disease Service
Singapore National Eye Center
and
Ocular Surface Research Group
Singapore Eye Research Institute
and
Office of Clinical Science
Duke-NUS Graduate Medical School
and
Department of Ophthalmology
Yong Loo Lin School of Medicine
National University of Singapore
Singapore

Tin Aung Tun
Singapore Eye Research Institute
Singapore National Eye Centre
Singapore

Hui Wang
Department of Mechanics
Henan University of Technology
Zhengzhou, People's Republic of China

Teerapot Wessapan
School of Aviation
Eastern Asia University
Pathumthani, Thailand

Tien Yin Wong
Department of Ophthalmology
Yong Loo Lin School of Medicine
National University of Singapore
and
Singapore Eye Research Institute
Singapore National Eye Centre
Singapore

Eva Yebra-Pimentel
Optometry Group
University of Santiago de Compostela
Santiago de Compostela, Spain

1

Retinal Vascular Imaging in Clinical Research

Mohammad Kamran Ikram, Shaun Sim, Yi Ting Ong, Carol Y. Cheung, and Tien Yin Wong

CONTENTS

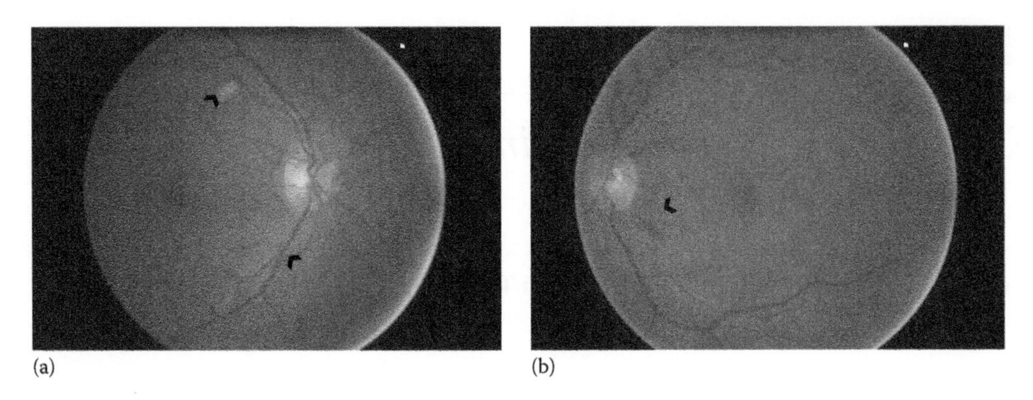

FIGURE 1.1
(See color insert.) Retinal photograph showing examples of retinal microvascular signs: (a) including cotton-wool spots (arrow head pointing to a bright spot) and arteriovenous nicking (arrow head pointing to a crossing of arteriole and venule) and (b) hemorrhage (arrow head pointing to a dark spot).

1.1 Introduction

Toward the end of the nineteenth century, the introduction of the ophthalmoscope in clinical practice provided an ideal opportunity to assess in vivo the human retina, including the microcirculation, noninvasively. The Scottish physician Robert Marcus Gunn, who in 1898 presented a series of observations from patients with stroke, recognized changes seen in the retinal blood vessels as *markers* of systemic disease [1,2]. These retinal signs included generalized arteriolar narrowing, arteriovenous nicking, cotton-wool spots, intraretinal hemorrhages, and papilledema. These signs subsequently became known as markers of hypertensive retinopathy (Figure 1.1). Subsequently, from the 1930s onward, several classification schemes for hypertensive retinopathy were proposed, and their relationship with a wide spectrum of cardiovascular diseases and mortality was described [3–7].

Despite the fact that these classifications provided new insights into the pathophysiology of hypertensive retinopathy, clinical application of these classifications proved tedious due to several reasons: First, the natural course of the development of hypertensive lesions was not clear (e.g., how many with mild stages progress to severe stages, and vice versa). Second, it was not clear that the classification stages were sequential. For example, optic disc papilledema, which is considered to be the most severe stage of hypertensive retinopathy, can develop in patients with malignant hypertension without showing any signs of less severe lesions, such as generalized arteriolar narrowing. Third, most of the initial research in the field of hypertensive retinopathy was done in clinic-based settings in a period prior to discovery of therapies for hypertension [2,8,9]. Finally, direct clinical ophthalmoscopy has been shown to be subjective and less reliable in the detection of hypertensive retinopathy lesions [1,10–12].

1.2 Retinal Vascular Imaging

In the last few decades, there have been three major advances in the field of assessment of these *hypertensive retinopathy* lesions. First, the invention of the fundus (retinal) camera allowed easy collection of retinal images, which could be analyzed, stored, and reanalyzed. It allowed the collection of retinal images over time to determine changes in retinal signs. Second, the move from film-based to digital retinal photography allowed images to be analyzed by computer systems. Finally, the application of modern computer software allowed the development of novel techniques, which have revolutionized the field of ophthalmology in terms of both clinical practice and research.

With respect to the retinal microcirculation, retinal photography captures a large segment of the retina and allows a more objective documentation of major retinal vessels and its branches [12]. Over the years, these new methods have been applied to large general population cohorts and have demonstrated moderate to excellent reproducibility for the detection of the different retinopathy signs (kappa values ranging from 0.80 to 0.99 for microaneurysms and retinal hemorrhages to 0.40–0.79 for focal retinal arteriolar narrowing and arteriovenous nicking) [12]. Furthermore, both hospital-based and population-based studies have shown that these qualitative retinopathy signs, as documented from photographs, are related to the risk of cardiovascular diseases [2]. However, up until the end of the twentieth century, quantitative assessment of the retinal microcirculation remained difficult.

In this respect, since the 1970s, several attempts had been made to develop semi-objective methods based on retinal photography or slide projection systems to measure vessel diameters. These methods relied on obtaining a ratio between arteriolar and venular calibers as a marker of generalized arteriolar narrowing. In 1974, Parr and Spears developed such a method for evaluation of generalized arteriolar narrowing [13,14]. They measured all retinal arteriolar blood column diameters in an area between half a disc diameter and one disc diameter from the optic disc margin. This region was selected because its vessels unequivocally are arterioles instead of arteries [2,12]. Furthermore, in the specified area, there was less overlap between the blood vessels than near or on the optic disc making the measurements more reliable. The measured arteriolar calibers were converted into one sum value representing the caliber of the retinal artery, named the *central retinal artery equivalent* (CRAE) [12–14]. In the 1990s, Hubbard et al. applied this Parr's method also to venules and summarized these as *central retinal vein equivalent* (CRVE) [12]. Using this technique, a semi-automated system was developed to measure reliably and accurately retinal vascular caliber from retinal photographs. Hubbard et al. developed formulae to generate summarized measures of retinal arteriolar and venular calibers, as well as their dimensionless ratio (arteriovenous ratio [AVR]) [12]. Furthermore, Knudtson et al. made further refinements based on the six largest arterioles and venules to compute these summarized retinal vascular measures [15]. Subsequently, these retinal vascular indices have been used in several large-scale epidemiological studies, which demonstrated excellent reproducibility for these quantitative measures of retinal vascular calibers (intraclass correlation coefficient ranged from 0.80 to 0.99) [12], suggesting that retinal photography may offer an accurate way of assessing structural changes in the retinal microcirculation (Figure 1.2) [16–18].

1.3 Which Factors Influence Retinal Vascular Calibers?

1.3.1 Age

One of the most important factors influencing retinal vascular calibers is age. Several studies have examined retinal vascular calibers among children of different ages. A study reported retinal vascular calibers among infants born at term with normal

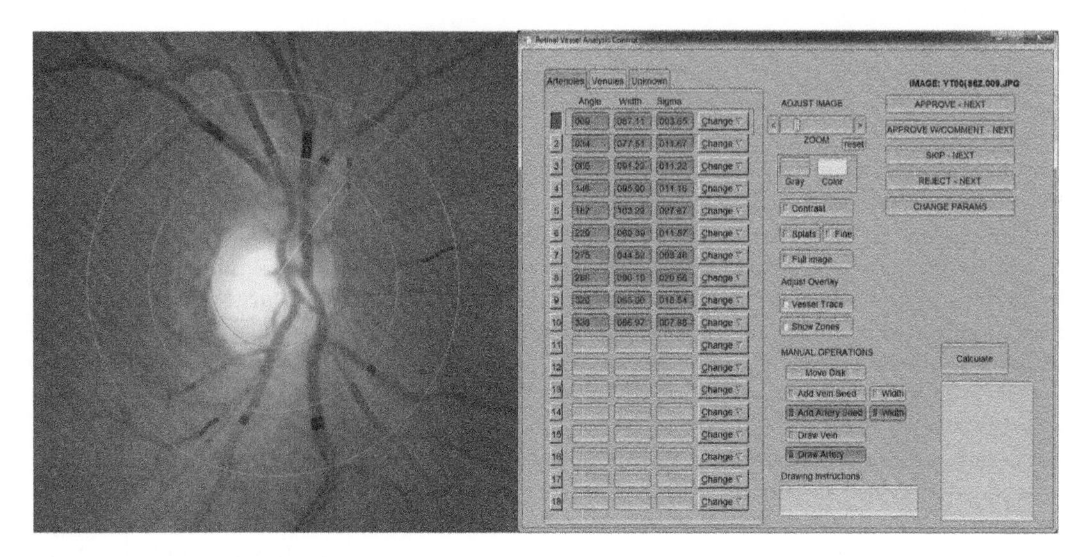

FIGURE 1.2
(See color insert.) Retinal fundus photograph assessed quantitatively by the Interactive Vessel Analysis software. The measured area of retinal vascular parameters was standardized as the region from 0.5 to 1.0 disc diameters away from the disc margin. Retinal arteriolar and venular calibers were summarized as CRAE and the CRVE, respectively, from retinal fundus photograph. CRAE and CRVE were defined based on the revised Knudtson–Parr–Hubbard formula.

birth weight [19]: mean retinal arteriolar caliber was 85.5 μm and mean venular one was 130.0 μm [19]. Results from the Sydney Childhood Eye Cohort showed that retinal arteriolar and venular calibers nearly doubled by the time a child is 6 years old with a mean retinal arteriolar caliber of 165.6 μm and venular caliber of 232.0 μm [20]. In contrast, over the same period of time, the body weight of these children would have increased by more than fivefold. Furthermore, data from adult populations showed that while retinal venular caliber remained approximately the same from the age of 6 onward, the retinal arteriolar caliber continued to increase from infancy to adulthood to a mean of 202.3 μm in those above 43 years old [20]. These data suggest that retinal arteriolar caliber increases at a different pace compared to retinal venular caliber. Finally, among middle-aged and elderly subjects, data from all large population-based studies have shown a converse association between retinal vascular calibers and age, namely, that older persons have both smaller retinal arteriolar and venular calibers. Nevertheless, despite the consistency of these associations, the absolute differences in calibers among persons above 80 years compared to those who are 55–60 years are only in the order of magnitude of 10–15 μm [12,21,22]. Overall, these data suggest that after an initial increase in retinal vascular calibers with increasing age, from middle age onward, there is a decrease in these calibers.

1.3.2 Blood Pressure and Hypertension

With respect to systemic diseases, one of the strongest associations has been found between retinal vascular calibers and hypertension [12,22–25]. It has long been recognized that retinal arteriolar narrowing is one of the earliest signs of hypertension, resulting from both acute and chronic exposures to increased blood pressure. More recently, multiple population-based studies have provided evidence in support of this link between blood pressure and retinal vascular calibers [12,22–25]. A recent meta-analysis of five cross-sectional studies comprising of 19,633 subjects showed that for every 10 mmHg increase in arterial blood pressure, the retinal arteriolar caliber decreased by 3.1 μm (95% confidence interval [CI]: 2.4–3.7 μm) [26].

Furthermore, longitudinal studies have shown that retinal arterial narrowing might even precede the development of hypertension [26]. A recent meta-analysis based on four population-based studies including 6247 participants (follow-up periods: from 3 to 7 years) showed that smaller arteriolar caliber was associated with an increased risk of incident hypertension (meta-analysis relative risk [RR], 1.91; 95% CI, 1.56–2.34) [26]. These longitudinal cohort studies provide evidence that narrower arteriolar calibers preceded the development of clinical hypertension and were not purely a secondary response to established hypertension [27–31].

1.3.3 Diabetes Mellitus

Microvascular pathology plays an important role in the pathophysiology of diabetes mellitus [32,33]. Prospective data from the Atherosclerosis Risks in Communities (ARIC) Study and Beaver Dam Eye Study showed that subjects without diabetes mellitus at baseline with smaller AVR had 50%–70% higher risk of developing incident diabetes, independent of other cardiovascular risk factors [17,34]. However, these studies did not report these associations for arteriolar and venular calibers separately. In contrast, investigators from the Rotterdam Eye Study proposed to examine these calibers separately and reported that the association between AVR and diabetes may be due to retinal venular dilatation rather than arteriolar narrowing. Also, they found that larger retinal venular caliber was associated with the development of impaired fasting glucose [35]. Subsequently, other studies also found an association between wider retinal arteriolar calibers and diabetes [36,37]. Data from Asian populations including Chinese, Malay, and Indians also reported a link between wider retinal arteriolar caliber and diabetes status [38,39]. Although the exact mechanisms leading to retinal venular dilatation and the observed associations with diabetes remain unknown, experimental studies have shown that the administration of intravenous dextrose can cause dilatation of retinal venules in normoglycemic patients [40]. Other mechanisms—including endothelial dysfunction and inflammatory processes leading to reduced vascular reactivity—may also underlie the development of wider retinal arteriolar and venular calibers in diabetes [41].

1.3.4 Obesity and Physical Activity

Thus far, retinal vascular manifestations of obesity are poorly understood [42]. Several cross-sectional studies showed that changes in retinal vascular caliber may be associated with several markers of obesity. Several individual studies showed that larger venular caliber, but not arteriolar caliber, was related to greater body mass index, waist–hip ratio, and dyslipidemia (higher levels of plasma triglyceride and low-density lipoprotein [LDL] cholesterol and lower levels of high-density lipoprotein [HDL] cholesterol) [22,43–45]. More recently, a meta-analysis of over 44,000 individuals showed that higher levels of body mass index were related not only to larger retinal venular caliber but also to smaller retinal arteriolar caliber, while controlling for traditional cardiovascular risk factors [46]. Furthermore, prospective data from the Blue Mountains Eye study showed that larger retinal venular caliber may predict the incidence of obesity, suggesting that microvascular dysfunction might play a role in the pathogenesis of obesity [47]. The lack of regular moderate-to-vigorous intensity physical activity, which is closely related to obesity and is a well-known modifiable risk factor for cardiovascular diseases, has been consistently shown to be related to wider retinal venular caliber [48–50]. Potential pathways including inflammation, oxidative stress, hyperleptinemia, and nitric oxide dysregulation have all been implicated in the link between larger retinal venules and obesity.

1.3.5 Atherosclerosis, Inflammation, and Endothelial Function

Several population-based studies have examined the association between retinal vascular calibers and markers of atherosclerosis [22,43,45,51–53]. However, the association between retinal vascular caliber and these markers of atherosclerosis has not been consistently demonstrated. In the ARIC study, smaller AVR was associated with carotid artery plaque but not intima-media thickness (IMT) [51], whereas the Rotterdam Study found an association between smaller AVR and carotid artery IMT [22]. Moreover, smaller AVR has also been independently associated with increased carotid artery stiffness, an early marker of atherosclerosis [22]. In terms of arteriolar and venular calibers separately, it has been shown that these associations were largely explained due to larger retinal venular calibers [22,52]. In contrast, data from the Cardiovascular Health Study (CHS) revealed no independent association between smaller AVR and markers of atherosclerosis [54]. Other markers of atherosclerosis that have been examined in relationship to retinal vascular caliber include coronary artery calcifications, left ventricular hypertrophy, and peripheral artery disease as measured by the ankle-arm index. In the Multi-Ethnic Study of Atherosclerosis (MESA), smaller retinal arteriolar caliber was related to left ventricular concentric remodeling and myocardial blood flow [55,56], whereas retinal vascular caliber was not associated with coronary artery calcifications [57]. Furthermore, larger venular caliber has been associated with a lower ankle-arm index [22].

The relationship between retinal vascular caliber and other markers of subclinical cardiovascular diseases such as inflammation and endothelial dysfunction has also been examined. Larger retinal venular caliber was related to various inflammatory markers, including C-reactive protein and leucocyte count [22,58,59]. Furthermore, markers of endothelial dysfunction, including soluble intercellular adhesion molecule-1 and serum E-selectin, were also shown to be associated with larger retinal venular caliber [59]. More recently, brachial flow-mediated dilatation examination or dynamic vessel analysis of the retinal vessel [60,61], as a marker for endothelial dysfunction, showed reduced responses in patients with larger venular calibers. These observations are in agreement with experimental studies showing an increase in retinal venules, but not arterioles, after administration of lipid hydroperoxide into the vitreous of rats [62]. These data suggest that both inflammation and endothelial dysfunction might have a crucial role underlying the association between retinal venular dilatation and systemic diseases.

1.3.6 Genetics

It has been noted that retinal vascular calibers were more highly correlated between relatives than between unrelated individuals [63]. This is in accordance with findings from a twin study showing that genetic factors accounted for 70% of the variance in retinal arteriolar caliber and 83% of the variance in retinal venular caliber [64]. More recently, a genome-wide linkage scan provided further support for a role of genetic factors in determining retinal vascular calibers [65]. Furthermore, the linkage regions for retinal vascular calibers overlapped with regions that have previously been linked with hypertension, coronary heart disease, endothelial dysfunction, and vasculogenesis [65,66]. Finally, a genome-wide association study demonstrated four novel loci (19q13, 6q24, 12q24, and 5q14) associated with retinal venular caliber. Of these four loci, the locus on 12q24 was also associated with coronary heart disease and hypertension [67]. While the currently available data are limited, there are nevertheless clear indications that genetic factors play a role in determining the retinal vascular calibers.

1.3.7 Birth Weight

According to the Barker hypothesis, children with low birth weight are at an increased risk of developing cardiovascular diseases during their adult life. However, in this association, the role of the microcirculation is not clear [68]. Over the last few years, several studies have used retinal imaging to assess the microcirculation in children with a low birth weight. It has been reported that the mean retinal arteriolar caliber narrowed by 2 μm per 1 kg reduction in birth weight [20,69]. In contrast, data from the Singapore Cohort Study of the Risk Factors for Myopia (SCORM) and the Avon Longitudinal Study showed that neither low birth weight nor preterm birth was associated with narrowed retinal arterioles [70,71]. However, ocular magnification errors and small sample sizes may have limited the ability to detect any association. Overall, there is increasing amount of evidence showing that low birth weight might result in microcirculatory structural changes.

1.4 Retinal Vascular Imaging and Brain Diseases

1.4.1 Stroke

The retinal microcirculation shares many features with the cerebral circulation including embryological origin and anatomical and physiological characteristics (such as blood–tissue barrier). Therefore, it has been suggested that the retinal vascular caliber could provide key insights into cerebrovascular pathology [72]. Smaller retinal AVR was reported to be associated with increased risk of stroke, including cerebral infarction [16,73]. In the Wisconsin Epidemiologic Study of Diabetic Retinopathy (WESDR), among persons with diabetes, smaller retinal arteriolar and larger venular calibers were related to the risk of stroke mortality [74]. The association of stroke with wider retinal venular caliber was confirmed in the Rotterdam Study, whereas retinal arteriolar caliber was not related to the risk of stroke [75]. Finally, a meta-analysis including data from 20,798 participants showed that retinal venular caliber, but not retinal arteriolar caliber, was related to an increased risk of stroke (RR per 20 μm increase in venular caliber, 1.15; 95% CI, 1.05–1.25) [76]. With respect to stroke subtypes, so far, studies have mainly focused on cerebral infarction, which comprises up to 80% of all strokes. With respect to the second most common subtype intracerebral hemorrhage, only one study showed that larger retinal venular caliber was related to this subtype [77].

1.4.2 Cerebral Small Vessel Disease

In several population-based studies, retinal vascular changes including retinopathy signs and retinal vascular calibers were associated not only with incident stroke [16,73–76] but also with subclinical MRI-defined changes, including cerebral infarction, white matter lesions, and atrophy [73,78–82]. Furthermore, data from the Rotterdam Scan Study showed that persons with larger retinal venular caliber were at a higher risk of progression in periventricular/subcortical white matter lesions and incident lacunar infarcts [83]. Subsequently, other population-based and clinic-based studies confirmed the association between retinal vascular calibers and lacunar infarcts [84,85].

1.4.3 Cognitive Decline and Dementia

Several large population-based studies have shown that retinal vascular changes are associated with cognitive impairment [86–92]. Furthermore, it was observed that larger retinal venular caliber was associated with an increased risk of dementia and in particular vascular dementia, which is in line with observations in stroke and cerebral small vessel disease [93]. Overall, these data suggest that the retinal microcirculation provides an ideal opportunity to explore the possibilities of elucidating the pathophysiology of age-related brain diseases including stroke and dementia.

1.4.4 Other Rare Brain Diseases

Apart from common age-related brain diseases such as dementia and stroke, retinal vascular abnormalities have also been examined in patients with rare brain conditions, such as cerebral autosomal dominant arteriopathy with subcortical infarcts and leukoencephalopathy (CADASIL) [94,95]. Clinically, patients present with symptoms such as migraine with aura, recurrent strokes, and cognitive decline. CADASIL is an inherited small arteriolar disease caused by *Notch 3* gene mutations and is pathologically characterized by degeneration of vascular smooth muscle cells of arterioles. One study reported that generalized arteriolar narrowing and arteriovenous nicking are the most common retinal findings in these patients. However, future studies with large sample sizes are needed to elucidate the exact link between retinal vascular abnormalities and cerebral lesions in CADASIL.

1.5 Retinal Vascular Imaging and Heart Diseases

Several population-based studies have examined the role of retinal vascular imaging in heart diseases. In the ARIC Study, smaller AVR was associated with increased risk of incident coronary heart disease (CHD) and acute myocardial infarction in women but not men [96,97]. In the CHS, both larger retinal venular and smaller arteriolar calibers were independently associated with an increased risk of incident CHD, especially in women [98]. In the Blue Mountains Eye Study, middle-aged persons of 49–75 years with larger venular caliber had a twofold increased risk of CHD mortality after adjusting for traditional risk factors. Additionally, in women, smaller arteriolar caliber was associated with 1.5 times higher risk of CHD mortality [99]. In combined analysis of the Blue Mountains Eye Study and the Beaver Dam Eye Study, smaller arterioles and larger venules were associated with an increased risk of CHD mortality [100]. Another meta-analysis comprising of 22,159 participants found that retinal vascular caliber changes of both wider venules and narrower arterioles were associated with increased risk of CHD in women, but not in men [101].

These studies suggest that retinal vascular caliber predicts CHD more strongly in women than men, possibly reflecting the greater contribution of microvascular disease to CHD development in women [96].

Finally, studies have shown that in the general population, smaller retinal arteriolar caliber was associated with left ventricular concentric remodeling, determined from cardiac MRI, even after adjusting for traditional risk factors [55,56]. These findings suggest that retinal vascular caliber may even provide insights into early subclinical myocardial abnormalities.

1.6 Retinal Vascular Imaging and Kidney Diseases

Thus far, few studies have examined the association between retinal vascular abnormalities and kidney disease [102–104]. These findings suggest that retinopathy and nephropathy may share common pathophysiological mechanisms. Smaller retinal arteriolar caliber was associated with a higher risk of developing chronic kidney disease [105–107]. Furthermore, studies among patients with diabetes mellitus type 1 showed that changes in retinal vascular calibers were related to both incidence of gross proteinuria and morphological parameters obtained from renal biopsy specimens [108,109]. However, further studies are needed to elucidate the exact link between changes in retinal vascular calibers and kidney disease [110].

1.7 Retinal Vascular Imaging and Other Systemic Diseases

1.7.1 Rheumatoid Arthritis and Osteoarthritis

Rheumatoid arthritis (RA) is a systemic inflammatory disease of a joint's connective tissues, such as the synovial membranes, and mostly affects the smaller joints of the hands, wrists, and feet. Furthermore, it is associated with endothelial dysfunction and increased cardiovascular morbidity and mortality. Other forms of arthritis include osteoarthritis (OA), which is caused by the breakdown of joint cartilage with age and affects largely the large weight-bearing joints. Also, people with OA have a higher prevalence of vascular diseases. With respect to the role of microvascular pathology, both these forms of arthritis have been examined in relationship to retinal vascular calibers. Two recent studies have shown that retinal venular caliber was significantly wider in patients with RA and OA compared to age- and gender-matched controls [111,112]. These findings provide novel insights into the role of microvascular pathology in the pathophysiology of both RA and OA and warrant further work.

1.7.2 Acquired Immunodeficiency Syndrome

Although persons with acquired immunodeficiency syndrome (AIDS) are known to be at increased risk for cardiovascular morbidity, the link with retinal vascular caliber has not been extensively examined. One study has shown that variations in retinal vascular caliber among persons with AIDS were related to the level of immunodeficiency as reflected by CD4+ T lymphocyte count and use of highly active antiretroviral drug therapy (HAART) [113]. Specifically, smaller retinal arteriolar caliber is related to increasing duration of HAART and with a higher HIV viral load [114]. Longitudinal studies are required to confirm these findings and explore the possible role of the caliber measurements as a tool in HIV-related assessment of vascular risk.

1.7.3 Lung Diseases

Chronic obstructive pulmonary disease (COPD) is currently one of the leading causes of death in the United States. Smoking is the major risk factor for the development of COPD. It has been hypothesized that smoking-related microvascular damage through endothelial dysfunction and inflammatory reactions may contribute to the pathogenesis of COPD. Data from the MESA study showed that larger retinal venular caliber was independently related to a decrease in spirometric measures such as FEV1 (forced expiratory volume in 1 s) [115]. In contrast, venular caliber was not related to CT lung density (lung attenuation area [%LAA] measured from CT scans). Furthermore, retinal arteriolar caliber was not associated with any of the lung parameters [115]. These data suggest that microvascular damage—as reflected by retinal venular caliber—may play a role in the development of COPD, but further confirmation is needed.

1.8 Retinal Vascular Imaging and Ocular Diseases

1.8.1 Diabetic Retinopathy

Presently, there is limited data on the relationship between retinal vascular calibers and the risk of diabetic retinopathy. In patients with type 1 diabetes, larger retinal venular caliber was associated with progression of mild to more severe levels of diabetic retinopathy, including proliferative retinopathy [116,117]. In contrast, findings from patients with type 2 diabetes are inconclusive [118]. Future research is needed to establish whether retinal vascular caliber measures provide clinically useful information in predicting incident diabetic retinopathy [119].

1.8.2 Age-Related Macular Degeneration

Thus far, several studies have also examined the association between retinal vascular caliber and age-related macular degeneration (AMD) [120–122]. Data from the Singapore Malay Eye Study revealed that wider venular caliber was independently associated with early AMD, whereas no association was found between retinal arteriolar caliber and AMD [120]. The Handan Eye Study showed that wider retinal arteriolar caliber was related to early AMD and venular caliber was not related to AMD [121]. In contrast to these studies, both cross-sectional and prospective studies could not confirm an association between retinal vascular calibers and incident AMD [122,123]. Finally, in eyes with neovascular AMD treated with intravitreal ranibizumab, larger baseline retinal venular caliber was significantly associated with a poorer response to treatment [124].

1.8.3 Open-Angle Glaucoma

Few studies, thus far, looked at the relationship between retinal vascular caliber and primary open-angle glaucoma (POAG). Several studies have shown that patients with POAG have been reported to have significantly smaller arteriolar calibers than age-matched control persons [125–127]. Furthermore, retinal vascular caliber changes were related to a decreased retinal nerve fiber layer thickness as measured with optical coherence tomography [128]. In contrast, other studies found no differences in retinal arteriolar or venular calibers in OAG patients compared to control persons [129]. Finally, data from the Rotterdam Study using prospective data did not show an association between baseline retinal vascular caliber and 6-year incidence of POAG [130]. In contrast, prospective data from the Blue Mountains Eye Study showed that smaller retinal arteriolar caliber was associated with the long-term risk of POAG (10-year incidence of OAG). These data support the concept that early microvascular changes are involved in the pathogenesis of OAG [131].

Normal-tension glaucoma (NTG) is defined as OAG with an intraocular pressure that always measures within the statistically normal range, although it remains controversial whether NTG and high-tension glaucoma differ in their pathogenesis. Vascular mechanisms have also been implicated in the pathogenesis of NTG. Several studies have shown that retinal arteriolar caliber is smaller in NTG patients compared with controls [128]. It remains unclear whether these differences are a cause or consequence of NTG.

1.8.4 Retinal Vein Occlusion

Finally, one study examined the association between retinal vascular caliber and retinal vein occlusion among 10,890 participants [132]. Persons who had a retinal vein occlusion had both narrower retinal arteriolar and venular calibers compared to age- and gender-matched controls. Future studies are needed to confirm these findings in patients with retinal vein occlusion.

1.9 Limitations of Retinal Vascular Caliber Measurements

The clinical application of retinal vascular imaging is currently limited due to several limitations:

First, research using retinal vascular imaging has largely focused on differences between groups. Before retinal vascular imaging could be used as a potential risk stratification tool, studies must produce results that allow an assessment of absolute risk in individual patients. One of the most important components is the measurement of absolute retinal vascular caliber, which requires addressing the issue of magnification effect from retinal photography [22]. While several methods have been proposed to adjust for magnification using ocular biometric data, its applicability in a clinical setting is unknown.

Second, current population-based studies have used retinal caliber measurements obtained from one retinal image. However, it has been shown that retinal caliber may vary up to 15% depending on the moment in the cardiac cycle, when the image was taken [133]. Further standardization is required to improve the accuracy of these measurements.

Third, despite an enormous wealth of data on retinal vascular measurements from various population-based studies, there is lack of normative data for these measurements. For a clinical tool development, it is crucial to define what is normal and abnormal. One of the problems in compiling normative datasets has been the confounding effect of systemic (e.g., hypertension, diabetes, smoking, medications) processes on retinal vascular caliber measurements. Alternatively, performing retinal vascular caliber measurements in healthy young adults, who are generally free of these confounding factors, may provide better normative datasets.

Finally, the retinal vascular caliber measurements do not reflect the 3D structure or the functional aspects of the retinal microcirculation. Therefore, the full potential of retinal image analysis in relationship to the prediction of cardiovascular diseases remains undetermined.

1.10 Future Directions

Efforts are currently underway to quantify novel retinal vascular parameters. These include both local and global vascular topographic features, including the branching angles of blood vessels, retinal vessel tortuosity, and fractal dimension [134]. These new retinal vascular parameters indicate how optimally designed and developed the retinal microvascular system is. Variations from the optimal geometry are known to occur in particular conditions, such as diabetes mellitus. Similar variations may occur in other cardiovascular diseases and need to be explored further. Finally, dynamic and functional aspects of the retinal microcirculation are being assessed with novel technologies, such as the laser Doppler flowmeter or dynamic vessel analysis of retinal vascular diameter in response to flickering light [135]. These novel parameters will complement the present static measurements in identifying early biomarkers for the prediction of cardiovascular diseases.

1.11 Conclusions

The retina provides an ideal opportunity to explore the role of microvascular pathology in the pathophysiology of cardiovascular diseases. Over the last decade, advances in retinal vascular imaging allowed the development of accurate and reliable quantitative parameters such as retinal vascular calibers. Using these parameters, several large population-based studies have shown that retinal vascular calibers are related to cardiovascular diseases. However, the full potential of these retinal image-analysis techniques remains undetermined. With the further advancement of retinal imaging techniques, there still remains a scope for improvement in the quantification of retinal microvascular parameters, which may be utilized as noninvasive biomarkers for cardiovascular diseases.

References

1. Walsh JB. 1982. Hypertensive retinopathy. Description, classification, and prognosis. *Ophthalmology* 89:1127–1131.
2. Wong TY, Klein R, Klein BE, Tielsh JM, Hubbard L, Nieto FJ. 2001. Retinal microvascular abnormalities and their relationship with hypertension, cardiovascular disease, and mortality. *Surv Ophthalmol* 46:59–80.
3. Keith NM, Wagener HP, Barker NW. 1974. Some different types of essential hypertension: Their course and prognosis. *Am J Med Sci* 268:336–345.
4. Scheie HG. 1953. Evaluation of ophthalmoscopic changes of hypertension and arteriolar sclerosis. *AMA Arch Ophthalmol* 49:117–138.
5. Leishman R. 1957. The eye in general vascular disease: Hypertension and arteriosclerosis. *Br J Ophthalmol* 41:641–701.
6. Wong TY, Mitchell P. 2004. Hypertensive retinopathy. *N Engl J Med* 351:2310–2317.
7. Tso MO, Jampol LM. 1982. Pathophysiology of hypertensive retinopathy. *Ophthalmology* 89:1132–1145.
8. Klein R, Klein BE, Moss SE, Wang Q. 1994. Hypertension and retinopathy, arteriolar narrowing, and arteriovenous nicking in a population. *Arch Ophthalmol* 112:92–98.
9. Yu T, Mitchell P, Berry G, Li W, Wang JJ. 1998. Retinopathy in older persons without diabetes and its relationship to hypertension. *Arch Ophthalmol* 116:83–89.
10. Dimmitt SB, West JN, Eames SM, Gibson JM, Gosling P, Littler WA. 1989. Usefulness of ophthalmoscopy in mild to moderate hypertension. *Lancet* 1:1103–1106.
11. Ikram MK, Borger PH, Assink JJ, Jonas JB, Hofman A, De Jong PT. 2002. Comparing ophthalmoscopy, slide viewing, and semiautomated systems in optic disc morphometry. *Ophthalmology* 109:486–493.
12. Hubbard LD, Brothers RJ, King WN, King WN, Clegg LX, Klein R, Cooper LS, Sharrett AR, Davis MD, Cai J. 1999. Methods for evaluation of retinal microvascular abnormalities associated with hypertension/sclerosis in the Atherosclerosis Risk in Communities Study. *Ophthalmology* 106:2269–2280.
13. Parr JC, Spears GF. 1974. Mathematic relationships between the width of a retinal artery and the widths of its branches. *Am J Ophthalmol* 77:478–483.
14. Parr JC, Spears GF. 1974. General caliber of the retinal arteries expressed as the equivalent width of the central retinal artery. *Am J Ophthalmol* 77:472–477.
15. Knudtson MD, Lee KE, Hubbard LD, Wong TY, Klein R, Klein BE. 2003. Revised formulas for summarizing retinal vessel diameters. *Curr Eye Res* 27:143–149.
16. Wong TY, Klein R, Couper DJ, Cooper LS, Shahar E, Hubbard LD, Wofford MR, Sharrett AR. 2001. Retinal microvascular abnormalities and incident stroke: The Atherosclerosis Risk in Communities Study. *Lancet* 358:1134–1140.
17. Wong TY, Klein R, Sharrett AR, Schmidt MI, Pankow JS, Couper DJ, Klein BE, Hubbard LD, Duncan BB; ARIC Investigators. 2002. Retinal arteriolar narrowing and risk of diabetes mellitus in middle-aged persons. *JAMA* 287:2528–2533.
18. Wong TY, Klein R, Sharrett AR, Duncan BB, Couper DJ, Tielsch JM, Klein BE, Hubbard LD. 2002. Retinal arteriolar narrowing and risk of coronary heart disease in men and women. The Atherosclerosis Risk in Communities Study. *JAMA* 287:1153–1159.
19. Kandasamy Y, Smith R, Wright IMR. 2011. Retinal microvasculature measurements in full-term newborn infants. *Microvasc Res* 82:381–384.
20. Mitchell P, Liew G, Rochtchina E, Wang JJ, Robaei D, Cheung N, Wong TY. 2008. Evidence of arteriolar narrowing in low-birth weight children. *Circulation* 118:518–524.
21. Wong TY, Knudtson MD, Klein R, Klein BE, Meuer SM, Hubbard LD. 2004. Computer-assisted measurement of retinal vessel diameters in the Beaver Dam Eye Study: Methodology, correlation between eyes, and the effect of refractive errors. *Ophthalmology* 111:1183–1190.

22. Ikram MK, De Jong FJ, Vingerling JR, Witteman JC, Hofman A, Breteler MMB, De Jong PT. 2004. Are retinal arteriolar or venular diameters associated with markers for cardiovascular disorders? The Rotterdam Study. *Invest Ophthalmol Vis Sci* 45:2129–2134.
23. Gepstein R, Rosman Y, Rechtman E, Koren-Morag N, Segev S, Assia E, Grossman E. 2012. Association of retinal microvascular caliber with blood pressure levels. *Blood Press* 21:191–196.
24. Sharrett AR, Hubbard LD, Cooper LS, Sorlie PD, Brothers RJ, Nieto FJ, Pinsky JL, Klein R. 1999. Retinal arteriolar diameters and elevated blood pressure: The Atherosclerosis Risk in Communities Study. *Am J Epidemiol* 150:263–270.
25. Wong TY, Klein R, Klein BE, Meuer SM, Hubbard LD. 2003. Retinal vessel diameters and their associations with age and blood pressure. *Invest Ophthalmol Vis Sci* 44:4644–4650.
26. Chew SK, Xie J, Wang JJ. 2012. Retinal arteriolar diameter and the prevalence and incidence of hypertension: A systemic review and meta-analysis of their association. *Curr Hypertens Rep* 14:144–151.
27. Wong TY, Klein R, Sharrett AR, Duncan BB, Couper DJ, Klein BE, Hubbard LD, Nieto FJ. 2004. Retinal arteriolar diameter and risk for hypertension. *Ann Intern Med* 140:248–255.
28. Wong TY, Shankar A, Klein R, Klein BE, Hubbard LD. 2004. Prospective cohort study of retinal vessel diameters and risk of hypertension. *BMJ* 329:79.
29. Smith W, Wang JJ, Wong TY, Rochtchina E, Klein R, Leeder SR, Mitchell P. 2004. Retinal arteriolar narrowing is associated with 5-year incident severe hypertension: The Blue Mountains Eye Study. *Hypertension* 44:442–447.
30. Ikram MK, Witteman JC, Vingerling JR, Breteler MM, Hofman A, De Jong PT. 2006. Retinal vessel diameters and risk of hypertension: The Rotterdam Study. *Hypertension* 47:189–194.
31. Kawasaki R, Cheung N, Wang JJ, Klein R, Klein BE, Cotch MF, Sharrett AR, Shea S, Islam FA, Wong TY. 2009. Retinal vessel diameters and risk of hypertension: The Multiethnic Study of Atherosclerosis. *J Hypertens* 27:2386–2393.
32. Tooke JE. 1995. Microvascular function in human diabetes. A physiological perspective. *Diabetes* 44:721–726.
33. Caballero AE, Arora S, Saouaf R, Lim SC, Smakowski P, Park JY, King GL, LoGerfo FW, Horton ES, Veves A. 1999. Microvascular and macrovascular reactivity is reduced in subjects at risk for type 2 diabetes. *Diabetes* 48:1856–1862.
34. Wong TY, Shankar A, Klein R, Klein BE, Hubbard LD. 2005. Retinal arteriolar narrowing, hypertension, and subsequent risk of diabetes mellitus. *Arch Intern Med* 165:1060–1065.
35. Ikram MK, Janssen JA, Roos AM, Rietveld I, Witteman JC, Breteler MM, Hofman A, Van Duijn CM, De Jong PT. 2006. Retinal vessel diameters and risk of impaired fasting glucose and diabetes: The Rotterdam Study. *Diabetes* 55:506–510.
36. Nguyen TT, Wang JJ, Sharrett AR, Islam FM, Klein R, Klein BE, Cotch MF, Wong TY. 2008. Relationship of retinal vascular caliber with diabetes and retinopathy: The Multi-Ethnic Study of Atherosclerosis (MESA). *Diabetes Care* 31:544–549.
37. Tikellis G, Wang JJ, Tapp R, Simpson R, Mitchell P, Zimmet PZ, Shaw J, Wong TY. 2007. The relationship of retinal vascular caliber to diabetes and retinopathy: The Australian Diabetes, Obesity and Lifestyle (AusDiab) study. *Diabetologia* 50:2263–2271.
38. Tsai AS, Wong TY, Lavanya R, Zhang R, Hamzah H, Tai ES, Cheung CY. 2011. Differential association of retinal arteriolar and venular caliber with diabetes and retinopathy. *Diabetes Res Clin Pract* 94:291–298.
39. Jeganathan VS, Sabanayagam C, Tai ES, Lee J, Lamoureux E, Sun C, Kawasaki R, Wong TY. 2009. Retinal vascular caliber and diabetes in a multiethnic Asian population. *Microcirculation* 16:534–543.
40. Falck A, Laatikainen L. 1995. Retinal vasodilation and hyperglycaemia in diabetic children and adolescents. *Acta Ophthalmol Scand* 73:119–124.
41. Nguyen TT, Wong TY. 2006. Retinal vascular manifestations of metabolic disorders. *Trends Endocrinol Metab* 17:262–268.
42. Cheung N, Wong TY. 2007. Obesity and eye diseases. *Surv Ophthalmol* 52: 180–195.

43. Sun C, Wang JJ, Mackay DA, Wong TY. 2009. Retinal vascular caliber: Systemic, environmental and genetic associations. *Surv Ophthalmol* 54:74–95.
44. Wong TY, Islam FM, Klein R, Klein BE, Cotch MF, Castro C, Sharrett AR, Shahar E. 2006. Retinal vascular caliber, cardiovascular risk factors, and inflammation: The multi-ethnic study of atherosclerosis (MESA). *Invest Ophthalmol Vis Sci* 47:2341–2350.
45. Liew G, Sharrett AR, Wang JJ, Klein R, Klein BE, Mitchell P, Wong TY. 2008. Relative importance of systemic determinants of retinal arteriolar and venular caliber: The Atherosclerosis Risk in Communities Study. *Arch Ophthalmol* 126:1404–1410.
46. Boillot A, Zoungas S, Mitchell P, Klein K, Klein B, Ikram MK, Klaver CC et al.; on behalf of the META-EYE Study Group. 2013. Obesity and the microvasculature: A systemic review and meta-analysis. *PLoS ONE* 8(2):e52708.
47. Wang JJ, Taylor B, Wong TY, Chua B, Rochtchina E, Klein R, Mitchell P. 2006. Retinal vessel diameters and obesity: A population-based study in older persons. *Obesity* 14:206–214.
48. Anuradha S, Healy GN, Dunstan DW, Tai ES, Van Dam RM, Lee J, Nang EE, Owen N, Wong TY. 2011. Associations of physical activity and television viewing time with retinal vascular caliber in a multiethnic Asian population. *Invest Ophthalmol Vis Sci* 52:6522–6528.
49. Tikellis G, Anuradha S, Klein R, Wong TY. 2010. Association between physical activity and retinal microvascular signs; the Atherosclerosis Risk in Communities (ARIC) Study. *Microcirculation* 17:381–393.
50. Anuradha S, Healy GN, Dunstan DW, Klein R, Klein BE, Cotch MF, Wong TY, Owen N. 2011. Physical activity, television viewing time, and retinal microvascular caliber: The multi-ethnic study of atherosclerosis. *Am J Epidemiol* 173:518–525.
51. Klein R, Sharrett AR, Klein BE, Chambless LE, Cooper LS, Hubbard LD, Evans G. 2000. Are retinal arteriolar abnormalities related to atherosclerosis? The Atherosclerosis Risk in Communities Study. *Arterioscler Thromb Vasc Biol* 20:1644–1650.
52. Van Hecke MV, Dekker JM, Nijpels G, Stolk RP, Henry RM, Heine RJ, Bouter LM, Stehouwer CD, Polak BC. 2006. Are retinal microvascular abnormalities associated with large artery endothelial dysfunction and intima-media thickness? The Hoorn Study. *Clin Sci* 110:597–604.
53. Liao D, Wong TY, Klein R, Jones D, Hubbard LD, Sharrett AR. 2004. Relationship between carotid artery stiffness and retinal arteriolar narrowing in healthy middle-aged persons. *Stroke* 35:837–842.
54. Wong TY, Klein R, Sharrett AR, Manolio TA, Hubbard LD, Marino EK, Kuller L et al. 2003. The prevalence and risk factors of retinal microvascular abnormalities in older persons: The Cardiovascular Health Study. *Ophthalmology* 110:658–666.
55. Cheung N, Bluemke DA, Klein R, Sharrett AR, Islam FM, Cotch MF, Klein BE, Criqui MH, Wong TY. 2007. Retinal arteriolar narrowing and left ventricular remodeling: The multi-ethnic study of atherosclerosis. *J Am Coll Cardiol* 50:48–55.
56. Wang L, Wong TY, Sharrett AR, Klein R, Folsom AR, Jerosch Herold M. 2008. Relationship between retinal arteriolar narrowing and myocardial perfusion: Multi-ethnic study of atherosclerosis. *Hypertension* 51:119–126.
57. Wong TY, Cheung N, Islam FM, Klein R, Criqui MH, Cotch MF, Carr JJ, Klein BE, Sharrett AR. 2008. Relation of retinopathy to coronary artery calcification: The multi-ethnic study of atherosclerosis. *Am J Epidemiol* 167:51–58.
58. Cheung CY, Wong TY, Lamoureux EL, Sabanayagam C, Li J, Lee J, Tai ES. 2010. C-reactive protein and retinal microvascular caliber in a multiethnic Asian population. *Am J Epidemiol* 171:206–213.
59. Klein R, Klein BE, Knudtson MD, Wong TY, Tsai MY. 2006. Are inflammatory factors related to retinal vessel caliber? The Beaver Dam Eye Study. *Arch Ophthalmol* 124:87–94.
60. Nguyen TT, Islam FM, Faroque HM, Klein R, Klein BE, Cotch MF, Herrington DM, Wong TY. 2010. Retinal vascular caliber and brachial flow-mediated dilation: The Multi-Ethnic Study of Atherosclerosis. *Stroke* 41:1343–1438.
61. Nguyen TT, Kawasaki R, Wang JJ, Kreis AJ, Shaw J, Vilser W, Wong TY. 2009. Flicker light-induced retinal vasodilation in diabetes and diabetic retinopathy. *Diabetes Care* 32:2075–2080.

62. Tamai K, Matsubara A, Tomida K, Matsuda Y, Morita H, Armstrong D, Ogura Y. 2002. Lipid hydroperoxide stimulates leukocyte–endothelium interaction in the retinal microcirculation. *Exp Eye Res* 75:69–75.
63. Lee KE, Klein BE, Klein R, Knudtson MD. 2004. Familial aggregation of retinal vessel caliber in the Beaver Dam Eye Study. *Invest Ophthalmol Vis Sci* 45:3929–3933.
64. Taarnhoj NC, Larsen M, Sander B, Kyvik KO, Kessel L, Hougaard JL, Sorensen TI. 2006. Heritability of retinal vessel diameters and blood pressure: A twin study. *Invest Ophthalmol Vis Sci* 47:3539–3544.
65. Xing C, Klein BE, Klein R, Jun G, Lee KE, Iyengar SK. 2006. Genome-wide linkage study of retinal vessel diameters in the Beaver Dam Eye Study. *Hypertension* 47:797–802.
66. Wang JJ, Wong TY. 2006. Genetic determinants of retinal vascular caliber: Additional insights into hypertension pathogenesis. *Hypertension* 47:644–645.
67. Ikram MK, Sim X, Jensen RA, Cotch MF, Hewitt AW, Ikram MA, Wang JJ et al. 2010. Four novel loci (19q13, 6q24, 12q24, 5q14) influence the microcirculation in vivo. *PLoS Genet* 6:e1001184.
68. Liew G, Wang JJ, Duncan BB, Klein R, Sharrett AR, Brancati F, Yeh HC, Mitchell P, Wong TY; Atherosclerosis Risk in Communities Study. 2008. Low birth weight is associated with narrower arterioles in adults. *Hypertension* 51:933–938.
69. Sun C, Ponsonby AL, Wong TY, Brown SA, Kearns LS, Cochrane J, MacKinnon JR et al. 2009. Effect of birth parameters on retinal vascular caliber: The Twins Eye Study in Tasmania. *Hypertension* 53:487–493.
70. Cheung N, Islam FM, Saw SM, Shankar A, de Haseth K, Mitchell P, Wong TY. 2007. Distribution and associations of retinal vascular caliber with ethnicity, gender, and birth parameters in young children. *Invest Ophthalmol Vis Sci* 48:1018–1024.
71. Tapp RJ, Wiliams C, Witt N, Chaturvedi N, Evans R, Thom SA, Hughes AD, Ness A. 2007. Impact of size at birth on the microvasculature: The Avon Longitudinal Study of Parents and Children. *Pediatrics* 120:1225–1228.
72. Patton N, Aslam T, MacGillivray T, Pattie A, Deary IJ, Dhillon B. 2005. Retinal vascular image analysis as a potential screening tool for cerebrovascular disease: A rationale based on homology between cerebral and retinal microvasculatures. *J Anat* 206:319–348.
73. Longstreth W Jr, Larsen EK, Klein R, Wong TY, Sharrett AR, Lefkowitz D, Manolio TA. 2007. Associations between findings on cranial magnetic resonance imaging and retinal photography in the elderly: The Cardiovascular Health Study. *Am J Epidemiol* 165:78–84.
74. Klein R, Klein BE, Moss SE, Wong TY. 2007. Retinal vessel caliber and microvascular and macrovascular disease in type 2 diabetes: XXI: The Wisconsin Epidemiologic Study of Diabetic Retinopathy. *Ophthalmology* 114:1884–1892.
75. Ikram MK, de Jong FJ, Bos MJ, Vingerling JR, Hofman A, Koudstaal PJ, de Jong PT, Breteler MM. 2006. Retinal vessel diameters and risk of stroke: The Rotterdam Study. *Neurology* 66:1339–1343.
76. McGeechan K, Liew G, Macaskill P, Irwig L, Klein R, Klein BE, Wang JJ et al. 2009. Prediction of incident stroke events based on retinal vessel caliber: A systematic review and individual-participant meta-analysis. *Am J Epidemiol* 170:1323–1332.
77. Wieberdink RG, Ikram MK, Koudstaal PJ, Hofman A, Vingerling JR, Breteler MM. 2010. Retinal vascular calibers and the risk of intracerebral hemorrhage and cerebral infarction: The Rotterdam Study. *Stroke* 41:2757–2761.
78. Wong TY, Klein R, Sharrett AR, Couper DJ, Klein BE, Liao DP, Hubbard LD, Mosley TH; ARIC Investigators. 2002. Atherosclerosis Risk in Communities Study. Cerebral white matter lesions, retinopathy, and incident clinical stroke. *JAMA* 288:67–74.
79. Wong TY, Mosley TH Jr, Klein R, Klein BE, Sharrett AR, Couper DJ, Hubbard LD; Atherosclerosis Risk in Communities Study. 2003. Retinal microvascular changes and MRI signs of cerebral atrophy in healthy, middle-aged people. *Neurology* 61:806–811.
80. Cooper LS, Wong TY, Klein R, Sharrett AR, Bryan RN, Hubbard LD, Couper DJ, Heiss G, Sorlie PD. 2006. Retinal microvascular abnormalities and MRI-defined subclinical cerebral infarction: The Atherosclerosis Risk in Communities Study. *Stroke* 37:82–86.

81. Kawasaki R, Cheung N, Mosley T, Islam AF, Sharrett AR, Klein R, Coker LH et al. 2010. Retinal microvascular signs and 10-year risk of cerebral atrophy: The Atherosclerosis Risk in Communities (ARIC) Study. *Stroke* 41:1826–1828.
82. Baker ML, Wang JJ, Liew G, Hand PJ, De Silva DA, Lindley RI, Mitchell P et al.; Multi-Centre Retinal Stroke Study Group. 2010. Differential associations of cortical and subcortical cerebral atrophy with retinal vascular signs in patients with acute stroke. *Stroke* 41:2143–2150.
83. Ikram MK, De Jong FJ, Van Dijk EJ, Prins ND, Hofman A, Breteler MM, De Jong PT. 2006. Retinal vessel diameters and cerebral small vessel disease: The Rotterdam Scan Study. *Brain* 129:182–188.
84. Lindley RI, Wang JJ, Wong MC, Mitchell P, Liew G, Hand P, Wardlaw J et al.; Multi-Centre Retina and Stroke Study (MCRS) Collaborative Group. 2009. Retinal microvasculature in acute lacunar stroke: A cross-sectional study. *Lancet Neurol* 8:628–634.
85. Cheung N, Mosley T, Islam A, Kawasaki R, Sharrett AR, Klein R, Coker LH et al. 2010. Retinal microvascular abnormalities and subclinical magnetic resonance imaging brain infarct: A prospective study. *Brain* 133:1987–1993.
86. Wong TY, Klein R, Sharrett AR, Nieto FJ, Boland LL, Couper DJ, Mosley TH, Klein BE, Hubbard LD, Szklo M. 2002. Retinal microvascular abnormalities and cognitive impairment in middle-aged persons: The Atherosclerosis Risk in Communities Study. *Stroke* 33:1487–1492.
87. Patton N, Pattie A, MacGillivray T, Aslam T, Dhillon B, Gow A, Starr JM, Whalley LJ, Deary IJ. 2007. The association between retinal vascular network geometry and cognitive ability in an elderly population. *Invest Ophthalmol Vis Sci* 48:1995–2000.
88. Baker ML, Marino Larsen EK, Kuller LH, Klein R, Klein BE, Siscovick DS, Bernick C, Manolio TA, Wong TY. 2007. Retinal microvascular signs, cognitive function, and dementia in older persons: The Cardiovascular Health Study. *Stroke* 38:2041–2047.
89. Ding J, Patton N, Deary IJ, Strachan MW, Fowkes FG, Mitchell RJ, Price JF. 2008. Retinal microvascular abnormalities and cognitive dysfunction: A systematic review. *Br J Ophthalmol* 92:1017–1025.
90. Liew G, Mitchell P, Wong TY, Lindley RI, Cheung N, Kaushik S, Wang JJ. 2009. Retinal microvascular signs and cognitive impairment. *J Am Geriatr Soc* 57:1892–1896.
91. Gatto NM, Varma R, Torres M, Wong TY, Johnson PL, Segal-Gidan F, Mack WJ. 2012. Retinal microvascular abnormalities and cognitive function in Latino adults in Los Angeles. *Ophthalmic Epidemiol* 19:127–136.
92. Lesage SR, Mosley TH, Wong TY, Szklo M, Knopman D, Catellier DJ, Cole SR et al. 2009. Retinal microvascular abnormalities and cognitive decline: The ARIC 14-year follow-up study. *Neurology* 73:862–868.
93. de Jong FJ, Schrijvers EM, Ikram MK, Koudstaal PJ, de Jong PT, Hofman A, Vingerling JR, Breteler MM. 2011. Retinal vascular caliber and risk of dementia: The Rotterdam study. *Neurology* 76:816–821.
94. Liu Y, Wu Y, Xie S, Luan XH, Yuan Y. 2008. Retinal arterial abnormalities correlate with brain white matter lesions in cerebral autosomal dominant arteriopathy with subcortical infarcts and leucoencephalopathy. *Clin Exp Ophthalmol* 36:532–536.
95. Roine S, Harju M, Kivela TT, Poyhonen M, Nikoskelainen E, Tuisku S, Kaimo H, Viitanen M, Summanen PA. 2006. Ophthalmologic findings in cerebral autosomal dominant arteriopathy with subcortical infarcts and leucoencephalopathy. *Ophthalmology* 113:1411–1417.
96. McClintic BR, McClintic JI, Bisognano JD, Block RC. 2010. The relationship between retinal microvascular abnormalities and coronary heart disease: A review. *Am J Med* 123:374.e1–374.e7.
97. Wong TY, Klein R, Sharrett AR, Duncan BB, Couper DJ, Tielsch JM, Klein BE, Hubbard LD. 2002. Retinal arteriolar narrowing and risk of coronary heart disease in men and women. The Atherosclerosis Risk in Communities Study. *JAMA* 287:1153–1159.
98. Wong TY, Kamineni A, Klein R, Sharrett AR, Klein BE, Siscovick DS, Cushman M, Duncan BB. 2006. Quantitative retinal venular caliber and risk of cardiovascular disease in older persons: The cardiovascular health study. *Arch Intern Med* 166:2388–2394.

99. Wang JJ, Liew G, Wong TY, Smith W, Klein R, Leeder SR, Mitchell P. 2006. Retinal vascular caliber and the risk of coronary heart disease-related death. *Heart* 92:1583–1587.
100. Wang JJ, Liew G, Klein R, Rochtchina E, Knudtson MD, Klein BE, Wong TY, Burlutsky G, Mitchell P. 2007. Retinal vessel diameter and cardiovascular mortality: Pooled data analysis from two older populations. *Eur Heart J* 28:1984–1992.
101. McGeechan K, Liew G, Macaskill P, Irwig L, Klein R, Klein BE, Wang JJ et al. 2009. Meta-analysis: Retinal vessel caliber and risk for coronary heart disease. *Ann Intern Med* 151:404–413.
102. Kaul K, Hodgkinson A, Tarr JM, Kohner EM, Chibber R. 2010. Is inflammation a common retinal–renal–nerve pathogenic link in diabetes? *Curr Diabetes Rev* 6:294–303.
103. Edwards MS, Wilson DB, Craven TE, Stafford J, Fried LF, Wong TY, Klein R, Burke GL, Hansen KJ. 2005. Associations between retinal microvascular abnormalities and declining renal function in the elderly population: The Cardiovascular Health Study. *Am J Kidney Dis* 46:214–224.
104. Wong TY, Coresh J, Klein R, Muntner P, Couper DJ, Sharrett AR, Klein BE, Heiss G, Hubbard LD, Duncan BB. 2004. Retinal microvascular abnormalities and renal dysfunction: The atherosclerosis risk in communities study. *J Am Soc Nephrol* 15:2469–2476.
105. Yau JW, Xie J, Kawasaki R, Kramer H, Shlipak M, Klein R, Klein B, Cotch MF, Wong TY. 2011. Retinal arteriolar narrowing and subsequent development of CKD Stage 3: The Multi-Ethnic Study of Atherosclerosis (MESA). *Am J Kidney Dis* 58:39–46.
106. Sabanayagam C, Tai ES, Shankar A, Lee J, Sun C, Wong TY. 2009. Retinal arteriolar narrowing increases the likelihood of chronic kidney disease in hypertension. *J Hypertens* 27:2209–2217.
107. Sabanayagam C, Shankar A, Koh D, Chia KS, Saw SM, Lim SC, Tai ES, Wong TY. 2009. Retinal microvascular caliber and chronic kidney disease in an Asian population. *Am J Epidemiol* 169:625–632.
108. Wong TY, Shankar A, Klein R, Klein BE. 2004. Retinal vessel diameters and the incidence of gross proteinuria and renal insufficiency in people with type 1 diabetes. *Diabetes* 53:179–184.
109. Klein R, Knudtson MD, Klein BE, Zinman B, Gardiner R, Suissa S, Sinaiko AR et al. 2010. The relationship of retinal vessel diameter to changes in diabetic nephropathy structural variables in patients with type 1 diabetes. *Diabetologia* 53:1638–1646.
110. Ooi QL, Tow FK, Deva R, Alias MA, Kawasaki R, Wong TY, Mohamad N, Colville D, Hutchinson A, Savige J. 2010. The microvasculature in chronic kidney disease. *Clin J Am Soc Nephrol* 6:1872–1878.
111. Van Doornum S, Strickland G, Kawasaki R, Xie J, Wicks IP, Hodgson LAB, Wong TY. 2011. Retinal vascular caliber is altered in patients with rheumatoid arthritis: A biomarker of disease activity and cerebrovascular risk? *Rheumatology* 50:939–943.
112. Davies-Tuck ML, Kawasaki R, Wluka AE, Wong TY, Hodgson L, English DR, Giles GG, Cicuttini F. 2012. The relationship between retinal vessel caliber and knee cartilage and BMLs. *BMC Musculoskeletal Disord* 13:255.
113. Pathai S, Weiss HA, Lawn SD, Peto T, D'Costa LM, Cook C, Wong TY, Gilbert CE. 2012. Retinal arterioles narrow with increasing duration of anti-retroviral therapy in HIV infection: A novel estimator of vascular risk in HIV? *PLoS ONE* 7:e51405.
114. Gangaputra S, Kalyani PS, Fawzi AA, Van Natta ML, Hubbard LD, Danis RP, Thorne JE, Holland GN; on behalf of the studies of the ocular complications of AIDS research group. 2012. Retinal vessel caliber among people with acquired immunodeficiency syndrome: Relationships with disease-associated factors and mortality. *Am J Ophthalmol* 153:434–444.
115. Harris B, Klein R, Jerosch-Herold M, Hoffman EA, Ahmed FS, Jacobs Jr DR, Klein BEK et al. 2012. The association of systemic microvascular changes with lung function and lung density: A cross-sectional study. *PLoS ONE* 7:e50224.
116. Klein R, Klein BE, Moss SE, Wong TY, Hubbard L, Cruickshanks KJ, Palta M. 2003. Retinal vascular abnormalities in persons with type 1 diabetes: The Wisconsin Epidemiologic Study of Diabetic Retinopathy: XVIII. *Ophthalmology* 110:2118–2125.
117. Klein R, Klein BE, Moss SE, Wong TY, Hubbard L, Cruickshanks KJ, Palta M. 2004. The relation of retinal vessel caliber to the incidence and progression of diabetic retinopathy: XIX: The Wisconsin Epidemiologic Study of Diabetic Retinopathy. *Arch Ophthalmol* 122:76–83.

118. Klein R, Klein BE, Moss SE, Wong TY, Sharrett AR. 2006. Retinal vascular caliber in persons with type 2 diabetes: The Wisconsin Epidemiological Study of Diabetic Retinopathy: XX. *Ophthalmology* 113:1488–1498.
119. Antonetti DA, Klein R, Gardner TW. 2012. Diabetic retinopathy. *N Engl J Med* 366:1227–1239.
120. Jeganathan VSE, Kawasaki R, Wang JJ, Aung T, Mitchell P, Saw SM, Wong TY. 2008. Retinal vascular caliber and age-related macular degeneration: The Singapore Malay Eye Study. *Am J Ophthalmol* 146:954–959.
121. Yang K, Zhan SY, Liang YB, Duan X, Wang F, Wong TY, Sun LP, Wang NL. 2012. Association of dilated retinal arteriolar caliber with early age-related macular degeneration: The Handan Eye Study. *Graefes Arch Clin Exp Ophthalmol* 250:741–749.
122. Klein R, Klein BE, Tomany SC, Wong TY. 2004. The relation of retinal microvascular characteristics to age-related eye disease: The Beaver Dam Eye Study. *Am J Ophthalmol* 137:435–444.
123. Ikram MK, van Leeuwen R, Vingerling JR, Hofman A, de Jong PT. 2005. Retinal vessel diameters and the risk of incident age-related macular disease: The Rotterdam Study. *Ophthalmology* 112:548–552.
124. Wickremasinghe SS, Busija L, Guymer RH, Wong TY, Qureshi S. 2012. Retinal venular calibre predicts visual outcome after intravitreal ranibizumab injection treatments for neovascular AMD. *Invest Ophthalmol Vis Sci* 53:37–41.
125. Jonas JB, Nguyen XN, Naumann GO. 1989. Parapapillary retinal vessel diameter in normal and glaucoma eyes. I. Morphometric data. *Invest Ophthalmol Vis Sci* 30:1599–1603.
126. Mitchell P, Leung H, Wang JJ, Rochtchina E, Lee AJ, Wong TY, Klein R. 2005. Retinal vessel diameter and open-angle glaucoma: The Blue Mountains Eye Study. *Ophthalmology* 112:245–250.
127. Angelica MM, Sanseau A, Argento C. 2001. Arterial narrowing as a predictive factor in glaucoma. *Int Ophthalmol* 23:271–274.
128. Chang M, Yoo C, Kim SW, Kim YY. 2011. Retinal vessel diameter, retinal nerve fiber layer thickness, and intraocular pressure in Korean patients with normal-tension glaucoma. *Am J Ophthalmol* 151:100–105.
129. Arend O, Remky A, Plange N, Martin BJ, Harris A. 2002. Capillary density and retinal diameter measurements and their impact on altered retinal circulation in glaucoma: A digital fluorescein angiographic study. *Br J Ophthalmol* 86:429–433.
130. Ikram MK, deVoogd S, Wolfs RC, Hofman A, Breteler MM, Hubbard LD, deJong PT. 2005. Retinal vessel diameters and incident open-angle glaucoma and optic disc changes: The Rotterdam study. *Invest Ophthalmol Vis Sci* 46:1182–1187.
131. Kawasaki R, Wang JJ, Rochtchina E, Lee AJ, Wong TY, Mitchell P. 2013. Retinal vessel caliber is associated with the 10-year incidence of glaucoma. *Ophthalmology* 120:84–90.
132. Youm DJ, Ha MM, Chang Y, Song SJ. 2012. Retinal vessel caliber and risk factors for branch retinal vein occlusion. *Curr Eye Res* 37:334–338.
133. Knudtson MD, Klein BE, Klein R, Wong TY, Hubbard LD, Lee KE, Meuer SM, Bulla CP. 2004. Variation associated with measurement of retinal vessel diameters at different points in the pulse cycle. *Br J Ophthalmol* 88:57–61.
134. Cheung CY, Tay WT, Mitchell P, Wang JJ, Hsu W, Lee ML, Lau QP et al. 2011. Quantitative and qualitative retinal microvascular characteristics and blood pressure. *J Hypertens* 29:1380–1391.
135. Nguyen TT, Kawasaki R, Wang JJ et al. 2009. Flicker light-induced retinal vasodilation in diabetes and diabetic retinopathy. *Diabetes Care* 32:2075–2080.

2

*Detection, Modeling, and Analysis of the Major Temporal Arcade in Fundus Images of the Retina**

Faraz Oloumi, Rangaraj M. Rangayyan, and Anna L. Ells

CONTENTS

* This chapter is a revised and expanded version of Oloumi, F., Rangayyan, R.M., and Ells, A.L., Parabolic modeling of the major temporal arcade in retinal fundus images, *IEEE Transactions on Instrumentation and Measurement (TIM)*, 61(7):1825–1838, July 2012.

2.1 Introduction

2.1.1 Posterior Vascular Changes in the Retina

Changes in the vascular structure of the retina can indicate the presence of several types of pathology, such as hypertension, arteriosclerosis, proliferative diabetic retinopathy (PDR), myopia, and retinopathy of prematurity (ROP). The vessels in the retina are modified in terms of their width, shape, and tortuosity by the diseases listed in the preceding sentence [1–5]. Changes in the architecture of the major temporal arcade (MTA), in the form of a decrease in the angle of insertion as well as straightening, have been cited as manifestations of at least two types of pathology [1,5]: as a sequela of ROP and as an indicator of the severity of myopia [1,5]. The architecture of the MTA is also known to be affected by PDR due to tractional retinal detachment.

The angle of insertion of the MTA has been loosely defined as the angle between the superior and inferior temporal arcades (STA and ITA) as they diverge from the optic nerve head (ONH) and extend toward the periphery of the retina. This angle, also called the arcade angle, has been used as an indicator of the structural integrity of the macular region [3,5–7]. Despite the clinical importance of abnormal changes in the architecture of the MTA, only the angle of insertion of the MTA has been quantified in only a few studies: a study dealing with myopia [5] and two studies dealing with ROP [6,7].

2.1.2 Changes in the Angle of Insertion of the MTA

Fledelius and Goldschmidt [5] measured the angle between the STA and the ITA and correlated its decrease to progression of myopia based on follow-up data over a 38-year period. They defined the arcade angle by manually marking cardinal points at the first or the second major arteriole–venule crossing away from the ONH (decided subjectively to represent the direction of the temporal arcade vessels and not just the venule), with the vertex of the angle being at the center of the ONH. The cardinal points were used as landmarks from image to image. Two lines were drawn from the center of the ONH to the marked cardinal points on the ITA and the STA. The angle between the two lines was measured using a transparent angle meter. Fledelius and Goldschmidt [5] reported a decrease of more than 4° in the arcade angle in 25% (6 of 24) of the cases with high and stable myopia and in 60% (12 of 20) of the cases with high and progressive myopia. The change in the arcade angle of the progressive myopia group as compared to the stable myopia group was shown to be statistically highly significant ($p < 0.01$). For the high and progressive myopia group, the change in the arcade angle was shown to be correlated with the degree and increase of myopia.

Change in the angle of insertion of the MTA has also been featured in the classification of retrolental fibroplasia [8] and more recently in the classification of ROP [1]; it has also been used in the evaluation of structural changes following cryotherapy [9]. The Cryotherapy for Retinopathy of Prematurity Cooperative Group [9] evaluated the arcade angle by manually tracking the MTA in 30° sectors; however, the normal range of the arcade angle was not defined.

Wilson et al. [6] defined the angle of insertion of the MTA as follows: the center of the ONH and the fovea are manually marked by two independent observers. A line is drawn through the manually marked center of the ONH and the fovea; this is the retinal raphe. The image is rotated so that the retinal raphe is horizontal. A line perpendicular

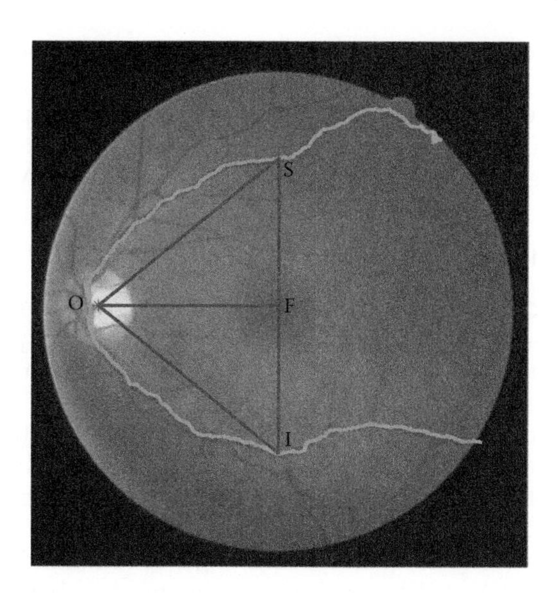

FIGURE 2.1
Image 21 of the DRIVE database illustrating the procedure for measuring the angle of insertion of the MTA as proposed by Wilson et al. [2]. The MTA, as traced by a retinal specialist (see Section 2.2.1), is highlighted. The points O and F represent the center of the ONH and the fovea marked by a retinal specialist. The points S and I represent the intersection of the normal (SI) to the retinal raphe (OF) with the STA and ITA, respectively. The angle ∠SOF is the SAA, the angle ∠IOF is the IAA, and the angle ∠SOI is the TAA. Hence, TAA = SAA + IAA, where $SAA = \arctan(SF/OF)$ and $IAA = \arctan(IF/OF)$. (Reproduced with permission from Oloumi, F., Rangayyan, R.M., and Ells, A.L., Parabolic modeling of the major temporal arcade in retinal fundus images, *IEEE Trans. Instrum. Meas.*, 61(7), 1825–1838, © July 2012 IEEE.)

to the retinal raphe is drawn from the fovea until it intersects the ITA and the STA. From the intersections, two lines are drawn to the center of the ONH. The total arcade angle (TAA) is defined as the sum of the inferior and the superior arcade angles (IAA and SAA), as shown in Figure 2.1. Wilson et al. [6] reported a high degree of interocular symmetry with a mean TAA of 82° for both eyes. They indicated that interocular asymmetry of above 14°–20° between the two eyes of a patient should be treated with suspicion. A significant level of acuteness in the IAA of the left eye was associated between stage 0 and 1, stage 1 and 2, and stage 1 and 3 of ROP (higher numbers indicate higher severity of ROP).

In a related follow-up study by Wong et al. [7], semiautomated measurements were made of four different angles of the temporal and the nasal venules and arterioles. The procedures required manual editing of automatically detected vessels; this step required 10–15 min per image. The vertex of all measured angles was set at the center of the ONH, and the other two points were obtained automatically as the intersection of a circle of radius 60 pixels with the previously marked major arteriole and venule branches on both the temporal and the nasal sides. As compared to the previous related study of Wilson et al. [6], the angles were measured using reference points selected closer to the center of the ONH. The nasal angles were found to have no statistically significant differences between normal cases and ROP of various stages. The angles of the temporal venules and arterioles were found to have statistically significant differences between normal cases and stage 3 ROP. However, when all stages of ROP were combined, only the angle of the temporal arterioles indicated statistically significant difference as compared to the normal cases.

By combining time series of fundus images into short video clips, Ells and MacKeen [10,11] illustrated that the changes that occur in the MTA in the presence of progressive ROP are dynamic as they alter the posterior architecture of the MTA.

2.1.3 Detection and Modeling of the MTA

Because the MTA originates from the ONH and follows a curved, almost parabolic, path toward the macula, it can be used to detect or estimate the position of the ONH. Furthermore, relative to the location of the ONH, the macular region can also be estimated or detected [12–18].

Using an estimate of the ONH location and a binarized image of the vasculature, Tobin et al. [13] proposed to apply a parabolic model to the statistical distribution of a set of points given by a morphologically skeletonized vascular image to find an estimate of the retinal raphe. A parabola of the form $ay^2 = |x|$ was modified to accommodate for the shifted vertex at the most likely ONH location and the angle of rotation of the retinal raphe, β. The resulting model and the skeletonized image were used with a least-squares method to estimate the parameters a and β. Even though Tobin et al. estimated the openness of the parabolic model, it was only used to draw a parabola on the image.

Using steerable filters and color thresholding, Kochner et al. [16] extracted edge points on the main blood vessels. An ellipse was then fitted to these points using the generalized Hough transform (GHT). The end of the long axis of the ellipse was taken as an estimate of the location of the ONH.

Using an active shape model and defining a point distribution model, Li and Chutatape [14] proposed a method to detect the boundary of the ONH and the main course of the blood vessels. Using the active shape model and principal component analysis, the location of the ONH was estimated. A modified active shape model was used to extract the main course of the blood vessels. Thirty landmark points on the main course of the vessels were used to derive the point distribution model. The Hough transform and linear least-squares fitting methods were combined to estimate a parabolic model.

Niemeijer et al. [18] used a point distribution model to represent the ONH, the fovea, and the MTA. The point distribution model consisted of 16 points, where different sets of points were constrained to represent different structures; a set of 10 points was used to mark the MTA. Five hundred retinal images were used to train an optimization algorithm to minimize a cost function and obtain a set of parameters. The cost function employed was based on two global terms, vessel width and orientation, and one local term, structure measurement around the model points. The optimization procedure was performed in both the parameter space and in the image space. The set of obtained parameters was used with the same optimization algorithms to minimize the cost function, given an image, to obtain a point distribution model. The methods were tested using another set of 500 images. However, since the MTA model consisted of only 10 points, the results of modeling of the MTA were evaluated visually. If all 10 points were lying on the correct vessel, as indicated by a human observer, the result was considered to be a complete detection; if only the ITA or the STA was detected, the result was labeled as partial detection. The result was considered to be a failure if neither the former nor the latter was true. Niemeijer et al. reported 93.2% complete detection of the MTA, 5.6% partial detection, and 1.2% complete failure to detect the MTA in 500 images of the retina.

By using the supremum of openings operator on an enhanced grayscale image of blood vessels, Welfer et al. [19] extracted the STA and the ITA to locate the ONH. A set of 24 linear structuring elements of length 80 pixels was used to extract the MTA. The resulting image was binarized, skeletonized, and pruned to obtain a binary image that represented the STA and the ITA.

Foracchia et al. [12] proposed a method for the detection of the ONH by defining a directional model for the vessels, assuming that the main vessels originate from the ONH and extend in paths that can be geometrically modeled as parabolas. A directional model was defined using the parabolic formulation and assuming that the preferred direction of the vessels is tangential to the parabolas themselves. With the model and data indicating the center points, direction, and caliber of the vessels, by using a residual sum of squares method, the parameters of the model were identified.

Fleming et al. [15] proposed a method to extract the MTA by means of vessel enhancement and semielliptical curve fitting using the GHT. First, the vessels were enhanced to get a magnitude image and a phase image of the vascular architecture. Assuming that, having an edge map and knowing the orientation of the arcade, a reference point can only be at one of a few locations, the GHT was applied to a skeletonized image of the vasculature. The Hough-space dimension was set to be five, with variables for inclination, horizontal axis length, left or right opening, and the location of the center of the ellipse. Anatomical restrictions were applied to the variables to limit the number of semiellipses generated by the method. The global maximum in the Hough space was selected as the closest fit to the MTA.

Ying and Liu [17] obtained a vascular topology map using an energy function defined as the normalized product of the local blood vessel width and density. A quantile threshold was used on the vascular topology map to extract the pixels in a high-energy band. A circle-fitting method was applied to the extracted pixels to model the MTA as a circle, which was then used to localize the macula.

The previously published methods to measure the angle of insertion of the MTA, as explained in Section 2.1.2, may not properly reflect the changes that occur in the structure of the MTA, as they only define the openness of the MTA based on three points. Furthermore, only the location of the vertex of the arcade angle has been consistently defined as the center of the ONH; the locations of the other two points have been defined in different manners, as mentioned in Section 2.1.2. Even though the structure of the MTA has been used to estimate the ONH and the macula in previously reported works, only Tobin et al. [13] modeled the arcade for parameterization of its openness; however, they used the openness parameter only to draw the parabolic model on the image.

The parabolic profile of the MTA allows for effective modeling using a form of the GHT [20–23]. In such a model, changes in the architecture of the MTA could be expected to be reflected as changes in the openness parameter of the parabola: this approach forms the basis for the present work [20–23].

2.2 Methods

2.2.1 Database and Annotation of the MTA

The proposed methods were tested with retinal fundus images from the Digital Retinal Images for Vessel Extraction (DRIVE) database [24], which contains 40 retinal images of adults. Each image is of size 584 × 565 pixels, with a field of view (FOV) of 45° and spatial resolution of approximately 20 μm per pixel. The DRIVE database includes 33 images with no abnormal signs and 7 images with signs of diabetic retinopathy, such as exudates, hemorrhages, and pigment epithelium changes. For the purpose of evaluation of the performance of the proposed methods, the STAs and the ITAs in all of the 40 images were traced separately by an expert ophthalmologist and retinal specialist (A.L.E.), by magnifying the original image by 145% using the software ImageJ [25]. Only the main venule, the thickest branch, was traced within the FOV. At each branching point, the larger branch was followed. The availability of separate traces of the STA and the ITA facilitates the assessment of the accuracy of the dual-parabolic modeling procedure as described in Section 2.2.8. The hand-drawn traces of the STA and the ITA can be combined to obtain the trace of the MTA.

The foveas in all of the 40 images were also marked, using the same setup, by the same specialist. The centers of the ONH in all of the images were also marked by A.L.E., as described in a related report [26] (see Figure 2.1 for an example of an annotated image). The manual markings of the ONH centers and the foveas were used to correct for any rotation existing between the retinal raphe and the horizontal axis of a given image, as described in Section 2.2.7.

2.2.2 Overview of the Image Processing Methods

There are three main steps involved in the detection of the MTA. The first step of the proposed algorithm is only presented in point form, because it has been described in detail in one of our previous publications [27]. The second step is outlined briefly in Section 2.2.3 as it also has been presented in detail in our previous related study [20]. The third step is discussed in detail in Section 2.2.5. The three steps are as follows:

1. Preprocessing of images [27]
   a. Normalizing each color component in the original image
   b. Computing the luminance component
   c. Thresholding the luminance component to obtain the effective area
   d. Extending the luminance component beyond the effective area to avoid the detection of its edges
2. Obtaining the skeletons of the MTA, the ITA, and the STA [20,22,23] (see Sections 2.2.3 and 2.2.8)
   a. Obtaining the Gabor-magnitude response using 180 Gabor filters over the range of [−90°, 90°] to represent the MTA [27]
   b. Separating the Gabor-magnitude response image into its superior and inferior parts to represent the STA and the ITA, respectively
   c. Binarizing the Gabor-magnitude response images of the MTA, the ITA, and the STA
   d. Skeletonizing the binary images
   e. Applying the morphological process of area open to filter the skeletons
3. Detecting parabolas and semiparabolas using the GHT [20–23] (see Sections 2.2.5 and 2.2.8)
   a. Rotating each skeleton image by 180°, if the MTA opens to the left (i.e., the image is of the right eye)
   b. Cropping each skeleton image horizontally

c. Applying the GHT to the preprocessed skeleton images of the MTA, the STA, and the ITA
d. Rotating the Hough spaces by 180°, if the MTA opens to the left, and obtaining the parameters of the best-fitting parabolas

2.2.3 Detection of the MTA Using Gabor Filters

Gabor filters are sinusoidally modulated Gaussian functions. A Gabor filter is defined by the standard deviation (STD) values of the Gaussian function in the x and y directions (σ_x and σ_y) and the frequency, f_0, of the modulating sinusoid as [27,28]

$$g(x,y)=\frac{1}{2\pi\sigma_x\sigma_y}\exp\left[-\frac{1}{2}\left(\frac{x^2}{\sigma_x^2}+\frac{y^2}{\sigma_y^2}\right)\right]\cos(2\pi f_0 x). \tag{2.1}$$

To simplify the design procedure, a variable named τ, representing the average thickness of the vessels to be detected, is introduced in the design of the Gabor filter. The value of σ_x is defined in relation to τ as $\sigma_x=\tau/\{2\sqrt{2\ln 2}\}$. The value of f_0 is defined as $f_0=1/\tau$. The parameter σ_y is set as $\sigma_y=2\sigma_x$. In the present work, we use $\tau=16$ pixels (0.32 mm).

A set of 180 Gabor filters spanning the range [–90°, 90°] is prepared by rotating the basic Gabor function in Equation 2.1. A magnitude response image is created by using the maximum value of the responses of the 180 Gabor filters for each pixel. The Gabor-magnitude response image is then thresholded at 0.0095 of the normalized intensity to obtain a binarized image. The binarized image is skeletonized [29] and undesired short segments are removed by using the area open procedure [30]. The skeletonization procedure uses the concept of pixel connectedness [31] to delete unwanted pixels and retains lines of single-pixel thickness without altering the structure of the objects. The morphological operation of area open procedure also uses the concept of pixel connectedness [31] to detect segments of connected pixels having less than 70 pixels (as specified in the present work) and removes them.

2.2.4 Hough Transform

The Hough transform has long been recognized as a powerful image processing method for the detection of curves, shapes, and motion in images with noisy and irrelevant or even missing data [32,33]. Hough [34] originally proposed the method for the detection of straight lines in bubble-chamber photographs. The method has since been modified and extended, in many different ways, to detect lines, circles, and parabolic and hyperbolic curves; for estimation of 2D and 3D motion; for object recognition; and for the detection of arbitrary shapes [32,33,35]. The Hough transform either refers to the general process of detection of shapes or to the original method to detect straight lines and its different variations; the GHT refers to all other methods that employ the Hough transform process but detect other shapes and curves, instead. Both the Hough transform and the GHT have been used in industrial settings as well as in image processing hardware algorithms for rapid detection of lines and other curves [32]. One of the earliest applications of the GHT in biomedical image processing was demonstrated by Wechsler and Sklansky [36]; they applied the GHT for the detection of parabolas in X-ray images of the chest to detect the rib cage. Different forms and variations of the GHT have since been used in various biomedical image processing applications [37–40].

The Hough transform has several important properties that make it desirable for shape detection and modeling:

1. The Hough transform recognizes partial or slightly misshaped curves and lines, which can pose problems for other shape detection methods.
2. The Hough transform detects shapes in the presence of random and unrelated data.
3. The Hough transform detects several variations of the same shape in the given image in one operation.
4. The Hough transform processes each pixel independently; hence, parallel processing of data is possible for fast hardware implementation.

It should be noted that unwanted data that are similar to the shape to be detected could have an effect on the outcome of the Hough transform and should be treated with care.

The Hough transform reduces a global shape detection problem in the spatial domain to a simpler peak detection problem in a parameter space. Every spatial point that belongs to the pattern leads to a vote on different combinations of parameters that could have caused its presence, if it were part of the shape to be detected. An accumulator matrix is used to store and count the votes; the final count for each accumulator cell indicates the likelihood of the shape, described by the corresponding parameter values of the accumulator cell, belonging to the given pattern in the spatial domain. The size of the accumulator matrix is determined by the number of parameters and their limits.

The Hough transform is said to be similar to template-matching methods, but it is more efficient and advantageous [32,33,41]. Template matching is implemented entirely in the spatial domain, whereas the Hough transform is implemented in a parameter domain or the Hough space. In template matching, different templates are generated by shifting and reflecting a basic template and then trying to determine how well the image points match the template points. However, in many instances, corresponding points do not exist in the image domain, which makes the template-matching algorithm inefficient; the Hough transform assumes a match between a given template and an image point and then attempts to determine the transformation parameters that relate the two. The Hough transform does not generate the inessential data that are generated by a template-matching algorithm. Further restrictions on the limits of the Hough-space parameters can make the Hough transform even more efficient.

Specific forms of the Hough transform have also been shown to have similarities to other estimation methods such as the Radon transform and the generalized maximum-likelihood estimators. The Hough transform for line-segment detection has some qualitative properties that are similar to the Radon transform. However, the Radon transform cannot provide all of the different variations that are possible to be achieved by the Hough transform [32,33,40]. Depending on the kernel function used to relate the image in the spatial domain to the parameter space, the Hough transform can take on different forms of the class of maximum-likelihood estimators. A quadratic kernel function, for example, implies that the Hough transform could behave like a least-squares estimator in the continuous domain; the concept can be extended to the discrete domain [33].

2.2.5 Generalized Hough Transform for the Detection of Parabolas

Fleming et al. [15] and Kochner et al. [16] assumed semielliptic and elliptic profiles for the MTA, respectively. However, the MTA diverges away from the ONH toward the macula and then converges down into the macular region. Furthermore, after the second or third branching point, it becomes difficult to distinguish between the original arcade and the new branch as they are both similar in diameter and can branch erratically. The second and third branching points occur approximately over the macula. If one were to use a parametric curve to fit a model to the entire MTA, it would be difficult to define a specific model; an ellipse appears to be the best estimate to the overall vascular structure, but not a specific arcade.

The fact that posterior changes occur close to the ONH, along with a priori knowledge of the center of the ONH, and the observation that the macula is situated approximately two ONH diameters (ONHD) temporal to the ONH [42] are used in the present work to guide the modeling procedure and reduce the computational cost of the algorithm. The average ONHD is about 1.6 mm [42,43]. The MTA has a parabolic shape up to the macula, so we only need a skeleton of the MTA from the ONH to the macular region for parabolic modeling. There appears to be no useful information on the nasal side of the ONH; thus, this part may also be eliminated. Hence, in the present work, the skeleton image is horizontally limited from $0.25 \times$ ONHD nasal to $2 \times$ ONHD temporal with respect to the center of the ONH. Using the average ONHD and given the spatial resolution of the DRIVE database [24], the width of the image is automatically limited to the range $\left[O_x - 20,\ O_x + 160\right]$, where O_x denotes the x-coordinate of the automatically detected center of the ONH using Gabor filters and phase portrait analysis as described by Rangayyan et al. [26].

The general formula defining a parabola with its directrix parallel to the y-axis and its symmetrical axis parallel to the x-axis is

$$(y - y_0)^2 = 4a(x - x_0), \tag{2.2}$$

where

(x_0, y_0) is the vertex of the parabola
the quantity $4a$ is known as the latus rectum [44]

The absolute value of a defines the aperture or openness of the parabola and its sign indicates the direction of the opening of the parabola; for a positive a value, the parabola opens to the right (see Figure 2.2a). The parameters (x_0, y_0, a) define the parameter domain or the Hough space, represented by an accumulator matrix, A. For every nonzero pixel in the image domain, there exists a parabola in the Hough space for each value of a; a single point in the Hough space defines a parabola in the image domain (see Figure 2.2b through d).

For the DRIVE images, the size of each (x_0, y_0) plane in the Hough space was defined to be the same as the horizontally cropped skeleton image (584×180 pixels). In the present work, the value of a is restricted by physiological limits on the MTA and the size of the image. For the DRIVE database, $|a|$ was confined to the range [35, 120]. In order not to make the accumulator too large, only positive values of a were defined. If an image had the MTA opening to the left (i.e., an image of the right eye), it was rotated by 180° so that the MTA would open to the right in the image used for the subsequent steps. Thus, the number of planes in the Hough space for the parameter a was defined to be 86. To make further use of the possible anatomical restrictions, the vertex location (x_0, y_0) of the parabolas represented in the Hough space was restricted to be within $0.25 \times$ ONHD of the automatically detected center of the ONH.

For each nonzero pixel in the given vascular skeleton, the parameter a was computed for each (x_0, y_0) in the Hough space, and the corresponding accumulator cell was incremented

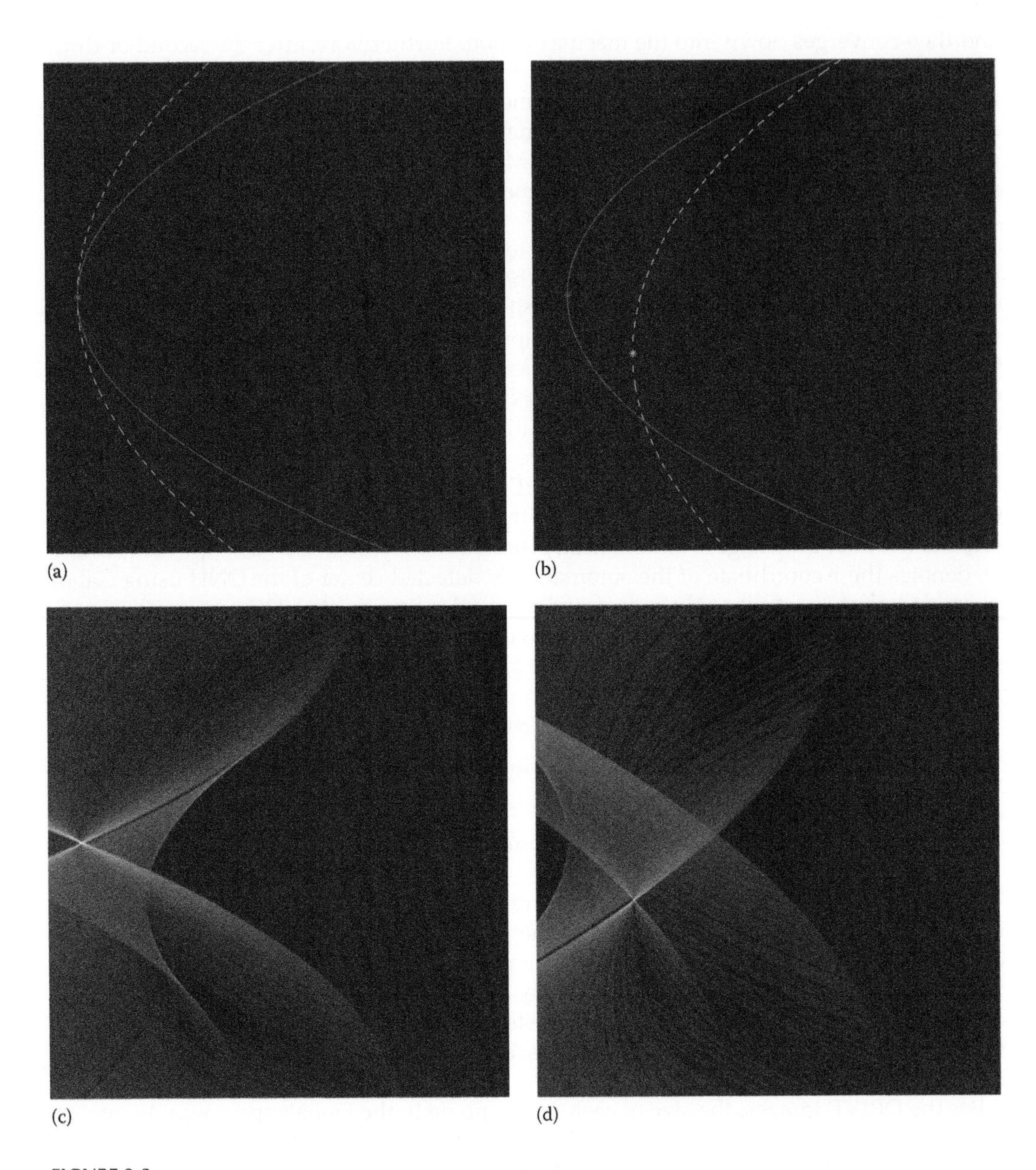

FIGURE 2.2
(a) A test image of size 584 × 565 pixels, showing two parabolas with different openness parameters; the line parabola has $a = 60$ and the dashed-line one has $a = 120$. Both parabolas share the same vertex for the sake of comparison of their openness. (b) The same parabolas as in (a) but with different vertices; the solid-line parabola has its vertex at (40, 280) and the dashed-line parabola has its vertex at (120, 350); the top-left corner of the image is represented by the coordinates (1, 1). (c) The Hough-space plane for $a = 60$ for the image in part (b), showing the detected vertex (41, 280) for the parabola with the smaller aperture as the point with the highest value. (d) The Hough-space plane for $a = 120$ for the image in part (b), showing the detected vertex (120, 351) for the parabola with the larger aperture. The detected vertex coordinates, along with the corresponding a value, define the parabolic model. (Reproduced with permission from Oloumi, F., Rangayyan, R.M., and Ells, A.L., Parabolic modeling of the major temporal arcade in retinal fundus images, *IEEE Trans. Instrum. Meas.*, 61(7), 1825–1838, ©July 2012 IEEE.)

by unity if the value of a was within the specified range. Usually, a binarized skeleton image of only the MTA is used in the GHT. However, we can use the Gabor-magnitude response of the blood vessels to provide a larger weight to the pixels that belong to the MTA; the higher the Gabor-magnitude response of a pixel on the skeleton, the more likely it belongs to the MTA (for the Gabor parameters used in the present work). Thus, in a variation of the GHT, instead of incrementing each accumulator cell by unity, it was incremented by the Gabor-magnitude response of the same pixel. The point in the resulting Hough space with the highest value was selected to obtain the parameters (x_0, y_0, a) of the best-fitting parabolic model to the MTA.

2.2.6 Selection of Candidates from the Hough Space

The global maximum in the Hough space may not always present the best-fitting model. Hence, a procedure based on the mean distance to the closest point (MDCP) [45] was implemented to select the best fit among the top 10 Hough-space candidates. The MDCP measures the closeness of two given contours based on the mean of the distance to the closest point (DCP) from one of the contours (the model) to the other (the reference). Given a model, $M = \{m_1, m_2, \ldots, m_N\}$, and a reference, $R = \{r_1, r_2, \ldots, r_K\}$, the DCP for a single point m_i on M is defined as

$$\text{DCP}(m_i, R) = \min(\| m_i - r_j \|), \quad j = 1, 2, \ldots, K, \tag{2.3}$$

where $||\cdot||$ is a norm operator, such as the Euclidean norm. The MDCP is computed as

$$\text{MDCP}(M, R) = \frac{1}{N} \sum_{i=1}^{N} \text{DCP}(m_i, R). \tag{2.4}$$

The smaller the MDCP value, the closer the fit is to the reference. The MDCP values were calculated for each of the top 10 parabolic fits with the automatically detected vascular skeleton serving as the reference. The fit with the smallest MDCP value was selected as the best-fitting model to the MTA. To compare the effects of the vertex restriction and the updating of the accumulator by the Gabor-magnitude response, four versions of the GHT were tested: the unity-updated GHT, the unity-updated GHT with the vertex restriction, the Gabor-magnitude-updated GHT, and the Gabor-magnitude-updated GHT with the vertex restriction.

2.2.7 Correction of the Retinal Raphe Angle

Any rotation that might exist between the retinal raphe and the horizontal axis of the given image could affect the modeling procedure. The manual markings of the fovea and the center of the ONH were used to determine the rotation angle and correct the image by the same amount. Given (F_x, F_y) and (O_x, O_y) as the coordinates of the fovea and the center of the ONH, respectively, the raphe angle, θ, is defined as

$$\theta = \arctan\left(\frac{F_y - O_y}{F_x - O_x}\right). \tag{2.5}$$

Figure 2.3a shows an image before and after raphe-angle correction as explained. All of the 40 DRIVE images were rotated, using bilinear interpolation, by their calculated

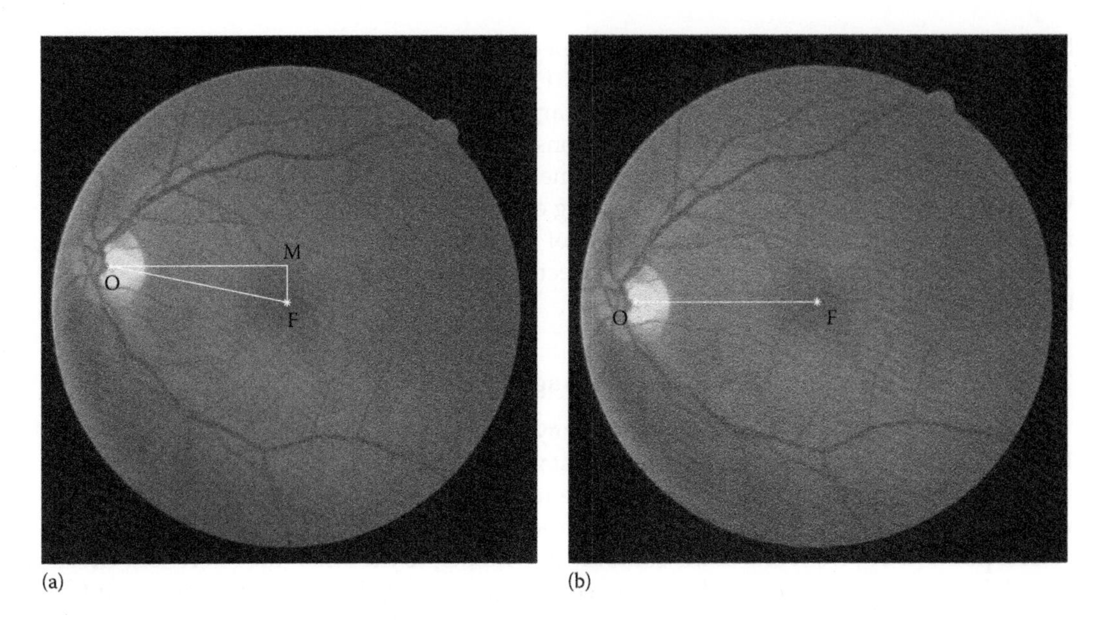

FIGURE 2.3
(a) Image 21 of the DRIVE database (584 × 565 pixels) showing the manually marked fovea (F) and the center of the ONH (O). The line OF represents the retinal raphe. The line OM is parallel to the horizontal axis of the image. The retinal raphe angle is defined as $\theta = \arctan(MF/OF)$. (b) The image in (a) with the raphe angle corrected. (Reproduced with permission from Oloumi, F., Rangayyan, R.M., and Ells, A.L., Parabolic modeling of the major temporal arcade in retinal fundus images, *IEEE Trans. Instrum. Meas.*, 61(7), 1825–1838, © July 2012 IEEE.)

θ values. The same procedures outlined in Section 2.2.2 were also applied to all of the 40 DRIVE images with correction for the retinal raphe angles.

2.2.8 Dual-Parabolic Modeling

The ITA and the STA are often asymmetric; thus, a single-parabolic model may match either one of the arcades, but not both. Modeling each part of the arcade separately may be a more suitable option. For this purpose, the automatically detected center of the ONH was used to separate the Gabor-magnitude response image into its superior and inferior parts. To represent the ITA, any information in the range $y \in [1, O_y]$ was eliminated in the Gabor-magnitude response image. Any information within the range $y \in [(O_y + 1), 584]$ was eliminated in the Gabor-magnitude response image to obtain a representation of the STA. The same procedures as in Section 2.2.3 were applied to the superior and inferior Gabor-magnitude response images to obtain the vascular skeletons of the STA and ITA, respectively. When modeling each arcade separately, it is essential to restrict the vertex of the resulting parabolas in the Hough space. For this reason, the Gabor-magnitude-updated GHT with the vertex restriction along with the raphe-angle correction and the MDCP-based selection procedures were applied to the skeleton images obtained of the STA and the ITA. The part of the fit to the STA in the range $y \in [1, V_y]$ was taken as the STA model, where V_y is the y-coordinate of the detected vertex of the parabola. The ITA model was taken as the fit to the ITA in the range $y \in [V_y, 584]$. This form of modeling results in two openness parameters: a_{STA} and a_{ITA}. Separate analysis of the openness of each arcade (ITA and STA) may be more beneficial as shown by the correlation of the stages of ROP with only the changes in the IAA in the work of Wilson et al. [6].

The ITA and the STA converge within the ONH, but not necessarily at a single point. Indeed, the arcades drawn by the expert ophthalmologist (A.L.E.) for the images of the DRIVE database indicate different points of convergence of the ITA and the STA into the ONH. For these reasons, no restriction was placed on the vertices of the two parabolas in the dual-parabolic modeling procedure other than being located within a distance of $0.25 \times \text{ONHD}$ of the automatically detected center of the ONH.

2.2.9 Measures of Performance

In order to evaluate the accuracy of the automatically detected vascular skeleton and the parabolic model derived thereof (*Auto*), as compared to the hand-drawn MTA traces, the unity-updated GHT with the vertex restriction was applied to the hand-drawn traces (*Hand*). The parameters obtained for the hand-drawn traces were compared to the parameters of the parabolic fits from the four GHT versions applied to the vascular skeleton. The Euclidean distance between the two detected vertices, given as

$$d = \sqrt{\left(x_{oHand} - x_{oAuto}\right)^2 + \left(y_{oHand} - y_{oAuto}\right)^2}, \tag{2.6}$$

was used as an error measure for each image. As a second measure, the correlation coefficient, r, between the two sets of values of the parameter a (for the 40 DRIVE images) was calculated as

$$r = \frac{C(a_{Hand}, a_{Auto})}{\sqrt{C(a_{Auto}, a_{Auto}) - C(a_{Hand}, a_{Hand})}}, \tag{2.7}$$

where C is the covariance. A correlation coefficient close to unity and a vertex error close to zero would indicate that an accurate vascular skeleton image was obtained over the entire set of images. These measures are used in the present work only to assess the performance of the procedure to derive the vascular skeleton.

To assess the accuracy of the parabolic model for each image, the MDCP was obtained as one measure (see Section 2.2.6). The MDCP was measured from the parabolic model, obtained using each of the variations of the four different GHTs, to the corresponding hand-drawn trace of the MTA, the latter being treated as the reference. In the case of the dual-parabolic modeling procedure, the MDCP was measured from the STA and the ITA models to the hand-drawn traces of the STA and the ITA, respectively; hence, two separate measures were obtained for the results of the dual-parabolic modeling procedure. The lower the MDCP value, the more accurate is the parabolic model. The MDCP measure was restricted to $2 \times \text{ONHD}$ distance from the ONH center (as explained in Section 2.2.5).

The Hausdorff distance [46] was used as another measure to assess the accuracy of the parabolic models. The Hausdorff distance is comparable to the MDCP as it first finds the DCP from each point on the parabolic fit (model) to the corresponding hand-drawn trace (reference) of the MTA. However, instead of taking the mean of all the DCPs, the Hausdorff distance takes their maximum. Given the model, $M = \{m_1, m_2, \ldots, m_N\}$, and the reference, $R = \{r_1, r_2, \ldots, r_K\}$, the DCP for a single point m_i on M is defined using Equation 2.3. The Hausdorff distance, H, from M to R is computed as

$$H(M,R) = \max\{\mathrm{DCP}(M,R)\}, \tag{2.8}$$

where DCP(M,R) is an $N \times 1$ vector representing the DCPs for each point on M. It should be noted that the Hausdorff distance is not symmetric, that is, $H(M,R) \neq H(R,M)$. The Hausdorff distance indicates how much the longest distance is from the model to the reference. In the present work, the Hausdorff distance was obtained using the same setup as used to measure the MDCP.

2.3 Results

The methods were tested using a desktop computer with an Intel Core i7 (hyperthreaded quad-core) 2.8 GHz processor, 8 MB level 3 cache, 8 GB DDR3 RAM, running 64-bit Windows 7 Professional, and using a 64-bit version of MATLAB®. The computation time was 27 s to run all of the three steps listed in Section 2.2.2 for one image. The original image 24 from the DRIVE database is shown in Figure 2.4a. The inverted and preprocessed grayscale image used for Gabor filtering is shown in Figure 2.4b. The magnitude response of the Gabor filters is shown in Figure 2.4c. The thresholded binary image of the blood vessels, which was skeletonized and filtered using the area open procedure, is shown in Figure 2.4d; this result mostly contains the main temporal venule. However, small parts of the main arteriole are also present. The minor vessels are removed by the thresholding step because of their low response due to the large value of the thickness parameter used for the Gabor filters ($\tau = 16$ pixels).

The skeleton and the Gabor-magnitude images were automatically clipped horizontally up to the macula, as shown in Figure 2.4e and f. The restricted skeleton image was analyzed using the four different variations of the GHT described in Section 2.2.5. The restricted Gabor-magnitude image was used in the two Gabor-magnitude-updated versions of the GHT.

The Hough-space plane for $a = -64$ is shown in Figure 2.4g, which contains the global maximum in the case of the unity-updated GHT without the vertex restriction. The Gabor-magnitude-updated GHT had its global maximum in the $a = -66$ plane, as shown in Figure 2.4h. The use of the Gabor-magnitude response to update the Hough-space cells increases the intensity for parabolas originating from the thickest branch. Hence, it produces a less crowded Hough space with large values only close to the ONH. For the case of the Gabor-magnitude-updated GHT with the vertex restriction, the global maximum was in the $a = -75$ plane, as shown in Figure 2.4i. The Hough space was only updated if (x_0, y_0), as in Equation 2.2, was located within a circle with diameter $= 0.5 \times$ ONHD positioned at the automatically detected center of the ONH. This forces a parabolic fit close to the posterior pole.

The hand-drawn trace of the MTA for the image in Figure 2.4a and its parabolic fit, obtained using the unity-updated GHT with the vertex restriction, are shown in Figure 2.5a. The global maximum was used to determine the three parabolic fits resulting from the unity-updated GHT without vertex restriction, the Gabor-magnitude-updated GHT without vertex restriction, and the Gabor-magnitude-updated GHT with vertex restriction, as shown in Figure 2.5b through d, respectively.

The correlation coefficients of the parameter a and the vertex errors of the parabolic fits for the results of the four versions of the GHT, as compared to the parameters of the fits to the corresponding hand-drawn arcades using the unity-updated GHT with vertex

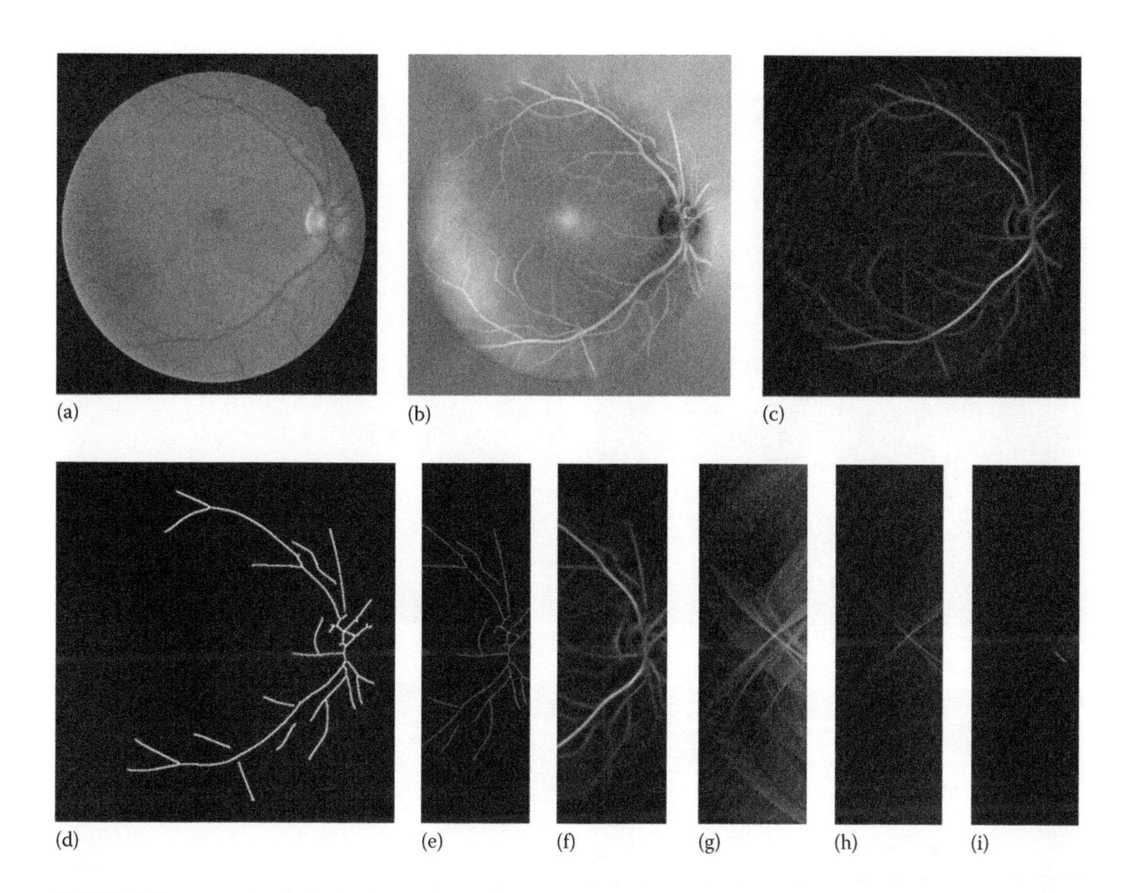

FIGURE 2.4
(See color insert.) (a) Image 24 of the DRIVE database (584 × 565 pixels). (b) The inverted and preprocessed grayscale image. (c) The Gabor-magnitude response. (d) The skeletonized and filtered image obtained from the result in (c). (e) The automatically limited skeleton image used in the GHT procedure (584 × 180 pixels). (f) The automatically limited Gabor-magnitude image used to update the Hough space. (g) The Hough space for $a = -64$ using the unity-updated GHT without vertex restriction. (h) The Hough space for $a = -66$ using the Gabor-magnitude-updated GHT without vertex restriction. (i) The Hough space for $a = -75$ using the Gabor-magnitude-updated GHT with vertex restriction. (Reproduced with permission from Oloumi, F., Rangayyan, R.M., and Ells, A.L., Parabolic modeling of the major temporal arcade in retinal fundus images, *IEEE Trans. Instrum. Meas.*, 61(7), 1825–1838, © July 2012 IEEE.)

restriction, are given in Table 2.1. The Gabor-magnitude-updated GHT with the vertex restriction has led to the highest correlation of the openness parameter a, whereas the unity-updated GHT with the vertex restriction has provided the lowest error in the positions of the detected vertices.

Figure 2.6a through d illustrates the DCP errors for the results of the four GHT versions without raphe-angle correction and MDCP-based selection for image 2 of the DRIVE database. The DCP, from the parabolic model to the hand-drawn MTA, is drawn in the illustrations only for every fifth point on the model. Figure 2.6e shows the DCP errors for the result of the Gabor-magnitude-updated GHT with vertex restriction and raphe-angle correction. The DCP for the Gabor-magnitude-updated GHT with vertex restriction, raphe-angle correction, and MDCP-based selection is shown in Figure 2.6f. The lower MDCP errors for the results in Figure 2.6e and f as compared to the result in Figure 2.6d are apparent by visual inspection.

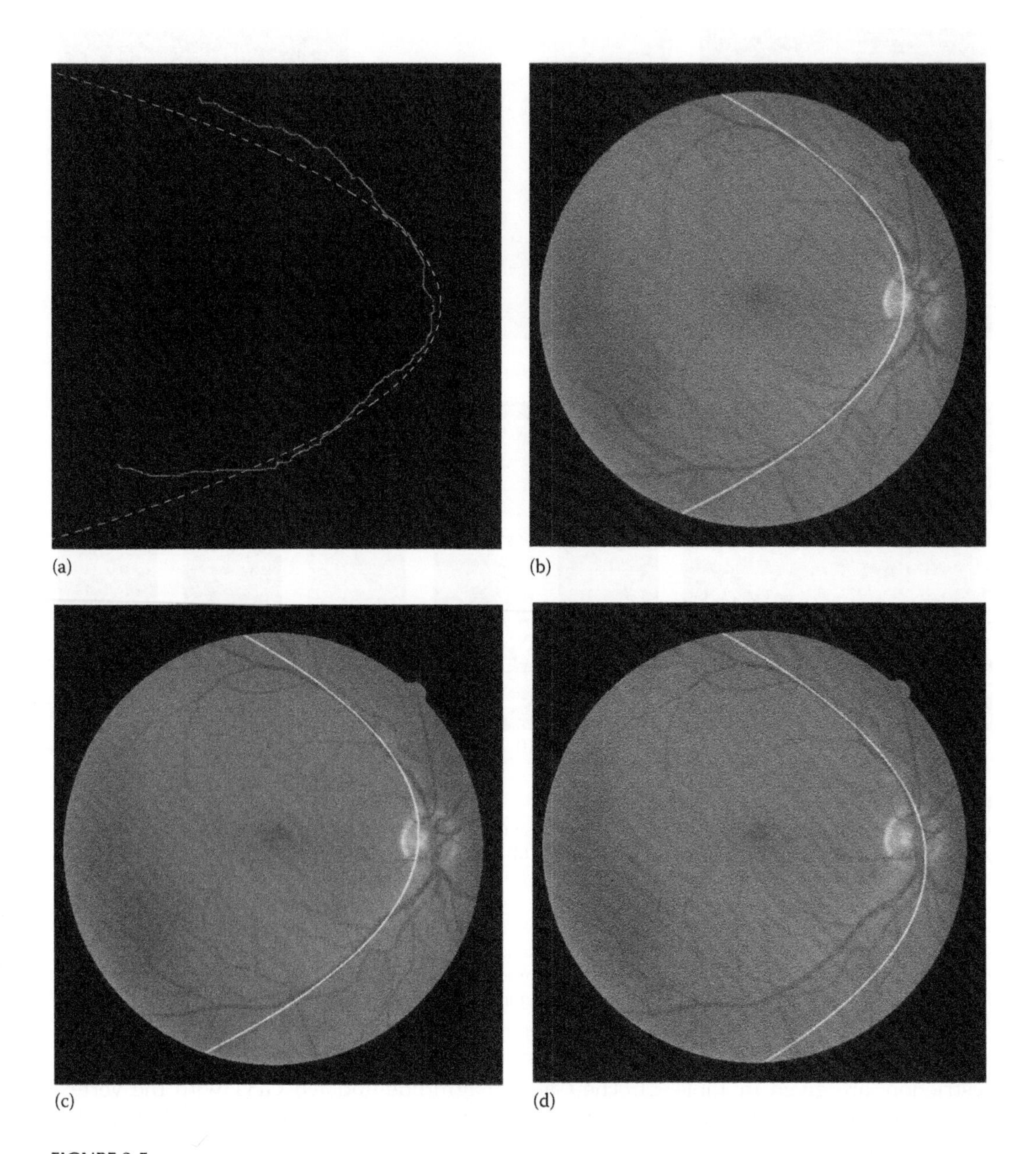

FIGURE 2.5
All of the parabolic fits shown in this figure were obtained by taking the global maximum in their corresponding Hough spaces. (a) Hand-drawn trace of the MTA (solid line) for the image in Figure 2.4a and its parabolic fit (dashed-line) obtained using the unity-updated GHT with vertex restriction. The parameters of the parabola are (494, 291, –41). (b) The best-fitting parabola obtained from the unity-updated GHT without vertex restriction, with the parameters (463, 279, –64). (c) The best-fitting parabola obtained from the Gabor-magnitude-updated GHT without vertex restriction; the parameters are (460, 279, –66). (d) The best-fitting parabola obtained from the Gabor-magnitude-updated GHT with vertex restriction, having the parameters (489, 314, –75). Although the models in (b) and (c) may appear to be similar, the detected vertices and the a parameters are different. (Reproduced with permission from Oloumi, F., Rangayyan, R.M., and Ells, A.L., Parabolic modeling of the major temporal arcade in retinal fundus images, *IEEE Trans. Instrum. Meas.*, 61(7), 1825–1838, © July 2012 IEEE.)

TABLE 2.1

Correlation Coefficients and the Average Vertex Position Errors between the Parameters of the Parabolas Obtained with the Four Different GHT Versions Compared to the Parameters of the Unity-Updated GHT Applied to the Hand-Drawn Arcades for All 40 DRIVE Images

GHT Version	Correlation Coefficient	Vertex Error, Mean ± STD (Pixels)
Unity-updated	0.91	37.65 ± 35.17
Unity-updated with vertex restriction	0.96	10.61 ± 8.18
Gabor-magnitude-updated	0.92	36.82 ± 25.18
Gabor-magnitude-updated with vertex restriction	0.97	12.53 ± 9.2

Source: Reproduced with permission from Oloumi, F., Rangayyan, R.M., and Ells, A.L., Parabolic modeling of the major temporal arcade in retinal fundus images, *IEEE Trans. Instrum. Meas.*, 61(7), 1825–1838, © July 2012 IEEE.

Note: The average vertex errors and their STDs are in terms of pixels, where each pixel is approximately 20 μm.

Figure 2.7a shows an example of modeling the ITA and STA separately: The brighter semiparabola is the fit to the STA and the darker semiparabola is the fit to the ITA; the models do not share the same vertex and have different a parameters. Figure 2.7e illustrates the DCP errors for the ITA model as compared to the hand-drawn trace of the ITA. Similarly, Figure 2.7f shows the DCP errors for the STA model as compared to the hand-drawn trace of the STA. By comparing Figure 2.7e and f to b through d, it is obvious that the dual-parabolic modeling procedure produces more accurate fits than the single-parabolic modeling procedure. Figure 2.8 demonstrates the DCP errors for the results of dual-parabolic modeling for image 19 of the DRIVE database; for the sake of comparison of the ITA and the STA fits, both models are combined in one image. It can be observed that the STA has a semiparabolic shape, whereas the ITA resembles an exponential curve; this point is reinforced by the low MDCP for the STA model as compared to the above-average MDCP for the ITA model.

The average MDCP and Hausdorff distances of the parabolic fits for the results of the four different versions of the GHT and the dual-parabolic modeling procedure, as compared to the hand-drawn arcades for all of the 40 DRIVE images, are listed in Tables 2.2 and 2.3, respectively. Both of the measures were also used to assess the performance of the modeling methods with the added procedures of raphe-angle correction and MDCP-based selection, separately and combined together. The dual-parabolic modeling procedure provides separate models for the ITA and the STA; hence, the MDCP and the Hausdorff measures were obtained for each of the ITA and STA models separately as compared to their corresponding hand-drawn traces. Combining the ITA and the STA models to obtain the MDCP and the Hausdorff measures, for the sake of comparison to the results of the other GHT versions, is not appropriate as it may bias the final results. Therefore, direct comparison of the results of single-parabolic modeling to the results of dual-parabolic modeling may not be meaningful in the case of MDCP. However, since the Hausdorff distance is an indicator of the possibility of getting large distances on the average, a direct comparison of the Hausdorff distances for the results of the dual-parabolic modeling procedure to the Hausdorff distances for the results of the single-parabolic modeling procedures is acceptable.

Among the four different versions of the GHT for single-parabolic modeling (see Table 2.2), the two Gabor-magnitude-updated procedures have lower MDCP, on the

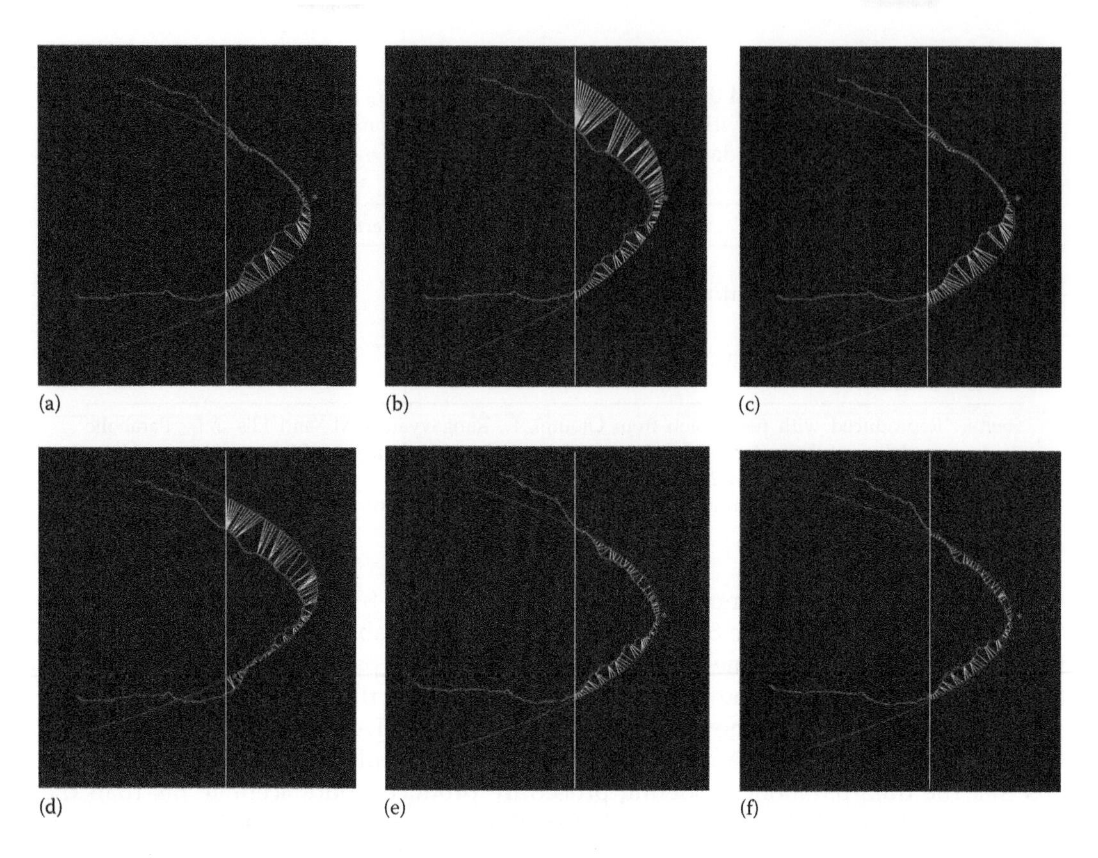

FIGURE 2.6
In each case, the smooth line represents the parabolic model and the rougher trace represents the hand-drawn arcade. The * indicates the automatically detected center of the ONH. The vertical line indicates the automatically determined horizontal extent of MDCP measurement from the ONH. The lines connecting the model to the hand-drawn arcade are the DCPs. Neither raphe-angle correction nor MDCP-based selection was applied in cases (a)–(d). The MDCP values for the various models obtained are as follows: (a) the unity-updated GHT = 17.63 pixels (0.35 mm); (b) the unity-updated GHT with vertex restriction = 38.19 pixels (0.76 mm); (c) the Gabor-magnitude-updated GHT = 17.63 pixels (0.35 mm); (d) the Gabor-magnitude-updated GHT with vertex restriction = 25.04 pixels (0.5 mm); (e) the Gabor-magnitude-updated GHT with vertex restriction and raphe-angle correction = 12.63 pixels (0.25 mm); and (f) the Gabor-magnitude-updated GHT with vertex restriction, raphe-angle correction, and MDCP-based selection = 12.33 pixels (0.24 mm). (Reproduced with permission from Oloumi, F., Rangayyan, R.M., and Ells, A.L., Parabolic modeling of the major temporal arcade in retinal fundus images, *IEEE Trans. Instrum. Meas.*, 61(7), 1825–1838, © July 2012 IEEE.)

average, with and without the raphe-angle correction and the MDCP-based selection being used, as compared to the unity-updated GHT procedures. The results of the dual-parabolic modeling procedure for the STA have a higher MDCP, on the average, as compared to the results of modeling of the ITA, which can be partly attributed to the high MDCP produced by several oddly shaped STAs in the DRIVE images, also evident from the high STD in the MDCP of the STA models. The added procedures of raphe-angle correction and MDCP-based selection have less impact when used separately; combining the two appears to have a bigger influence on the results of the unity-updated GHTs as compared to the Gabor-magnitude-updated GHTs. The raphe-angle correction and MDCP-based selection methods have a minor effect when applied to the dual-parabolic modeling procedure as compared to the single-parabolic modeling procedures. The Hausdorff distances

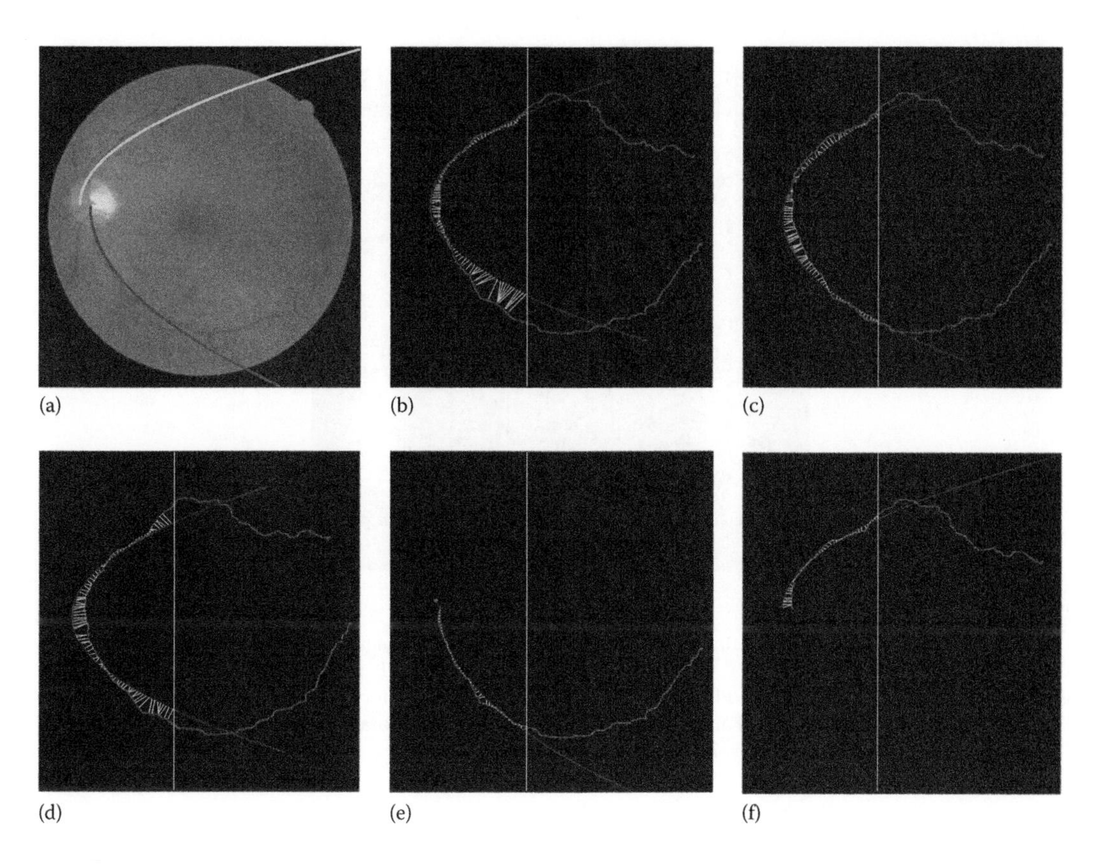

FIGURE 2.7
An example of the dual-parabolic modeling procedure with image 9 of the DRIVE database; the ITA and STA are modeled separately. (a) The STA and the ITA models, the brighter and darker semiparabolas, respectively, obtained with the Gabor-magnitude-updated GHT with vertex restriction. (b) The MDCP for a single-parabolic model obtained using Gabor-magnitude-updated GHT with vertex restriction = 12.22 pixels (0.24 mm). (c) The MDCP for a single-parabolic model obtained using the Gabor-magnitude-updated GHT with vertex restriction and raphe-angle correction = 8.61 pixels (0.17 mm). (d) The MDCP for a single-parabolic model obtained using the Gabor-magnitude-updated GHT with vertex restriction, raphe-angle correction, and MDCP-based selection is 11.50 pixels (0.23 mm). (e) The MDCP for the ITA model in (a) is 2.16 pixels (0.04 mm) and (f) for the STA model in (a) is 4.26 pixels (0.08 mm). (Reproduced with permission from Oloumi, F., Rangayyan, R.M., and Ells, A.L., Parabolic modeling of the major temporal arcade in retinal fundus images, *IEEE Trans. Instrum. Meas.*, 61(7), 1825–1838, © July 2012 IEEE.)

(see Table 2.3) indicate that the dual-parabolic modeling procedure produces lower errors, on the average, for both the ITA and the STA models as compared to all four of the single-parabolic modeling procedures.

In order to test the statistical significance of the differences in the MDCP of the results provided by the various modeling options, the p-values for many selected pairs of sets of MDCP values were computed. The differences between the MDCPs obtained using raphe-angle correction by itself, as compared to the single-parabolic modeling procedures without any options, have no statistical significance; the same is true when only using the MDCP-based selection option. When both raphe-angle correction and MDCP-based selection are combined, only the difference between the MDCP for Gabor-magnitude-updated GHT with vertex restriction with and without both options is statistically significant ($p = 0.0252$).

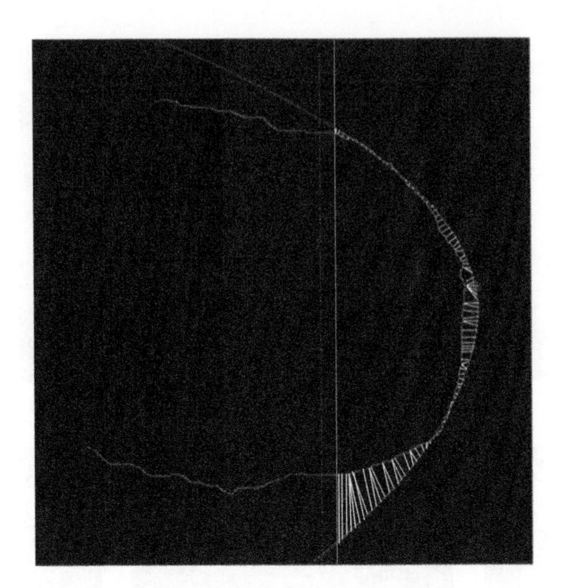

FIGURE 2.8
Illustration of the DCPs for the result of dual-parabolic modeling for image 19 of the DRIVE database using the Gabor-magnitude-updated GHT with vertex restriction. The MDCP for the STA model is 5.53 pixels (0.11 mm). The MDCP for the ITA model is 20.58 pixels (0.41 mm). (Reproduced with permission from Oloumi, F., Rangayyan, R.M., and Ells, A.L., Parabolic modeling of the major temporal arcade in retinal fundus images, *IEEE Trans. Instrum. Meas.*, 61(7), 1825–1838, © July 2012 IEEE.)

TABLE 2.2

Average MDCP (in Pixels, where Each Pixel is Approximately 20 μm) of the Parabolic Fits for the Four Versions of the GHT and the Dual-Parabolic Modeling Procedure, as Compared to the Hand-Drawn MTAs for All 40 DRIVE Images

GHT Version	MDCP, Mean ± STD	With Raphe-Angle Correction	With MDCP-Based Selection	With Raphe-Angle Correction and MDCP-Based Selection
Unity-updated	18.35 ± 11.40	16.62 ± 9.42	16.26 ± 9.93	14.20 ± 7.07
Unity-updated with vertex restriction	16.27 ± 8.84	15.09 ± 7.85	15.15 ± 8.13	13.45 ± 7.54
Gabor-magnitude-updated	14.08 ± 9.93	13.93 ± 9.20	12.68 ± 8.80	12.79 ± 8.63
Gabor-magnitude-updated with vertex restriction	16.06 ± 9.05	12.64 ± 6.39	14.59 ± 8.00	12.10 ± 6.16
Gabor-magnitude-updated with vertex restriction, ITA model	12.07 ± 8.88	12.33 ± 11.02	10.90 ± 8.71	10.64 ± 8.76
Gabor-magnitude-updated with vertex restriction, STA model	15.01 ± 16.32	14.09 ± 15.28	14.52 ± 16.71	13.93 ± 16.06

Source: Reproduced with permission from Oloumi, F., Rangayyan, R.M., and Ells, A.L., Parabolic modeling of the major temporal arcade in retinal fundus images, *IEEE Trans. Instrum. Meas.*, 61(7), 1825–1838, © July 2012 IEEE.

Note: The MDCP values for the procedures with raphe-angle correction, MDCP-based selection in the Hough space, and both combined are also provided.

TABLE 2.3

Average Hausdorff Distance (in Pixels, where Each Pixel is Approximately 20 μm) of the Parabolic Fits for the Four Versions of the GHT and the Dual-Parabolic Modeling Procedure, as Compared to the Hand-Drawn MTAs for All 40 DRIVE Images

GHT Version	Hausdorff Mean ± STD	With Raphe-Angle Correction	With MDCP-Based Selection	With Raphe-Angle Correction and MDCP-Based Selection
Unity-updated	53.14 ± 34.42	49.17 ± 31.10	50.17 ± 34.27	42.50 ± 24.82
Unity-updated with vertex restriction	45.49 ± 22.33	40.94 ± 18.61	43.12 ± 20.78	36.75 ± 17.70
Gabor-magnitude-updated	45.82 ± 34.52	46.05 ± 32.50	42.32 ± 29.29	43.55 ± 33.62
Gabor-magnitude-updated with vertex restriction	46.72 ± 26.49	36.28 ± 15.63	42.51 ± 21.60	34.90 ± 16.60
Gabor-magnitude-updated with vertex restriction, ITA model	34.19 ± 15.70	35.25 ± 20.46	30.18 ± 15.73	29.80 ± 16.46
Gabor-magnitude-updated with vertex restriction, STA model	39.66 ± 31.51	38.06 ± 30.25	37.38 ± 32.27	36.36 ± 31.29

Source: Reproduced with permission from Oloumi, F., Rangayyan, R.M., and Ells, A.L., Parabolic modeling of the major temporal arcade in retinal fundus images, *IEEE Trans. Instrum. Meas.*, 61(7), 1825–1838, © July 2012 IEEE.

Note: The Hausdorff distance values for the procedures with raphe-angle correction, MDCP-based selection, and both combined are also provided.

In the case of dual-parabolic modeling, the differences between the MDCP with and without raphe-angle correction and MDCP-based selection (separately and combined) were found to have no statistical significance. The difference between the MDCP of dual-parabolic modeling with MDCP-based selection and single-parabolic modeling using the unity-updated GHT is statistically significant with $p = 0.0242$.

The differences between the MDCPs of a few other pairs of options, such as the unity-updated GHT as compared with the Gabor-magnitude-updated GHT (without any other option), the Gabor-magnitude-updated GHT with and without vertex restriction, and Gabor-magnitude-updated GHT with and without all of the options listed in Table 2.2, were found to have no statistical significance.

2.4 Graphical User Interface

By providing user guidance over a few of the variables used in the detection and modeling procedures, it may be possible to reduce the modeling error and improve the accuracy of the related measures [47]. The present section provides a description of the design of a graphical user interface (GUI) for such a purpose. The GUI is being developed and tested in consultation with a pediatric ophthalmologist and retinal specialist (A.L.E.) and adheres to the main principles of GUI development, such as human factors, knowledge of the user's requirements and expectations, ease of use, intuitiveness, error handling capabilities, and proper documentation [47,48].

The GUI (see Figure 2.9) was designed using MATLAB's GUI development environment. All of the underlying code to run the various modules of the GUI was written in the form of MATLAB functions. The GUI is deployable as a stand-alone installation package.

The GUI contains a separate module for each of the three main steps involved in the detection and modeling of the MTA, as further described in Sections 2.4.1 through 2.4.3. The GUI also contains a module for measurement of the angle of insertion of the MTA, as explained in Section 2.4.4. Figure 2.9 shows a screenshot of the GUI.

2.4.1 Detection of Blood Vessels

The user has the option of manually specifying the Gabor filter parameters (thickness (τ), elongation (l), and number of filters (K)); however, by default, the GUI uses ($\tau = 16, l = 2$, and $K = 45$) to emphasize the presence of the MTA (see Ref. [27] for more details on Gabor filters). By default, the GUI uses the luminance component (Y of the YIQ color space) for Gabor filtering; however, the user has the option of using the green component of the RGB color space, instead. The resulting Gabor-magnitude response image is then displayed within the internal display area of the GUI.

2.4.2 Binarization of the Detected Vessels

The Gabor-magnitude response image can be thresholded using a sliding threshold. An editable text field indicates the selected threshold value, which could also be used to type in a specific threshold for binarization. The internal display area of the GUI is automatically updated with the resulting binary image every time the threshold is changed. As explained in Section 2.2.2, in order to remove unwanted small vessel segments that may remain even after the thresholding step, the user can specify the maximum number of connected pixels to be removed (via the morphological operation of area open) in the corresponding editable text field provided. The internal display area is updated with the new binary image.

2.4.3 Modeling of the MTA

The modeling module requires a binary image in order to perform the GHT procedure, which can be obtained by using the two previously described modules. The user has to first indicate if the current image is an image of the right or the left eye. (Information is provided under the *Help* tab in the menu bar on how to distinguish between images of the left and right eye.) Starting the modeling procedure prompts the user to mark the approximate location of the ONH in a separate window by clicking on the image. After marking the ONH, the user has the option of marking the location again or continuing with the modeling procedure.

By default, the GUI performs single-parabolic modeling; however, the user has the option of obtaining a dual-parabolic model. The Gabor-magnitude-updated version of the GHT with vertex restriction is used in the proposed GUI (see Section 2.2.5 for more information). The parabolic model is then overlaid on the binary image displayed within the internal display area of the GUI. The user has the option of viewing the model on the original color image or the binary image in a separate window, using the *View* tab in the menu bar. All original, preprocessed, processed, and resulting images can also be viewed in separate windows using the *View* tab. After the modeling procedure is performed, the

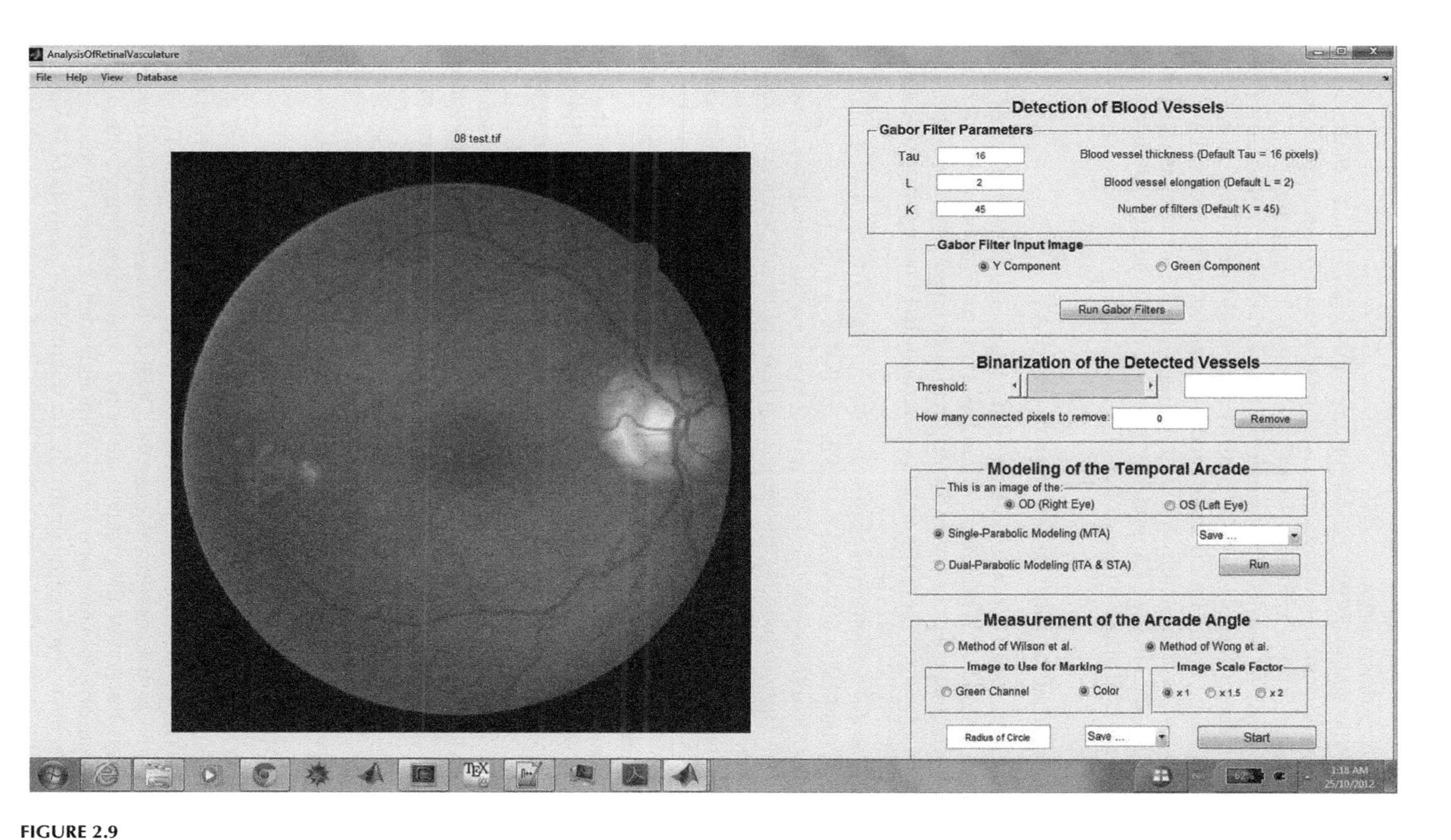

FIGURE 2.9
The main GUI window showing a selected retinal image.

user has the option of saving the model parameters (single model, ITA model, and STA model) using a drop-down menu.

The results of the dual-parabolic modeling procedure via the GUI, obtained with 40 images of the DRIVE database, as compared with hand-drawn traces of the STA and ITA, indicate low-average MDCP values of 9.3 and 9.9 pixels (<0.2 mm) for the STA and ITA models, respectively. The results of the single-parabolic modeling procedure indicate an average MDCP value of 13.0 pixels (0.26 mm), as compared to the hand-drawn traces of the MTA. The average errors for all three models obtained using the GUI are lower as compared to the results of the automated method (see Table 2.2 for comparison). The largest improvement is seen in the STA models. More details on the semiautomated modeling method via the GUI are provided in Ref. [47].

2.4.4 Measurement of the Angle of Insertion of the MTA

The GUI contains a module for measurement of the angle of insertion of the MTA using two methods as defined by Wilson et al. [6] and Wong et al. [7]. The user has the option of using the green component image or the original color image to perform the required markings for the measurement of the angle of insertion. The image can also be scaled up to 1.5 or 2 times its original size [48].

Choosing the method of Wilson et al. prompts the user to mark the location of the center of the ONH and the fovea by clicking on the image that is opened in a separate window. After the two landmarks are identified, the retinal raphe and its normal are drawn on the image to assist the user in marking the remaining two points needed for computation of the TAA; see Figure 2.10a. Next, the user is asked to mark the point of intersection of the normal to the retinal raphe with the STA and ITA; the TAA is measured as the sum of the SAA and IAA, as shown in Figure 2.10a. Note that the implementation of the method of Wilson et al. as discussed earlier does not require the angle of the retinal raphe to be corrected, as explained in Section 2.1.2.

Choosing the method of Wong et al. prompts the user to mark the center of the ONH on the image, after which a circle with a specific radius is drawn on the image. The user has the option of specifying the radius of the circle; however, by default, the GUI uses a circle of radius $r = 120$ pixels. Next, the user is asked to mark the points of intersection of circle with the superior and inferior vessels. The TAA is measured as the angle between the three marked points with the center of the ONH being the vertex, as shown in Figure 2.10b, using $\arctan [(m_1 - m_2)/(1 + m_1 m_2)]$, where m_1 and m_2 are the slopes of the two lines and $m_2 > m_1$.

2.5 Clinical Application

In addition to ROP and myopia, PDR is also known to affect the structure of the retinal vasculature [49,50]. When considering the consequences of diabetes, it is only in the presence of PDR that the architecture of the MTA is known to be affected [49,50]. Fibrovascular proliferation of the pathological tissue near the ONH as well as contraction of the retinal surface causes traction of the arcades, tractional retinal detachment, macular dragging, and subsequently, loss of vision [49,50]. Although such changes in the architecture of the MTA have been observed qualitatively, no quantitative analysis of the abnormal architecture of the MTA in the presence of PDR has been reported. The present section

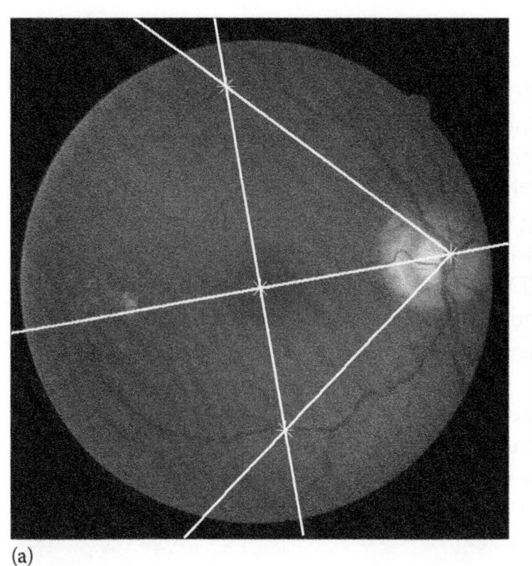
(a)

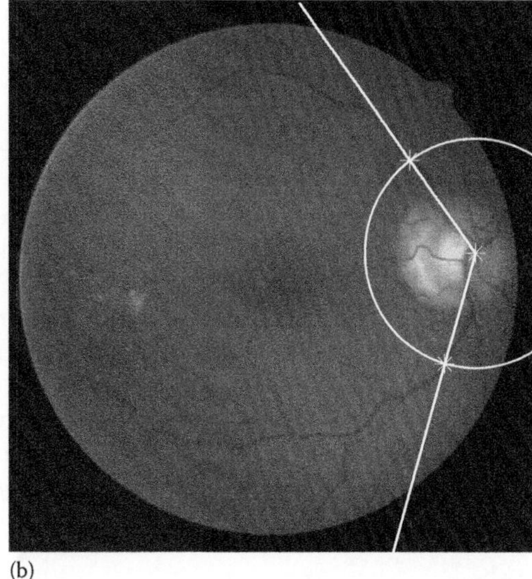
(b)

FIGURE 2.10
(a) After marking the center of the ONH and the fovea, the retinal raphe and its normal are automatically drawn on the image to aid the user in marking the points of intersection of the normal with the STA and the ITA. The measured angle based on the user's inputs: MTA angle = 81.9°. (b) After marking the center of the ONH, a circle of a specified radius (120 pixels in this illustration) is automatically drawn on the image to aid the user in marking the points of intersection of the circle with the superior and the inferior arcades. The measured angle is 127.9°.

summarizes the results of a pilot study on computer-aided diagnosis of PDR [51] by quantitative measurement of the changes in the openness of the arcades due to PDR via single- and dual-parabolic modeling of the MTA, STA, and ITA, as well as comparative analysis with arcade angles via the GUI as described in Section 2.4 [48,51,52].

The methods were tested with images from the STructured Analysis of the REtina (STARE) database [53]. Eleven cases of PDR and 11 normal cases were obtained. The STARE database has 22 cases of PDR; however, 11 cases were not used because either the major vessels were not distinguishable or the MTA was not in the FOV. The 11 images of normal cases were selected starting from the lowest image number in the subset of images of the STARE database that are used for the detection of the ONH; cases that either did not clearly show the entire MTA or possessed poor contrast within the FOV were not selected. The PDR cases are not part of the publicly available subset of images of the STARE database and were provided by Dr. A. Hoover (Clemson University) upon request. In recent years, there has been an increase in the number of publicly available databases of retinal images of non-PDR cases; however, the STARE database is the only available database that includes cases of PDR. For this reason, the number of fundus images used in the present pilot study to explore clinical application of our methods is limited.

For all of the images used in the present work, $l = 2$ and $K = 45$ were used to detect the MTA. The range of values of τ used is [16,26], which was needed due to the large variability of vessel thickness in the STARE images. A different threshold was selected using the sliding threshold, provided by the GUI, to obtain a binary image containing only the MTA for each original image. Varying numbers of connected pixels were removed for each image to ensure that no vessel other than the MTA would influence the modeling procedure.

On the average, it took about 1½ min to obtain the parabolic models (single and dual) for an image via the GUI using a Lenovo ThinkPad T510, equipped with an Intel Core i7 (hyper-threaded dual-core) 2.67 GHz processor, 4 MB of level 2 cache, and 8 GB of DDR3 RAM, running 64-bit Windows 7 Professional, and using 64-bit MATLAB software.

For the arcade angle measurements, the method of Wong et al. [7], using a circle of radius 120 pixels, was used on all images [48]. On the average, it took about 30 s to obtain the arcade angle measure for a single image using the same system as explained earlier [51,52].

Figure 2.11 illustrates the results of dual-parabolic modeling and arcade angle measurement for a normal case as well as a PDR case. There are large differences between the values of the arcade angle measure for the normal case as compared to the PDR case; the same is true for the values of the openness parameters of the dual models obtained (see Figure 2.11 for the actual values).

The differences between the absolute values of the openness parameters of the MTA ($|a_{MTA}|$) and the ITA ($|a_{ITA}|$) models for the normal cases as compared to the PDR cases were found to be statistically significant (p-value < 0.05). The same was true for the

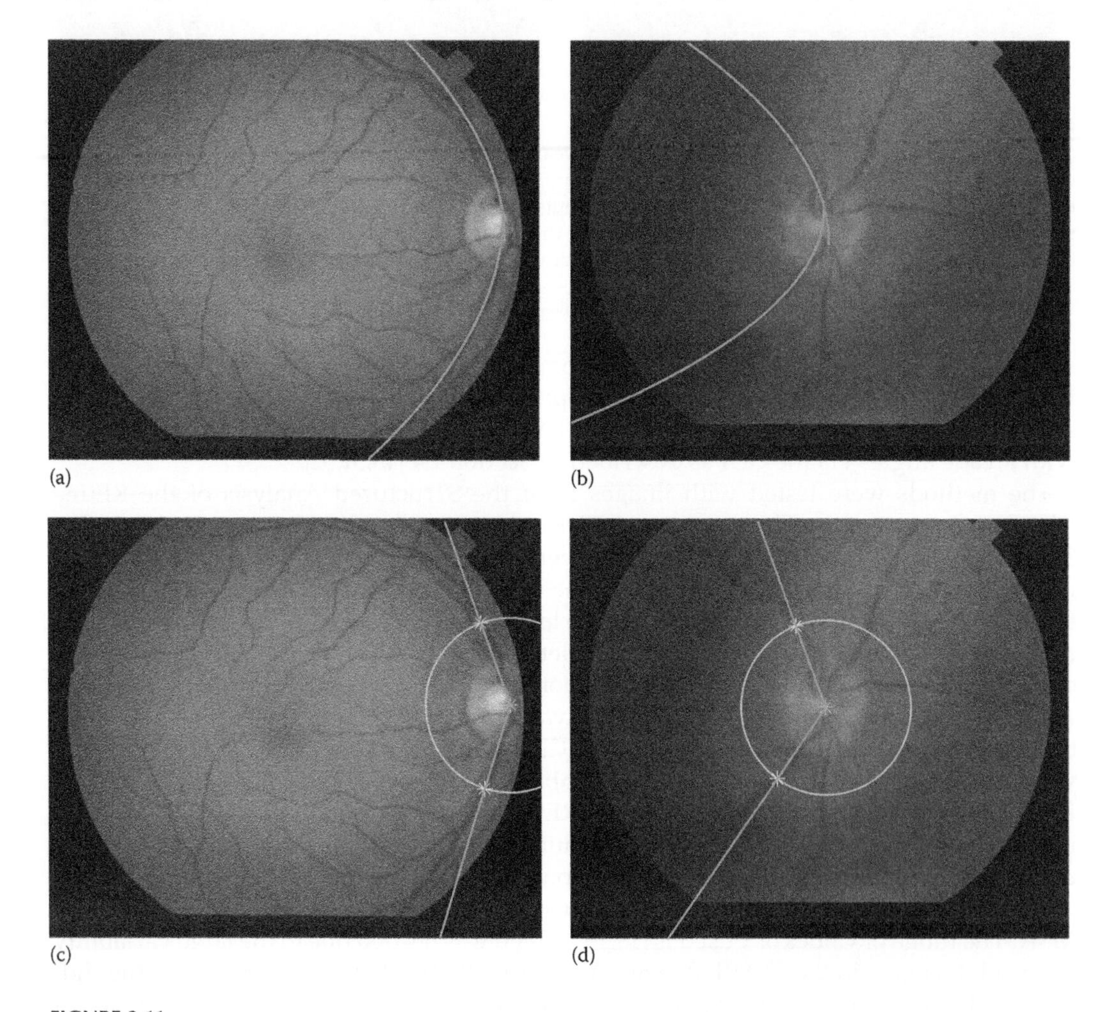

FIGURE 2.11
Dual-parabolic models for (a) a normal case ($a_{STA} = -136$, $a_{ITA} = -160$) and (b) a PDR case ($a_{STA} = -96$, $a_{ITA} = -60$). Arcade angle measures for the same cases as in (a) and (b), with (c) TAA = 142.7° and (d) TAA = 124.3°.

differences between the arcade angle measures for the normal cases as compared to the PDR cases. The areas under the receiver operating characteristic curves (A_z) obtained indicate high diagnostic accuracy for detection of PDR using $|a_{\mathrm{MTA}}|$, $|a_{\mathrm{ITA}}|$, and the arcade angle measures, in decreasing order, with $A_z = 0.87$, 0.82, and 0.80, respectively.

Although the results of the pilot study are encouraging, more cases of PDR are needed for further analysis. This is the first study to use quantification of changes in the overall architecture of the MTA to perform diagnostic discrimination between normal cases and cases of PDR. Further work is in progress to evaluate the proposed methods with larger databases of cases of PDR as well as ROP and to assess the statistical significance of the differences between the A_z values related to the various parameters.

2.6 Discussion

In comparison with our earlier studies [20–22], the addition of the anatomical restrictions on the vessel map and the search area in the Hough space as well as the use of Gabor-magnitude-weighted increments have significantly improved the results. By limiting the search area for the vertex to be close to the automatically detected center of the ONH, the Hough procedure is forced to fit the parabolic model to the posterior part of the MTA. By restricting the vessel map up to the macula, the parabolic profile of the appropriate portion of the MTA is emphasized. Updating the Hough space with the Gabor-magnitude response reduces the influence of smaller vessels on the result. This is also confirmed by the lower-average MDCP values for the results of the Gabor-magnitude-updated GHTs as compared to those of the unity-updated GHTs (see Tables 2.2 and 2.3).

The high correlation between the values of the parameter a obtained automatically and from the hand-drawn MTAs indicates that the automatically obtained vessel skeleton maps are accurate.

The MDCP-based selection procedure, applied to the raphe-angle-corrected images, helps to improve the accuracy of the models. The addition of raphe-angle correction and the MDCP-based selection procedures to the single-parabolic modeling procedures appears to have the same impact as the dual-parabolic modeling procedure without the use of raphe-angle correction and MDCP-based selection. The addition of raphe-angle correction and the MDCP-based selection options provides no statistically significant improvement over the results of the dual-parabolic modeling procedure. The dual-parabolic modeling procedures are more reliable as they are less likely to result in a large error as shown by the lower Hausdorff distances, on the average, as compared to the single-parabolic modeling procedures.

Although the results obtained are encouraging, there are still limitations that need to be addressed. If the major arteriole arcade is adequately thick, it may not get eliminated in the binarization step and could affect the modeling procedure. A method to distinguish between venules and arterioles could be used to eliminate the arterioles [54,55].

It is possible to reduce the number of Gabor filters used by considering the orientation range of the MTA, the computational cost, and the required detection accuracy [56], as shown in Section 2.4.1.

The present work is concerned with quantitative representation of the architecture of the MTA; the previously published modeling methods (see Section 2.1.3) have not modeled the MTA for quantitative analysis of its architecture. Even though the GHT has many similarities with other modeling methods (see Section 2.2.4), a comparison of the single-parabolic modeling procedure with the modeling methods mentioned in Section 2.1.3 (in terms of accuracy and execution time) could be beneficial as a separate study. However, such a comparison with the dual-parabolic modeling procedure is not feasible.

The raphe angles of the 40 images of the DRIVE database have an average of approximately 6°. Hence, in the present work, manual markings of the fovea and the ONH centers were used to obtain precise measurements of the raphe angles and to demonstrate the effects of raphe-angle correction on the modeling procedures. An automated method [13,14,17] may be used to detect the fovea and the results could be used along with the automatically detected center of the ONH [26] to correct for raphe-angle rotation. However, as indicated in the discussion in Section 2.3, using the raphe-angle correction option makes no statistically significant difference in the results of single- and dual-parabolic modeling procedures (for the DRIVE images). Hence, manual marking or automatic detection of the fovea is not essential for modeling of the MTA if the variations in the raphe angle are comparable to those found in the DRIVE images.

Retinal fundus images of preterm infants typically lack a clear depiction of the fovea; as shown by Chiang et al. [57], there is significant variability between ROP experts in the identification of the fovea in wide-angle retinal images of preterm infants at risk of ROP. This fact may preclude the application of the method of Wilson et al. [2] for the measurement of the arcade angle, which is dependent on the location of the fovea. The methods developed in the present work require only the location of the ONH (for which an automatic method has been proposed by Rangayyan et al. [26]) and provide the advantage of requiring a single landmark.

The present work is concerned with modeling and parametric representation of the MTA. The nasal arcade has a shorter distance to the ora serrata than the MTA and, hence, is less vulnerable to distortion. Furthermore, as shown by Wong et al. [7], the changes in the nasal arcade angles have no statistical significance in the presence of ROP.

Possible changes in the thickness and tortuosity of retinal blood vessels that are expected to occur in the presence of plus disease have been found to be not consistently correlated to the stages of ROP [2,58,59]. Moreover, detection accuracy of changes in the thickness and tortuosity of the blood vessels can be affected by low quality and presence of artifacts in images of preterm infants [7]. Detection and analysis of architectural parameters of the MTA, as proposed in the present work, could improve the diagnosis, staging, decision making for surgical treatment, and clinical management of ROP.

Parabolic modeling, as proposed in the present work, characterizes the architecture of the MTA up to the macular region, whereas the procedure of Wilson et al. [2] quantifies an angle based on the location of the ONH and two specific points on the ITA and STA that reflect the location of the fovea (see Figure 2.1). This observation implies that the two measures are fundamentally different from each other; this point was confirmed by low correlation (0.65, 0.63, and 0.42) between the automatically measured values of the TAA, the IAA, and the SAA using the procedure described by Wilson et al. [2] and the automatically obtained openness parameters, a_{MTA}, a_{ITA}, and a_{STA}, respectively. The method of Wong et al. [7] provides more accurate representation of the arcade angle as compared to the method of Wilson et al. [7]. As shown by Ells and MacKeen [10,11], analyzing the overall architecture of the MTA is more desirable than analyzing the variations in the angle of insertion of the MTA in the presence of progressive ROP.

Retinal fundus images of pediatric cases differ from those of adult cases in color and relative size of the features, mainly the blood vessels. Detection and analysis of the openness of the MTA in fundus images of preterm infants should be possible by fine-tuning the parameters of the Gabor filters and the GHT procedures. There is no publicly available annotated database of retinal images related to ROP. Application of the methods proposed in the present work to a database of fundus images of cases of ROP [60] is planned after the database is annotated with clinical interpretation in terms of stages of ROP and hand-drawn traces of the MTA.

Even though the dual-parabolic modeling approach improves the results, it can still be biased if the ITA or the STA has nonlinear rates of divergence (see Figure 2.8). A parabola has a linear divergence rate controlled by the parameter a. The approximate shape of the overall architecture of the MTA may appear to be parabolic or semielliptical; however, upon close inspection, it becomes clear that, first, the STA and the ITA are asymmetric and, second, more accurate modeling of each arcade may be possible by applying higher-order models. A high-order curve fitting method may provide more accurate results in terms of modeling and parameterization of the STA and ITA.

More inter- and intrauser testing of the GUI is needed to further assess the usability of the GUI in a clinical setting. Although the results of the pilot study with a small number of cases of PDR are promising, the methods need to be evaluated with large databases of cases of various types of retinal pathology that affect the MTA.

2.7 Conclusion

We have proposed parabolic modeling methods using the GHT to detect, measure, and parameterize the architecture of the MTA in retinal fundus images. The two anatomical restrictions imposed on the width of the image as well as the search area for the vertex of the parabolic model have improved the performance of the modeling procedure. The global maximum in the Hough space does not always provide the best-fitting model, as shown by the improved results of modeling by using MDCP-based selection in the Hough space. Correction of the retinal raphe angle provides no statistically important difference in the results of single- and dual-parabolic modeling procedures (with the DRIVE database). The fact that the fully automatic dual-parabolic modeling procedure provides the highest improvement in the modeling results makes it the most important option among the modeling procedures presented. Higher-order models fitted to the STA and the ITA separately should provide more accurate models. We propose to test the methods on time series of fundus images of preterm infants and correlate the changes in the model parameters to the different stages of ROP. The proposed methods could assist in quantitative analysis of the architecture of the MTA in terms of its openness or narrowing and lead to improved diagnosis and clinical management of not only PDR but also ROP and myopia.

Acknowledgments

This work was supported by the Natural Sciences and Engineering Research Council of Canada.

We thank Dr. A. Hoover and April Ingram for their help with the STARE and TROPIC images, respectively.

References

1. International Committee for the Classification of Retinopathy of Prematurity. The international classification of retinopathy of prematurity revisited. *Archives of Ophthalmology*, 123:991–999, 2005.
2. Wilson CM, Cocker KD, Moseley MJ, Paterson C, Clay ST, Schulenburg WE, Mills MD et al. Computerized analysis of retinal vessel width and tortuosity in premature infants. *Investigative Ophthalmology and Visual Science*, 49(1):3577–3585, 2008.
3. Jelinek HF and Cree MJ. Introduction. In Jelinek HF and Cree MJ, eds., *Automated Image Detection of Retinal Pathology*, pp. 1–26. CRC Press, Boca Raton, FL, 2010.
4. Patton N, Aslam TM, MacGillivray T, Deary IJ, Dhillon B, Eikelboom RH, Yogesan K, and Constable IJ. Retinal image analysis: Concepts, applications and potential. *Progress in Retinal and Eye Research*, 25(1):99–127, 2006.
5. Fledelius HC and Goldschmidt E. Optic disc appearance and retinal temporal vessel arcade geometry in high myopia, as based on follow-up data over 38 years. *Acta Ophthalmologica*, 88(5):514–520, 2010.
6. Wilson C, Theodorou M, Cocker KD, and Fielder AR. The temporal retinal vessel angle and infants born preterm. *British Journal of Ophthalmology*, 90:702–704, 2006.
7. Wong K, Ng J, Ells AL, Fielder AR, and Wilson CM. The temporal and nasal retinal arteriolar and venular angles in preterm infants. *British Journal of Ophthalmology*, 95(12):1723–1727, 2011.
8. Reese AB, King MJ, and Owens WC. A classification of retrolental fibroplasia. *American Journal of Ophthalmology*, 36:1333–1335, 1953.
9. Cryotherapy for Retinopathy of Prematurity Cooperative Group. Multicenter trial of cryotherapy for retinopathy of prematurity: Ophthalmological outcomes at 10 years. *Archives of Ophthalmology*, 119:1110–1118, 2001.
10. Ells AL and MacKeen LD. Retinopathy of prematurity—The movie. *Journal of American Association for Pediatric Ophthalmology and Strabismus*, 8(4):389, 2004.
11. Ells AL and MacKeen LD. Dynamic documentation of the evolution of retinopathy of prematurity in video format. *Journal of American Association for Pediatric Ophthalmology and Strabismus*, 12(4):349–351, 2008.
12. Foracchia M, Grisan E, and Ruggeri A. Detection of optic disc in retinal images by means of a geometrical model of vessel structure. *IEEE Transactions on Medical Imaging*, 23(10):1189–1195, 2004.
13. Tobin KW, Chaum E, Govindasamy VP, and Karnowski TP. Detection of anatomic structures in human retinal imagery. *IEEE Transactions on Medical Imaging*, 26(12):1729–1739, December 2007.
14. Li H and Chutatape O. Automated feature extraction in color retinal images by a model based approach. *IEEE Transactions on Biomedical Engineering*, 51(2):246–254, 2004.
15. Fleming AD, Goatman KA, Philip S, Olson JA, and Sharp PF. Automatic detection of retinal anatomy to assist diabetic retinopathy screening. *Physics in Medicine and Biology*, 52:331–345, 2007.
16. Kochner B, Schuhmann D, Michaelis M, Mann G, and Englmeier KH. Course tracking and contour extraction of retinal vessels from color fundus photographs: Most efficient use of steerable filters for model based image analysis. In *SPIE Medical Imaging*, Vol. 3338, pp. 755–761, San Diego, CA, February 1998.
17. Ying H and Liu JC. Automated localization of macula-fovea area on retina images using blood vessel network topology. In *IEEE International Conference on Acoustics Speech and Signal Processing*, pp. 650–653, Dallas, TX, March 2010.
18. Niemeijer M, Abràmoff MD, and van Ginneken B. Segmentation of the optic disk, macula and vascular arch in fundus photographs. *IEEE Transactions on Medical Imaging*, 26(1):116–127, 2007.
19. Welfer D, Scharcanski J, Kitamura CM, Dal Pizzol MM, Ludwig LWB, and Marinho DR. Segmentation of the optic disk in color eye fundus images using an adaptive morphological approach. *Computers in Biology and Medicine*, 40(2):124–137, 2010.

20. Oloumi F and Rangayyan RM. Detection of the temporal arcade in fundus images of the retina using the Hough transform. In *31st Annual International Conference of the IEEE Engineering in Medicine and Biology Society (EMBS)*, pp. 3585–3588, Minneapolis, MN, September 2009.
21. Oloumi F, Rangayyan RM, and Ells AL. Parametric representation of the retinal temporal arcade. In *10th IEEE International Conference on Information Technology and Applications in Biomedicine (ITAB)*, pp. 1–4, paper no. 64 in CD-ROM, Corfu, Greece, November 2010.
22. Oloumi F, Rangayyan RM, and Ells AL. Dual-parabolic modeling of the superior and the inferior temporal arcades in fundus images of the retina. In *IEEE International Symposium on Medical Measurements and Applications (MeMeA)*, pp. xxxix–xliv, Bari, Italy, June 2011.
23. Oloumi F, Rangayyan RM, and Ells AL. Parabolic modeling of the major temporal arcade in retinal fundus images. *IEEE Transactions on Instrumentation and Measurement (TIM)*, 61(7):1825–1838, July 2012.
24. Digital Retinal Images for Vessel Extraction (DRIVE). www.isi.uu.nl/Research/Databases/DRIVE/download.php, accessed on June 21, 2011.
25. Image Processing and Analysis in Java. http://rsbweb.nih.gov/ij/, accessed on September 3, 2008.
26. Rangayyan RM, Zhu X, Ayres FJ, and Ells AL. Detection of the optic nerve head in fundus images of the retina with Gabor filters and phase portrait analysis. *Journal of Digital Imaging*, 23(4):438–453, August 2010.
27. Rangayyan RM, Ayres FJ, Oloumi F, Oloumi F, and Eshghzadeh-Zanjani P. Detection of blood vessels in the retina with multiscale Gabor filters. *Journal of Electronic Imaging*, 17:023018:1–023018:7, April–June 2008.
28. Ayres FJ and Rangayyan RM. Design and performance analysis of oriented feature detectors. *Journal of Electronic Imaging*, 16(2):023007:1–023007:12, 2007.
29. Arcelli C and Sanniti di Baja G. Skeletons of planar patterns. In Kong TY and Rosenfeld A, eds., *Topological Algorithms for Digital Image Processing*, Vol. 19 of *Machine Intelligence and Pattern Recognition*, pp. 99–143. North-Holland, Amsterdam, the Netherlands, 1996.
30. Acton ST. A pyramidal algorithm for area morphology. In *Proceedings of IEEE International Conference on Image Processing*, pp. 10–13, Vancouver, British Columbia, Canada, 2000.
31. Kong TY and Rosenfeld A. Digital topology: Introduction and survey. *Computer Vision, Graphics, and Image Processing*, 48:357–393, 1989.
32. Illingworth J and Kittler J. A survey of the Hough transform. *Computer Vision, Graphics, and Image Processing*, 44:87–116, 1988.
33. Princen J, Illingworh J, and Kittler J. A formal definition of the Hough transform: Properties and relationships. *Journal of Mathematical Imaging and Vision*, 1:153–168, 1992.
34. Hough PVC. Method and means for recognizing complex patterns. US Patent 3,069,654, December 18, 1962.
35. Jafri MZM and Deravi F. Efficient algorithm for the detection of parabolic curves. In *Proceedings of SPIE Vision Geometry III*, Vol. 2356(1), pp. 53–62, Boston, MA, 1995.
36. Wechsler H and Sklansky J. Finding the rib cage in chest radiographs. *Pattern Recognition*, 9:21–30, January 1977.
37. Lu W. Hough transforms for shape identification and applications in medical image processing. PhD thesis, University of Missouri, Columbia, MO, 2003.
38. Maalmi K, El Ouaazizi A, Benslimane R, Lew Yan Voon LFC, Diou A, and Gorria P. Detecting parabolas in ultrasound B-scan images with genetic-based inverse voting Hough transform. In *2010 IEEE International Conference on Acoustics, Speech, and Signal Processing*, Vol. 4, pp. IV-3337–IV-3340, Orlando, FL, May 2002.
39. Park KS, Yi WJ, and Paick JS. Segmentation of sperms using the strategic Hough transform. *Annals of Biomedical Engineering*, 25:294–302, 1997.
40. Rangayyan RM. *Biomedical Image Analysis*. CRC Press, Boca Raton, FL, 2005.
41. Sklansky J. On the Hough technique for curve detection. *IEEE Transactions on Computers*, C-27(10):923–926, 1978.
42. Larsen HW. *The Ocular Fundus: A Color Atlas*. Munksgaard, Copenhagen, Denmark, 1976.

43. Lalonde M, Beaulieu M, and Gagnon L. Fast and robust optic disc detection using pyramidal decomposition and Hausdorff-based template matching. *IEEE Transactions on Medical Imaging*, 20(11):1193–1200, 2001.
44. Wolfram MathWorld: Parabola. http://mathworld.wolfram.com/Parabola.html, accessed on December 22, 2013.
45. Xu J, Chutatape O, and Chew P. Automated optic disk boundary detection by modified active contour model. *IEEE Transactions on Biomedical Engineering*, 54(3):473–482, 2007.
46. Rogers CA. *Hausdorff Measures*. Cambridge University Press, Cambridge, U.K., 1970.
47. Oloumi F, Rangayyan RM, and Ells AL. A graphical user interface for measurement of the openness of the retinal temporal arcade. In *Proceedings of IEEE International Symposium on Medical Measurements and Applications (MeMeA)*, pp. 238–241, Budapest, Hungary, May 2012.
48. Oloumi F, Rangayyan RM, and Ells AL. A graphical user interface for measurement of temporal arcade angles in fundus images of the retina. In *Proceedings of IEEE Canada 25th Annual Canadian Conference on Electrical and Computer Engineering (CCECE)*, pages 4 on CD-ROM, Montreal, Quebec, Canada, April 2012.
49. Meier P and Wiedemann P. Vitrectomy for traction macular detachment in diabetic retinopathy. *Graefe's Archive for Clinical and Experimental Ophthalmology*, 235:569–574, 1997.
50. Danis RP and Davis MD. Proliferative diabetic retinopathy. In Duh EJ, ed., *Diabetic Retinopathy, Contemporary Diabetes*, pp. 29–65. Humana Press, Totowa, NJ, 2008.
51. Oloumi F, Rangayyan RM, and Ells AL. Computer-aided diagnosis of proliferative diabetic retinopathy. In *34th Annual International Conference of the IEEE Engineering in Medicine and Biology Society (EMBS)*, pp. 1438–1441, San Diego, CA, August 2012.
52. Oloumi F, Rangayyan RM, and Ells AL. Computer-aided diagnosis of proliferative diabetic retinopathy via modeling of the major temporal arcade in retinal fundus images. *Journal of Digital Imaging*, 26(6):1124–1130, 2013.
53. Structured Analysis of the Retina. http://www.ces.clemson.edu/~ahoover/stare/, accessed on January 2012.
54. Narasimha-Iyer H, Beach JM, Khoobehi B, and Roysam B. Automatic identification of retinal arteries and veins from dual-wavelength images using structural and functional features. *IEEE Transactions on Biomedical Engineering*, 54:1427–1435, 2007.
55. Grisan E and Ruggeri A. A divide et impera strategy for automatic classification of retinal vessels into arteries and veins. In *25th Annual International Conference of the IEEE Engineering in Medicine and Biology Society*, Vol. 1, pp. 890–893, Cancún, Mexico, September 2003.
56. Kalliomäki I and Lampinen J. On steerability of Gabor-type filters for feature detection. *Pattern Recognition Letters*, 28(8):904–911, 2007.
57. Chiang MF, Thyparampil PJ, and Rabinowitz D. Interexpert agreement in the identification of macular location in infants at risk for retinopathy of prematurity. *Archives of Ophthalmology*, 128(9):1153–1159, September 2010.
58. Heneghan C, Flynn J, O'Keefe M, and Cahill M. Characterization of changes in blood vessels width and tortuosity in retinopathy of prematurity using image analysis. *Medical Image Analysis*, 6(1):407–429, 2002.
59. Swanson C, Cocker KD, Parker KH, Moseley MJ, and Fielder AR. Semiautomated computer analysis of vessel growth in preterm infants without and with ROP. *British Journal of Ophthalmology*, 87(12):1474–1477, 2003.
60. Hildebrand PL, Ells AL, and Ingram AD. The impact of telemedicine integration on resource use in the evaluation ROP–Analysis of the telemedicine for ROP in Calgary (TROPIC) database. *Investigative Ophthalmology and Visual Sciences*, 50:3151, 2009 (E-Abstract).

3

Application of Higher-Order Spectra Cumulants for Diabetic Retinopathy Detection Using Digital Fundus Images

Roshan Joy Martis, Karthikeyan Ganesan, U. Rajendra Acharya, Chua Kuang Chua, Lim Choo Min, E.Y.K. Ng, Augustinus Laude, and Jasjit S. Suri

CONTENTS

3.1 Introduction

Diabetes mellitus (DM) is a condition of the body arising from improper insulin metabolism. This results in an elevated level of blood glucose, which in turn leads to a number of complications in the body. One such serious complication is diabetic retinopathy (DR). DR is a major cause of concern in the developed world since it is a leading cause of blindness in people above 55 years of age [1]. There are treatments for DR, which include laser photocoagulation and corticosteroid injections [1]. But for any treatment to be effective, the diagnosis must be done at an early stage to prevent permanent vision loss. As a result, the World Health Organization recommends regular screening of diabetic patients for signs of DR to treat the condition at an early stage [1]. But one major problem with this recommendation is the requirement for a large number of ophthalmologists who will have to be put in place for handling an increased inflow of patients who come in for regular screening. This would be practically impossible in many countries due to the shortage of qualified and trained medical professionals. Hence, in order to eliminate the need for a large number of professionals, research is in progress to automate the procedure of DR screening. Automation of the procedure can also help to reduce interobserver and intraobserver errors in the screening process and can act as an adjunct tool for ophthalmologists. DR is quite easy to identify with several symptoms appearing, which include red lesions, such as microaneurysms, intraretinal microvascular abnormalities, and hemorrhages, and bright lesions like hard exudates and soft exudates or cotton-wool spots [2].

A short description of different features used to identify DR is given below:

1. Microaneurysms: These grow out of capillaries of the eyes. These are one of the first symptoms that indicate the onset of retinopathy. They usually appear as tiny indiscernible dots on a fundus image [3].
2. Hard exudates: It is a condition where proteins of the eye leaking through blood vessels weakened by worsening of diabetes [3].
3. Hemorrhages: This occurs when capillaries of the eye rupture. They appear as tiny dots or large blots on the retina [3].
4. Cotton-wool spots: This is a condition caused by reduced supply of oxygen to certain regions of the eye. This results in some areas of the retina displaying a grayish-white spot with fluffy white edges [3].
5. Venous beading: This is an advanced stage of cotton-wool spots with several *beads* of grayish-white spots being formed in bead-like structures all over the retina in small loops [3].

Based on the occurrence of these different features, DR is usually categorized into several stages as listed in the following:

1. Nonproliferative diabetic retinopathy (NPDR): This is the first stage of DR characterized by the presence of microaneurysms, hard exudates, and tiny infarctions [4]. This stage is further classified into three stages: mild, moderate, and severe NPDR.
   a. Mild and moderate NPDR: This is an early symptom of the onset of DR with microaneurysms, intraretinal hard exudates, and hemorrhages being widespread in many cases [4].
   b. Severe NPDR: Widespread intraretinal hard exudate formation and cotton-wool spots aggravating to venous beading can be found in patients with moderate to severe NPDR [4].
2. Proliferative diabetic retinopathy (PDR): This is an advanced stage of DR with the optic disc having several branchings of existing blood vessels. They form structures all over the retina and build pressure inside the eye. This results in the blood vessels becoming thinner and more fragile resulting in vessel rupture, ultimately leading to vision loss [4]. This vision loss can progress from partial to complete.

Automated detection of DR is done by making use of these symptoms by using them as features in the identification process. In the current study, we use these features to classify digital fundus images into normal and DR images. For an objective evaluation, we consider the entire image for analysis in order to capture all subtle features of the fundus image. Since we use Radon transform (RT) in our study, we strongly believe that utilizing the entire image for extracting effective features would prove to be useful since RT is an effective line integral that can capture subtle information from different angles of the image. Further, higher-order spectra (HOS) of the RT information would help in extracting relevant information for the classification of our dataset into normal and DR images. A study close to ours was performed by Giancardo et al., who worked on microaneurysm detection using RT [5]. But the study did not experiment with further processing of the line integrals obtained through RT. In the current study, we study not just microaneurysm detection but fundus image classification as a whole using RT followed by HOS-based feature extraction techniques followed by classification.

One of the earliest methods for automated diagnostic procedures for DR detection was done by simple gray-level thresholding as discussed in [6,7]. But gray-level thresholding has a blatant problem in the sense that the results are not consistent due to uneven illumination of the hard exudates [8]. But the problem was easy to counter with the introduction of edge detection and mixture model algorithms discussed by Sanchez et al. [8]. Apart from edge detection techniques, region growing and Bayesian-based approach applied to adaptive region growing were tried and tested by Kose et al. [9]. This technique was shown to be effective for segmentation of lesions in fundus images for automated DR screening. Moving on from the aforementioned techniques, Marwan and Saleh [10] worked on thresholding and shape features for microaneurysm and hemorrhage detection. This gave good results in automated DR diagnosis and grading. But as seen in the case of thresholding [8], uneven illumination often results in a need to adopt advanced techniques of processing and analysis.

Garcia et al. [11] tested an advanced set of neural networks to find the ability of several types of neural networks to classify digital fundus images. This study proved that neural networks were indeed capable of differentiating different types of fundus images. But the accuracy levels obtained in this study were not very high with an average of 86%. But other types of algorithms based on combination techniques such as an ensemble-based system with a pyramidal decomposition, edge detector, and Hough transform were used by Qureshi et al. [12] to obtain higher accuracy rates. This study was used to detect the macula and optic disc in digital fundus images as a precursor for DR diagnosis. In a similar study, Sanchez et al. [13] used probability maps and wavelet analysis to detect exudates in fundus images. In another study with similar goals, a simple technique of Fisher linear discriminant analysis (Fisher LDA) was used to obtain an accuracy rate of 100% for hard exudate detection. This study used color images, which shows that color images have previously been used in literature to obtain good accuracy rates. In a study close to ours, Gaussian mixture models (GMMs) and support vector machine (SVM) were used to classify shape and statistical features for microaneurysm detection [14]. Multiple-instance learning frameworks have been used by Quellec et al. [15] for a two-class classification of normal and DR digital fundus images. Similarly, dictionary learning and sparse representation classifier (SRC) were used by Zhang et al. [16] for microaneurysm detection and blood vessel identification in digital fundus images. Our group had previously tested nonlinear HOS features with SVM kernels for a five-class DR classification problem for automatic detection of mild, moderate, and severe PDR and NPDR classes with an accuracy rate of 86% [17]. In the current study, we intend to extend the previous work by including RT in the algorithm along with HOS cumulants for classifying DR stages in a more effective and precise way.

Our proposed system is shown in Figure 3.1. After contrast enhancement and intensity correction, we use RT to form a transformed image in a 2D space, from which we extract

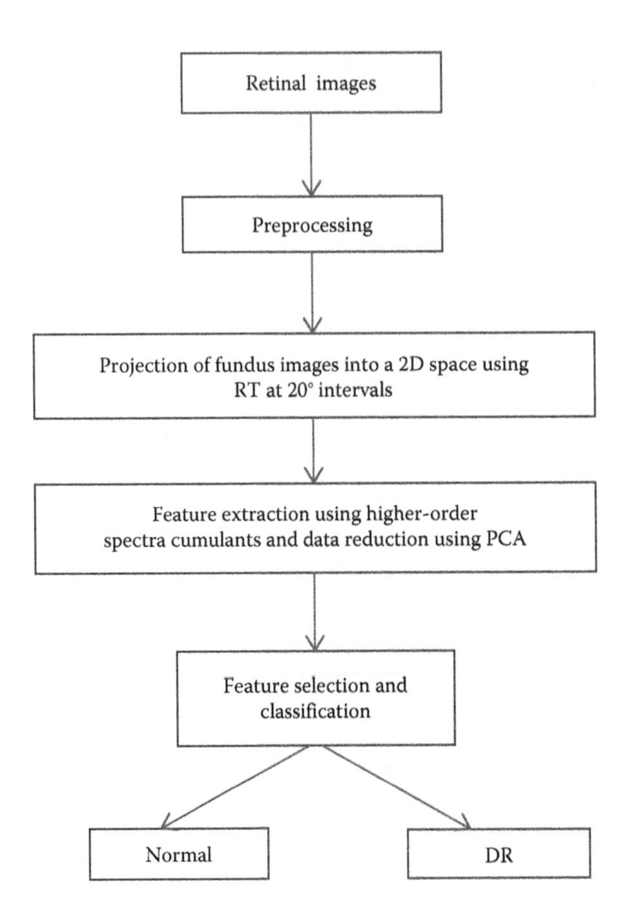

FIGURE 3.1
The proposed system.

HOS cumulants. The cumulant coefficients are subjected to principal component analysis (PCA). We classify these features into normal and DR classes using several classifiers including SVM with linear, quadratic, polynomial, and radial basis function (RBF) kernels and *k*-nearest neighbor (*k*-NN) classifier.

3.2 Materials and Methods

3.2.1 Image Database

The data used in this work were obtained from the Department of Ophthalmology, Kasturba Medical College, Manipal, India. The images were acquired using a TOPCON nonmydriatic retinal camera to provide a 3.1-megapixel retinal image. For the purpose of this study, 170 normal images and 170 DR images were used. Out of the 170 abnormal images, 23 were mild NPDR images, 52 were moderate NPDR images, 30 were severe NPDR images, and 65 were PDR images. The age group of patients considered for the study was 24–57 years. Typical normal and DR images are shown in Figure 3.2.

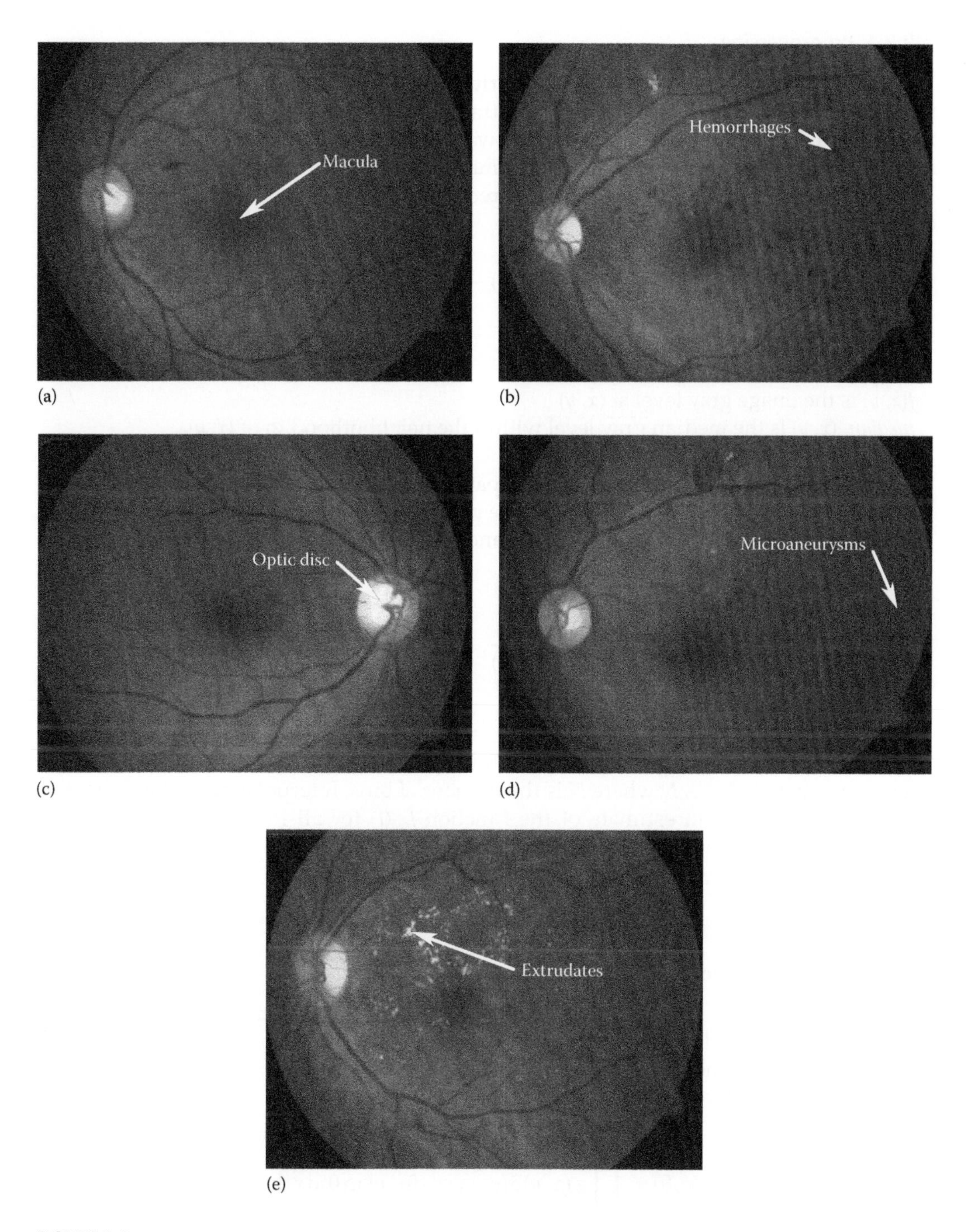

FIGURE 3.2
(See color insert.) Sample retinal images of (a) normal, (b) mild NPDR, (c) moderate NPDR, (d) severe NPDR, and (e) PDR.

3.2.2 Methods

3.2.2.1 Preprocessing

The color scale RGB images are first converted into grayscale for efficient computation. Since the exudates are visible with more contrast in grayscale, this mode was preferred for further analysis. An equalization procedure was performed on the images to obtain a local contrast that is approximately equal at all image intensities. In this method, a neighborhood $\wp$ of an image location (x, y) is considered. The local contrast of this neighborhood is estimated as

$$c(x,y) = f(x,y) - median_{\wp}(x,y) \tag{3.1}$$

where

$c(x, y)$ is the estimated local contrast
$f(x, y)$ is the image gray level at (x, y)
$median_{\wp}(x, y)$ is the median gray level within the neighborhood $\wp$ of (x, y)

Equation 3.1 can be equated to a high-pass spatial filter. The local contrast provides a measure of the high-frequency image noise. The noise associated with each image gray level I can be measured by the local contrast standard deviation $\sigma_c(I) \equiv \sigma\{c(I)\}$. The contrast enhancement function is then defined as

$$f_{ceq}(I_i) = \begin{cases} \dfrac{\sigma(I_i)}{\sigma_c(I_i)}, & \text{if } \sigma_c(I_i) > 0 \\ 0, & \text{otherwise} \end{cases} \tag{3.2}$$

While executing the contrast enhancement function, the grayscale is divided into several overlapping bins $i = 1, \ldots, N$ where N is the number of bins. Interpolation of the estimated $f_{ceq}(I_i)$ values provides an estimate of the function $f_{ceq}(I)$ for all image intensities I. This method of contrast enhancement is a nonlinear gray-level rescaling technique. This transfer function $f_{ceq}(I_i)$ is then normalized such that the total value adds up to 1, the same way it is done in the case of a probability density function.

3.2.2.2 Radon Transform

RT is a method of transformation to convert a 2D image into a domain where the image becomes an aggregated line integral obtained from various angles of image. This property of the transformation helps in applications where detection of features along line integrals plays an important role. The RT is defined as

$$g(\rho,\theta) = \int_{-\infty}^{\infty}\int_{-\infty}^{\infty} g(x,y)\delta(\rho - x\cos\theta - y\sin\theta)\,dx\,dy \tag{3.3}$$

where

θ is the angles at which the line integrals are calculated
$\rho = x\cos\theta + y\sin\theta$ with δ being the Kronecker-delta function

In this study, we use the standard form of RT as seen in Equation 3.3 for every 20° angles. The transformed images from all these angles are in turn combined and HOS cumulants are calculated using the procedure described in the following section.

3.2.2.3 Higher-Order Spectra Cumulants

HOS cumulants are higher-order correlations of signals. It captures the higher-order interrelations that are not captured by first- and second-order statistics. It models deviation of the distribution from a Gaussian process and is effective for nonlinear signals. Suppose if $\{X(k)\}$ is a sampled digital signal where $k=0, \pm1, \pm2, \ldots$ and if its moments up to order n exist, then the nth-order moment function is given by [18,19]

$$m_n^X(\tau_1, \tau_2, \ldots, \tau_{n-1}) = E\{x(k)x(k+\tau_1)\cdots x(k+\tau_{n+1})\} \tag{3.4}$$

This moment function depends only on time differences or time lags $\tau_1, \tau_2, \ldots, \tau_{n-1}, \tau_i = 0, \pm1, \pm2, \ldots$ for all i. The second-order moment m_2^X is the autocorrelation sequence of the time series $\{X(k)\}$. The third-order and the fourth-order moments are $m_3^X(\tau_1, \tau_2)$ and $m_4^X(\tau_1, \tau_2, \tau_3)$, respectively. $E\{\cdot\}$ is the statistical expectation operator. Using the nth-order moments, the nth-order cumulant can be computed as [18,19]

$$C_n^X(\tau_1, \tau_2, \ldots, \tau_{n-1}) = m_n^X(\tau_1, \tau_2, \ldots, \tau_{n-1}) - m_n^G(\tau_1, \tau_2, \ldots, \tau_{n-1}) \tag{3.5}$$

where
$m_n^X(\tau_1, \tau_2, \ldots, \tau_{n-1})$ is the nth-order moment function
$m_n^G(\tau_1, \tau_2, \ldots, \tau_{n-1})$ is the nth-order moment of an equivalent Gaussian process

Using the definition given by (3.4), the first fourth-order cumulants for a zero mean process are given by [18,19]

$$C_1^X = m_1^X \tag{3.6}$$

$$C_2^X(\tau_1) = m_2^X(\tau_1) \tag{3.7}$$

$$C_3^X(\tau_1, \tau_2) = m_3^X(\tau_1, \tau_2) \tag{3.8}$$

$$C_4^X(\tau_1, \tau_2, \tau_3) = m_4^X(\tau_1, \tau_2, \tau_3) - m_2^X(\tau_1)m_2^X(\tau_2 - \tau_3) - m_2^X(\tau_2)m_2^X(\tau_3 - \tau_1) - m_2^X(\tau_3)m_2^X(\tau_1 - \tau_2) \tag{3.9}$$

In the current study, the third-order cumulant is computed on the RT of the images. The cumulant plots and their contour representations of normal and DR images can be seen in Figures 3.3 and 3.4, respectively.

3.2.2.4 Principal Component Analysis

Principal component analysis (PCA) is a linear dimensionality reduction method [20,21]. It computes the directions of highest variability and projects the data onto them. It uses eigenvectors of covariance matrix as the basis vectors for these directions. The covariance

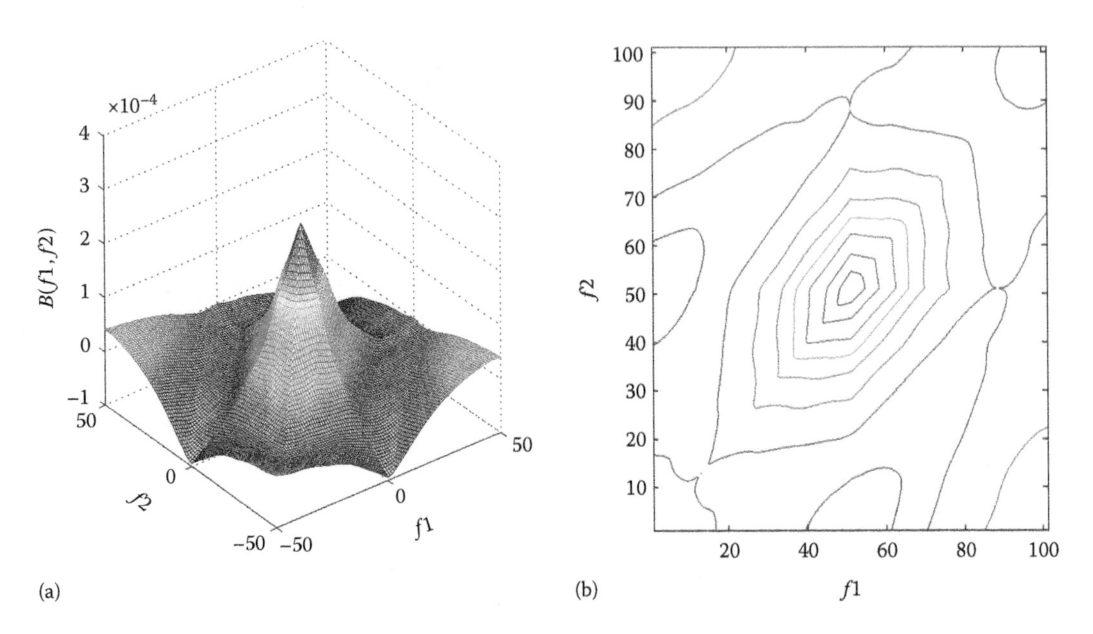

FIGURE 3.3
(a) The cumulant plot of normal images and (b) its contour representation.

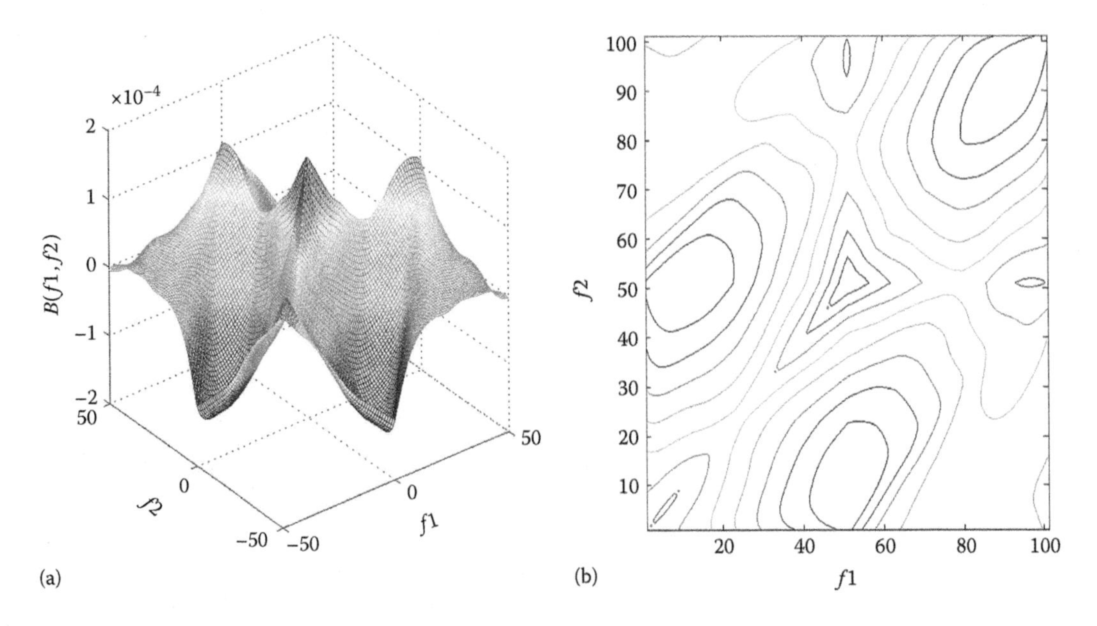

FIGURE 3.4
(a) The cumulant plot of abnormal images and (b) its contour representation.

matrix is decomposed using eigenvalue decomposition to get eigenvalues and eigenvectors. A threshold on the total variability contained by the considered principal components is used to choose the number of components. The systematic procedure of PCA is as follows [20,21]. We obtain 10 principal components from every HOS cumulant at 20° intervals. Hence, we have a total of 90 principal components.

Algorithm 3.1 Procedure for PCA [22]

Step 1: Compute the covariance matrix of order $N \times N$ for the signal under consideration as $\sum = (1/(N-1))(X-\bar{X})(X-\bar{X})^T$, where N is the number of features in the pattern space before application of PCA and $\bar{X} = (1/M)\sum_{i=1}^{N} x(i)$ is the mean of the ith feature.

Step 2: Compute the eigenvalue matrix D and the eigenvector matrix V as $V^{-1}\Sigma V = D$.

Step 3: Arrange the eigenvectors in terms of descending order of eigenvalues present in D.

Step 4: Compute the cumulative energy present in each component, which is the amount of variation in the component.

Step 5: Project the data present in the original pattern space onto the sorted eigenvectors and choose the number of components based on cumulative energy.

A scree plot of PCA carried out on our feature set (HOS cumulants) can be seen in Figure 3.5.

3.2.2.5 Feature Ranking and Selection

An important step in pattern recognition is identification of features, which contribute to the process of classification. Though there are several features that might be extracted using different techniques, it is essential to identify features that discriminate the classes well. In other words, it is necessary to rank and eliminate features that are not effective in the classification process. This requires us to reduce a high-dimensional feature vector d into a lower-dimensional feature vector m, which consists of features that are ranked in the order of their discriminatory capacity [20]. It is also essential to choose and rank the features in such a way that the chosen feature vector m represents the set of features that are the most effective representatives of the dataset. This process by which these representatives

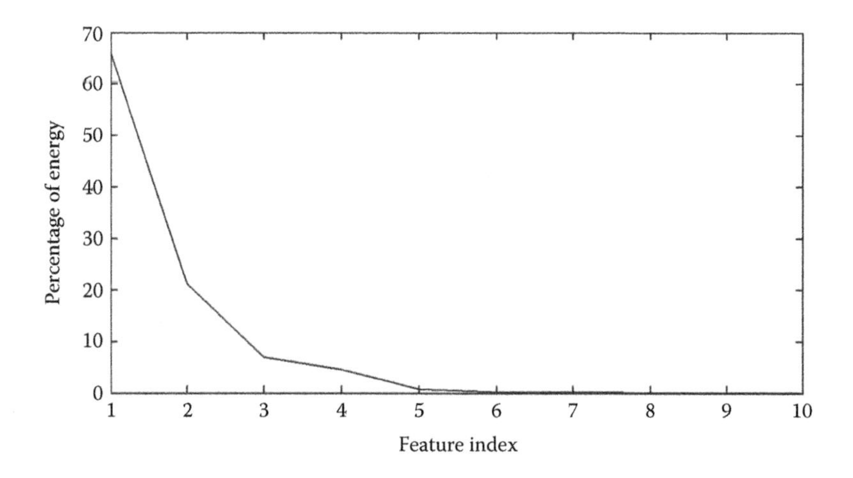

FIGURE 3.5
The scree plot for PCA.

are chosen is called as feature ranking and selection [20]. In this study, we rank features by finding a transformation from a d-dimensional feature vector into an m-dimensional feature space by using a forward feature selection technique with Mahalanobis distance measure in an unsupervised selection space.

3.2.2.6 Classification

Classification was performed using SVM with linear, quadratic, polynomial, and RBF kernels and k-NN classifier.

3.2.2.6.1 Support Vector Machine Classifier

SVM is a nonlinear classifier and has higher generalization ability in the sense that it can classify unseen data correctly [23,24]. It minimizes the structural risk unlike other classifiers that minimize empirical risk. It optimizes the class separation boundary such that the distance from the patterns of both (normal and DR) classes to the class separating hyperplane is maximum simultaneously [25]. If (x_i, y_i) are the patterns, where $i=1, 2, \ldots, N$, then x_i is the ith input and y_i is the corresponding pattern label. If c_+ and c_- are the class mean vectors of normal and abnormal classes, respectively, then the SVM classifier output is given by

$$y_i = sign\{(x_i - c)w\} = sign\{x_i c_+ - x_i c_- + b\} \tag{3.10}$$

where w is the unit vector of a perpendicular line on the class separating hyperplane, which needs to be determined by the optimization process and

$$b = \frac{1}{2}\{\| c_- \|^2 - \| c_+ \|^2\} \tag{3.11}$$

We need to find the optimal hyperplane that will separate the two classes such that Equations 3.10 and 3.11 are satisfied. Such a hyperplane is obtained by solving the following optimization problem:

$$minimize_{w,b} \frac{1}{2} \| w \| \tag{3.12}$$

Equation 3.12 is to be minimized in such a way that $y_i(wx_i+b) > 1, i=1, 2, \ldots, N$.

The problem defined by Equation 3.12 is a quadratic optimization problem, where one must find the saddle point using Lagrange multipliers as

$$L_p(w,b,\alpha) = \frac{1}{2} \| w \| - \sum \alpha_i \{y_i(w^T x_i + b) - 1\} \tag{3.13}$$

The linear SVM is solved using the objective function given by Equation 3.13. When the data are linearly inseparable, the data are first projected into a new space using a kernel transformation and then the optimization is carried in the kernel space [23,24]. Commonly used kernel functions are quadratic, polynomial, and RBF. Polynomial kernel of degree d is given by

$$k(x_i, x_j) = (x_i^T x_j + 1)^d \tag{3.14}$$

We have used a quadratic and polynomial kernel of order 3. For quadratic kernel, $d=2$, and for polynomial kernel, $d=3$. The RBF kernel transformation is given by

$$k(x_i, x_j) = exp\left(\frac{\| x_i - x_j \|}{2\sigma^2}\right) \tag{3.15}$$

where σ is the width parameter of RBF kernel.

3.2.2.6.2 k-Nearest Neighbor Classifier

k-NN is an example of instance-based learning and a nonparametric classification technique, which is one of the simplest and most effective classifiers in a clustering scheme [26]. In this classifier, the data points in the test feature space are compared with the training feature space to study the nearest neighbor of the dataset in question [26]. Once the value of this data point is studied, the classifier simply assigns this point to the class of its nearest neighbor depending upon the value of k chosen by the user. For instance, if $k=2$, the classifier compares the value of two neighbors before assigning the data point in consideration a class. We opted for the classifier since we wanted an objective evaluation by comparing the performance of our technique on a complex classifier like SVM and a simple clustering classifier like *k*-NN.

3.3 Results

In the current study, we obtained high accuracy for classification of digital fundus images into normal and DR classes. The accuracies reported in Table 3.1 are average values of sensitivity, specificity, positive predictive value (PPV) and accuracies during 10-fold cross-validation scheme performed on the entire dataset. As seen from Table 3.1, our accuracy rates are quite high compared to existing literature discussed in Table 3.2. We obtained a maximum accuracy of 97.06% with linear SVM kernel for 58 HOS cumulant features. We have shown that our technique of using HOS to calculate the moments and cumulants of images transformed using RT has provided very good results. Our results are better than the results obtained by Usman Akram et al. [14] who used a classification methodology that utilized

TABLE 3.1

Classification Performance of Different Classifiers with Optimal Number of Features

	Sensitivity (%)	Specificity (%)	PPV (%)	Accuracy (%)	Optimal Number of Features
SVM linear	98.70	95.31	95.35	97.06	58
SVM quadratic	96.64	89.65	90.78	93.24	10
SVM polynomial	95.44	86.25	87.54	90.88	32
SVM-RBF	82.82	94.85	95.02	88.82	10
k-NN	88.12	89.82	90.05	88.82	34

TABLE 3.2
Summary of Studies on Automated DR Screening

Authors	Feature Detected	Features and Classifiers	Accuracy (%)
Sanchez et al. [8]	Hard exudates	Color information and Fisher LDA	100
Kose et al. [9]	Image pixel information	Inverse segmentation using region growing, adaptive region growing, and Bayesian approaches	90
Garcia et al. [11]	Red lesions	Image and shape features using neural networks	86
Qureshi et al. [12]	Identifying macula optic disc	Ensemble combined algorithm of edge detectors, Hough transform, and pyramidal decomposition	95.33
Giancardo et al. [27]	Exudates in fundus images	Exudate probability map and wavelet analysis	94
Quellec et al. [15]	Abnormal patterns in fundus images	Multiple-instance learning	88.1
Zhang et al. [16]	Microaneurysms and blood vessel detection	Dictionary learning and SRC	84.67
Sanchez et al. [13]	Hard exudates	Edge detection and mixture models	95
Usman Akram et al. [14]	Image shape and statistics	GMMs and SVM	99.53
Noronha et al. [28]	Image pixel and color information	Wavelet transforms and SVM kernels	99
The current study	RT and HOS cumulants	SVM kernels, *k*-NN	88.82–97.06

features extracted directly from RT. This shows that the application of HOS after extracting RT features provides information about subtle changes in images. This can be seen from a well-differentiated scatterplot of normal and DR representative features shown in Figure 3.7.

Though SVM linear kernels provided the best classification accuracy, the other kernels such as quadratic, RBF, and polynomial also performed well. Their accuracy rates varied from 88.82% to 93.24% (Figure 3.6). Considering the fact that we operated on the entire image instead of a segmented area of interest, these classification accuracies prove that our technique can be used to classify images that are difficult to differentiate using normal texture measures.

In order to obtain an objective comparison of classification accuracies, we used another classifier, namely, *k*-NN, in order to compare the performance of our technique with a clustering algorithm. As seen from Table 3.1, *k*-NN provided a classification accuracy that was on par with SVM kernels. The average accuracies of a 10-fold cross-validation scheme for all the classifiers for an increasing number of features can be seen in Figure 3.6.

3.4 Discussion

The proposed algorithm that uses HOS to extract relevant features from Radon-transformed 2D digital fundus images has not been tested in literature yet. So far, the closest work in this field of research has been done by Giancardo et al. [5] who used a direct implementation of RT on digital fundus images followed by classifiers to detect microaneurysms. From the results obtained in this study, we have shown a clear superiority of our proposed

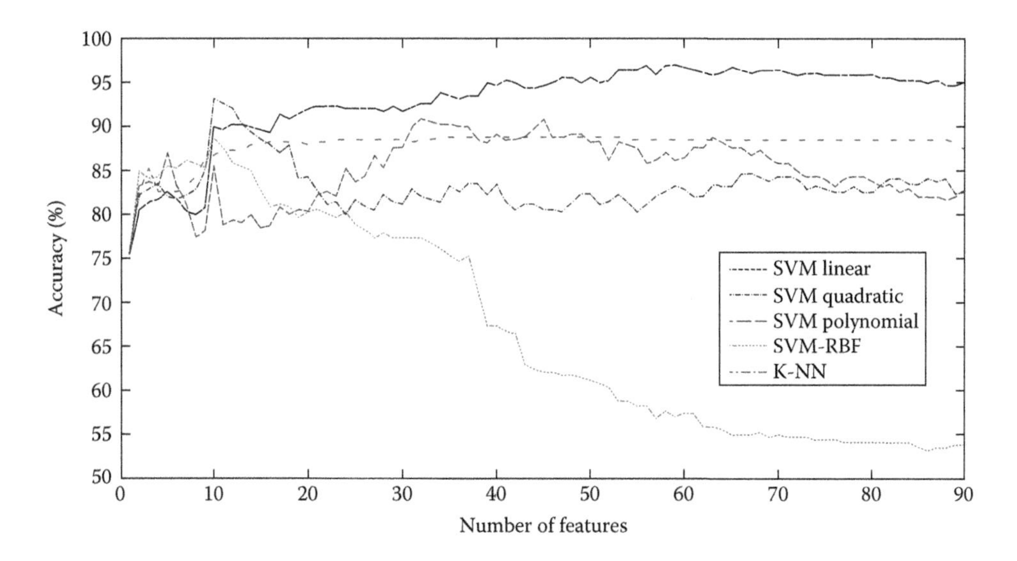

FIGURE 3.6
Average classification accuracy of 10-fold for different classifiers for varying number of features.

technique over existing studies. A list of literatures that might be of interest in providing a comparison to our current study can be seen in Table 3.2. From this list of literature, we can see that the proposed algorithm is comparable or even better than most of the existing techniques. This said, we must also take into consideration the fact that the current study is performed for a two-class classification problem and results might vary when it is extended to a multiclass problem. But this should not be a hindrance since we have obtained good results in a two-class and extension of this into a multiclass problem is only a matter of mathematical interpretation. Also, from the scatterplots seen in Figure 3.7, we realize that the features are very well separated. This is due to the fact that HOS is a technique that is not affected by noise in the original data and can adapt itself well to noisy data. Also, it is an extremely efficient way to increase between-class scatter and reduce within-class scatter. Since the main goal of any pattern recognition problem is to increase between-class scatter and reduce within-class scatter, we can use HOS in an effective way to separate our features for further classification. This can be very well seen in the feature scatterplots of Figure 3.7. An extension of the current study to a multiclass problem is definitely possible considering the fact that we have obtained very good accuracy rates for all the classifiers we have tested the algorithm on.

3.5 Conclusion

A new pipeline for classification of digital fundus images into normal and DR images has been proposed. In this study, we have improved upon an already existing study [5] that uses RT for microaneurysm detection in fundus images. We have proposed the usage of HOS to extract features from RT of the images in order to get a valid and objective feature space to build our classification model. As a start, we tested our algorithm on a two-class fundus image classification problem to classify normal and DR images. From the results,

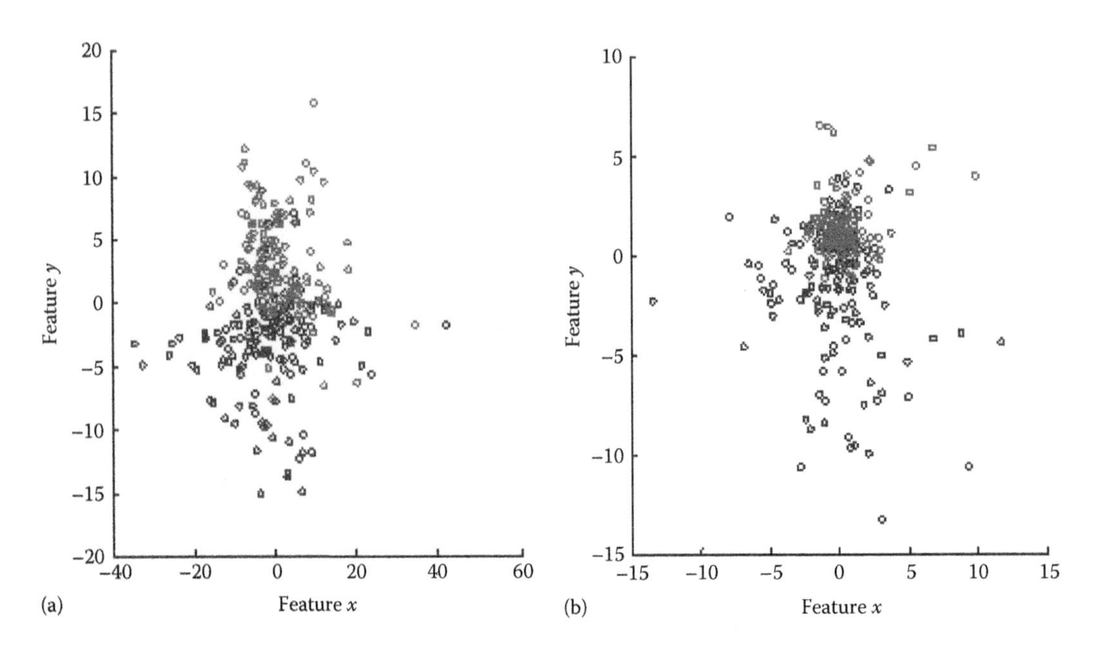

FIGURE 3.7
Scatterplot of two sets of representative features for normal (dark dots) and DR images (light dots).

we see that the technique works very well for the given problem in hand. This can also be viewed visually by looking at the representative scatterplots (Figure 3.7) of the feature set, which shows that the normal and DR images are well defined and well separated. Various kernels of SVM classifier provided equally good results with SVM linear kernel giving the best result. An objective comparison of *k*-NN classifier proved positive with equally good classification accuracy. We are confident that with promising results in hand, we can now test the proposed algorithm for a multiclass problem.

References

1. World Health Organisation. Prevention of blindness from diabetes mellitus: Report of a WHO consultation in Geneva, Switzerland. Geneva, Switzerland: WHO Library Cataloguing-in-Publication Data, 2005.
2. M. Garcia, C.I. Sanchez, M.I. Lopez, D. Abasolo, R. Hornero. Neural network based detection of hard exudates in retinal images, *Computer Methods and Programs in Biomedicine*, 93(1), 9–19, January 2009, ISSN: 0169-2607, doi: 10.1016/j.cmpb.2008.07.006.
3. A.A. Alghadyan. Diabetic retinopathy—An update, *Saudi Journal of Ophthalmology*, 25(1), 99–111, 2011.
4. F. Harney. Diabetic retinopathy, *Medicine*, 34(3), 95–98, 2006.
5. L. Giancardo , F. Meriaudeau, T.P. Karnowski, Y. Li, K.W. Tobin, E. Chaum. Microaneurysm detection with radon transform-based classification on retina images. In: *2011 Annual International Conference of the IEEE Engineering in Medicine and Biology Society, EMBC*, Boston, MA, pp. 5939, 5942, August 30–September 3, 2011, doi: 10.1109/IEMBS.2011.6091562.

6. R. Philips, J. Forrester, P. Sharp. Automated detection and quantification of retinal exudates, *Graefe's Archive for Clinical and Experimental Ophthalmology*, 231(2), 90–94, 1993.
7. D. Kavitha, S.S. Devi. Automatic detection of optic disk and exudates in retinal images. In: *Proceedings of the International Conference in Intelligent Sensing and Information Processing*, Chennai, India, pp. 501–506, 2005.
8. C.I. Sanchez, M. Garcia, A. Mayo, M.I. Lopez, R. Hornero. Retinal image analysis based on mixture models to detect hard exudates, *Medical Image Analysis*, 13(4), 650–658, August 2009, ISSN: 1361-8415, doi: 10.1016/j.media.2009.05.005.
9. C. Kose, U. Şevik, C. İkibaş, H. Erdol. Simple methods for segmentation and measurement of diabetic retinopathy lesions in retinal fundus images, *Computer Methods and Programs in Biomedicine*, 107(2), 274–293, August 2012, ISSN: 0169-2607, doi: 10.1016/j.cmpb.2011.06.007.
10. M.D. Saleh, C. Eswaran. An automated decision-support system for non-proliferative diabetic retinopathy disease based on MAs and HAs detection, *Computer Methods and Programs in Biomedicine*, 108(1), 186–196, October 2012, ISSN: 0169-2607, doi: 10.1016/j.cmpb.2012.03.004.
11. M. Garcia, M.I. Lopez, D. Alvarez, R. Hornero. Assessment of four neural network based classifiers to automatically detect red lesions in retinal images, *Medical Engineering & Physics*, 32(10), 1085–1093, December 2010, ISSN: 1350-4533, doi: 10.1016/j.medengphy.2010.07.014.
12. R.J. Qureshi, L. Kovacs, B. Harangi, B. Nagy, T. Peto, A. Hajdu. Combining algorithms for automatic detection of optic disc and macula in fundus images, *Computer Vision and Image Understanding*, 116(1), 138–145, January 2012, ISSN: 1077-3142, doi: 10.1016/j.cviu.2011.09.001.
13. C.I. Sanchez, R. Hornero, M.I. Lopez, M. Aboy, J. Poza, D. Abasolo. A novel automatic image processing algorithm for detection of hard exudates based on retinal image analysis, *Medical Engineering & Physics*, 30(3), 350–357, April 2008, ISSN: 1350-4533, doi: 10.1016/j.medengphy.2007.04.010.
14. M. Usman Akram, S. Khalid, S.A. Khan. Identification and classification of microaneurysms for early detection of diabetic retinopathy, *Pattern Recognition*, 46(1), 107–116, January 2013, ISSN: 0031-3203, doi: 10.1016/j.patcog.2012.07.002.
15. G. Quellec, M. Lamard, M.D. Abramoff, E. Decenciere, B. Lay, A. Erginay, B. Cochener, G. Cazuguel. A multiple-instance learning framework for diabetic retinopathy screening, *Medical Image Analysis*, 16(6), 1228–1240, August 2012, ISSN: 1361-8415, doi: 10.1016/j.media.2012.06.003.
16. B. Zhang, F. Karray, Q. Li, L. Zhang. Sparse Representation Classifier for microaneurysm detection and retinal blood vessel extraction, *Information Sciences*, 200, 78–90, October 2012, ISSN: 0020-0255, doi: 10.1016/j.ins.2012.03.003.
17. U.R. Acharya, C.K. Chua, E.Y.K. Ng, W. Yu, C. Chee. Application of higher order spectra for the identification of diabetes retinopathy stages, *Journal of Medical Systems*, 32(6), 481–488, December 2008.
18. C.L. Nikias, J.M. Mendel. Signal processing with higher-order spectra, *IEEE Signal Processing Magazine*, 10, 10–37, 1993.
19. J.M. Mendel. Tutorial on higher-order statistics (spectra) in signal processing and system theory: Theoretical results and some applications, *Proceedings of the IEEE*, 79, 278–305, 1991.
20. R. Andrew. *Webb, Statistical Pattern Recognition*, 2nd edn., John Wiley & Sons, Chichester, U.K., 2002, ISBN: 0470845147.
21. R.O. Duda, P.E. Hart, D.G. Stork. *Pattern Classification*, 2nd edn., John Wiley & Sons, New York, 2001.
22. R.O. Duda, P.E. Hart, D.G. Stork. *Pattern Classification*, John Wiley & Sons, 2012.
23. N. Cristianini, J. Shawe-Taylor. *An Introduction to Support Vector Machines and Other Kernel-Based Learning Methods*, Cambridge University Press, Cambridge, U.K., 2000.
24. B. Scholkopf, A.J. Smola. *Learning with Kernels: Support Vector Machines, Regularization, Optimization and Beyond*, The MIT Press, Cambridge, MA, 2002.

25. K.R. Muller, S. Mika, G. Ratsch, K. Tsuda, B. Scholkopf. An introduction to kernel based learning algorithms, *IEEE Transactions on Neural Networks*, 12(2), 181–201, 2001.
26. D. Coomans, D.L. Massart. Alternative k-nearest neighbour rules in supervised pattern recognition: Part 1. k-Nearest neighbour classification by using alternative voting rules, *Analytica Chimica Acta*, 136, 15–27, 1982, doi: 10.1016/S0003-2670(01)95359-0.
27. L. Giancardo, F. Meriaudeau, T.P. Karnowski, Y. Li, S. Garg, K.W. Tobin Jr., E. Chaum. Exudate-based diabetic macular edema detection in fundus images using publicly available datasets, *Medical Image Analysis*, 16(1), 216–226, January 2012, ISSN: 1361-8415, doi: 10.1016/j.media.2011.07.004.
28. K. Noronha, U. Rajendra Acharya, S. Kamath, S.V. Bhandary, K.P Nayak. Decision support system for diabetic retinopathy using discrete wavelet transform, *Proceedings of the Institution of Mechanical Engineers, Part H: Journal of Engineering in Medicine*, 227(3), 251–261, 2013.

4

*Quality Measures for Retinal Images**

S.R. Nirmala, S. Dandapat, and P.K. Bora

CONTENTS

Retinal images have the potential to facilitate the early detection of retinal pathologies. The clinically important features of a retinal image are the *optic disc* (OD), the *macula*, and the *blood vessels*. The ophthalmologists examine these features for signs of various eye-related diseases. The retinal image should be of sufficient quality for reliable diagnosis. In some applications like telemedicine, these images need to be processed for efficient storage and transmission. Any such processing causes distortion and degrades the quality of the image. But the important question is: will the processed image be clinically useful as the original? If the answer is yes, then it is required that little distortion occurs to the clinical information in the processed images. Then the processed image is of similar quality as that of the original. How does one evaluate the quality? The image quality is an attribute that has many definitions and interpretations depending on

* *Sources:* Reprinted from *Biomed. Signal Process. Control*, 5(4), Nirmala, S.R., Dandapat, S., and Bora, P.K., Wavelet weighted blood vessel distortion measure for retinal images, 282–291, Copyright 2010, with permission from Elsevier; With kind permission from Springer Science+Business Media: *Signal, Image and Video Process.*, Wavelet weighted distortion measure for retinal images, 7(5), 2012, 1005–1014, Nirmala, S.R., Dandapat, S., and Bora, P.K.

the application. A pair of medical images may appear identical when viewed by common people, but a medical expert might find them different. Hence, image quality evaluation is an important issue.

4.1 Image Quality Measures

There are many approaches for evaluating the quality of processed images. Image quality evaluation can be done either subjectively or objectively. *Subjective image quality* evaluation is the most accurate and reliable way of assessing the quality of an image. However, this method is slow, inconvenient, and expensive for practical usage. Thus, *objective image quality* metrics that can automatically predict the perceived image quality are preferred. The most common computable objective measures of image quality are the average distortion-based *mean square error* (MSE) and the *peak signal to noise ratio* (PSNR). These measures are simple to compute and depends on pixelwise distortion. But the drawback of the squared error measures is that a slight spatial shift of an image may cause a high numerical distortion but no perceptible distortion. On the other hand, a small average distortion may result in severe visual artifacts if all the error is concentrated in a small important region. Therefore, their predictions of the image quality often do not agree well with the human visual perception. The perceived quality of images with the same PSNR can actually be very different. It is proved that a higher PSNR or equivalently a lower MSE may not necessarily imply a higher subjective image quality [1].

The limitations of conventional objective measures are illustrated using Figure 4.1. The figure shows four retinal images having the same value of MSE (≃12%). But the error in each image is due to distortions in different spatial locations including the diagnostic features and other regions. The distortion in different retinal features is significant, whereas distortion in the dark background region is diagnostically insignificant. The high values of error measures due to distortion in the dark background regions may mislead the quality evaluation of retinal image. These measures quantify the error globally and fail to characterize the error in local clinical features.

Image quality assessment can be improved by incorporating some models of human visual system (HVS) into the evaluation process [1]. In recent years, approaches based on HVS models are slowly replacing the classical numerical quality measures. The quality improvement that can be achieved using an HVS-based approach is significant and applies to a large variety of image processing applications. The image quality measures (IQMs) developed in [2,3] do not directly employ the HVS model but are inspired by the functioning of the HVS. The Structural SIMilarity (SSIM) index is a change in the fundamental assumption from the intensity error–based IQMs. This is considered to be the best state-of-the-art IQM. Previous approaches measure the perceptual image quality assuming that image intensity is the key component of the visual quality. This method often measures intensity error and then penalizes these errors according to their visibility. The main idea here is that human visual perception is built to understand a scene based on its structure, suggesting that this structural information is the key component of visual quality. The subjective scores and various objective measures discussed are originally developed for assessing the quality of TV and multimedia images. Some of the conventional IQMs are used for quality evaluation of different medical images [4] and retinal images [5]. But the issue of quantifying the clinical distortion in retinal images has not been addressed.

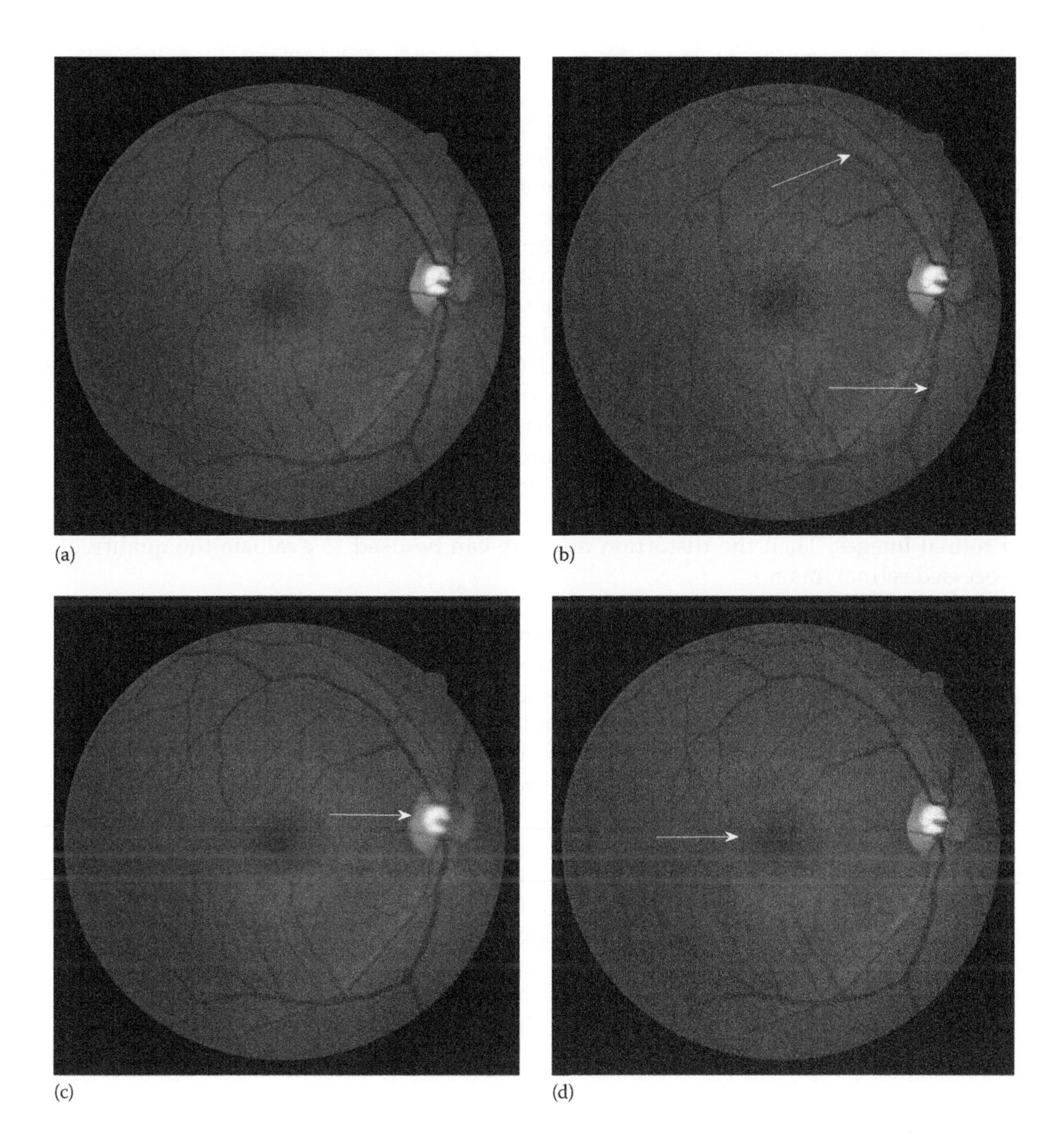

FIGURE 4.1
Retinal images with the same MSE but having distortion in the (a) dark background region, (b) thick blood vessels, (c) OD region, and (d) macula region (shown with white arrows).

For medical images, a distortion measure has to be defined from the diagnostic perspective. Such a measure should take proper account of the clinical nature of the images. Certain regions of a medical image are rich in clinical information and some regions are clinically nonsignificant. The distortion occurring in these clinically significant regions is more important than that in the background regions. The IQM is expected to emphasize any distortion in clinically important regions and give less importance to the effects in nonsignificant regions. Hence, measuring the distortion in clinical features is more meaningful than quantifying the error globally using the entire image. To incorporate the importance of distortion in clinically significant regions into the measure, it is required to segment the image into clinically important regions and the background. The accurate segmentation of clinical features in retinal image is relatively a difficult task. In this direction, alternate methods can be investigated to localize the retinal features. The spatial frequency localization and multiresolution analysis (MRA) properties of the discrete wavelet transform (DWT) present an efficient way of image representation. The multiresolution decomposition of a retinal image separates the image features into different frequency subbands in a specific direction and along a specific scale [6]. The multiscale property of the wavelet transform shows that the features that are difficult to detect at one scale may be easily detected at another scale. Hence, the DWT can be explored for localizing the retinal image components. The conventional compression techniques for medical images such as JPEG2000 and DICOM use the DWT. The DWT has been used in various biomedical image processing applications such as noise removal, enhancement, and detection of diagnostic features [7]. These attractive features of wavelet analysis give an insight that the distortion in retinal features can be now estimated by computing the error between subbands of original and processed images. This gives a motivation to develop a wavelet-based distortion measure to quantify the loss of clinical information in retinal images. Then the distortion measure can be used to evaluate the quality of processed retinal images.

There are three major discussions in this chapter. In the first, the effect of distortions in different wavelet subbands on clinical features is discussed. This investigation identifies the subbands that carry significant information about a retinal feature. Secondly, after identifying the clinically significant subbands, different weights are assigned to different subbands. The clinical information loss is quantified as a weighted sum of the root of normalized MSEs of the coefficients in all the subbands. The clinical distortion measure is computed for each retinal feature. A global clinical distortion measure is defined by combining the distortion measures for individual features. As a third topic, the performance of the distortion measure is investigated in predicting the quality of the retinal images with different artifacts. The statistical measures used for evaluation are the Pearson linear correlation coefficient (PLCC), the Spearman rank-order correlation coefficient (SROCC), the outlier ratio (OR), and the root mean square error (RMSE) between the subjective scores and the predicted subjective scores after nonlinear regression. It is shown with various experiments that the subband weighted distortion measure (SWDM) can effectively quantify the distortion in clinical features of processed retinal images.

4.2 Wavelet Subband Analysis of Retinal Features

The analysis of clinical features is important for the clinical use of retinal images. The wavelet transform is utilized in order to adequately represent these features. The MRA of the wavelet helps in producing localized image features with good space frequency resolution [6,7]. This spatial localization has proven to be useful in analyzing the local spectral properties of particular regions like the anatomical structures, which are of interest in an image. The multiscale property of the wavelet shows that features that are difficult to detect at one scale may be detected at another scale. The wavelet decomposition uses a linear transformation to split an image into subbands or subimages containing different frequency information. It allows the processing of different frequency information separately. The multiresolution property of the wavelet transform has been successfully used in many applications such as image denoising, compression [8,9], and singularity detection [10].

The choice of a suitable wavelet filter influences the image quality as well as the system design. Different mother wavelets are characterized by their regularity, which describes the smoothness of the wavelet. The performance of different wavelet filters is evaluated by decomposing the image into various levels using a wavelet filter and for different compression ratio. Various quality measures are used to quantify the effect of wavelet filters [8] along with the subjective evaluation. The optimum decomposition level and a best-suited wavelet filter for retinal image analysis can be then chosen from the comparative study and experimental observations [11]. The advantages of using the wavelet transform is that the signal features can be extracted in the wavelet domain [12]. The research works related to wavelet transform-based retinal image analysis focussed on the use of processed retinal image for different applications. But no systematic study has been made to evaluate the retinal features at various wavelet subbands. A multilevel decomposition is performed on the retinal images generating various *detail subbands* and one *approximation band*. Each subband contains information about the retinal image in a specific direction and along a specific scale/frequency [9]. The detail coefficients may provide vital information about the localized features of the retinal image. The approximation coefficients represent the slowly varying low-frequency background of the retinal image.

It is important to evaluate the significance of each subband from the point of view of presence of clinical information in that subband. For a particular diagnostic feature, it is expected that certain subbands may contain information that is relatively more significant than the other subbands. The diagnostic importance of each level subbands is examined by zeroing the coefficients of the subbands and keeping all other subband coefficients unchanged. The effect is analyzed by reconstructing the image using the distorted subbands. The original and the reconstructed images are visually examined to assess the image quality from the point of view of the blood vessels, the macula, and the OD. The distortions to different frequency subbands will have different impact on the quality of the image. These effects are also quantified by computing the SSIM index between the retinal features before and after the subband distortion. This study shows which of the subbands carry significant information of the features.

4.2.1 Blood Vessel Information

The blood vessels are major structure in the retinal image and have high diagnostic impact. It is required to analyze the significance of each wavelet subband from the point of view of blood vessel information in a retinal image. The blood vessels are darker compared to the background and their thickness varies as they travel radially out of the OD. The vascular network is thicker in the area near the OD and the vessel thickness gradually reduces leading to the thin end part. The main thick vessel splits into many small thin branches. The nonvessel region acts as background and is one with slowly varying pixel values. Based on the above information, the diagnostic importance of each detail subband is examined by zeroing the coefficients of the subband and keeping all other subbands undisturbed. The diagnostic quality of the retinal image is examined by reconstructing the image with the altered subbands.

To illustrate the importance of subbands at each decomposition level, the retinal images from digital retinal images for vessel extraction (DRIVE) database [13] are considered. The green channel images are extracted from original color retinal images and resized to 512 × 512. These images are wavelet decomposed to five levels using the biorthogonal filter. This generates 15 detail subbands and 1 approximation band. The 15 detail subbands can be put into 5 groups according to the level of transformation: level-1 (L1), level-2 (L2), level-3 (L3), level-4 (L4), and level-5 (L5). The images in Figure 4.2 show the effect of introducing distortion in different subbands. The blood vessels represent changes in intensity level and characterized by high-frequency subbands. The image in Figure 4.2b is obtained after zeroing the highest-frequency coefficients of decomposition L1 subbands H(1), V(1), and D(1). It is observed that the vessel structure

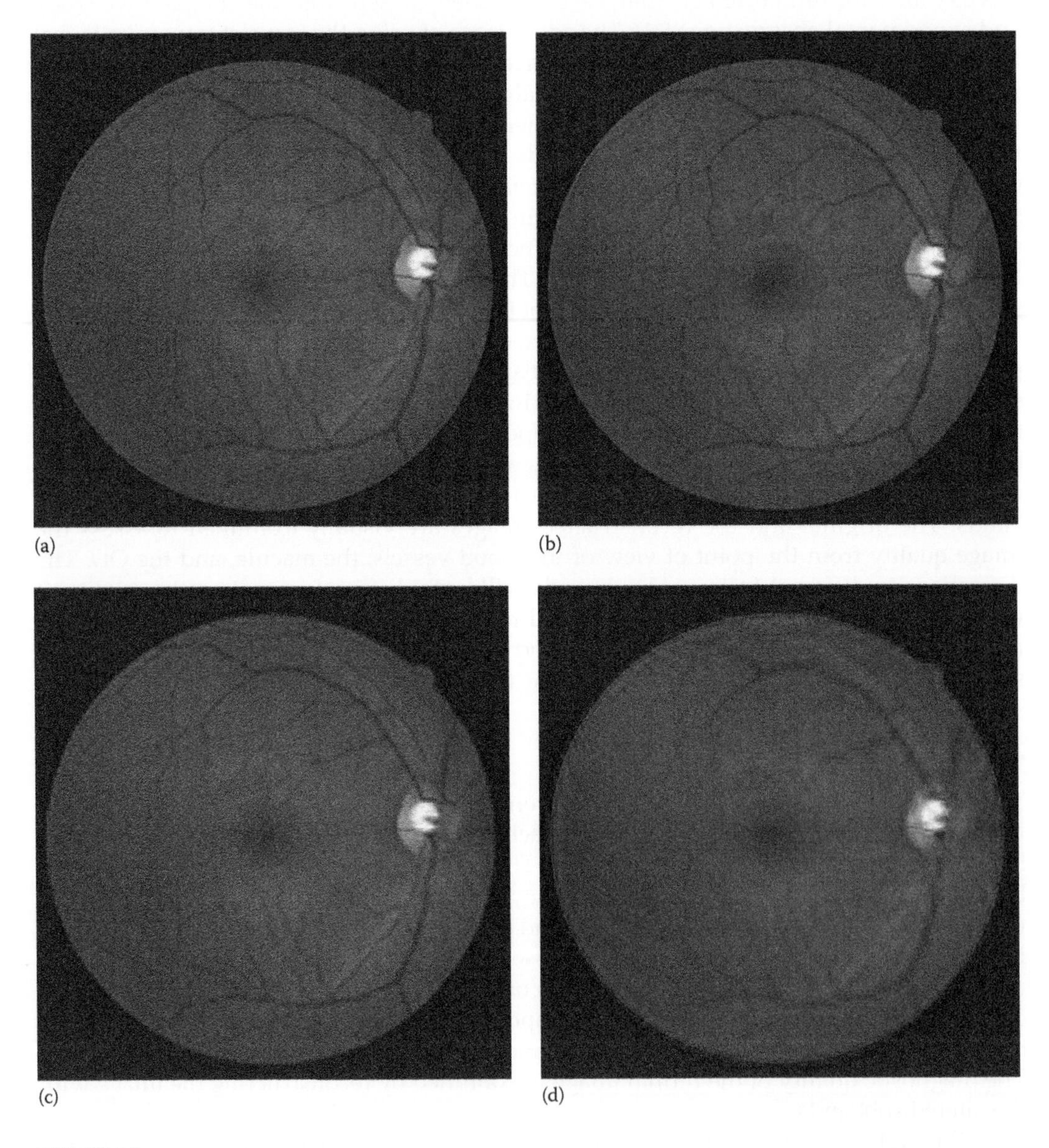

FIGURE 4.2
(a) Original image and reconstructed images when subband coefficients of (b) L1, (c) L2, and (d) L3 are made zero.

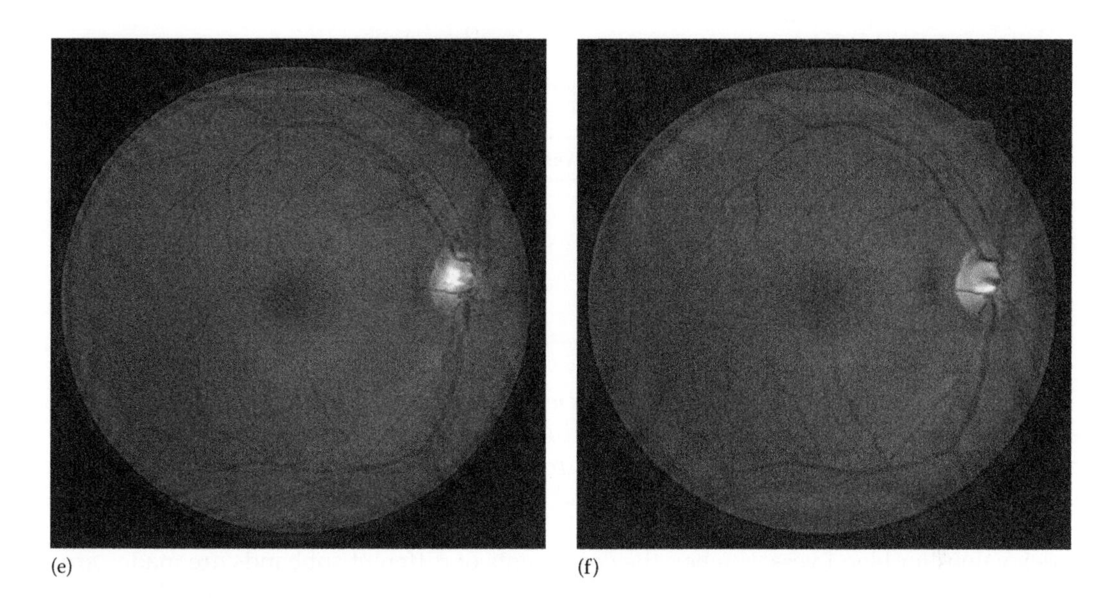

FIGURE 4.2 (continued)
Original image and reconstructed images when subband coefficients of (e) L4 and (f) L5 are made zero.

is well reconstructed and the overall image quality is close to the original image. This implies that subbands H(1), V(1), and D(1) do not carry significant blood vessel information. Generally, these subbands are considered to capture the high-frequency noise, and eliminating them does not affect the image features. The image in Figure 4.2c is produced after zeroing the coefficients of L2 subbands H(2), V(2), and D(2). In this image, the blood vessels look slightly smeared, but still the details of main vessels are retained. Most of the thin vessels have lost their sharpness by spreading into the surroundings and the faint end part of small branches has disappeared. It is observed that the quality of the image is not as good as that of Figure 4.2b. It shows that any alteration of L2 subband coefficients has more effect on the thin vessels, whereas there is a little effect on thick vessels. The thin vessels are considered to be of higher-frequency components as compared to the thick vessels. Hence, the L2 subbands are expected to have higher significance for thin vessels. The reconstructed image after zeroing the subband H(3), V(3), and D(3) coefficients is shown in Figure 4.2d. The image shows that the main thick vessels are smeared, and most of the thin vessels are preserved. It is observed that the image quality is low as compared to that of Figure 4.2c. This shows that thin vessels are less affected but thick vessels are more sensitive to changes in the L3 subband coefficients. The thick vessels constitute the low-frequency components of the image in relative to the thin vessels. This may be the reason for distortion in thick vessels when the L3 subband coefficients are altered. So the L3 subbands are important for thick vessels as compared to higher-frequency L2 subbands. Figure 4.2e shows the image after zeroing the coefficients of subbands H(4), V(4), and D(4) of L4. It is observed that the thin vessels are clear and little distortion in thick vessels. When the coarsest subband H(5), V(5), and D(5) coefficients are made zero, the reconstructed image in Figure 4.2f shows that the vessel pattern is well preserved. The image shows a thin ringlike appearance along the circular periphery of the image. The diagnostic quality of the image still be retained since these artifacts do not disturb the diagnostic features. The experiment is repeated for all images in the database.

TABLE 4.1

SSIM Index Values for Blood Vessels in Different Directions

Zeroed Band	Thick Vert. Vessels	Thin Vert. Vessels
V(1)=0	0.994	0.992
V(2)=0	0.977	0.957
V(3)=0	0.928	0.972
V(4)=0	0.925	0.998
V(5)=0	0.994	0.999

To quantify the effect of altering the coefficients of a subband on blood vessels, a simple experiment is performed. Small sections of thick and thin vessels in approximately vertical (Vert) orientation are picked from the original and the reconstructed images. The SSIM index for blood vessels is then computed and tabulated. When there is strong similarity, the SSIM index takes a value of one and it takes zero for no similarity. Table 4.1 shows SSIM index values for blood vessels when the coefficients of different subbands are made zero. Only the vertical subband coefficients from all decomposition levels are considered and their effect on blood vessels is observed. Thin vertical vessels get disturbed when the coefficients of subband V(2) are made zero. The thin vertical vessels show lower SSIM index value of 0.957, whereas the thick vertical vessels show SSIM index reading 0.977. This indicates that the thin vessels are significantly distorted compared to thick vessels. The third-row entries show the SSIM index values when coefficients of subband V(3) are zeroed. The SSIM index value in the second column of the third row, 0.928, indicates that the distortion of the thick vessel in the vertical direction is more significant. The thin vessels in the same direction are comparatively less disturbed as indicated by an SSIM index value of 0.972 in the same row. The result of the earlier experimental studies shows that the lower-frequency subbands (L3 and L4) carry thick vessel information. The higher-frequency (L2) subbands carry information about fine structures such as thin vessels. The L1 and L5 subbands have less clinical importance as they do not disturb the blood vessel structure. From the point of view of distortion in blood vessels, different subbands behave differently.

The results of visual quality investigation and SSIM index values are used to rank the clinical importance of subbands of different levels. In image processing applications, the distortion in the image is generally due to the attenuation of the high-frequency components. The thin vessels are composed of higher-frequency components and the distortions in them are perceived even at low compression rates. Hence, the L2 subbands are expected to have higher importance compared to the other subbands. With the increase in compression values, the next lower-frequency L3 subband coefficients start getting affected. For the blood vessel feature, now different subbands can be ranked in the descending order of their importance as L2, L3, L4, L5, and L1.

4.2.2 Optic Disc Information

The detection and analysis of OD has several potential clinical uses. The OD area is a slowly varying bright homogeneous region interrupted by blood vessels. The intensity variation between the OD and the retinal background is relatively high. The wavelet subbands of each level are examined from the point of view of the OD information. Since the OD and macula regions are small compared to the entire retinal image space, their characteristics are effectively studied considering a local region. A section that contains the OD is selected from the retinal image and shown in Figure 4.3a. The OD region of the reconstructed image in Figure 4.3b is obtained after zeroing the coefficients of L1 subbands. Compared to the original OD image (Figure 4.3a), it is observed that the OD structure is well reproduced. This shows that H(1), V(1), and D(1) subband coefficients carry little OD information. Figure 4.3c shows the reconstructed OD image after zeroing only the coefficients of L2 subbands. There is a sharp intensity transition from brighter OD region to the relatively darker background. This may constitute higher-frequency components represented by the L2 subbands. When coefficients of these subbands are zeroed, the sharp boundary (edge) of the OD changes to smooth variations and appears to be smeared. This shows that altering the

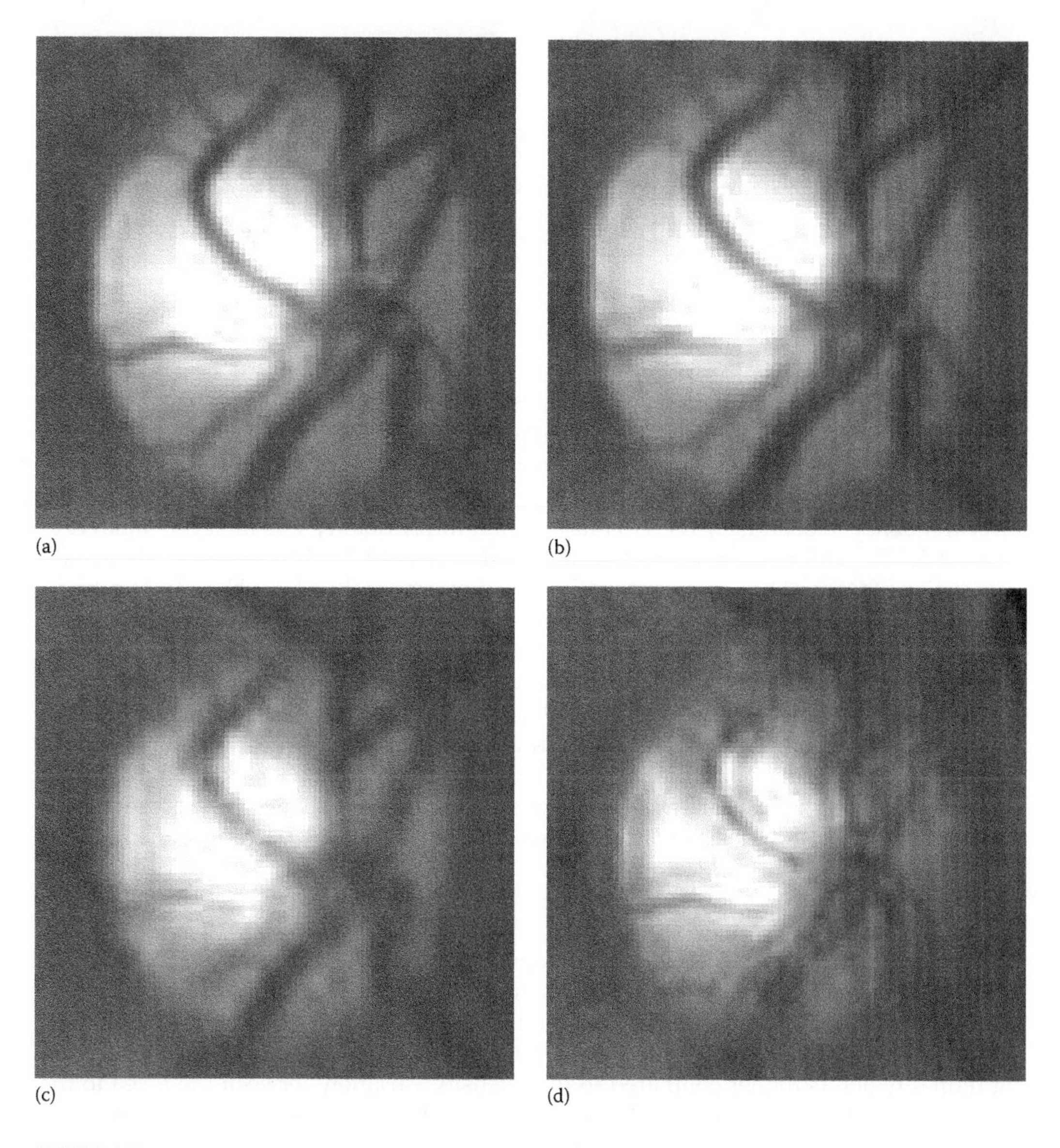

FIGURE 4.3
(a) Original and reconstructed OD images when subband coefficients of (b) L1, (c) L2, and (d) L3 are made zero.
(continued)

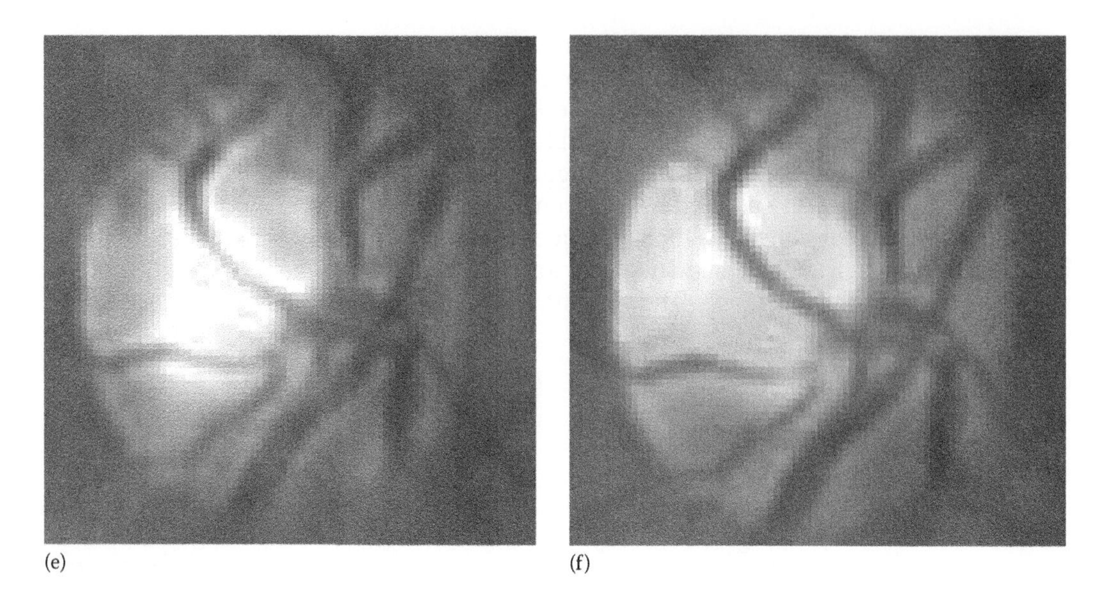

(e) (f)

FIGURE 4.3 (continued)
Original and reconstructed OD images when subband coefficients of (e) L4 and (f) L5 are made zero.

coefficients of L2 subbands has an impact on the OD properties. Figure 4.3d shows the OD image after zeroing the coefficients of L3 subbands. It is observed that the OD boundary is spread into the background and more distortion is observed inside the OD region. This may be due to the slow intensity changes inside the OD region captured by the relatively lower-frequency subbands of L3. This results in a lower quality OD image compared to Figure 4.3c. The observation shows that the coefficients of L3 subbands carry significant information of OD and has comparatively higher importance than L2 subbands. The modified coefficients of L4 subbands have little effect on OD structure as indicated by Figure 4.3e. Similarly, Figure 4.3f indicates that the coefficients of L5 subbands have minimum influence on OD information. This result shows that L4 and L5 subbands are less significant in carrying the information of the OD. Similar observations are made when tested with other retinal images. These effects can also be quantified by estimating the SSIM index values between the original and the reconstructed OD images [14,15]. The experimental results and the SSIM index values show that different subbands can be arranged in the descending order of their clinical information of the OD as L3, L2, L4, L5, and L1.

4.2.3 Macula Information

The macula is approximately a circular and specialized area of the retina. It is responsible for clear and detailed vision. It is detected as the dark region at the center of the retina and within the neighborhood of the OD. The macula has the darkest region at its center called the fovea. The relative intensity transition between the macula region and the surrounding retinal region is higher compared to the intensity variation between the fovea to the macular region [16]. A region from the retinal image that contains the macula is selected and shown in Figure 4.4a. The effect of making L1 subbands zero is shown in Figure 4.4b. It is observed that the fovea is less distorted, but the boundary of macula is spread into the background. This may be due to the sharp intensity change between the macula and the background, carried by these subbands. Figure 4.4c shows the reconstructed macula image after zeroing the coefficients of L2 subbands. It is observed that the intensity variations of both the macula and foveal region are smoothed out. Similar experiments on other retinal images show that the modified coefficients of L2 subbands result in macular distortion, but it is comparatively higher than the distortion that results by zeroing the L1 subbands. This may be due to the intensity variation of the macula region reflected in the high-frequency components of L2 subbands. The result of making the relatively lower-frequency L3 subband coefficients zero has a moderate effect as shown in Figure 4.4d.

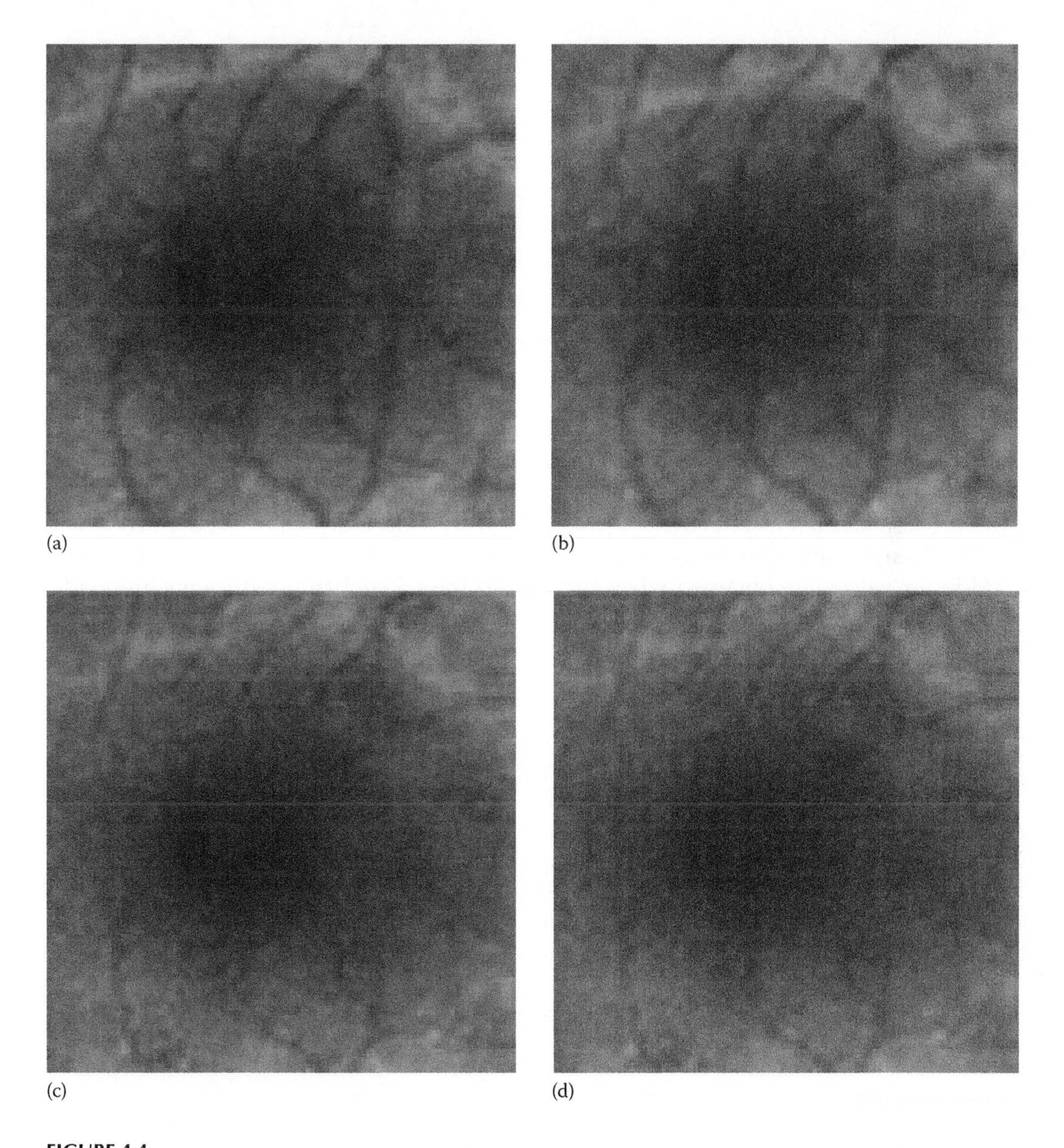

FIGURE 4.4
(a) Original macula image and reconstructed images when subband coefficients of (b) L1, (c) L2, and (d) L3 are made zero (images are contrast enhanced for better visualization).

(continued)

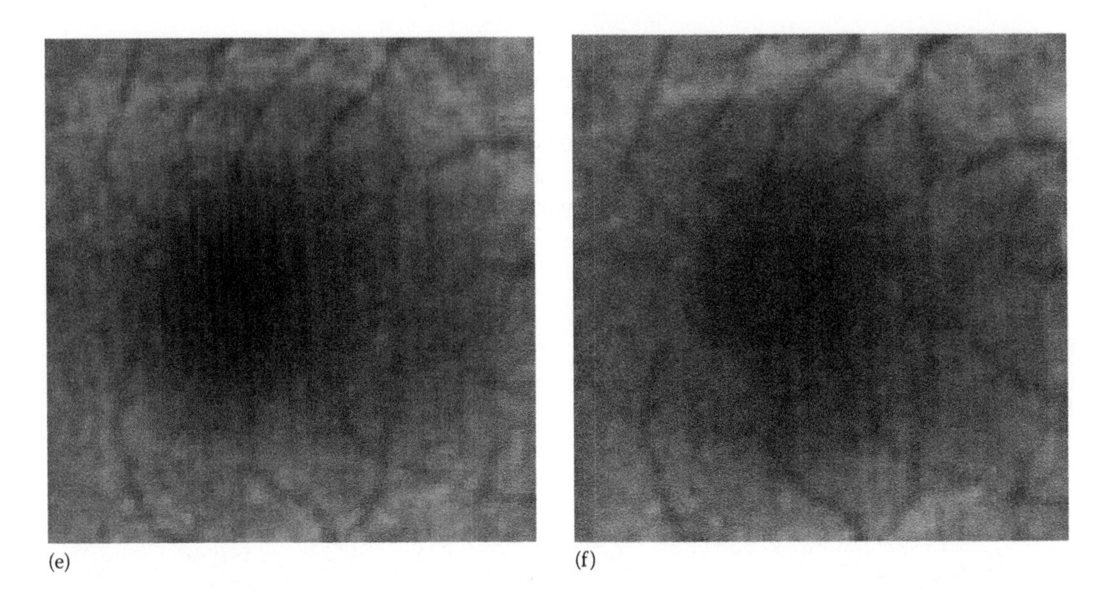

(e) (f)

FIGURE 4.4 (continued)
Original macula image and reconstructed images when subband coefficients of (e) L4 and (f) L5 are made zero (images are contrast enhanced for better visualization).

The lower-frequency coefficients of L4 and L5 subbands have minimum influence on the macular information as shown in Figure 4.4e and f.

Similar to the other cases, the SSIM index values can be computed between the original and the reconstructed macula images [15]. The lowest SSIM index value is obtained when the L2 subband coefficients are zeroed and indicates significant information loss. The high SSIM index values are obtained when the L4 and the L5 subband coefficients are made zero respectively. Now, different subbands can be arranged in the descending order of their importance with respect to the macula information, as L2, L1, L3, L4, and L5.

From the earlier experiments, it is found that different subbands have different diagnostic relevance. A distortion measure that can treat different subband errors differently will be more suitable in evaluating the clinical quality of the processed retinal images. Hence, wavelet subband weighted distortion measures (SWDMs) are defined to quantify the information loss in each of the retinal feature. The information loss is quantified as a weighted error between wavelet coefficients in each subband of the original and the degraded images. The error between the significant subbands is given a higher weight. The nonsignificant error is given a lower weight. In this way, the distortion measure can emphasize the clinically significant distortion. A global distortion measure is then defined by combining the individual distortion measures and can be used to evaluate the quality of the processed retinal images.

4.3 Subband Weighted Distortion Measures (SWDM)

After identifying the subbands that contain significant information about a retinal feature f, a distortion measure SWDM_f is defined in the wavelet domain as

$$\text{SWDM}_f = \left(\Delta_e^{1/2}\right)^T \frac{\Gamma_f}{tr\left[\Gamma_f\right]} \left(\Delta_e^{1/2}\right) \tag{4.1}$$

where

Γ_f is the diagonal matrix of subband weights for each of the diagnostic feature
Δ_e is an error vector with 15 elements

Each element of Δ_e is a measure of the error between coefficients of the same subband from the original and the processed image. They can be considered to be one of the DWT-based distortion measures. Various DWT-based distortion measures are wavelet subband MSE (WMSE), relative WMSE (Rel WMSE), and the root of the normalized WMSE (RNWMSE) [9,17]. The WMSE is expressed as the MSE between the subband coefficients of original image and subband coefficients of the processed image. The WMSE for a subband b with K number of coefficients and at any given decomposition level n ($1 \leq n \leq$ final decomposition level N) is defined as

$$\text{WMSE}_{(b,n)} = \frac{\sum_{k=1}^{K} \left(d_{(b,n)}(k) - \tilde{d}_{(b,n)}(k)\right)^2}{K} \tag{4.2}$$

where

d is the wavelet coefficient of original image subband
$\tilde{d}$ is the wavelet coefficient of processed image subband

The Rel WMSE is obtained by normalizing the WMSE with the sum of the WMSE of all subbands. It is given by

$$\text{Rel WMSE}_{(b,n)} = \frac{\text{WMSE}_{(b,n)}}{\sum_{b \in (H,V,D)} \sum_{n=1}^{N} \text{WMSE}_{(b,n)}} \times 100\%. \tag{4.3}$$

The RNWMSE is given as

$$\text{RNWMSE}_{(b,n)} = \sqrt{\frac{\sum_{k=1}^{K} \left(d_{(b,n)}(k) - \tilde{d}_{(b,n)}(k)\right)^2}{\sum_{k=1}^{K} \left(d_{(b,n)}(k)\right)^2}} \times 100\%. \tag{4.4}$$

These DWT-based distortion measures are computed directly from the wavelet coefficients of a subband, and they show the average global error. Since all the subbands are equally weighted, the error in the dark background that does not have any clinically relevant information is treated the same as the significant distortion. As a solution to this problem, different weights are assigned to different subbands according to their diagnostic importance.

4.3.1 Estimation of Subband Weights

The diagnostic importance differs for different subbands. The error in each subband contributes to the overall distortion. A measure can better quantify the diagnostic distortion by having different weights for different subband errors. These weighting factors play an important role in emphasizing the diagnostically significant errors from the nonsignificant errors. The weight values are calculated using the subband coefficients of the original image.

The weight factor for a detail subband b at decomposition level n with K number of coefficients may be estimated as the sum of the absolute values of wavelet coefficients $d_{(b,n)}$ within the subband. It is defined as

$$\omega_{(b,n)} = \sum_{k=1}^{K} \left| d_{(b,n)}(k) \right|. \tag{4.5}$$

There will be 15 different weights for 15 different wavelet subbands. When these weights are plotted graphically, just for better representation and to make the evaluation simple, the weights of H, V, and D bands of a decomposition level are added and considered as the weight value at that decomposition level. Now the weight matrix with the weight value for each decomposition level as its diagonal elements may be represented as

$$\Gamma_f = \begin{bmatrix} \omega_{L1} & 0 & 0 & 0 & 0 \\ 0 & \omega_{L2} & 0 & 0 & 0 \\ 0 & 0 & \omega_{L3} & 0 & 0 \\ 0 & 0 & 0 & \omega_{L4} & 0 \\ 0 & 0 & 0 & 0 & \omega_{L5} \end{bmatrix}.$$

Then each of the weight value is normalized by the sum of all the weight values.

The approximation band contains the average information about the image. In image processing applications, the approximation band coefficients are generally kept unaltered. Hence, in this distortion measure, the effect of approximation band coefficients is not considered and the total distortion is computed using only the detail subbands [17]. The distortion measure for each of the local clinical feature in the retinal image is discussed in the following sections.

4.3.2 Distortion Measure for Blood Vessels (SWDM$_v$)

A subband weighted blood vessel distortion measure (SWDM$_v$) is defined using Equation 4.1 to capture the distortion in blood vessels. The SWDM$_v$ is obtained by considering the feature f as blood vessels v in Equation 4.1, and Δ_e is the normalized wavelet subband error vector with 15 scalar components computed using Equation 4.4 [18]. This measure estimates different weights for different subband errors using Equation 4.5 to form the weight matrix Γ_v.

The L1 subbands have minimum effect on the blood vessels; they are expected to have small weight values. The L2 subbands are expected to have higher weight values compared to all other subbands. The L3 subband error is weighted less than the L2 subband error. The L4 and L5 subbands contribute little in carrying the vessel information and hence weighted less than the L3 subbands. With all these observations, the weight factor for different subbands is expected to have values in the order $\omega_{L2} > \omega_{L3} > \omega_{L4} > \omega_{L5} > \omega_{L1}$. Figure 4.5 shows the actual values of weight factor computed for an image (36 training). The decreasing trend of weight factor values from L2 to L5 can be accepted as this satisfies the order of diagnostic influence of subbands. The weight for L1 is expected to have minimum weight factor value

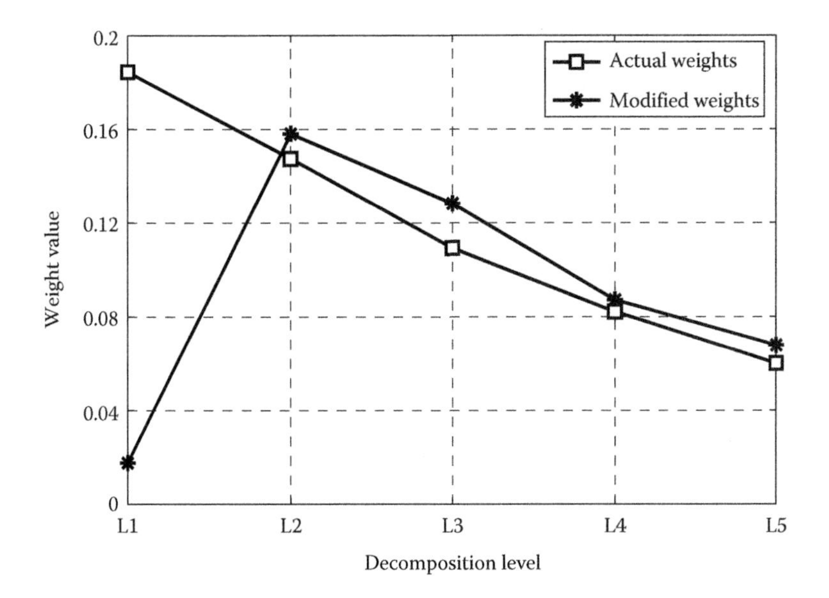

FIGURE 4.5
Characteristics of weight factor for blood vessels.

but shows a bigger weight value. This requires the correction of weight value for L1 subbands. The weight factors computed from Equation 4.5 are modified to make them follow the importance order. The weight values can be modified by using only the coefficients that are comparatively more significant than the other coefficients in a subband. The coefficients that fall within the circular periphery of the subband image (Figure 4.6b) are considered as significant coefficients. The coefficients outside this region represent the dark background and are diagnostically insignificant. They are made zero to reduce their influence on the distortion measure. The significant wavelet coefficients are arranged in the descending order of their absolute magnitude. A given number of coefficients are selected depending on the importance level of the subband. The higher number of coefficients are selected from those subbands having higher significance. The subbands of L2 are having the highest importance and more number of coefficients are selected from them. The absolute sum of the subband coefficients gives a large weight value for the subband. The L3 subbands are having the next higher importance. The number of coefficients selected is slightly less than the case of L1 subbands. This gives a smaller weight to L3 subbands compared to L2 subbands. The L1 is having the lowest importance and only few of the significant coefficients are considered from a large number of subband coefficients. Sum of these gives a smaller weight to the subbands. The number of coefficients considered to compute the weight may slightly vary depending on the image. After working with many retinal images from [13], the number of coefficients used for computing the weights is as follows:

For each subband of L2—90%–100%

For each subband of L3—70%–90%

For each subband of L4—30%–50%

For each subband of L5—8%–10%

For each subband of L1—2%–4%

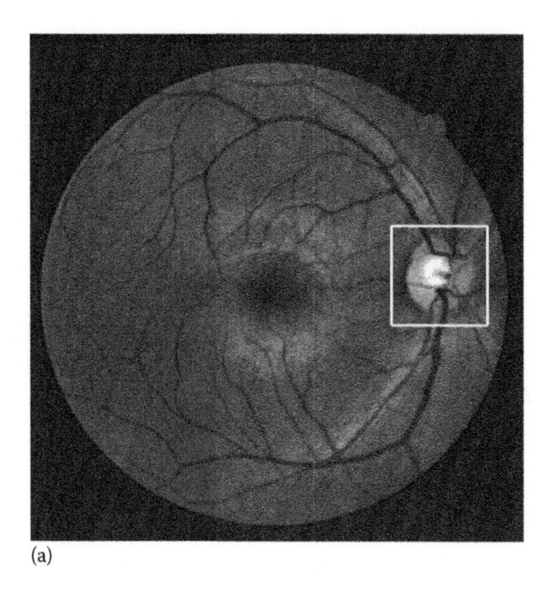

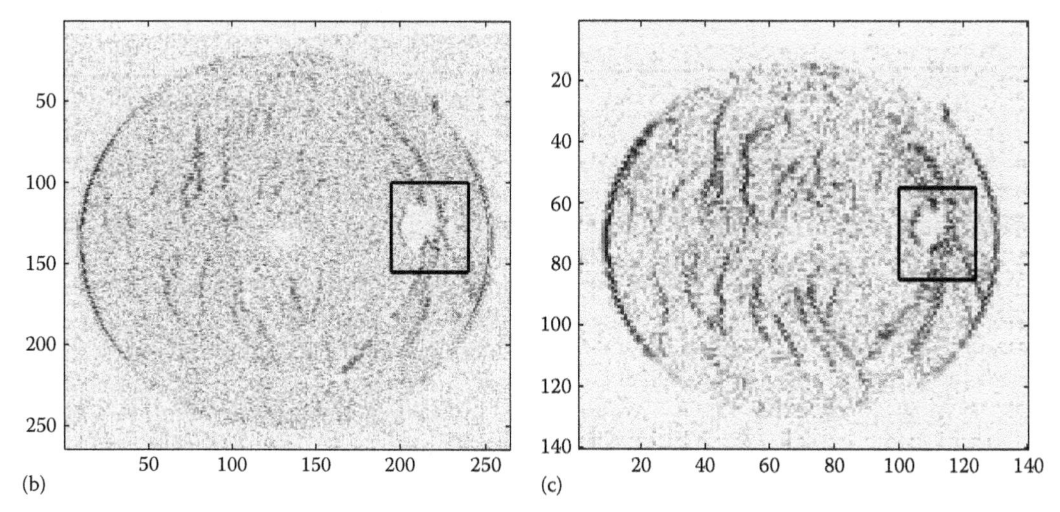

FIGURE 4.6
The OD regions (black square) in (a) original image, (b) subband V1, and (c) subband V2.

Figure 4.5 shows the values of modified weights for different subbands. It is observed that the modified weights satisfy the requirement of relative weight values of subbands. These modified weight values are expected to capture the distortion in blood vessel structure effectively.

4.3.3 Distortion Measure for the Optic Disc ($SWDM_d$)

This distortion measure is used to quantify the distortion in the OD of processed retinal images. In standard retinal images, a candidate area of approximately 100×100 pixels is considered as the OD region. The weights for different subbands are estimated using Equation 4.5 considering only those wavelet coefficients that lie within the OD region

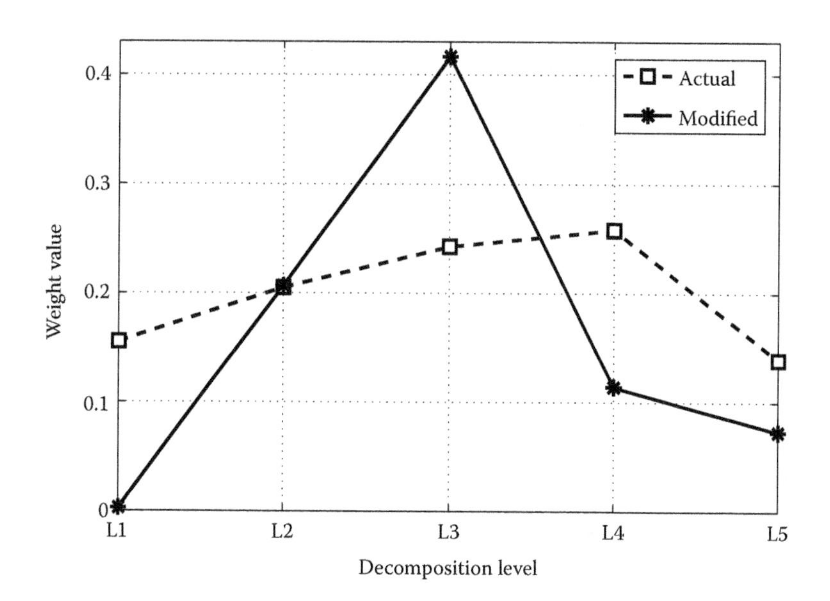

FIGURE 4.7
Characteristics of the actual and modified weight factors for the OD.

in each subband. Such regions are selected manually from each subband as shown in Figure 4.6b and c. The diagonal weight matrix Γ_d can be generated by putting the actual weight values as the diagonal elements. Figure 4.7 shows the weight values for different decomposition levels. It is observed that the actual weight of L4 subbands is high compared to the L2 and L3 subbands. The weight of L1 subbands is expected to be minimum but indicates a value higher than that of the L5 subbands.

These weight values do not follow the relative diagnostic importance order (L3, L2, L4, L5, and L1) for the OD discussed earlier. Therefore, the weight factors have to be modified to satisfy the order of diagnostic relevance. The weight values are modified by using only the coefficients that are comparatively more significant than the other coefficients in a subband. The wavelet coefficients belonging to the OD region in a subband are arranged in the descending order of their absolute magnitude. Similar to the previous case, the number of coefficients selected for computing the weights is decided depending on the significance of the subbands. The modified weight value Γ_d at each L for the same image is shown in Figure 4.7. The modified weight values for the whole set of images are calculated. Then average weight values are computed and found that they satisfy the order of relative diagnostic significance of subbands. These modified weight values may be more appropriate to quantify the distortion in the OD.

4.3.4 Distortion Measure for the Macula (SWDM$_m$)

The distortion measure (SWDM$_m$) is required to capture the changes in the macula of processed retinal images. A small region that contains the macula is considered in each subband. The weights are generated using only those wavelet coefficients that lie within this region. An example of a weight matrix Γ_m with actual weights computed for an image (36 training) having diagonal elements as weight values for each decomposition level is given by

$$\Gamma_m = \begin{bmatrix} 0.424 & 0 & 0 & 0 & 0 \\ 0 & 0.275 & 0 & 0 & 0 \\ 0 & 0 & 0.175 & 0 & 0 \\ 0 & 0 & 0 & 0.071 & 0 \\ 0 & 0 & 0 & 0 & 0.055 \end{bmatrix}.$$

These weight values are required to follow the relative importance order of subbands (L2, L1, L3, L4, and L5). It is observed that the actual weights for L3–L5 subbands satisfy the diagnostic order of the subbands. The weight value of L1 subbands is expected to be lower than L2 subbands, but the calculated weight shows a higher value. The modified weights are computed using only the significant coefficients as discussed for other cases. The weight matrix Γ_m with modified weight values and satisfying the relative importance order of subbands is given by

$$\Gamma_m = \begin{bmatrix} 0.163 & 0 & 0 & 0 & 0 \\ 0 & 0.278 & 0 & 0 & 0 \\ 0 & 0 & 0.061 & 0 & 0 \\ 0 & 0 & 0 & 0.045 & 0 \\ 0 & 0 & 0 & 0 & 0.034 \end{bmatrix}.$$

The average modified weight values at each L are computed and these new weights are expected to be more effective in emphasizing the macula distortion.

After computing the distortion measure for each retinal feature, a global distortion measure is defined as the linear combination of individual distortion measures [15]. This gives a wavelet SWDM defined as

$$\text{SWDM} = \sum_{f \in (v,d,m)} \text{SWDM}_f \tag{4.6}$$

where SWDM_f is the distortion measure for individual clinical feature.

4.3.5 Evaluation of Individual Distortion Measures

The distortion measure SWDM_f is expected to respond strongly when a particular retinal feature f is distorted and to be less sensitive for any changes in other features. The performance is evaluated by introducing distortion in different regions of the retinal image shown in Figure 4.8. The performance of the SWDM_f is investigated under different conditions:

1. Introducing distortion artificially into a particular f feature keeping the other features undisturbed.
2. Introducing distortion in other features while keeping a particular feature f undisturbed.
3. Introducing distortion in clinically nonsignificant regions.

The distortion considered in this study is smoothing of the retinal features. The smoothing of the image structures may occur during the process of lossy compression [19].

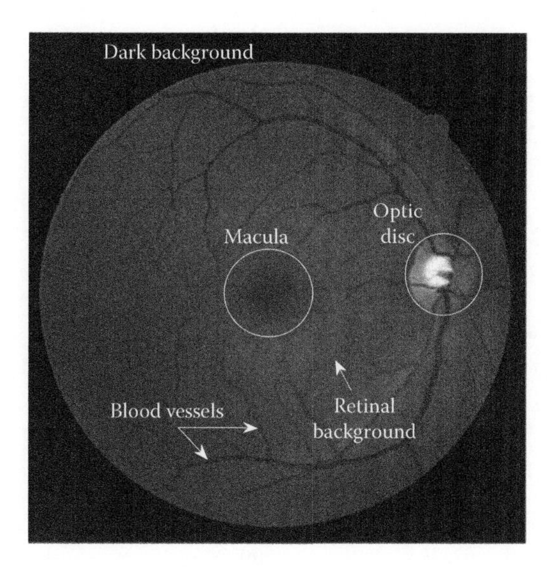

FIGURE 4.8
Retinal image showing different regions.

The process of compression involves truncation of high-frequency details. During quantization, the high-frequency wavelet coefficients are made zero. This results in the loss of details and smoothing of the image. Smoothing is also experienced during the process of image denoising. The smoothing distortion is introduced by using a Gaussian smoothing filter. The standard deviation σ of the Gaussian filter is varied to have different amount of smoothness. This gives the distorted images. Then the distortion is computed between the original image and the distorted image. To simplify the computation, the distortions computed for *H*, *V*, and *D* bands of a given decomposition level are summed up, and it is considered as the total distortion value at that decomposition level.

4.3.5.1 Results for $SWDM_v$

The $SWDM_v$ is required to highlight the distortion in blood vessels. The performance of the measure is investigated by introducing distortion in the blood vessels. Artificially distorting the vessel alters the size and contrast of the blood vessels. In this approach, the thick vessels are artificially distorted by Gaussian smoothing so that the vessels look blurred. This is tested for different levels of smoothing. Figure 4.9a shows a section of the thick blood vessel from the original image. Figure 4.9b shows the same vessel from the distorted image, obtained after Gaussian smoothing of the vessel. All the distortion measures are computed for each case of smoothing. Then it is investigated which level reflects comparatively more error by showing a high distortion value. When this experiment was performed on several retinal images, the obtained result pointed comparatively more error in the L3 subbands, proving that it is due to the distortion in thick vessel. Similar procedure is repeated for some thin vessels also. The thin vessels are altered so that the sharpness gradually reduces and gets blended with the background. In this case, large error is expected to appear at L2 and then in L3. Table 4.2 shows the values of weighted WMSE (wWMSE), weighted relative WMSE (wRel WMSE), and $SWDM_v$. The wWMSE and wRel WMSE show that the total distortion is contributed by all the subbands from L2 to L5. This indicates that the distortion is distributed among these subbands and fails to

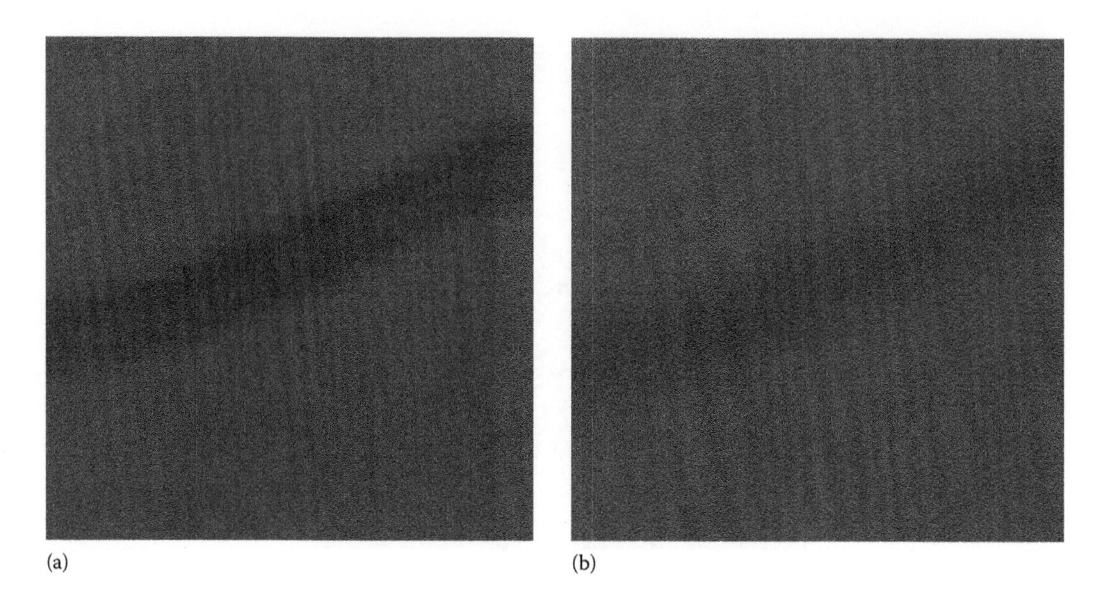

(a) (b)

FIGURE 4.9
(a) A section of thick vessel (original) and (b) thick vessel after smoothing (reconstructed).

TABLE 4.2
Performance of the $SWDM_v$ When Only Thin Vessels Are Distorted

Distortion Measure	Distortion Computed at Each L					Total Distortion
	L1	L2	L3	L4	L5	
wWMSE	0.001	0.195	0.253	0.194	0.128	0.771
wRel WMSE (%)	0.004	0.712	0.921	0.694	0.475	2.806
$SWDM_v$ (%)	0.094	2.253	0.792	0.254	0.121	3.514

highlight the distortion in thin blood vessels. The $SWDM_v$ shows the significant distortion in L2 and L3 subbands emphasizing the distortion in thin vessels.

The $SWDM_v$ is also required to give less importance to distortion in the regions with no vessels. Such regions are the retinal background regions. To investigate the efficiency of the distortion measure, those regions are distorted by Gaussian smoothing resulting in a distorted image.

Table 4.3 shows the error values obtained using wRel WMSE, $SWDM_v$, and SSIM computed between the original and the distorted image. The wRel WMSE shows a high value contributed by L2 and L3 subbands. This gives an impression that some blood vessels are distorted. But the proposed $SWDM_v$ gives low values for all the levels and a small total value. This reflects a small distortion in clinically significant features. The SSIM index shows a good similarity, which is true as all the diagnostic features are well preserved.

The $SWDM_v$ is also evaluated when vessel features are not distorted, but other features such as the OD and macula are distorted with Gaussian smoothing. The observations are recorded in Table 4.4. The $SWDM_v$ reads smaller values of 1.319 and 1.283. For the case of approximately same quantity of distortion in few of the thin vessels, it shows a high value of 3.139 contributed by L2 subbands.

TABLE 4.3

Distortion in Clinically Nonsignificant Regions

Distortion Measure	Distortion Computed at Each L					Total Distortion
	L1	L2	L3	L4	L5	
wRel WMSE (%)	0.034	2.557	0.812	0.235	0.085	3.723
$SWDM_v$ (%)	0.051	0.793	0.137	0.032	0.011	1.024
SSIM	—	—	—	—	—	0.9989

TABLE 4.4

Performance of the Proposed $SWDM_v$ When Other Features of Retinal Image Are Distorted

Distortion in	Distortion Computed at Each L					Total Distortion
	L1	L2	L3	L4	L5	
Thin vessels	0.631	1.784	0.522	0.149	0.053	3.139
OD	0.035	0.785	0.344	0.092	0.063	1.319
Macula region	0.044	0.923	0.255	0.046	0.015	1.283

All these observations suggest that the $SWDM_v$ shows high error values in appropriate level subbands when the blood vessels are distorted. The measure indicates low values for the distortion in other retinal features. It was also observed that the measure is less sensitive to the distortion in the nondiagnostic regions. Thus this measure is more suitable in emphasizing the distortion in the blood vessels.

4.3.5.2 Results for $SWDM_d$

The performance of the $SWDM_d$ is evaluated and compared with that of the other weighted wavelet-based distortion measures. The distortion is introduced in the OD region of different retinal images by Gaussian smoothing. All the distortion measures are computed between the original image and the reconstructed image having distortion in the OD. The results are shown in Table 4.5. The wWMSE and wRel WMSE show high values for L3 and L4. But L4 is less important compared to L2 for the OD feature. The $SWDM_d$ emphasizes the significant error at appropriate levels, L3 and L2, and shows lower values at other levels.

The $SWDM_d$ is also evaluated under distortion in different features and the experimental results are shown in Table 4.6. All the distorted images considered in the experiment

TABLE 4.5

Performance of the Distortion Measure $SWDM_d$ When Only the OD Is Distorted

Distortion Measure	Distortion Computed at Each L					Total Distortion
	L1	L2	L3	L4	L5	
wWMSE	0.002	0.767	5.345	2.239	0.152	8.505
wRel WMSE (%)	0.001	0.711	4.949	2.075	0.142	7.878
$SWDM_d$ (%)	0.074	4.585	6.895	0.878	0.112	12.544

TABLE 4.6

Performance of the Proposed $SWDM_d$ for Different Cases

	Distortion Measures (%)	
Distortion in	**wRel WMSE**	**$SWDM_d$**
Thin vessels	7.3934	2.2645
Thick vessels	7.0934	1.7288
Macula	9.0226	2.1373
Clinically nonsig. region	5.5612	1.2932

are having approximately the same MSE. The first row gives the distortion values when some of the thin vessels are distorted but the OD region is not disturbed. In this situation, the distortion measures are expected to show smaller values. But the wRel WMSE shows a high value. This large error is contributed mainly by the L3 and L2 subbands. These subbands are considered as significant subbands from the OD point of view. This may give an impression that the OD region is having distortion. But the $SWDM_d$ shows comparatively a low value. This low value is contributed by L2 subbands, which are relatively less significant and thus indicate very little distortion in the OD. The same conclusion holds for the case of distortion in other retinal features such as the thick vessels and the macula. These verifications and comparisons demonstrate that $SWDM_d$ gives a high value when the OD is distorted indicating a significant distortion of clinically relevant feature. When approximately the same amount of distortion is introduced in other diagnostic features, the $SWDM_d$ shows low values compared to wRel WMSE. Hence, it is more suitable to quantify the distortion of the OD in retinal images.

4.3.5.3 Results for $SWDM_m$

The efficacy of this measure is evaluated to emphasize the distortion in macular region and give less importance to the distortion in other regions. Table 4.7 presents the distortion computed by different measures when the macula is subjected to a distortion of Gaussian smoothing. The wWMSE and wRel WMSE show more distortion in L2 subbands but fail to highlight the next significant error in subbands of L1. They show higher values in L3 subbands, which are relatively less significant than L1 subbands. The $SWDM_m$ records high values in L2 and L1 subbands, respectively, and shows low values in subbands of L3, L4, and L5, satisfying the order of importance. The distortion measure is also tested when the distortion is present in other regions and features. The results of this investigation are given in [15]. The wRel WMSE shows a high value supplied by different subbands,

TABLE 4.7

Performance of the Distortion Measure $SWDM_m$ When Only the Macula Is Distorted

	Distortion Computed at Each L					
Distortion Measure	**L1**	**L2**	**L3**	**L4**	**L5**	**Total**
wWMSE	0.094	1.752	1.135	0.391	0.123	3.495
wRel WMSE (%)	0.147	2.782	1.769	0.603	0.241	5.542
$SWDM_m$ (%)	1.752	3.551	0.601	0.113	0.024	6.041

which are considered as significant from the macula point of view. This may indicate that the macular region is altered, which is not the actual situation. But the SWDM_m results in a considerably low value indicating little distortion in the macula. This suggests that the distortion measure can effectively be used to estimate the distortion of the macular region in retinal images.

Similar methods can be followed to evaluate the performance of the global distortion measure SWDM. The local distortion measures help improve the performance of the SWDM in predicting the image quality. A comparison of SWDM with other weighted measures is given in [15].

4.4 Evaluating the Quality of Retinal Images with Different Artifacts

A good objective measure should reflect the distortion introduced in the image due to different types of image processing. Validation is an important step toward successful development of image quality measurement systems. The most standard form of validation is to compare objective quality measures with the ratings by human subjects on a set of distorted images. This section presents the qualitative and quantitative evaluation of the global distortion measure SWDM in predicting the clinical quality of the processed retinal images by correlating it with subjective scores. The reference images are derived from [13]. The distorted images are created by distorting the reference retinal images. Four types of image distortions commonly encountered in image processing applications are considered in this experiment. The compression artifacts are generated by two compression algorithms: the discrete cosine transform (DCT)-based JPEG and the wavelet-based set partitioning in hierarchical trees (SPIHT) [20]. The other types of distortions are the Gaussian blur (Gblur) and the addition of white Gaussian noise (WGN) for various values of the standard deviation. The level of distortion is adjusted manually so that the images with minimum to significant distortion are generated.

The subjective evaluation is a method to measure the quality of a distorted image relative to a reference image. The subjective quality rating or mean opinion score (MOS) is obtained using a *double-stimulus continuous quality scale* (DSCQS) procedure [21,22]. The subjective MOS values are obtained from retinal specialists and research scholars working in different areas of signal and image processing. Then various state-of-the-art objective IQMs used to evaluate the quality of a distorted image are listed in Table 4.8. The global distortion measure SWDM is also considered along with other measures.

TABLE 4.8

IQMs under Test

IQM	Comment
MSE	Pixel difference based
SSIM	[2]
MS-SSIM	[3]
VSNR	[23]
IFC	[24]
VIF	[25]

4.4.1 Evaluation Metrics

After calculating the objective scores for all the distorted images, they can be correlated with the MOS using different statistical measures. There are four widely used metrics to evaluate the performance of IQMs [21]. The PLCC and the SROCC are used to evaluate the correlation between the objective and subjective scores. The other two metrics are the OR and RMSE between the actual and predicted subjective scores. The objective measures may not correlate linearly with the MOS. Hence, before calculating the correlation, the objective measures obtained from image quality metrics are passed through a nonlinear transformation function. A three-parameter logistic function recommended by [21] is used to transform the set of objective measure values to a set of predicted MOS values.

4.4.2 Performance Evaluation of Image Quality Measures

The objective scores given by different quality measures and the difference MOS (DMOS) values are used to evaluate the performance of the objective measures. The DMOS values are generated by taking the difference between the MOS for a reference image and the MOS for a distorted image. The scatterplots for various objective measures along with the best-fitted logistic regression curve are shown in Figure 4.10. The scatterplots can be used

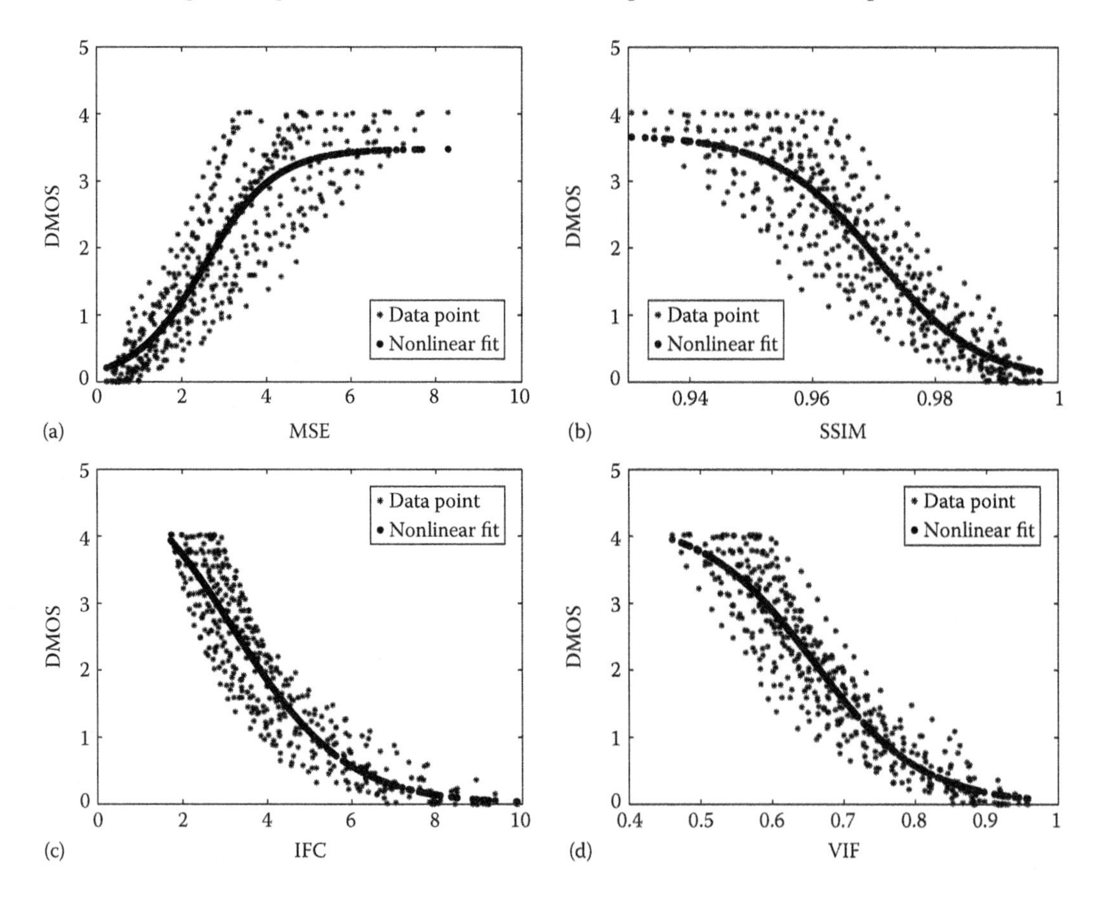

FIGURE 4.10
Scatterplots showing the nonlinear fit using the logistic function for the (a) MSE, (b) SSIM, (c) IFC, and (d) VIF, versus DMOS. Each data point represents one distorted image.

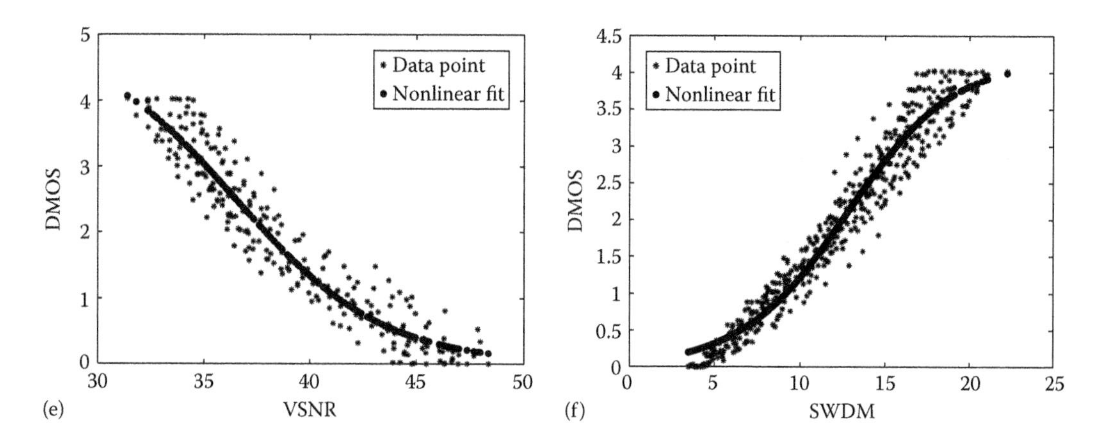

FIGURE 4.10 (continued)
Scatterplots showing the nonlinear fit using the logistic function for the (e) VSNR and (f) SWDM versus DMOS. Each data point represents one distorted image.

as a visual check on correlation between the two measures. Each data point in the scatterplot represents one distorted image. If the data points are clustered densely around the fitted line, then it implies the better consistency between subjective and objective quality evaluations. The scatterplots shown in Figure 4.10 are for the SPIHT compression type of distortion. The scatterplots of MSE, SSIM index, and MS-SSIM index show widely spread data points indicating a lower correlation with the subjective score. The scatterplots of IFC, VIF, and VSNR measures show less spread data points and improved correlation. By comparing the scatterplots of all the measures, it is observed that the new SWDM possesses a compact scatterplot with all the data points lying within a small range. This implies that the SWDM provides better quality estimation and is more consistent with the subjective scores as compared to the other measures.

After the nonlinear curve fitting process, different metrics are used to compute the correlation between the objective and the subjective scores. The performance of all objective quality measures in terms of the PLCC, the SROCC, the RMSE, and the OR metrics after nonlinear regression is evaluated. Different measures respond with differing sensitivities to artifacts and distortions. The evaluation metrics computed for SPIHT compression artifacts are shown in Table 4.9. The metrics for other artifacts and distortions can also be computed similarly [15].

In this chapter, new subband weighted distortion measures to quantify the information loss in retinal features are discussed. These measures are defined after carrying out the analysis of retinal image information in different wavelet subbands. It was found

TABLE 4.9

PLCC, SROCC, RMSE, and OR Computed after Nonlinear Regression for the SPIHT Compression Artifacts

Measures/Distortion	MSE	SSIM	MS-SSIM	VSNR	IFC	VIF	SWDM
PLCC	0.8714	0.8932	0.8911	0.9441	0.9143	0.9199	0.9662
SROCC	0.8737	0.8942	0.8943	0.9434	0.9155	0.9210	0.9659
RMSE	0.6038	0.5537	0.5591	0.4048	0.4989	0.4831	0.3173
OR	0.1454	0.1406	0.1410	0.1420	0.1586	0.1476	0.1167

that the significant information of a retinal feature is captured by only a few subbands. The distortion measures assign different weights for different subband errors to emphasize the loss of clinically significant information. A global distortion measure is defined by combining the individual distortion measures. This measure shows better prediction of image quality than the other most widely used quality measures in the image processing literature. The SWDM is simple and more effective to quantify the clinically significant distortions in processed retinal images.

References

1. Z. Wang and A. C. Bovik, Mean squared error: Love it or leave it? A new look at signal fidelity measures, *IEEE Signal Process. Mag.*, 26(1), 98117, 2009.
2. Z. Wang, A. C. Bovik, H. Sheikh, and E. P. Simoncelli, Image quality assessment: From error visibility to structural similarity, *IEEE Trans. Image Process.*, 13(4), 600–612, 2004.
3. Z. Wang, E. P. Simoncelli, and A. C. Bovik, Multi-scale structural similarity for image quality assessment, *Proceedings IEEE Asilomar Conference on Signals, Systems, and Computers*, Pacific Grove, CA, pp. 1398–1402. November 2003.
4. P. Cosman, R. M. Gray, and R. A. Olshen, Evaluating the quality of compressed medical images: SNR, Subjective Rating and Diagnostic accuracy, *Proc. IEEE*, 82(6), 919–932, 1994.
5. R. H. Eikelboom, K. Yogesan, C. J. Barry, I. J. Constable, M. T. Kearney, L. Jitskaia, and P. H. House, Methods and limits of digital image compression of retinal images for telemedicine, *Invest. Ophthalmol. Vis. Sci.*, 41(7), 1916–1924, 2000.
6. S. Mallat, *A Wavelet Tour of Signal Processing*, 2nd edn. San Diego, CA: Academic Press, 1999.
7. M. Unser and A. Aldroubi, A review of wavelets in biomedical applications, *Proc. IEEE*, 84, 626–638, 1996.
8. A. Thakur and R. S. Anand, Image quality based comparative evaluation of wavelet filters in ultrasound speckle reduction, *Digital Signal Process.*, 15, 455–465, 2005.
9. Z. Gao and Y. F. Zheng, Quality constrained compression using DWT-based image quality metric, *IEEE Trans. Circuits Syst. Video Technol.*, 18(7), 910–922, 2008.
10. S. Mallat and W. L. Hwang, Singularity detection and processing with wavelets, *IEEE Trans. Inform. Theory*, 38(2), 617–643, 1992.
11. S. R. Nirmala, S. Dandapat, and P. K. Bora, Performance evaluation of wavelet filters for compression of retinal images, *Proceedings of National Conference on Communication (NCC)*, Guwahati, India, January 2009.
12. R. S. Khandpur, *Handbook of Biomedical Instrumentation*, 2nd edn. New Delhi, India: Tata Mcgraw Hill Education Pvt Ltd, 2003.
13. J. J. Staal, M. D. Abramoff, M. Niemeijer, M. A. Viergever, and B. van Ginneken, Ridge based vessel segmentation in color images of the retina, *IEEE Transactions on Medical Imaging*, 23, 501–509, 2004.
14. S. R. Nirmala, S. Dandapat, and P. K. Bora, Wavelet weighted diagnostic distortion measure for the Optic disc, *Proceedings of 8th International Conference on Signal Processing and Communications (SPCOM)*, Bangalore, India, July 2010.
15. S. R. Nirmala, S. Dandapat, and P. K. Bora, Wavelet weighted distortion measure for retinal images, *Signal, Image Video Process.*, 7(5), 1005–1014, 2013.
16. S. Sekhar, W. Al-Nuaimy, and A. K. Nandi, Automated localisation of optic disk and fovea in retinal fundus images, *16th European Signal Processing Conference (EUSIPCO 2008)*, Lausanne, Switzerland, 2008.

17. E. Dumic, S. Grgic, and M. Grgic, New image-quality measure based on wavelets, *J. Electron. Imaging*, 19(1), 011–018, 2010.
18. S. R. Nirmala, S. Dandapat, and P. K. Bora, Wavelet weighted blood vessel distortion measure for retinal images, *Biomed. Signal Process. Control*, 5(4), 282–291, 2010.
19. H. F. Jelinek and M. J. Cree, eds., *Automated Image Detection of Retinal Pathology*. Boca Raton, FL: CRC Press/Taylor & Francis Group, 2010.
20. A. Said and W. A. Pearlman, A new fast and efficient image codec based on set partitioning in hierarchical trees, *IEEE Trans. Circuits Syst. Video Technol.*, 6(3), 243–250, 1996.
21. Video Quality Experts Group (VQEG), Final report from the video quality experts group on the validation of objective models of video quality assessment, phase II, 2003, http://www.vqeg.org.
22. ITU—R Recommendation B T 500-11, Methodology for the subjective assessment of the quality of the television pictures, International Telecommunication Union, Geneva, Switzerland, Zech. Rep., 2002.
23. D. M. Chandler and S. S. Hemami, VSNR: A wavelet-based visual signal-to-noise ratio for natural images, *IEEE Trans. Image Process.*, 16(9), 2284–2298, 2007.
24. H. R. Sheikh, A. C. Bovik, and G. de Veciana, An information fidelity criterion for image quality assessment using natural scene statistics, *IEEE Trans. Image Process.*, 14(12), 2117–2128, 2005.
25. H. R. Sheikh and A. C. Bovik, Image information and visual quality, *IEEE Trans. Image Process.*, 15(2), 430–444, 2006.

5

Graph Search Retinal Vessel Tracking

Enea Poletti and Alfredo Ruggeri

CONTENTS

5.1 Introduction

Most retinopathies, for example, from hypertension or diabetes, could be diagnosed early and treated if an accurate and objective analysis of symptoms at their initial onset could be performed. The analysis should be accurate enough to detect minor pathological signs and objective enough to be able to compare results with accepted clinical standards and with results obtained from the same patient at different times. This latter requirement is of paramount importance when assessing the effect of established therapeutic treatments and even more when evaluating in a quantitative way the efficacy of new drugs during their development.

Most of the early symptoms indicating the onset of retinopathies are related to morphological features of the retinal vascular tree [35]. When no major signs of retinal degeneration are present (such as cotton wool spots, hemorrhages, exudates), the clinical diagnostic procedure for retinopathy always starts with a careful evaluation of the main features of the network of retinal vessels, obtained from fundus camera images [18]. The clinically most relevant signs taken into account by expert ophthalmologists are in general vessel tortuosity, vessel caliber and its distribution among different vessels, presence of vessel caliber irregularities along the same vessel, and the Gunn and Salus signs, that is, local caliber reduction or local deviation of vessel direction at the crossings between artery and vein [18].

In order to detect and quantitatively describe these diagnostic signs, the information to be extracted from the vascular network is the layout and the dimension of all the relevant vessels contained in the image. This task is relatively easy for an expert ophthalmologist if performed at a qualitative level, but rather cumbersome, highly subjective, and error prone if a set of measurements is sought for [11,33].

5.1.1 Related Work

A vast number of research projects have been carried out to develop automatic computerized systems for the extraction of retinal vascular structure. For the sake of simplicity, we can divide them into three categories: global unsupervised, global supervised, and tracking techniques.

Global techniques consist in analyzing every pixel of the image and assign it the *vessel* or *nonvessel* label with some sort of classifier, supervised or not. Unsupervised methods' rationale is to define a *vesselness* measure, which is then compared with a threshold to identify actual vessel pixels. Most of the work is based on multiorientation and multiscale template matching techniques, where the vessel image is convolved with a bank of oriented and scaled kernels [6,8,14,17,21]. The main drawback of this method is the computational time required to process the image with a high number of filters [32]. An approach proposed in literature to speed up the search for filter orientation is the use of steerable filters, such as Hessian filters [19], but its major drawback is the possible overfitting of noise and of nonvascular structures. Other methods use mathematical morphology to exploit the a priori known vasculature shape features [24,40], such as being piecewise linear and connected.

As far as the supervised methods are concerned, classifiers are trained with data from manually labeled images. Back propagation multilayer neural network (NN) was proposed as classifier [4,15]: images were at first processed *via* equalization and edge detection, and then a square subimage centered on each pixel was evaluated by the NN. An NN scheme was also employed in [23], where seven-element feature vectors are composed of gray-level and moment invariant-based features for pixel representation. A k-nearest neighbor (kNN) classifier was proposed in [25], where the 31 features associated to each pixel were extracted with a Gaussian filter and its derivatives, up to order 2 at 5 different scales. A kNN classifier paired with sequential forward feature selection was employed in [34]: by assigning each pixel to its nearest line element (primitive based on ridges), the image is partitioned into patches, whose properties are employed to compute 27-element feature vectors. In [31], a Gaussian mixture model Bayesian classifier was proposed. Multiscale analysis was performed on the image by using the Gabor wavelet transform and the maximum responses considered as pixel features. Modified line detector transform was employed in [29] to derive three-element feature vectors, which were then used to feed a support vector machine (SVM) classifier. SVM is used also in [28], where features are computed by means of local multiscale texture analysis and local multiscale vesselness measures.

Unlike the global techniques, tracking-based methods analyze only local areas of the images. They have to start from a set of reliable points (seeds) placed on the vessels and then follow vessel centerlines, by deciding iteratively the most appropriate candidate pixel. Methods proposed in the literature to this end use matched filters [5], Kalman filters [7], optimization of Gaussian profiles [22], or classification techniques based on vessel profiles [16,37].

5.1.2 Motivation

Literature reports that, as far as accuracy and sensitivity are concerned, supervised methods generally outperform the others [23,25]. On the other hand, supervised methods have some cons. They need the manual annotation of an adequate number of images, which needs a long and tedious work and is useful only if performed in a very accurate way. Moreover, if a supervised method has to be employed on a new dataset exhibiting different features, manual segmentation of images from the new dataset has to be performed.

As far as global methods are concerned, being them supervised or nonsupervised, their most important hindrance is that they provide as result a binary image (vessel/nonvessel) that is not directly usable for the extraction of vessel features such as length, caliber, and tortuosity. Moreover, global techniques tend to be more time-consuming than tracking techniques, as every pixel in the image has to be processed. This difference becomes much more relevant when the image resolution increases, as the number of analyzed pixels grows with the square of the image dimensions.

The modularity of a segmentation method, that is, its usability/integrability as a module in a larger processing framework, is an underrated feature that sometimes is not considered. In our specific case, we wish a segmentation system that can be included in an editing graphical user interface (GUI) for the manual correction of the automatic segmentation's errors [30,39]. Ideally, a correction/editing procedure should require the minimal amount of manual intervention so to minimize the human operator's efforts. A fully manual procedure would require a higher number of interactions in order to draw a given vessel than a tracking-driven manual procedure that, for example, only needs a few key seed points in order to track the same vessel.

To sum up, a nonsupervised tracking algorithm that performs, as well as other global methods, would provide the following additional benefits:

1. *No need of manual annotation (ground truth)*, as new images with unexpected features can be tackled simply by retuning the algorithm's parameters
2. *Computational efficiency*, as the number of pixels involved in the computation does not have to be the totality of pixels in the image
3. *Modularity/integrability* with other programs such as GUIs for manual editing
4. *Direct control of the measure*, as the tracking itself is the assessment of the vessel's features, as opposed to methods that provide binary classification of pixels

5.1.3 Our Contribution

In this chapter, a fully automatic system for the extraction of retinal vessel is proposed and discussed. The method exploits the advantages of both global and tracking-based techniques, and at the same time, it overcomes some of their drawbacks. It independently manages vessel axis network extraction and vessel width evaluation.

The first task is performed by using a sparse tracking technique employing a multidirectional graph search approach to find vessel centerlines. In the following step, vessel calibers are detected by means of an innovative adaptive 1D matched filter approach.

5.2 Methods

The rationale of our method is to consider the image as a weighted unoriented sparse graph, where each node represents a pixel and the edges describe the eight-adjacency among pixels. Under the assumption that vessels are minimum cost paths connecting remote nodes, we employ a graph search approach in order to identify them [26,27].

As a first step, luminance and contrast drifts are removed from images using a correction method we had previously developed [13]. This preprocessing also ensures uniform interimage contrast and luminosity.

A seed point extraction identifies a set of points used as starting nodes for simultaneous searches, where the searches are carried out by means of search trees, each rooted at a seed point. Iteratively, the leave nodes of the trees are analyzed and the most promising one expanded. When two trees touch, the shortest path connecting them is recorded and considered as starting point for a new search. A final refinement step connects the vessel segments with a custom algorithm.

After the vessel axes have been identified, vessel diameter extraction is performed. Cross-sectional vessel profiles are extracted along every branch of the vessel network, orthogonally to the axis direction. They are then preprocessed with a monodimensional shift-invariant Gaussian filter, to reduce noise [12]. For each profile, a preliminary vessel width estimation is performed, in order to estimate the kernel scale for the monodimensional filtering. Caliber measurements that appear to be nonconsistent are fixed, either by changing the matched filter scale or by forcing them to a trustworthy value if a reliable caliber cannot be identified.

5.2.1 Seed Finding

An initial seed-finding algorithm, based on multiscale matched filters over regular grids, is run. The objective of this module is to extract a set of points (seeds) from which the tracking step can start. Since the whole point of the sparse tracking procedure is to ensure that even nonconnected vessels can be tracked, these seed points should be spread out in the image as much as possible. In order to achieve this, a number of equally spaced rows and columns of the image are analyzed. From each selected line, the gray-level profile is extracted and analyzed looking for patterns corresponding to candidate vessels: the profile is convolved with a discretized Laplacian of Gaussian function filter over multiple

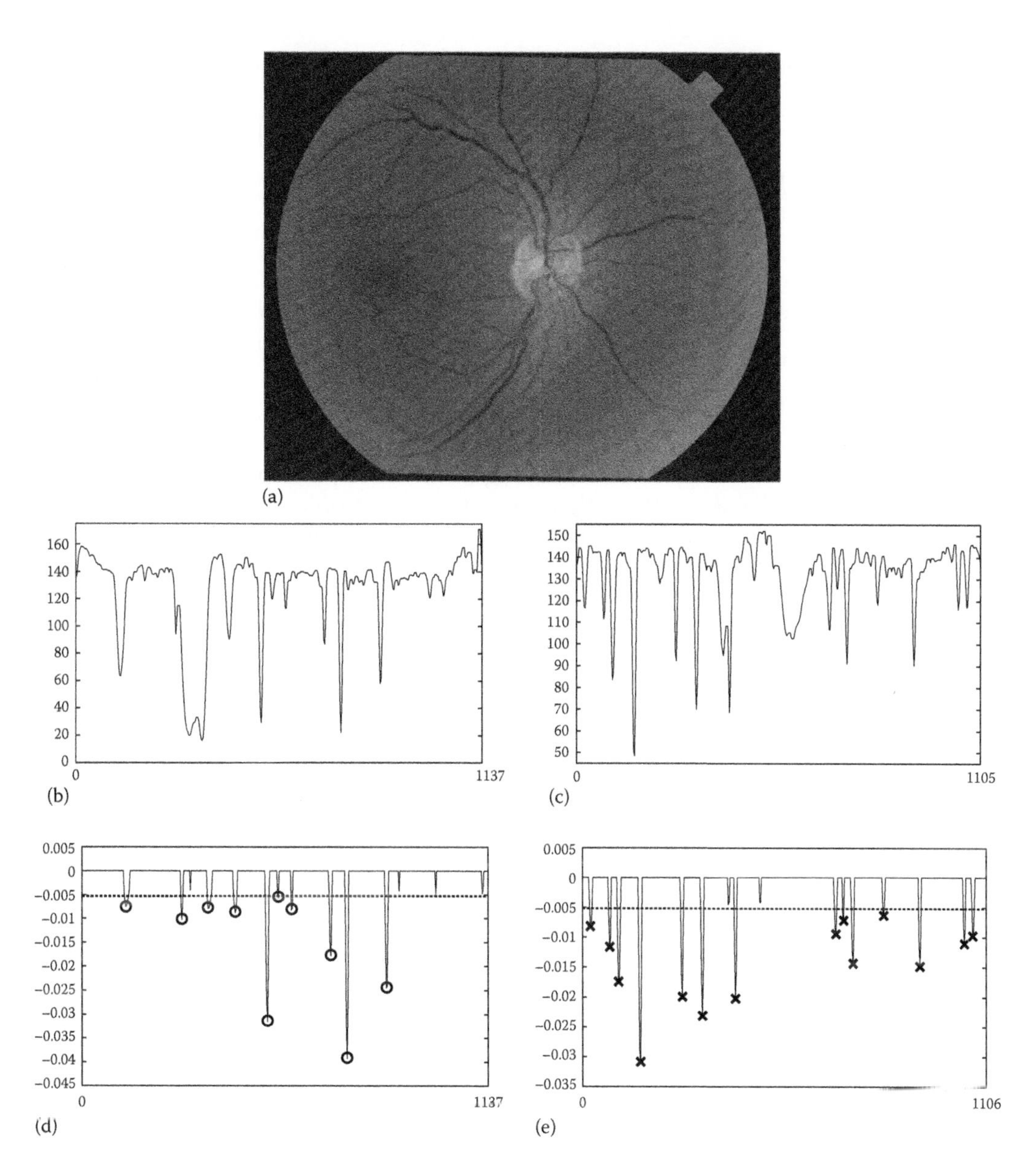

FIGURE 5.1
Seed points found by analyzing (a) the horizontal profile (b) and the vertical profile (c). After matched filtering (d and e), thresholding provides the set of points suggesting the presence of vessel: circles and crosses correspond to the seeds deployed in (a).

scales, and the maximum response among the output results is considered (Figure 5.1). In order to maximize the difference between vessels and background along the profile and to improve the seed extraction procedure, the grid lines need to be perpendicular to the vessels. We decided to use two regular grids: one of equally spaced rows and columns and a similar one rotated by 45°.

The zero-mean discrete filter used is described by the following equation:

$$kernel_{sc}(x) = \begin{cases} -1, & -\lfloor 3sc/2 \rfloor < x \leq -\lfloor sc/2 \rfloor \\ 2, & -\lfloor sc/2 \rfloor < x \leq \lfloor sc/2 \rfloor \\ -1, & \lfloor sc/2 \rfloor < x \leq \lfloor 3sc/2 \rfloor \\ 0, & \text{elsewhere} \end{cases} \quad (5.1)$$

where x and the scale sc are discrete values expressed in pixel. Given the profile, $p(x)$, the family of filter, $f_{sc}(x)$, and a set of scales, SC, the final filter response is given by

$$res(x) = \min\{p(x) \otimes kernel_{sc}(x) \mid sc \in SC\} \quad (5.2)$$

where $\otimes$ is the convolution operation. Looking at the most prominent local minima of $res(x)$, we derive a set $K = \{k_i, i \in \{1,\ldots,N_K\}\}$ of points on the profile suggesting the possible presence of vessels in the corresponding points of the image. From now on, $S = \bigcup K$ is the entire set of detected seed points.

It is worth noting that we favored the seed-finding procedure sensitivity (detected vessels over true vessels) rather than its specificity (nondetected vessels over nonvessel). As explained in Section 5.2.2.5, the efficacy of our algorithm is less affected by the presence of false seed points, that is, seeds not positioned over vessels, than by their absence in some regions of the image.

5.2.2 Multidirectional Graph Search Tracking

5.2.2.1 Background

In this section, some basic graph search concepts and definitions are given, while the description of the proposed algorithm is provided in Sections 5.2.2.2 through 5.2.2.6. Let us consider the undirected graph $G = (N, E)$ derived from the image I. Each node $i \in N$ is associated to the pixel in I having row $row(i)$, column $col(i)$, and gray level $g(i) = I(row(i), col(i))$. The edge $(i,j) \in E$ exists if $|row(i) - row(j)| \leq 1$ and $|col(i) - col(j)| \leq 1$. To each edge $(i,j) \in E$, a cost is associated by a real-value function $f: E \rightarrow \mathbb{R}^+$ that will be defined in Section 5.2.2.5. A path P in G is a sequence of nodes that are sequentially connected by edges in E. A path P connecting the nodes $a, b \in N$ is the shortest one if $\sum_{(i,j)\in P} f(i,j)$ is minimal among all paths connecting a to b.

Given a graph G and a node, s, the shortest path tree problem consists in finding a spanning directed tree T^* rooted at s such that the cost of all paths in T^* from s to all other nodes is minimal in G. Algorithms that compute T^* have a common scheme: starting from an initial tree $T(0) \subseteq T^*$, they iteratively update it until, at the iteration n, $T(n) = T^*$ is found. The problem can be solved by the Dijkstra's algorithm [10], which can also be used for finding the shortest path from two single vertices by early stopping the algorithm at the iteration n in which $T(n)$ meets the target vertex (without computing the entire T^*). This latter problem can be solved by a bidirectional search approach [9], which, for a running time profit, runs two simultaneous searches, one from the initial state and one from the goal, and stops when the two $T(n)$ meet.

The specific problem we are dealing with, however, requires connecting several nodes. The scheme of the proposed algorithm is to run multiple shortest path searches, each

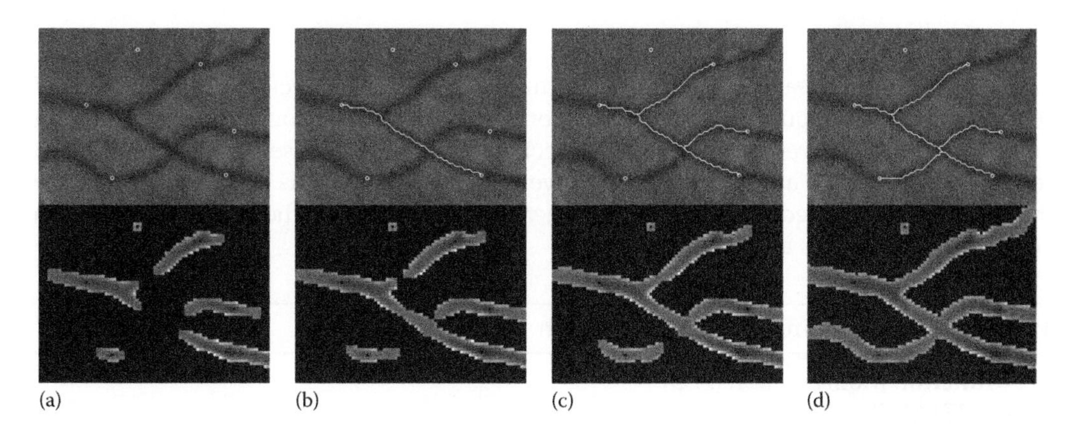

FIGURE 5.2
Example of exploration starting from six manually deployed seeds. Upper row: a particular of the original image with seeds and paths found. Lower row: images of the matrix storing the *distance* values, after 380 (a), 540 (b), 642 (c), and 1020 (d) iterations.

starting from one of the seeds found according to the procedure described in Section 5.2.1. When two trees meet, they provide the shortest path connecting their roots, but differently from the bidirectional approach, the algorithm does not stop. Instead, these two trees merge into a single new tree, from which the search goes on in successive iterations (Figure 5.2).

5.2.2.2 Initialization

Every seed $s \in S \subset G$ is considered the root of a different search tree T_s. Every node $i \in T_s$ carries four labeled values: *dist*, *pred*, *id*, and *state*. The *distance* $dist_i$ provides the cost of the path from i to s, $pred_i$ is the reference to the *predecessor* of i in T_s, id_i is an *identification tag* that univocally identifies the tree to which i belongs, and $state_i$ indicates whether i is a leave of T_i or has already been explored. At the first iteration, every T_s coincides with its root s: $dist_s$ is equal to zero for all $s \in S$, while for all other nodes of the graph *dist* is set to ∞.

Algorithm 5.1 Initialization

```
 1  function INITIALIZE (S, G)
 2     for all s ∈ S do                                   ▷ for all seeds
 3        dist_s ← 0                          ▷ distance from the source
 4        pred_s ← ∅                          ▷ predecessor in the tree
 5        id_s ← s                           ▷ tree's identification tag
 6        state_s ← leaf             ▷ exploration starts from leaves
 7     end for
 8     for all n ∈ N(G) \ S do                      ▷ for all other nodes
 9        dist_n ← ∞
10     end for
11  end function
```

5.2.2.3 Search

At each iteration, the leaf node i with the minimum distance is selected. Let J be the set of nodes reached by the outgoing edges of i. If one of these nodes belongs to a tree different from T_i, then the two trees are merged (see Section 5.2.2.4). Otherwise, the distance of each node in J is calculated as if its predecessor were i. If this distance is less (better) than the one previously recorded in the node $j \in J$, then j becomes part of the current exploration tree, and its four labels are updated.

Algorithm 5.2 Multidirectional Graph Search

```
1   function MULTISEARCH (S, G)
2   INITIALIZE (S,G)
3     P ← ∅                                              ▷ Set of the minimum paths
4     repeat
5       i ← argmin_i {dist_i | state_i = leaf, i ∈ N(G)}
6       state_i ← explored                              ▷ it will never be selected
7       for all j|(i,j) ∈ E(G) do
8         If id_j ≠ id_i and state_j = explored then
9           P ← P ∪ MERGE(i, j, G)
10        else if state_j ≠ explored then
11          newdistance ← COSTFUNCTION (i, j)
12          if new distance < d_j then
13            dist_j ← newdistance
14            pred_j ← i
15            id_j ← id_i
16            state_j ← leaf
17          end if
18        end if
19      end for
20      ec ← EVALUATEENDCONDITION (P, G)
21    until ec
22  return P
23  end function
```

5.2.2.4 Merging

The merging operation consists of two steps. First, the minimum path is reconstructed by exploiting the *predecessor* label, that is, step by step backward from node i and from node j along their tree, until a seed point $s \in S$ is reached or until a node belonging to a previously found path is reached (see Figure 5.2). Second, the two exploration trees are merged (i.e., the *identification tag* of their nodes is made the same).

5.2.2.5 Cost Function

We defined the cost function f associated to the edge (i, j) as follows:

$$f(i,j) = dist_i + k_{i,j} w_{i,j} \tag{5.3}$$

$$k_{i,j} = g(i)^{p_1} + |g(i) - g(j)|^{p_2} \tag{5.4}$$

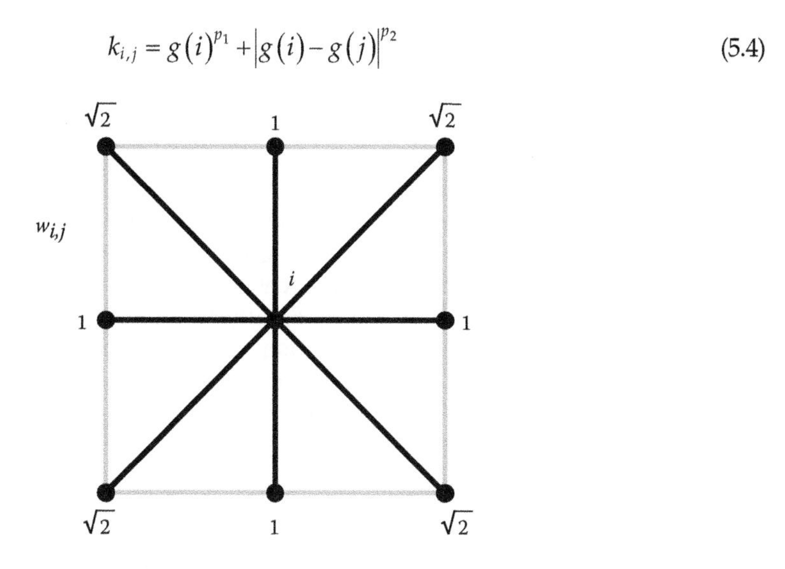

where $w_{i,j} = 1$ if i and j represent four-adjacent pixels, otherwise, $w_{i,j} = \sqrt{2}$. The first term of the sum in Equation 5.4, $g(i)^{p_1}$, penalizes the exploration of brighter pixels, while the second term, $|g(i) - g(j)|^{p_2}$, penalizes the transition from inside to outside the vessels and vice versa. The values of p_1 and p_2 have been chosen empirically on a small subset of images.

By means of the proposed f, the exploration from the true-vessel seeds evolves much faster than from the false-vessel ones. Indeed, as the number of iterations grows, only false seeds remain to be connected. To exploit this feature to minimize the occurrence of vessels detection, we defined a termination criteria based on two conditions.

The first one considers the degree of connectivity of the estimated vessel network after acyclic number of iterations. We considered the network as a set of trees in which the nodes correspond to the bifurcations and the leaves to the endpoints of the vessels. The more the iterations of the algorithm, the more the vessel network becomes connected, with the leaves-to-nodes ratio approaching the lower bound value 1/2. The termination condition is satisfied when that ratio reaches the empirically set value of 2.

After the first condition is met, every new path found is accepted only if the average gray level of its pixels significantly differs from the average background value of the preprocessed image. After three consecutive path rejections, the algorithm ends, since it is assumed that the remaining paths cannot be better than those already found.

5.2.2.6 Circular Path Fixing

The proposed algorithm allows to connect N given seed points with at most $N - 1$ paths, and it is intrinsically unable to find circular paths [36]. Since retinal vessels frequently overlap and cross each other delineating circular patterns, we had to design a fixing step in order to detect the missing vessel segments.

The rationale is to consider every endpoint of the current vessel network (termination tips of the vessels) and to search for a path that starts from it and connects it to the vessel network reconstructed so far. To this end, the algorithm presented in Section 5.2.2.3 is run once more, considering all the vessel tips as seeds and with the constraint to explore the region around the vessel prolongations, without being allowed to backtrack along the vessels already traced.

5.2.3 Vessel Caliber Extraction

5.2.3.1 Vessel Profile Setup

As far as the identification of the vessel width is concerned, each segment of the estimated vessel network is considered separately. It can be expressed as a curve $C(i)$ defined in the parametric curvilinear coordinate $i \in \{1,\ldots,N\}$. For every i, the profile $p_{C(i)}$, centered in $C(i)$ and orthogonal to the local direction of the vessel segment, is considered. The length of every profile is fixed to a value large enough to contain the widest vessel cross section. In order to smooth the digital noise, the average of three adjacent profiles $p_{C(i-1)}$, $p_{C(i)}$, and $p_{C(i+1)}$ is computed for every $i \in \{2, N-1\}$. Finally, to improve the profile SNR, the averaged profile is processed with a monodimensional version of the shift-invariant Gaussian filter proposed in [38]. This consists in a combination of domain and range filtering technique for edge-preserving smoothing. From now on, *FP* will be the profile after shift-invariant Gaussian filtering.

5.2.3.2 Border Point Extraction

The extraction of the border points for every profile $FP_{C(i)}$ is performed in two steps: first, a raw caliber value is estimated; second, the border points are detected by analyzing the response of a matched filter whose scale corresponds to the raw caliber estimation.

Starting from the local maximum closest to the center of the profile and moving away in both directions, the caliber estimation limits are set where the slope of the profile decreases below 1/2 of its current average value. If a central reflex is present, the vessel profile usually shows two peaks. In this case, if one of the two estimated limits erroneously ended up in the valley corresponding to the central reflex, it is moved to the nearest valley where the slope rule mentioned previously is met again.

Let *EC* be the resulting estimated caliber: the profile *FP* is convoluted with a monodimensional matched filter with scale *EC* (Equations 5.1 and 5.5):

$$MFP_{C(i)}(x) = FP_{C(i)}(x) \otimes kernel_{EC_{C(i)}}(x) \tag{5.5}$$

Border points are detected comparing the filtered profile *MFP* with a threshold (Figure 5.3) determined with a fuzzy *c*-means clustering method.

5.2.3.3 Adaptive Correction

A common drawback of all vessel tracking techniques is that they may fail in regions where vessels are not clearly detectable with respect to the background, for example, low-contrast regions and areas where two vessels cross, overlap, touch, or almost touch. The presence of lesions, such as hemorrhages, may also lead to errors in vessel detection. In all these situations, the local caliber estimation might be imprecise, causing the matched filter to use an inaccurate scale, hence potentially yielding inexact vessel border locations.

To overcome this problem, vessel segments are considered as tubular structures whose calibers have to satisfy continuity and regularity constraints. The distance of every matching pair of border points (Section 5.2.3.2) is compared with the median M computed on

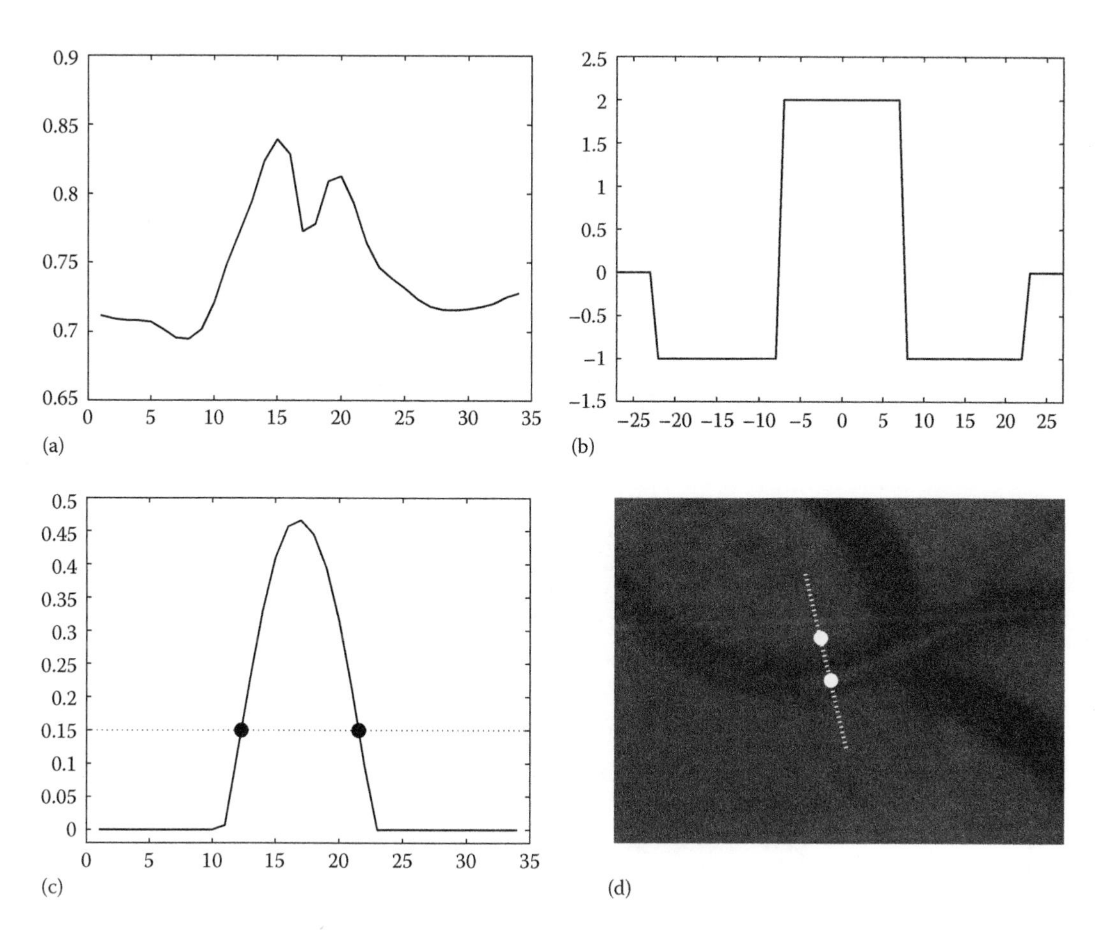

FIGURE 5.3
The starting FP_i^s profile (a), the kernel function $k_{EC_k^s}(x)$ centered in $x=0$ with $EC_k^s = 15$ as estimated scale (b), the output of the matched filter, with the threshold (dotted black) chosen by using a fuzzy two-mean clustering (c), and the final estimated border points (d).

the entire vessel. If this distance is narrower than $M/2$, the profile is reanalyzed with a matched filter using a larger scale; likewise, if the diameter is wider than $3M/2$, the filtering is performed with a smaller scale. With this diameter estimation/correction system, multiple scales are used only for critical profiles. In such a way, the accuracy provided by the matched filter technique is preserved, but at the same time, the computational effort is kept low.

If a reliable diameter cannot be found even after scale adjustment, the position of the border points is imposed, so that their distance matches M (Figure 5.4b). It should be mentioned that this latter solution is adopted in very critical situations only, in which the transition from vessel to background cannot be reliably identified.

Regularity of vessel borders is finally achieved by means of an interpolation function. The fact that vessels are continuous structures, at least with their first derivative, suggested the use of a cubic smoothing spline interpolation. Two final curves C^{left} and C^{right} lying on the vessel borders are computed. The vessel centerline is obtained by averaging the C^{left} and the C^{right} coordinates (Figure 5.4c).

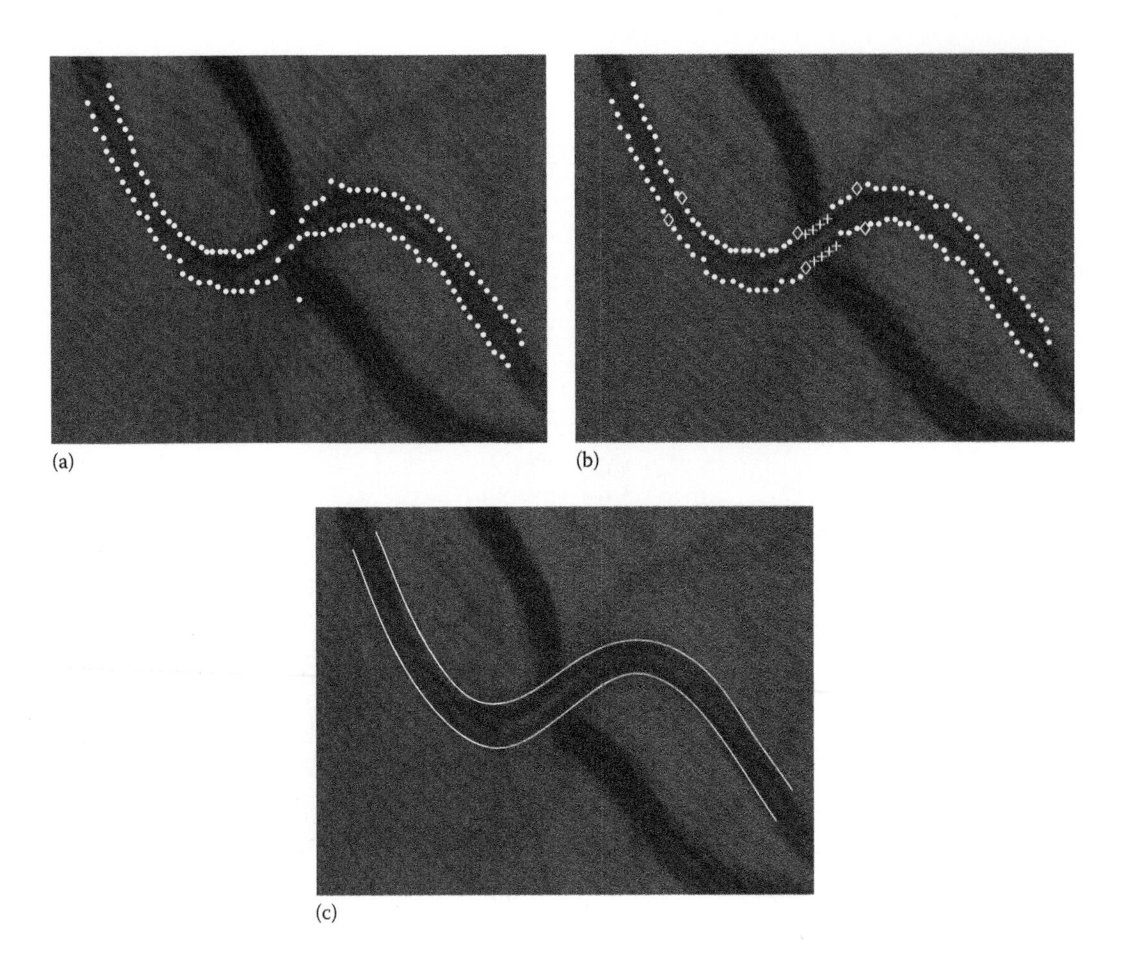

FIGURE 5.4
Border points evaluated before (a) and after (b) diameter correction, along with the final vessel segmentation (c). In the middle image, rhombus points were successfully corrected, while crosses were forced to the median caliber of the analyzed vessel segment.

5.3 Material

Ten color fundus images were acquired both in normal and in pathological subjects with a commercial fundus camera according to the NM1 standard [3]: 50° field focused centrally between the temporal margin of the optic disc and the center of the macula. Slides were then digitized at 24-bit color depth and 1360 dpi, yielding images of an approximate size of 1400×1200 pixels. An author (EP) and an external image expert independently performed a manual segmentation of the vessel network for each image, to produce what we considered the ground-truth and the second human observer's references. This so-called YARD, comprehensive of original images and manual segmentations, is publicly available for download at http://bioimlab.dei.unipd.it.

In order to provide also a comparison between the effectiveness of our method and those previously proposed by other authors, we run our algorithms also on the three public datasets: DRIVE [34], STARE [17], and REVIEW [2].

5.4 Results

5.4.1 Vessel Segmentation

To perform the comparison with other retinal vessel segmentation algorithms, specificity, sensitivity, and accuracy have been assessed. Sensitivity measures the proportion of vessel pixels that have been correctly identified as vessel, while specificity measures the proportion of background pixels that have been correctly identified as background. Accuracy is the ratio of the number of correctly classified pixels (both vessel and nonvessel) over the total number of pixels. The performance was assessed using the ground-truth references coming with each database (Figure 5.5).

Tables 5.1 through 5.3 present the average accuracy, sensitivity, and specificity calculated on YARD, DRIVE, and STARE dataset, respectively. In Tables 5.2 and 5.3, performance of our method is compared to those obtained with the best methods in literature [6,17,20,24,25,31], those of a second human observer (the first human observer segmentation is the ground-truth reference), and those obtained if all pixels were classified as background.

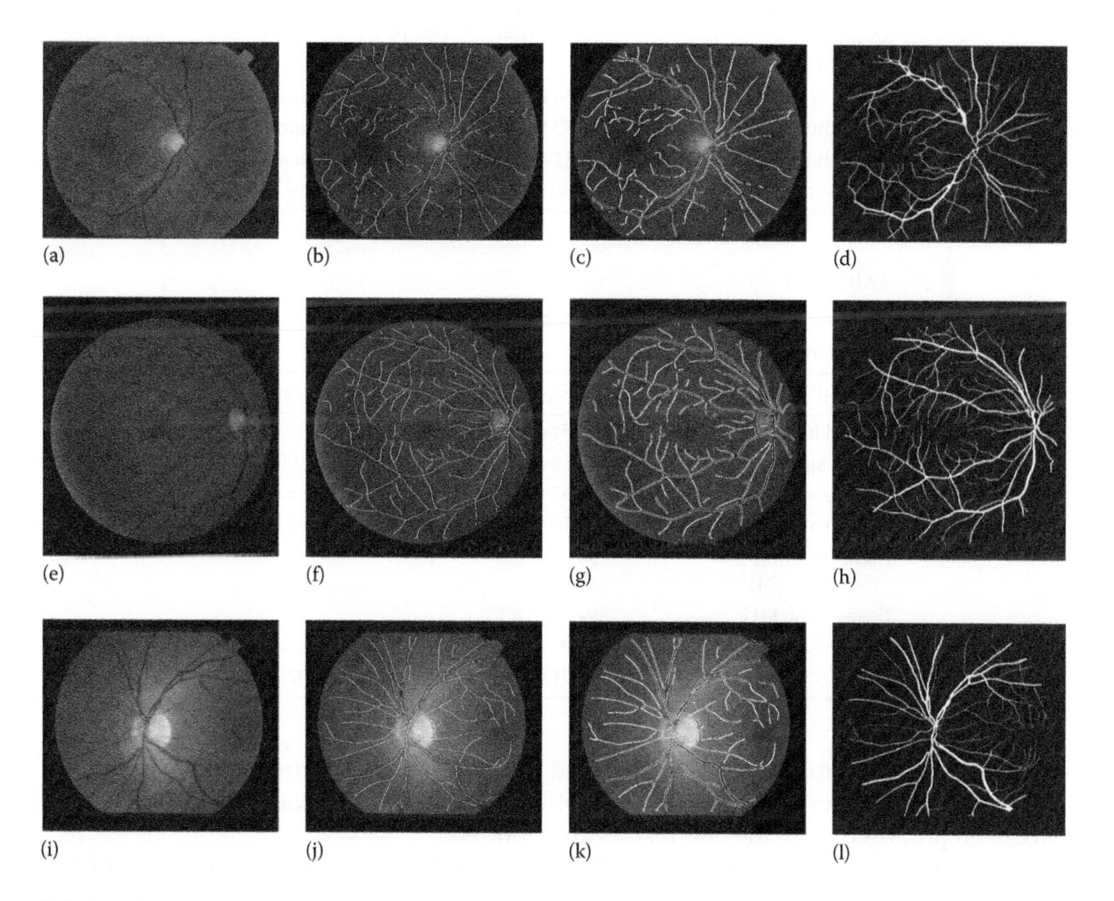

FIGURE 5.5
Original images (leftmost column), estimated vessel axis networks (second column), estimated vessel diameters (third column), and ground-truth references (rightmost column) from the YARD (a–d), DRIVE (e–h), and STARE (i–l) datasets.

TABLE 5.1

Performance Results of the Proposed Method on the YARD: Mean and Standard Deviation (%)

	Accuracy	Sensitivity	Specificity
Second human observer	96.44 (1.30)	75.99	98.32
All background	91.98 (1.67)	0.00	100.00
Our method	96.18 (1.54)	82.58	97.49

TABLE 5.2

Performance Results on the DRIVE Dataset: Mean and Standard Deviation (%)

Method	Accuracy	Sensitivity	Specificity
Second human observer [34]	94.93 (0.48)	77.61	97.25
All background	87.27 (1.23)	0.00	100.00
Staal et al. [34]	94.42 (0.65)	71.94	97.73
Niemeijer et al. [25]	94.17 (0.65)	68.98	97.96
Mendonça and Campilho [24]	94.63 (0.65)	73.15	97.81
Soares et al. [31]	94.66 (n.a.)	n.a.	n.a.
Chaudhuri et al. [6]	87.73 (2.32)	n.a.	n.a.
Jiang and Mojon [20]	89.11 (n.a.)	n.a.	n.a.
Our method	93.56 (0.69)	73.04	96.62

TABLE 5.3

Performance Results on the STARE Dataset: Mean and Standard Deviation (%)

Method	Accuracy	Sensitivity	Specificity
Second human observer [17]	93.54 (1.71)	89.49	93.90
All background	89.58 (n.a.)	0.00	100.00
Hoover et al. [17]	92.67 (0.99)	67.51	95.67
Staal et al. [34]	95.16 (n.a.)	69.70	98.10
Mendonça and Campilho [24]	94.63 (0.65)	73.15	97.81
Soares et al. [31]	94.80 (n.a.)	n.a.	n.a.
Jiang and Mojon [20]	90.09 (n.a.)	n.a.	n.a.
Our method	94.01 (1.60)	69.23	97.34

The performances for the methods [20] and [17] are the ones reported in [34], while the results for [6] are taken from [25]. Since in both [24] and [31] several variants of the method have been proposed, only the best results are reported.

The average run time of our MATLAB® implementation of the multidirectional graph searching algorithm, ran on a single image, is 15 s using an Intel Duo Core 2 PC (2.2 GHz, 4 GB of RAM).

The average run time of our MATLAB implementation of the diameter extraction step, ran on a single image, is 20 s using an Intel Duo Core 2 PC (2.2 GHz, 4 GB of RAM).

5.4.2 Caliber Estimation

We used three datasets from the REVIEW database to assess the diameter measurement performance (Table 5.4) [2]. These contain a number of retinal profiles (including center-points, width, and direction) marked up by three observers, with the mean width used as a ground truth. The high-resolution image set (HRIS) contains 2368 profiles from 90 segments from 4 images, resolution 2438 × 3584. These are downsampled by a factor of four before submission to the measurement algorithms, so that the vessels' widths are known to of a pixel, discounting human error. The vascular disease image set (VDIS) contains 2249 profiles from 79 segments from 8 images, resolution 1024 × 1360. Both HRIS and VDIS images contain a range of normal and diseased retinae, including diabetic retinopathies and an arteriosclerotic. The central light reflex image set (CLRIS) contains 285 profiles from 21 segments from 2 images, at a resolution of 1440 × 2169, representing early atherosclerotic changes with an exaggerated vascular light reflex.

Sometimes algorithms fail entirely to detect the vessel width at a given point (e.g., do not converge). We therefore report results as a success rate (i.e., a meaningful measurement was returned), together with the error variance of the successful measurements. The different algorithms may yield consistently different mean widths to one another, and observers. This bias is due to the different implicit width definitions in the algorithms and can easily be compensated for by subtraction of a bias constant. It is also worth noting that the key physiological feature of interest is a change in the width along a segment and consistent bias is irrelevant in the detection of changes. In contrast, variance in the estimation error cannot be compensated for. For this reason, the mean measurement error is ignored and the standard deviation of the measurement error is used to assess the performance of the algorithms. The width difference equals the following:

$$\chi_i = \omega_i - \psi_i \tag{5.6}$$

where

ω_i is the estimated width
ψ_i is the corresponding benchmark width

TABLE 5.4

Performance Results on the REVIEW Dataset: Success Rate (%) and Standard Deviation of the Width Difference

	HRIS		VDIS		CLRIS	
Number of Vessel Mean Diameter	**2343 4.35**		**3466 8.85**		**453 13.8**	
	%	σ_χ	%	σ_χ	%	σ_χ
Standard	100	—	100	—	100	—
O_1	100	0.285	100	0.669	100	0.566
O_2	100	0.256	100	0.621	100	0.698
O_3	100	0.288	100	0.543	100	0.567
Gregson	100	1.479	100	1.494	100	2.841
HHFW	88.3	0.926	78.4	0.879	0	—
1D G	99.6	0.896	99.9	2.110	98.6	4.137
2D G	98.9	0.703	77.2	1.328	26.7	6.016
Al-Diri et al. [1]	99.7	0.420	99.6	0.766	93.0	1.469
Our method	99.7	0.304	96.1	0.844	100	1.107

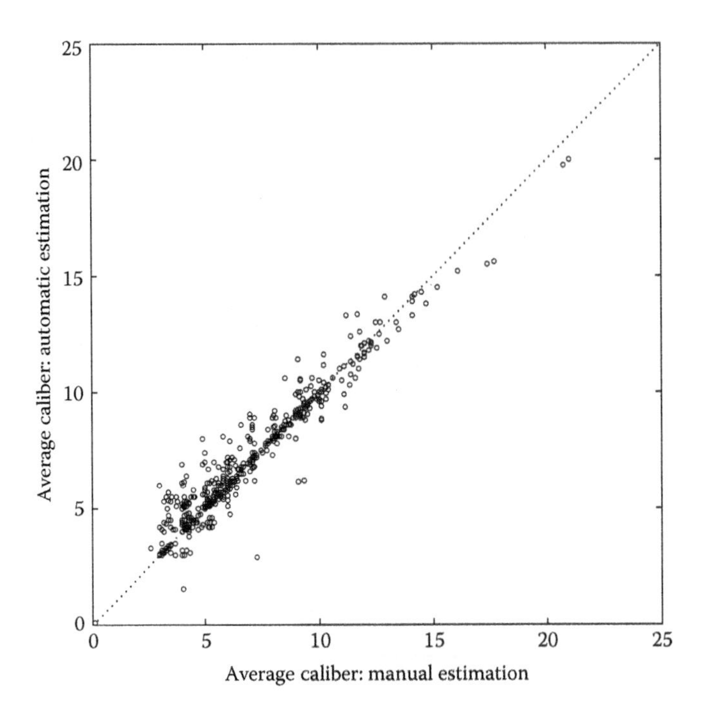

FIGURE 5.6
Average caliber: scatter plot of manual vs. automatic estimations.

The standard deviation of the width difference, σ_χ, is a useful measure of algorithm performance, as it is unaffected by correction for additive bias.

The caliber estimation method was also tested by analyzing a set of 739 vessel segments manually segmented by an external image expert on YARD. The vessel axis network, obtained by applying a skeletonization to the ground-truth binary image, was used as start point to evaluate vessel diameters and centerline. The algorithm performance was assessed by computing the correlation between automatic evaluation and manual evaluation of the average caliber of every vessel segment, resulting in $\rho = 0.97$. In Figure 5.6, the scatter plot of the average caliber values, from manual evaluation vs. automatic evaluation, is shown.

The whole evaluation required the analysis of 17,032 vessel profiles; 4,758 of them (27.9%) needed to be processed by the adaptive correction module (Section 5.2.3.3) in order to find a reliable diameter. A total of 2653 diameters were effectively recovered (55.8% of the profiles processed by the adaptive correction module), while the remaining 2105 were forced to the median caliber evaluated on the corresponding vessel segment.

5.5 Discussion

As shown in tables, the proposed system behaves differently in the three datasets. This is due to the different image features and the differences in the ground-truth manual labeling.

The images from different datasets have different fields of view and resolutions: YARD, 50°, 1400 × 1200 pixels; DRIVE, 45°, 768 × 584 pixels; and STARE, 35°, 605 × 700 pixels. In these last two datasets, the smallest capillaries manually segmented by human observers are 1 pixel wide, while in YARD, the smallest capillaries manually segmented are about 4 pixels wide. The proposed method showed some difficulties to detect these very small vessels mainly because the seed-finding procedure was not able to detect them. As we made the algorithm more sensible toward the small vessel of the DRIVE and STARE images, small capillaries and spurious grains not present in the ground-truth mask of YARD were found.

In the DRIVE dataset, the performance of our algorithm is perfectly aligned with all other automatic method results. The sensitivity is almost equal to the one reached in [24], and they are 1%–4% better than the other automated methods. Even in STARE dataset, the performance of our algorithm is in line with the results of the other methods; both accuracy and specificity are slightly better than those obtained by the second human observer.

Although the comparison between manual and automatic masks enables the comparison among gold standard, second human references, and performances of other algorithms, it must be noticed that it is not informative for what concerns the correlation between actual and estimated diameters. In fact, it is not possible to discern whether false negatives are due to wide vessel underestimation or small vessel undetection and whether false positives are due to vessel overestimation or detection of nonexistent vessels. For that reason in Section 5.4.2, the performance of the diameter estimation step was evaluated with a custom experiment setup. As it can be appreciated in Table 5.4, which shows performance assessment on the REVIEW dataset, our method, with respect to the one proposed in [1], has a better performance in both HRIS and CLRIS image sets, although being slightly worse in the VDIS image set. In Figure 5.6, manual average calibers are plotted against automatic estimations: their outstanding correlation proves the usefulness of the adaptive correction module, which processed 28% of the profiles.

In its present form, the described method has prove to be robust with respect to initial false-positive seeds and efficient in the tracking process. Its main drawbacks are the difficulty of detecting small capillaries of 1–3 pixel diameters and the different behavior in different datasets.

The system is made of two components: a vessel segmentation method able to estimate the central axis of the retina vessels and a vessel border detection step. The division of the segmentation process in two sequential and independent tasks provides some advantages. Two remarks can be made about this issue.

First, we could use a tracking method that does not require to identify the longitudinal cross section of the vessel and thus not require to detect the vessel diameters, allowing us to choose a technique that analyzes fewer pixels. The method proposed here uses the Dijkstra's algorithm, revised and expanded in order to connect multiple source points. The Dijkstra's algorithm has been widely studied, it is well known, and its implementation can be highly optimized for both computational cost and memory occupancy. Since it is at the core of the tracking algorithm, the whole system benefits from its efficiency.

The second remark concerns the edge detection step efficiency. The rationale of the method consists in exploiting the features provided by the vessel axis as prior information. Each point of the vessel axis is analyzed by coupling a matched technique both with the information of the vessel local direction and with a roughly estimated scale of the vessel diameter, to reduce the dimensionality of the problem.

Results from [24,25,31,34] are in some cases slightly better than our results, as these are supervised methods, which often show slightly higher performance with respect to the unsupervised ones. On the other hand, their drawback is the need of manually segmented images (ground truth) in order to extract a training set. On the contrary, an important advantage of the proposed method is that it is completely unsupervised, so there is no need for manually labeled images. Another advantage is the minimum number of parameters used, as well as its simplicity and easy implementation.

5.6 Conclusion

This chapter describes a new automatic system to extract the vessel structure in retinal images, based on a multidirectional graph search algorithm coupled with an efficient matched filtering approach. In order to assess the performance of the method, we provided two different analyses: in the first one, we assessed accuracy, sensitivity, and specificity of the binary classification task by comparing the automatic segmentations of the vessel network with the ground-truth ones, from three different datasets. Although performances slightly differ among the different datasets, overall the method provided accuracy, sensitivity, and specificity that are comparable to those obtained by the second human observers, as well as the ones obtained by other algorithms. In the second analysis, we computed the correlation between true diameters and estimated diameters in a set of highly accurate manual segmented vessels. Calibers estimated with the proposed method are highly correlated with those measured on the manually segmented images. The satisfactory results obtained with this algorithm suggest the possibility of using it to identify the retinal vascular structures for clinical purposes.

Acknowledgment

We would like to thank Enrico Grisan (Department of Information Engineering, University of Padova) for having kindly provided the second human reference manual segmentation of the YARD.

References

1. B. Al-Diri, A. Hunter, and D. Steel. An active contour model for segmenting and measuring retinal vessels. *IEEE Transactions on Medical Imaging*, 28(9):1488–1497, September 2009.
2. B. Al-Diri, A. Hunter, D. Steel, M. Habib, T. Hudaib, and S. Berry. Review—A reference data set for retinal vessel profiles, In *Proceedings of 30th Annual International Conference of the IEEE*, Vancouver, BC, pp. 2262–2265, August 2008.
3. S.E. Bursell, J.D. Cavallerano, A.A. Cavallerano, A.C. Clermont, D. Birkmire-Peters, L.P. Aiello, and L.M. Aiello. Stereo nonmydriatic digital-video color retinal imaging compared with Early Treatment Diabetic Retinopathy Study seven standard field 35-mm stereo color photos for determining level of diabetic retinopathy. *Ophthalmology*, 108(3):572–585, 2001.

4. H.L. Cook, C. Sinthanayothin, J.F. Boyce, and T.H. Williamson. Automated localisation of the optic disc, fovea and retinal blood vessels from digital colour fundus images. *British Journal of Ophthalmology*, 83:902–910, 1999.
5. A. Can, H. Shen, J.N. Turner, H.L. Tanenbaum, and B. Roysam. Rapid automated tracing and feature extraction from retinal fundus images using direct exploratory algorithms. *IEEE Transactions on Information Technology in Biomedicine*, 3(2):125–138, 1999.
6. S. Chaudhuri, S. Chatterjee, N. Katz, M. Nelson, and M. Goldbaum. Detection of blood vessels in retinal images using two-dimensional matched filters. *IEEE Transactions on Medical Imaging*, 8(3):263–269, September 1989.
7. O. Chutatape, L. Zheng, and S.M. Krishnan. Retinal blood vessel detection and tracking by matched Gaussian and Kalman filters. In *Proceedings of the 20th Annual International Conference of the IEEE Engineering in Medicine and Biology Society*, Hong Kong, vol. 6, pp. 3144–3149, 1998.
8. M.G. Cinsdikici and D. Aydın. Detection of blood vessels in ophthalmoscope images using MF/ant (matched filter/ant colony) algorithm. *Computer Methods and Programs in Biomedicine*, 96(2):85–95, 2009.
9. D. de Champeaux and L. Sint. An improved bidirectional heuristic search algorithm. *The Journal of the ACM*, 24(2):177–191, 1977.
10. E. Dijkstra. A note on two problems in connection with graphs. *Numerische Mathematik*, 1:269–271, 1959.
11. P.H. Eichel, E.J. Delp, K. Koral, and A.J. Buda. A method for a fully automatic definition of coronary arterial edges from cineangiograms. *IEEE Transactions on Medical Imaging*, 7(4):313–320, 1988.
12. D. Fiorin, E. Poletti, E. Grisan, and A. Ruggeri. Fast adaptive axis-based segmentation of retinal vessels through matched filters. In *World Congress on Medical Physics and Biomedical Engineering*, September 7–12, 2009, Munich, Germany, pp. 145–148, 2009.
13. M. Foracchia, E. Grisan, and A. Ruggeri. Luminosity and contrast normalization in retinal images. *Medical Image Analysis*, 9(3):179–190, 2005.
14. A.F. Frangi, W.J. Niessen, K.L. Vincken, and M.A. Viergever. Multiscale vessel enhancement filtering. In *Medical Image Computing and Computer-Assisted Interventation (MICCAI'98)*, Springer, Berlin, Heidelberg, vol. 1496, pp. 130–137, 1998.
15. T.H. Williamson, G.G. Gardner, D. Keating, and A.T. Elliott. Automatic detection of diabetic retinopathy using an artificial neural network: A screening tool. *British Journal of Ophthalmology*, 80:940–944, 1996.
16. E. Grisan, A. Pesce, A. Giani, M. Foracchia, and A. Ruggeri. A new tracking system for the robust extraction of retinal vessel structure. In *26th Annual International Conference of the IEEE Engineering in Medicine and Biology Society (IEMBS'04)*, San Francisco, CA, vol. 1, pp. 1620–1623, 2004.
17. A.D. Hoover, V. Kouznetsova, and M. Goldbaum. Locating blood vessels in retinal images by piecewise threshold probing of a matched filter response. *IEEE Transactions on Medical Imaging*, 19(3):203–210, March 2000.
18. L.D. Hubbard, R.J. Brothers, W.N. King, L.X. Clegg, R. Klein, L.S. Cooper, A.R. Sharrett, M.D. Davis, and J. Cai. Methods for evaluation of retinal microvascular abnormalities associated with hypertension/sclerosis in the Atherosclerosis Risk in Communities Study. *Ophthalmology*, 106(12):2269, 1999.
19. M. Jacob and M. Unser. Design of steerable filters for feature detection using canny-like criteria. *IEEE Transactions on Pattern Analysis and Machine Intelligence*, 26(8): 1007–1019, 2004.
20. X. Jiang and D. Mojon. Adaptive local thresholding by verification-based multi-threshold probing with application to vessel detection in retinal images. *IEEE Transactions on Pattern Analysis and Machine Intelligence*, 25(1):131–137, January 2003.
21. S.M. Kay. *Fundamentals of Statistical Signal Processing: Detection Theory*, Prentice Hall PTR, vol. 2, pp. 345–349, 1998.
22. H. Li, W. Hsu, M.L. Lee, and H. Wang. A piecewise Gaussian model for profiling and differentiating retinal vessels. In *Proceedings of the International Conference on Image Processing*, vol. 1, pp. 1069–1072. Citeseer, 2003.

23. D. Marn, A. Aquino, M.E. Gegundez-Arias, and J.M. Bravo. A new supervised method for blood vessel segmentation in retinal images by using gray-level and moment invariants-based features. *IEEE Transactions on Medical Imaging*, 30(1):146–158, 2011.
24. A.M. Mendonça and A. Campilho. Segmentation of retinal blood vessels by combining the detection of centerlines and morphological reconstruction. *IEEE Transactions on Medical Imaging*, 25(9):1200–1213, September 2006.
25. M. Niemeijer, J.J. Staal, B. van Ginneken, M. Loog, and M.D. Abramof. Comparative study of retinal vessel segmentation methods on a new publicly available database. In J. Michael Fitzpatrick and M. Sonka, eds., *SPIE Medical Imaging*, San Diego, CA, vol. 5370, pp. 648–656. SPIE, 2004.
26. E. Poletti, D. Fiorin, E. Grisan, and A. Ruggeri. Retinal vessel axis estimation through a multi-directional graph search approach. In *World Congress on Medical Physics and Biomedical Engineering*, September 7–12, 2009, Munich, Germany, pp. 137–140, 2009.
27. E. Poletti , D. Fiorin, E. Grisan, and A. Ruggeri. Automatic vessel segmentation in wide-field retina images of infants with retinopathy of prematurity. In *2011 Annual International Conference of the IEEE Engineering in Medicine and Biology Society (EMBC)*, Boston, MA, pp. 3954–3957. IEEE, 2011.
28. E. Poletti and A. Ruggeri. Segmentation of vessels through supervised classification in wide-field retina images of infants with retinopathy of prematurity. In *25th International Symposium on Computer-Based Medical Systems (CBMS), 2012*, Rome, Italy, pp. 1–6. IEEE, 2012.
29. E. Ricci and R. Perfetti. Retinal blood vessel segmentation using line operators and support vector classification. *IEEE Transactions on Medical Imaging*, 26(10):1357–1365, 2007.
30. A. Ruggeri, E. Poletti, D. Fiorin, and L. Tramontan. From laboratory to clinic: The development of web-based tools for the estimation of retinal diagnostic parameters. In *2011 Annual International Conference of the IEEE Engineering in Medicine and Biology Society (EMBC)*, Boston, MA, pp. 3379–3382. IEEE, 2011.
31. J.V.B. Soares, J.J.G. Leandro, R.M. Cesar, H.F. Jelinek, and M.J. Cree. Retinal vessel segmentation using the 2-d gabor wavelet and supervised classification. *IEEE Transactions on Medical Imaging*, 25(9):1214–1222, September 2006.
32. M. Sofka and C.V. Stewart. Retinal vessel centerline extraction using multiscale matched filters, confidence and edge measures. *IEEE Transactions on Medical Imaging*, 25(12):1531–1546, 2006.
33. M. Sonka, M.D. Winniford, and S.M. Collins. Robust simultaneous detection of coronary borders in complex images. *IEEE Transactions on Medical Imaging*, 14(1):151–161, 1995.
34. J.J. Staal, M.D. Abramof, M. Niemeijer, M.A. Viergever, and B. van Ginneken. Ridge based vessel segmentation in color images of the retina. *IEEE Transactions on Medical Imaging*, 23(4): 501–509, 2004.
35. A.V. Stanton, B. Wasan, A. Cerutti, S. Ford, R. Marsh, P.P. Sever, S.A. Thom, and A.D. Hughes. Vascular network changes in the retina with age and hypertension. *Journal of Hypertension*, 13(12 Pt 2):1724, 1995.
36. C. Sun and S. Pallottino. Circular shortest path in images. *Pattern Recognition*, 36(3):709–719, 2003.
37. Y.A. Tolias and S.M. Panas. A fuzzy vessel tracking algorithm for retinal images based on fuzzy clustering. *IEEE Transactions on Medical Imaging*, 17(2):263–273, 1998.
38. C. Tomasi and R. Manduchi. Bilateral filtering for gray and color images. In *Proceedings of the Sixth International Conference on Computer Vision*, Bombay, India, vol. 846, pp. 839–846. Citeseer, 1998.
39. L. Tramontan, E. Poletti, D. Fiorin, and A. Ruggeri. A web-based system for the quantitative and reproducible assessment of clinical indexes from the retinal vasculature. *IEEE Transactions on Biomedical Engineering*, (99):1–1, 2011.
40. F. Zana and J.C. Klein. Segmentation of vessel-like patterns using mathematical morphology and curvature evaluation. *IEEE Transactions on Image Processing*, 10(7):1010–1019, 2001.

6

Fundus Autofluorescence Imaging: Fundamentals and Clinical Relevance

Yasir J. Sepah, Abeer Akhtar, Yamama Hafeez, Humzah Nasir, Brian Perez, Narissa Mawji, Mohammad Ali Sadiq, Diana J. Dean, Daniel Araújo Ferraz, and Quan Dong Nguyen

CONTENTS

6.1 Introduction

Fundus autofluorescence (FAF) is a relatively new, noninvasive imaging modality that has been developed over the past decade. The autofluorescence (AF) images are obtained through the use of confocal scanning laser ophthalmoscopy (cSLO). It uses the fluorescent properties of lipofuscin (LP) to generate images that provide information beyond that is acquired by utilizing more conventional imaging methods such as fluorescein angiography, fundus photography, and regular optical coherence tomography (OCT). FAF has been an area of interest in ophthalmic research for over 40 years. However, it has only recently become clinically relevant because of various important technological advances. FAF has proved to be helpful in understanding the pathophysiological mechanisms, diagnostics, and identification of predictive markers for disease progression and for monitoring of novel therapies.

6.2 Principle of Autofluorescence Imaging and Interpretation of FAF Images

6.2.1 Retinal Pigment Epithelium and Lipofuscin

Retinal pigment epithelium (RPE) is a single layer of polygonal-shaped cells, which separates the choroid from the neurosensory retina. This epithelial layer plays a critical role in the normal functioning of the retina. It is responsible for phagocytosis and lysosomal breakdown of pigmented outer segments of photoreceptors, which allows the renewal process necessary to maintain photoreceptor excitability. Over the course of a lifetime, each RPE cell will phagocytose three billion outer segments [1]. With aging, incomplete or partial breakdown of these segments in the postmitotic RPE cells causes the accumulation of LP. LP is composed of several different molecules, most important of which is *N*-retinyl-*N*-retinylidene ethanolamine (A2E) (Figure 6.1). A2E is not recognized by lysosomal enzymes and therefore is incompletely broken down and accumulates in the lysosomes. An increased accumulation of this degraded material in the lysosomal compartment of the RPE cells is considered a hallmark of the aging process in the eye. In fact, a quarter of the RPE cytoplasm is composed of LP and melano-lipofuscin in persons over the age of 70. Excessive LP deposition is considered pathologic and is associated with visual loss. There are significant clinical and experimental evidences demonstrating that accumulation of LP above a certain threshold can cause functional loss of cells and lead to apoptosis.

Another component of LP, a toxic aldehyde known as all-*trans*-retinal, is produced in the outer segments of the photoreceptor when exposed to light. Photoreceptors lack *cis–trans* isomerase function for retinal and are unable to regenerate all-*trans*-retinal into 11-*cis*-retinal after transduction of light energy (Figure 6.2) into electrical impulses [2]. The excess

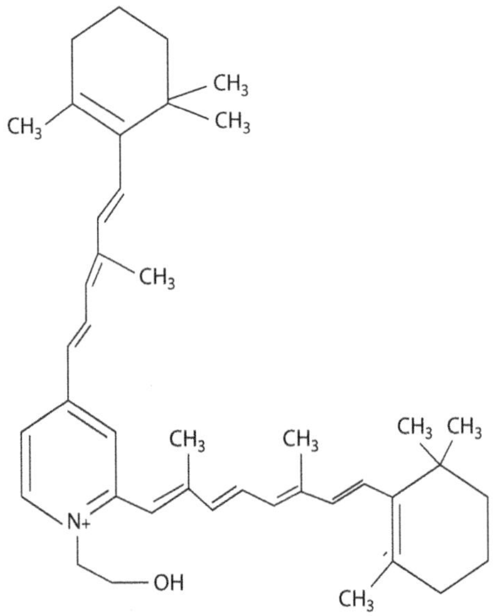

CH_3 CH_3 CH_3 CH_3 CH_3 CH_3 CH_3 CH_3 CH_3 CH_3 N+ OH

FIGURE 6.1
Chemical structure of A2E.

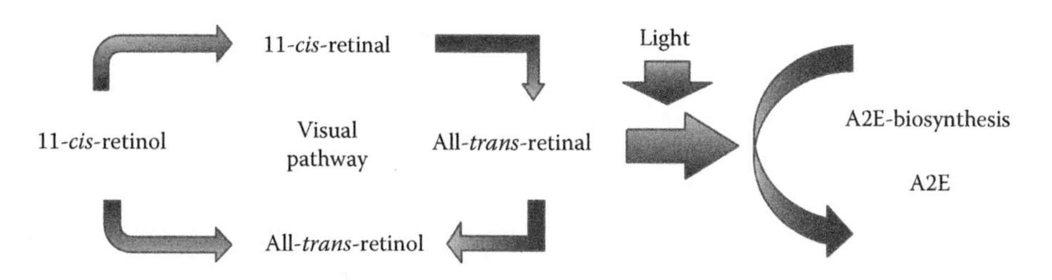

FIGURE 6.2
Biochemical pathway representing the various steps involved in the metabolism of LP.

all-*trans*-retinal accumulates within the photoreceptor, forming bisretinoids, which upon oxidation contribute to LP production [3].

6.2.2 Typical Findings in the Retina Using Fundus Autofluorescence

FAF images demonstrate a spatial distribution corresponding to the intensity of the signal emitted, where dark pixel values correspond to low intensities of emission and bright pixel values correspond to high intensities of emission [1]. The naturally occurring AF of the ocular fundus is known to be of low intensity such that the distribution of FAF in normal eyes demonstrates a consistent pattern in which the optic nerve head typically appears dark due to the absence of LP in this area [1]. Retinal vessels are characterized by a reduced FAF signal due to the absorption by blood [1]. FAF signal is also reduced in the macular area, particularly around the fovea due to the absorption of the luteal pigment [1]. It can be noted that even though the signal in the parafoveal area tends to be higher, it presents with a relatively reduced intensity when compared to the background signal in the more peripheral areas of the retina. This observation is thought to be caused by an increased concentration of melanin and decreased concentration of LP granules in central RPE cells [1].

However, the distinction between the optic disc and the macula is reversed if the wavelength of the excitation source is changed (e.g., devices using blue light will give you the former pattern on the FAF images, while devices using the green light will give you the latter) (Figure 6.3). Green light FAF is relatively new and has not been available commercially until recently. Hence, there is a lack of information as to how various diseased retinas would appear when scanned with a device utilizing a green light as the fluorophore excitation source.

6.2.3 Interpretations of the Fundus Autofluorescence Images

FAF imaging is used to record fluorescence that may occur naturally in ocular structures or as a by-product of a disease process. This technique allows the topographic mapping of LP distribution in the RPE [1]. The intensity portrayed by FAF corresponds to the accumulation of LP, which increases with aging, RPE cell dysfunction, or an abnormal metabolic load on the RPE.

When evaluating an FAF image, any deviation from the normal should be thoroughly investigated to identify a possible cause. Reasons for a reduced FAF signal may include but are not limited to RPE loss or atrophy, intraretinal fluid, reduction in RPE LP density, fibrosis, or the presence of luteal pigment [1]. Causes for increased FAF signal may include but are also not limited to drusen in the subpigmented epithelial space, excessive RPE

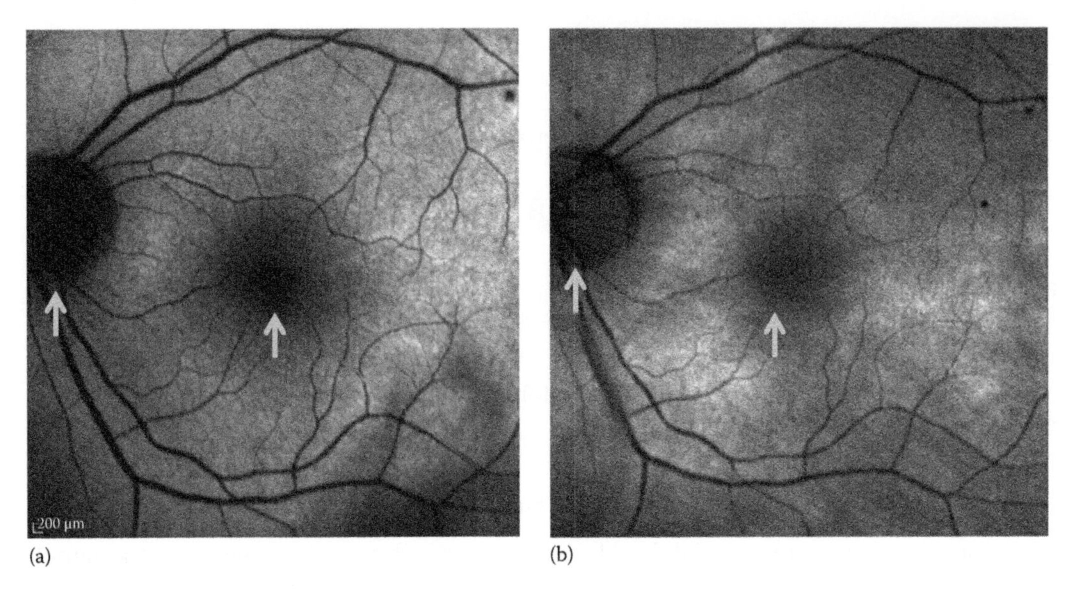

FIGURE 6.3
FAF and wavelength. Blue light (a) and green light (b) FAF images of a 28-year-old woman with visual acuity of 20/20 and without known eye disease. The FAF images show noticeable differences in the foveal and optic disc AF signal. Arrows represent corresponding areas of the same eye showing different AF signal when imaged with two different optical systems.

LP accumulation, age-related macular degeneration (AMD), or occurrence of fluorophores anterior or posterior to the RPE cell monolayer [1]. However, it is to be noted that the quality of the image may be affected by the opacity of the vitreous, lens, cornea, or anterior chamber and thus influence the identification of abnormalities. Thinner areas of retina adhere to the *window effect* meaning that they exhibit increased AF otherwise known as hyperautofluorescence [4].

6.3 Clinical Applications of Fundus Autofluorescence Imaging

Various histopathological studies have demonstrated the accretion of autofluorescent material and deposits in the RPE in various retinal dystrophies. Since FAF imaging enables the visualization of changes in LP distribution in the RPE [5], it can be useful in providing information about retinal dystrophies in which the health of the RPE is an important factor. FAF imaging has proven to be useful in regards to understanding and providing new perspectives concerning various pathophysiological mechanisms. FAF has also played a role in the monitoring of novel therapies of the retina and the identification of predictive markers for disease progression [1]. FAF allows for noninvasive mapping and documentation of metabolic change by noting the level of fluorescence, providing information that may otherwise not be clinically detectable. FAF findings have aided physicians in the identification of early retinal disease stages as well as phenotyping in retinal dystrophies such as retinitis pigmentosa. Additionally, FAF has recently been added to the imaging

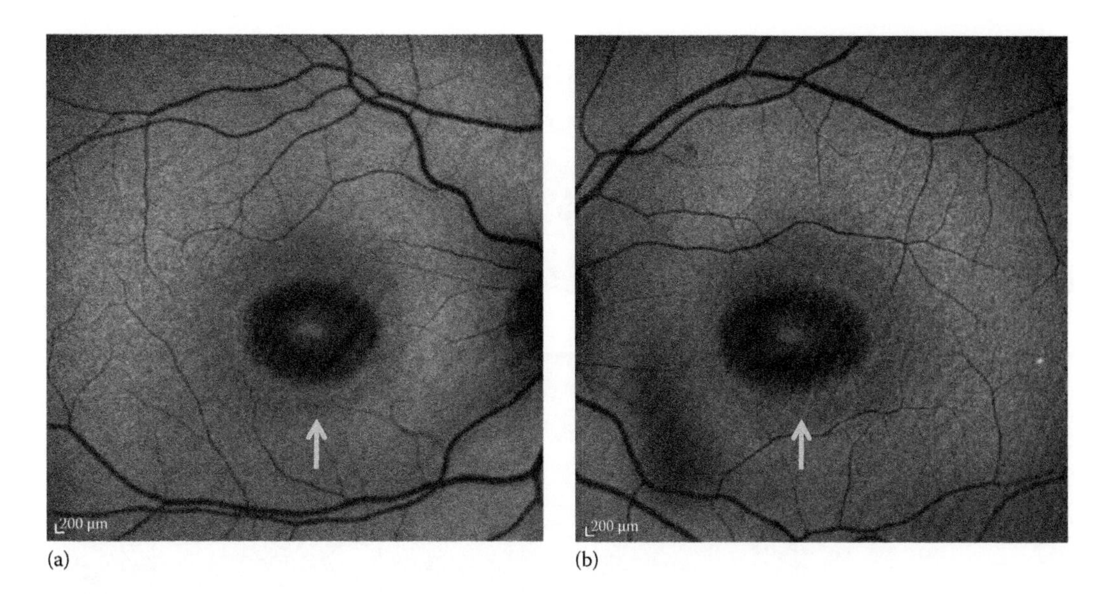

(a) (b)

FIGURE 6.4
Chloroquine maculopathy. Fovea surrounded by circular band of hypoautofluorescence with oculus sinister (OS) (b) effected to a greater extent than oculus dexter (OD) (a). Arrows point to the macular lesion of chloroquine toxicity.

studies recommended by the National Eye Institute (National Institutes of Health, United States) to investigate and follow patients suspected of chloroquine retinopathy that results in devastating visual loss (Figure 6.4). The future identification of high-risk characteristics or biomarkers can be useful in following patients and for performing clinical trial interventions in certain cases.

6.3.1 Age-Related Macular Degeneration

AMD is a progressive chronic pathology, which is considered the most common cause of legal blindness in industrialized countries [6]. Both environmental and genetic risk factors have been observed to influence the development of AMD [1,7]. The presence of drusen in color fundus photography is considered pathognomonic of AMD [8].

Since the accumulation of LP in postmitotic RPE cells has been postulated to play an important role in the pathogenesis of AMD [7,9], the monitoring of the metabolic integrity of the RPE with FAF imaging is useful to the clinician monitoring disease progression in AMD. Increased FAF is seen due to excessive accumulation of LP within the lysosomal compartment of RPE, and decreased FAF is characteristic in patients with geographic atrophy (GA) due to the absence of LP granules in the RPE [8] (Figures 6.5 and 6.6).

FAF has been described as a prognostic marker of GA. While FAF has been described as a marker for progression of the disease, some authors did not find any correlation between abnormal FAF and progression of GA [9]. Nevertheless, there is evidence that increased AF in the 500 µm margin around areas of GA could be used to distinguish between fast and slow progression of the disease [10].

Different patient classification systems have been proposed for describing FAF imaging findings in AMD. In 2005, Bindewald et al. proposed a classification to describe FAF as focal, banded, patchy, and diffuse in patients with GA [11]. Additionally, another

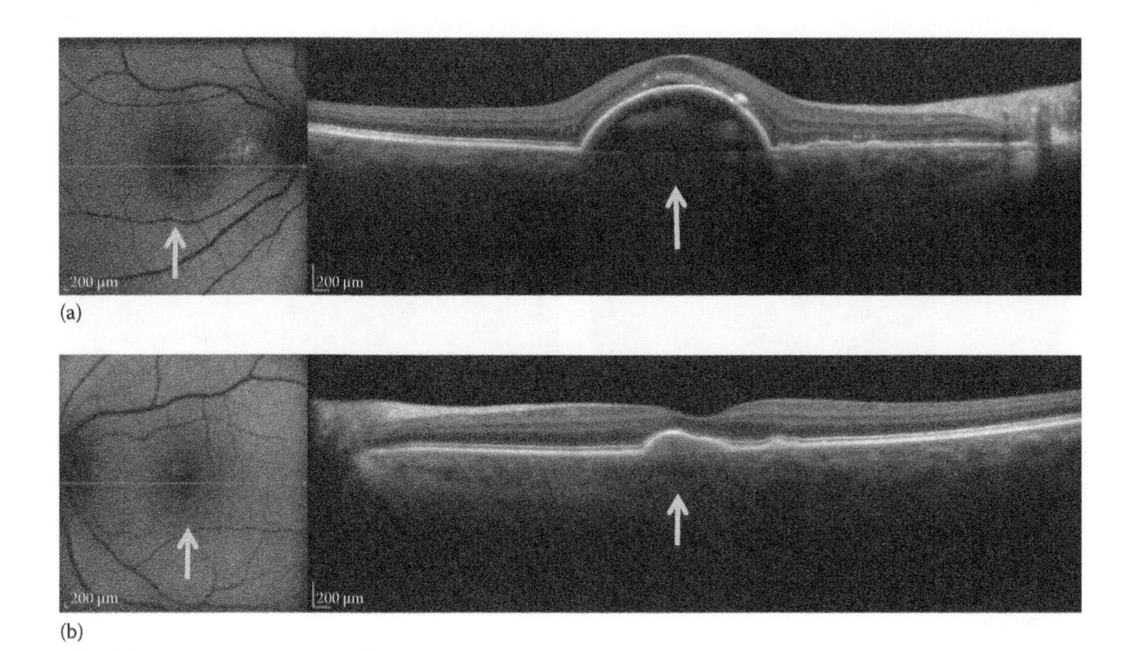

FIGURE 6.5
(See color insert.) Neovascular AMD, right eye (a) with more advanced disease compared to left eye (b). Fovea surrounded by a band of hypoautofluorescence corresponding to the site of neovascularization shown by OCT. Both arrows in (a) and (b) are pointing towards the disease process surrounding the fovea.

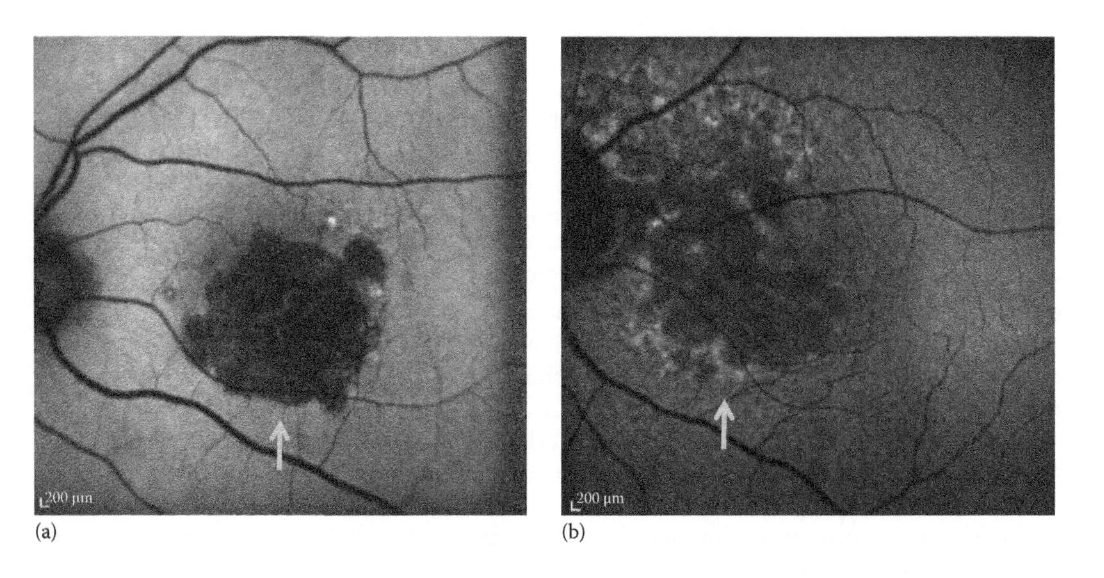

FIGURE 6.6
GA. (a) Well-circumscribed area of hypoautofluorescence. (b) Area of hypoautofluorescence surrounded at the edges by hyperautofluorescence as shown by the arrow. Arrow points to the boundary of the GA lesion.

kind of classification in patients with early AMD was proposed by Bindewald to describe early AMD as normal, minimal change, focal, increased, patchy, linear, lacelike, reticular, and speckled [12]. In 2002, Lois had proposed to describe FAF as focal, increased, reticular, combined, and homogeneous [9,13]. As distinctions between the classifications in these studies are hazy, standardized terminology is greatly needed to describe pathologic patterns of FAF [9].

Midena et al. studied the relationship between microperimetry and FAF of the macular region with drusen and pigment abnormalities in early AMD and found that microperimetry and FAF can be helpful for monitoring the progression of AMD before changes in visual acuity are observed [14].

6.3.2 Retinal Artery Occlusion

Retinal artery occlusions are blockages in the small arteries that carry blood to the retina. In most patients, the central retinal artery provides the only blood supply for the retina [15]. Historically, complications such as occlusions have generated poor visual outcomes, as vast majority do not regain vision [15]. However, FAF has proven to be a useful tool in pointing out areas of retinal artery occlusion. Occlusions inhibit proper AF of the RPE due to increased thickness resulting in a decrease in FAF [4]. Such property allows the identification of areas of the retina that are ischemic and of lower AF intensity (Figure 6.7). Hence, the technique can be used to objectively assess response to therapy or a natural reduction in the severity of the disease. It has been shown that the level of FAF exhibited in a particular area of the retina is proportional to the thickness of that area, thus proving useful in imaging retinal artery occlusions. In theory, FAF would allow for better measurement of the progression or regression of the disease as compared to the current standards of measurement, which include visual acuity.

6.3.3 White Dot Syndromes

White dot syndromes refer to a constellation of rare inflammatory disorders affecting the retina, RPE, and choroid [16,17]. Diagnosis of a white dot syndrome in a patient is often challenging due to the similarities in the presentation among different disorders. FAF could prove a valuable diagnostic tool in helping with this diagnostic challenge [18].

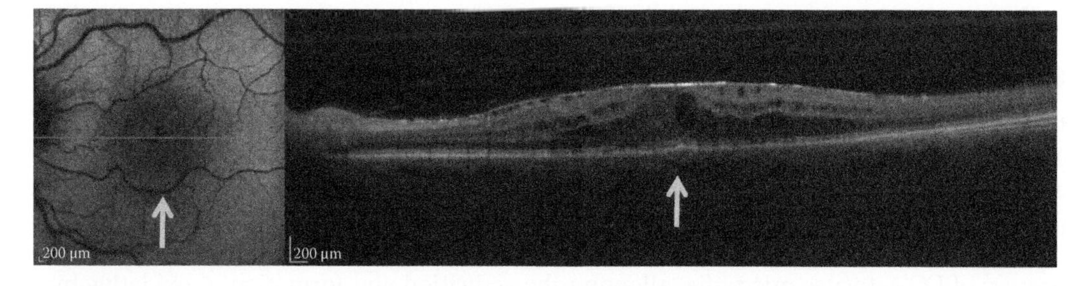

FIGURE 6.7
A diffuse area of hypoautofluorescence area involving the fovea and the surrounding area in an eye with cystic macular edema associated with central retinal vein occlusion. Arrow on the left side of the image is pointing towards the area of hypoautofluorescence and arrow on the right side is pointing towards cystic changes in the macula.

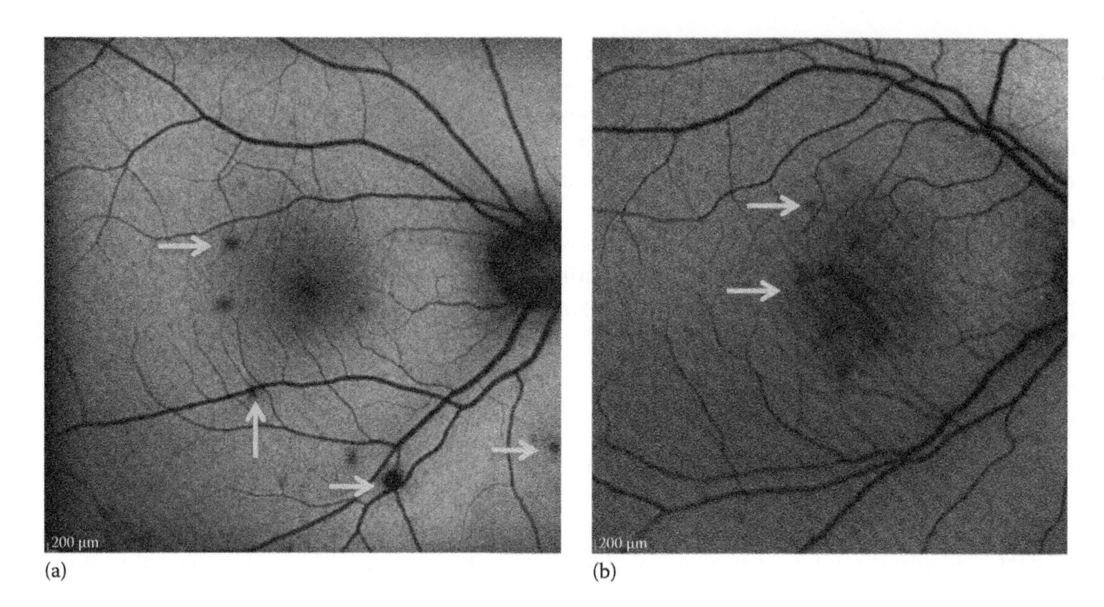

FIGURE 6.8
Well-circumscribed lesions of multifocal choroiditis within and outside the arcades as shown by the arrows in a stable eye showing hypoautofluorescence (a). Similar lesions of PIC located within the arcades as indicated by the arrows showing hypoautofluorescence (b).

Not all forms of white dot syndromes actually produce white dots, but they all do express lesions in the fundus [17]. The ones that do produce white dots, such as multifocal choroiditis and punctate inner choroidapathy (PIC), may exhibit hyper- or hypoautofluorescence on FAF in the lesions and the areas around the dots (Figure 6.8) [19]. In a study conducted by Yeh et al., it was found that FAF hypofluorescence around the foveal area was positively correlated with poorer visual acuity [18]. Such correlation provides important evidence, as hypofluorescence caused by inflammation of the RPE is associated with decreased vision.

AF as a diagnostic tool may therefore provide more accurate information than visual acuity on the status of a patient with white dot syndrome, as there are many other impediments that can affect visual acuity.

6.3.4 Diabetic Retinopathy

In diabetic retinopathy (DR), the mechanism of accumulation of LP in the retina is different as compared to AMD. LP is composed of different products of peroxidation of lipids and proteins; for this reason, LP is considered a marker of oxidative processes in the retina [20]. Xu et al. showed that accumulation of LP in mice might be found in greater proportion in microglia than in the RPE [21]. As is currently understood, the pathophysiologic process of DR activates microglia, allowing the activation and formation of oxidative byproducts and therefore formation of LP granules, which can be detected by FAF imaging (Figure 6.9) [20,21]. Currently, not a lot of work has been done to exploit the usefulness of FAF imaging in DR patients. However, based on animal studies and small clinical studies, FAF has shown tremendous potential, and it is expected to become an important imaging technique in caring for patients with DR.

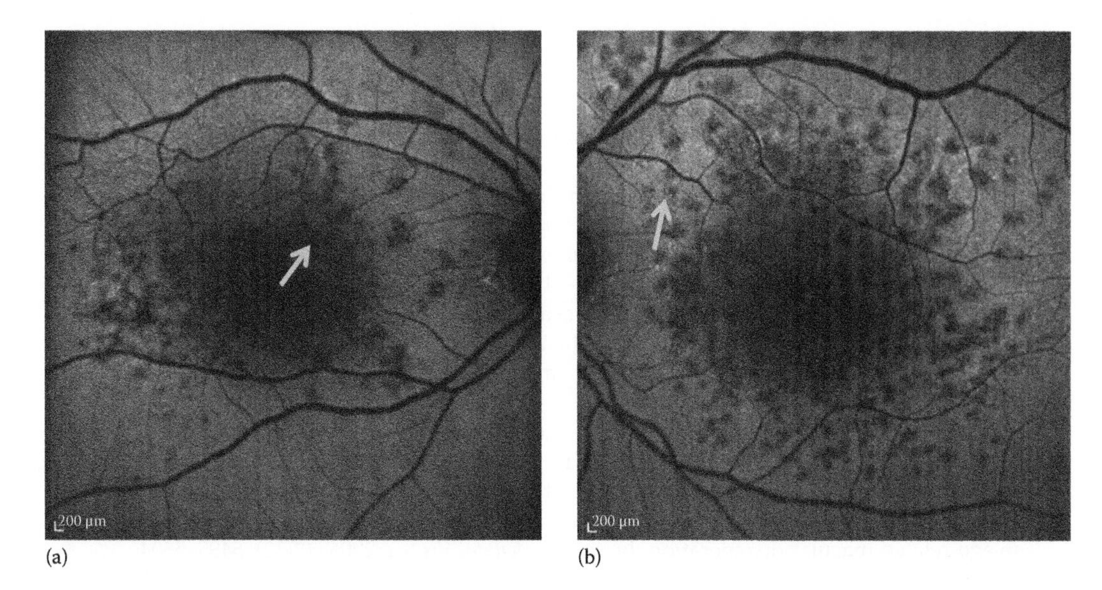

(a) (b)

FIGURE 6.9
Numerous small well-circumscribed areas of hypoautofluorescence (marked by the arrows), left eye (b) more than the right eye (a) in eyes with diabetic macular edema representing leakage from microaneurysms.

6.4 Limitations and Future Directions

The use of FAF to map natural or pathological presence of fluorophores has influenced our understanding and interpretation of various kinds of retinal diseases. The future of this imaging technique may allow further understanding of retinal diseases as certain aspects of this technique begin to be greater understood. It may also be used in patients with retinal dystrophies to access the potential functional preservation of the outer retina, which would therefore have implications in monitoring or evaluation of treatments for this in the future [19]. At present, most limitations arise from the fluorescent properties of other ocular structures, as well as the resolution of the image and the time taken to acquire a good quality image [1,18]. The optical media and the lens, which may present confounding background noise, can influence the intensity of fluorescence coming from the retina. Improving the acquisition method of this technique can increase the resolution and reduce the background noise in the topographic mapping of fluorophores [1,18]. With increasing age, fluorescent properties of the lens also change, which makes the uses of FAF in older patients more difficult to interpret. Presently, scanning laser ophthalmoscopy (SLO) addresses the limitations of reduced intensities of AF and the fluorescent crystalline lens; yet, this technique is limited by the optical properties of the eye. Therefore, further advancements in AF using SLO need to address these limitations in order to improve image resolution [1,18]. In the attempt to reduce background noise and improve image contrast, new developments are currently being made. Such developments include real-time averaging, where mean images are obtained to effectively reduce background noise. In addition, 55° wide-field view image acquisition with the use of a new lens highlights recent developments in FAF [1]. Thus, the applications of FAF most likely will remain protean, with future advancements confirming (or disproving) the use of this technology in the management of ocular diseases.

References

1. Schmitz-Valckenberg, S. et al., Fundus autofluorescence imaging: Review and perspectives. *Retina*, 2008. **28**(3): 385–409.
2. Strauss, O., The retinal pigment epithelium in visual function. *Physiol Rev*, 2005. **85**: 845–881. doi:10.1152/physrev.00021.2004.
3. Lambris, J.D. and A.P. Adamis, *Inflammation and Retinal Disease: Complement Biology and Pathology*. New York: Springer, 2010. pp. 63–74 (Print).
4. Mathew, R., E. Papavasileiou, and S. Sivaprasad, Autofluorescence and high-definition optical coherence tomography of retinal artery occlusions. *Clin Ophthalmol*, 2010. **4**: 1159–1163.
5. Boon, C.J. et al., Fundus autofluorescence imaging of retinal dystrophies. *Vision Res*, 2008. **48**(26): 2569–2577.
6. Schmitz-Valckenberg, S. et al., Fundus autofluorescence and progression of age-related macular degeneration. *Surv Ophthalmol*, 2009. **54**(1): 96–117.
7. Lim, L.S. et al., Age-related macular degeneration. *Lancet*, 2012. **379**(9827): 1728–1738.
8. Smith, R.T. et al., Autofluorescence characteristics of early, atrophic, and high-risk fellow eyes in age-related macular degeneration. *Invest Ophthalmol Vis Sci*, 2006. **47**(12): 5495–5504.
9. Hopkins, J., A. Walsh, and U. Chakravarthy, Fundus autofluorescence in age-related macular degeneration: An epiphenomenon? *Invest Ophthalmol Vis Sci*, 2006. **47**(6): 2269–2271.
10. Bearelly, S. et al., Use of fundus autofluorescence images to predict geographic atrophy progression. *Retina*, 2011. **31**(1): 81–86.
11. Bindewald, A. et al., Classification of abnormal fundus autofluorescence patterns in the junctional zone of geographic atrophy in patients with age related macular degeneration. *Br J Ophthalmol*, 2005. **89**(7): 874–878.
12. Bindewald, A. et al., Classification of fundus autofluorescence patterns in early age-related macular disease. *Invest Ophthalmol Vis Sci*, 2005. **46**(9): 3309–3314.
13. Lois, N. et al., Fundus autofluorescence in patients with age-related macular degeneration and high risk of visual loss. *Am J Ophthalmol*, 2002. **133**(3): 341–349.
14. Midena, E. et al., Microperimetry and fundus autofluorescence in patients with early age-related macular degeneration. *Br J Ophthalmol*, 2007. **91**(11): 1499–1503.
15. Sharma, S., Ophthaproblem. Central retinal arterial occlusion. *Can Fam Physician*, 1997. **43**: 1513–1520.
16. Abu-Yaghi, N.E. et al., White dot syndromes: A 20-year study of incidence, clinical features, and outcomes. *Ocul Immunol Inflamm*, 2011. **19**(6): 426–430.
17. Matsumoto, Y., S.P. Haen, and R.F. Spaide, The white dot syndromes. *Compr Ophthalmol Update*, 2007. **8**(4): 179–200; discussion 203–204.
18. Yeh, S. et al., Fundus autofluorescence imaging of the white dot syndromes. *Arch Ophthalmol*, 2010. **128**(1): 46–56.
19. Penha, F.M. et al., Fundus autofluorescence in multiple evanescent white dot syndrome. *Case Rep Ophthalmol Med*, 2011. **2011**: 807565.
20. Vujosevic, S. et al., Diabetic macular edema: Fundus autofluorescence and functional correlations. *Invest Ophthalmol Vis Sci*, 2011. **52**(1): 442–448.
21. Xu, H. et al., Age-dependent accumulation of lipofuscin in perivascular and subretinal microglia in experimental mice. *Aging Cell*, 2008. **7**(1): 58–68.

7

Needs/Requirements and Design of Retinal Imaging and Image Processing Methods for Diabetic Retinopathy in the Indian Context

Sudipta Mukhopadhyay, Amod Gupta, and Reema Bansal

CONTENTS

7.1 Diabetes in India

Diabetes is a major public health disease globally. About 6.6% (285 million people) of the world's population is affected by diabetes mellitus (DM), and according to the International Diabetes Federation, this number is expected to increase to 380 million by 2025.[1] Nearly 80% of people with diabetes are in developing countries, mainly India and China. India tops the list with 40.9 million diabetics (followed by China with 39.8 million) and is called the *diabetes capital of the world*.[2] India constitutes about 15% of the global burden of diabetes. By 2025, this number is expected to be 70 million. Every fifth diabetic in the world is an Indian. The first phase of a national study to determine the prevalence of diabetes and prediabetes (impaired fasting glucose and/or impaired glucose tolerance) in India estimated that in 2011, Maharashtra would have 6 million individuals with diabetes, Tamil Nadu 4.8 million, Jharkhand 0.96 million, and Chandigarh 0.12 million.[3]

7.2 Diabetic Retinopathy

Diabetic retinopathy (DR) is a vascular disorder affecting the microvascular system of retina due to prolonged hyperglycemia. If left untreated, it results in irreversible blindness. It affects both type 1 and type 2 diabetes patients. Epidemiological studies have shown that nearly all with type 1 and 75% of type 2 diabetics will develop DR after 15 years duration of diabetes.[4,5] Visual morbidity from DR is a major public health problem globally. It is largely preventable and treatable, if detected in time.

7.3 Diabetic Retinopathy in India

In Indian subcontinent, the prevalence rate of DR is reported to be 12% to 37% in type 2 DM. It is the sixth common cause of blindness in India. Asymptomatic nature of DR in its early stage prevents an early visit to an ophthalmologist, and hence, the occurrence of DR goes undetected until a late stage when the patient becomes visually symptomatic. The progression to the advanced stage of the disease occurs due to ignorance among both the people and the physicians. Although laser photocoagulation largely treats moderate visual loss in DR (sight-threatening retinopathy), prognosis is usually poor in further advanced stages. Majority of the hospitals that treat diabetes do not treat DR and do not even screen diabetic patients for DR. Screening all the patients with DM for early detection and timely treatment is the only way to preserve vision in these patients. Fundus screening for evaluation of DR is a valuable and necessary cost-effective health strategy for prevention of blindness. Fundus images at different stages of DR are shown in Figure 7.1.

Although diabetes is known to largely affect the affluent, it is fast becoming a problem of the poor Indians due to various lifestyle modifications and urbanization. Further, they are more prone to complications that lead to blindness due to poor access to healthcare facilities and lack of knowledge about the presence of diabetes and the need for visiting an eye specialist.

7.4 Healthcare Model

From Figure 7.2, we get that the present that is traditional healthcare system is manual in nature. It is inefficient as we take action only when the pain or discomfort forces us to visit the doctor. As the disease has already crept in by that time, the recovery is slow and the disease management becomes costly. In summary, we can tell the traditional healthcare model is (1) manual, (2) inefficient, (3) slow, and (4) costly (*MISC* model).

On the other hand, the proposed healthcare model focuses on prevention. It leverages the advancement in automation and thereby depends on periodic monitoring. The cost of health management is brought down as the corrective action is done in a planned manner using a network of knowledgebase, doctors and paramedics. In summary, we can say that the proposed healthcare model is (1) preventive in nature, (2) automated, (3) inexpensive, and (4) planned (*PAIP* model).

7.5 Screening for DR

In the PAIP model, the first step is to screen the entire risk group of the country for DR. To scan the entire risk group, we need to take the help of automation in the form

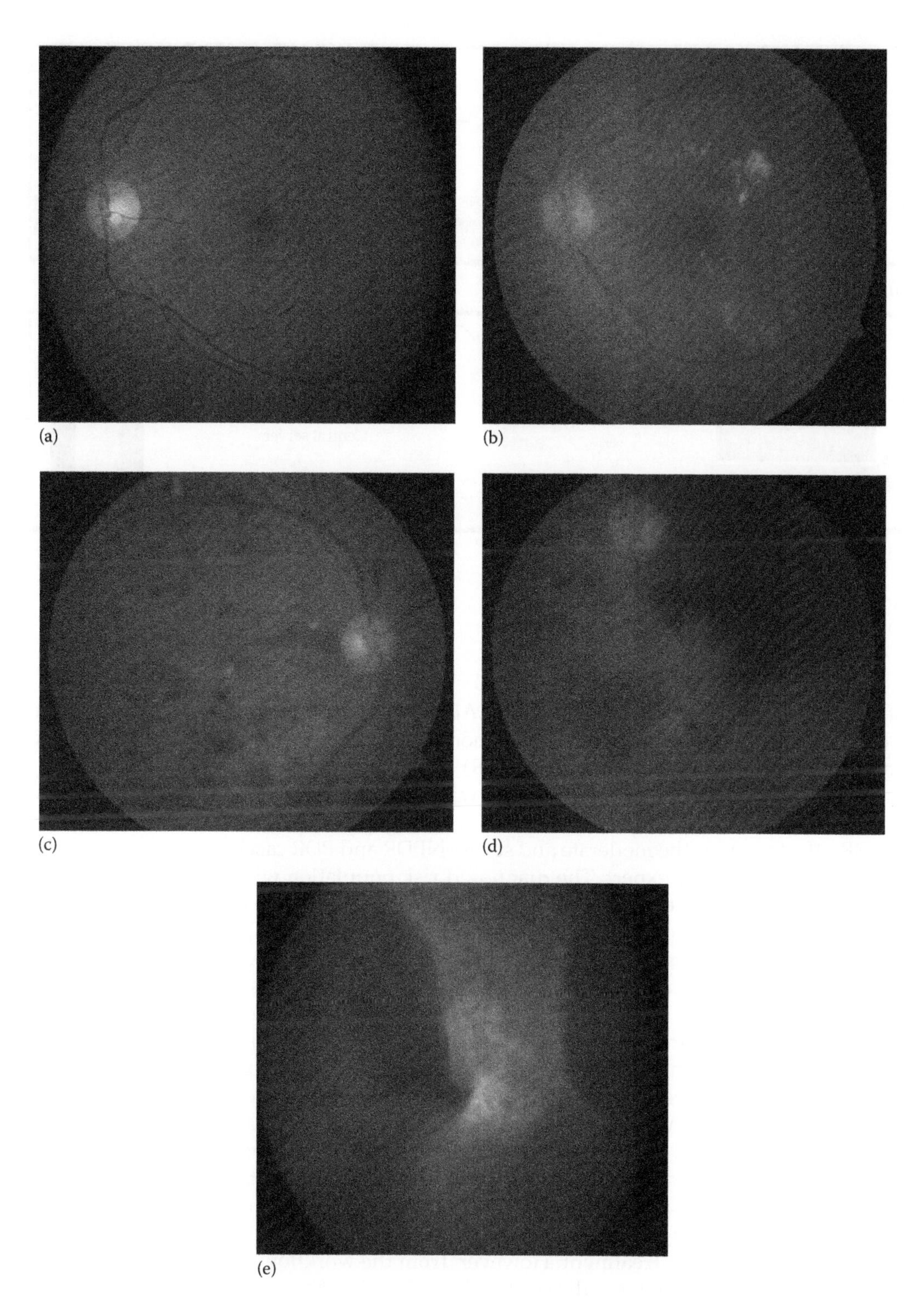

FIGURE 7.1
(See color insert.) Different stages of DR: (a) early NPDR, (b) moderate NPDR, (c) severe NPDR, (d) PDR with vitreous and subhyaloid hemorrhage, and (e) PDR with tractional retinal detachment.

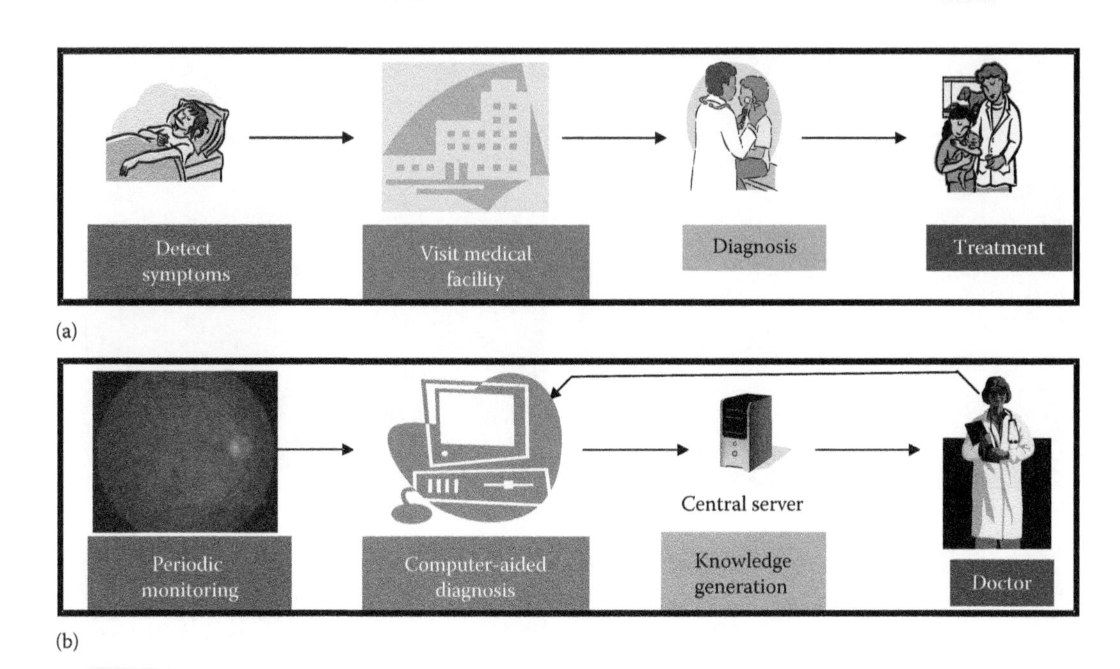

FIGURE 7.2
(a) Traditional (b) and preventive healthcare models.

of computer-aided diagnosis (CAD). The CAD should differentiate the no DR and mild DR cases from the moderate and severe nonproliferative diabetic retinopathy (NPDR) and proliferative diabetic retinopathy (PDR) cases. Staging of disease will further help the treatment. Output of the captured data will be analyzed to find pattern of the spread of disease across the geographical location for planning and to send the fundus images of the DR-affected cases (the moderate and severe NPDR and PDR cases) to the nearest health center with retinopathy expert. The diagnosed risk population will also be asked to visit the nearest retinopathy expert for treatment, where the reports are sent.

The gold standard for evaluating DR is the seven-standard stereoscopic 30° field photographs.[6] The American Diabetes Association and the American Academy of Ophthalmology recommends screening through a dilated fundus examination with stereoscopic evaluation of the posterior pole on slit lamp biomicroscopy.[7,8] Direct ophthalmoscopy through an undilated pupil, nonstereoscopic 45° retinal photography through an undilated pupil, and nonstereoscopic 45° retinal photography through a dilated pupil are the alternative methods used for screening. Digital photography is preferred to screen DR because the images can be stored and retrieved for analysis and review as and when required. In India mydriatic cameras are regularly used for screening and diagnosis. The paramedics will capture the image using mydriatic camera followed by diagnosis by the retina specialists. The workflow of screening is captured in Figure 7.3. After capturing the image, we can run it through the CAD system to identify the population needing immediate treatment. However, from the workflow, it is clear that even for the first person on the queue will require about 40 min of stay in the hospital premise. It will not only make the screening very slow and unattractive to the population, it will also demand a huge infrastructure to accommodate the participants in the screening program.

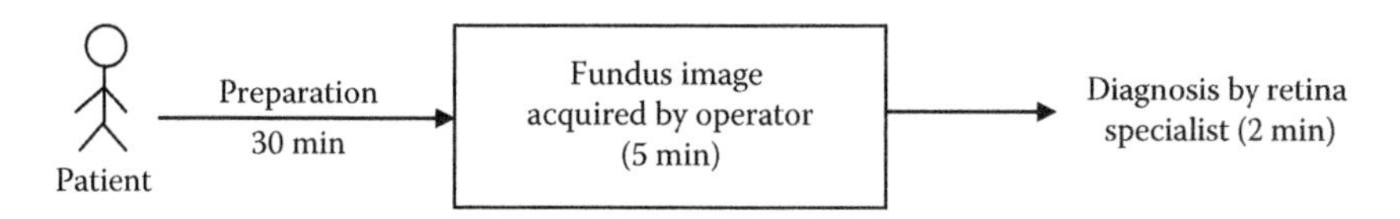

FIGURE 7.3
Block diagram of present DR screening protocol using mydriatic camera.

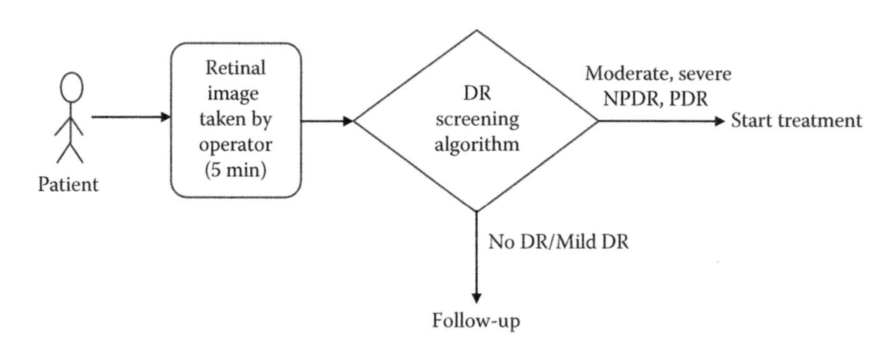

FIGURE 7.4
Block diagram of proposed DR screening tool using nonmydriatic camera.

Nonmydriatic cameras have been used for the last 25 years for assessing DR.[9,10] The need for dilating the pupil for photographing the fundus is eliminated due to their infrared focusing system. Using nonmydriatic camera, the screening time will reduce from 37 to 6 min as shown in Figure 7.4. In United States of America and Europe, regular screening of DR using nonmydriatic fundus camera is being widely recommended. Although this new generation of nonmydriatic cameras is an ideal tool for screening for DR, limited data are available regarding its use in the developing countries.

In our experience, although majority of the patients attending diabetic clinic could be photographed on the same visit with the nonmydriatic camera for detecting any level of DR, a significant proportion of them had poor quality fundus images that could not be graded in an undilated pupil (unpublished data). The need for dilation in these eyes increased the number of visits required by the patient just to be screened for assessing DR, and also increased the number of photographs taken and stored in the system. In Indian eyes, the nonmydriatic camera had a poor sensitivity and a high rate of ungradeable images, thereby limiting its use as a perfect screening tool in the population. This is largely attributed to the dark color of the iris in Indian eyes. Patients with dark colored iris are known to have a faster and stronger pupillary contraction as compared to those with light colored iris and are more uncomfortable with the flash of the fundus camera than those with light iris.

The other option of routinely dilating the pupil for screening purposes is discouraging to the patient as it disturbs daily activities and decreases patient compliance for attending the screening test. The concept of targeted mydriasis in some of the patients undergoing screening was proposed to achieve gradable diabetic screening photographs by identifying certain clinical variables.[11] To overcome these challenges, we need to have an imaging system that could have an increased sensitivity to detect DR at the earliest so as to prevent vision threatening complications of DR.

While in western countries, diabetes usually affects older people, it is much more common in young to middle-aged adults in Asian countries,[12] affecting the nation's health and economy in an adverse manner.

7.6 Telemedicine in India

The major limitations of currently available tools are artifacts and poor resolution. An ideal ophthalmic imaging system should be able to capture both anterior and posterior segments of the eye. It should be a wide-angle imaging system, with at least 50° of the fundus captured in a single image. The machine or the apparatus placed in the base hospital should be simple to operate, so that it can be handled easily by an operator with only a basic training of ophthalmic photography. It should be comfortable and convenient for the patient as well. The technology needs to be cost-effective, with low maintenance cost to be placed in rural settings, and should have broadband connectivity. While transferring the fundus images to the remote centers, it should be possible to compare the patient's images with standard graded photographs to allow grading or staging of the disease. Another important prerequisite is an early and prompt identification of the patient's fundus image among the several images available in the database for retrieval purpose. This could be facilitated by providing all possible templates for the various stages of the disease.

A community-based telemedicine unit (vision center) should be made available for a cluster of about 7–10 villages, covering a population of about 70,000–100,000. Ideally, the basic equipment for the photographer/technician should have a camera with a computer desk, a printer, and a broadband connectivity. The base hospital should have at least a server, broadband connection, software for image analysis, and facility for remote printing. The remote centers should have a printer, automated software for image analysis and interpretation without human intervention, and facility for audiovisual teleconferencing. A public–private collaboration is necessary to implement a perfect screening imaging system.

7.7 Social and Cultural Aspects of Retinal Imaging in India

A large proportion of DR incidence can be averted if there is early diagnosis and appropriate treatment. However, there are numerous barriers to the compulsory eye examination in all diabetics, such as socioeconomic factors, lack of referrals, poor access to healthcare system, lack of knowledge among people, insufficient number of ophthalmologists, and lack of networking between physicians, diabetologists and ophthalmologists. Although most diabetic patients often visit a healthcare facility for their multisystem involvement, their eye disease remains undetected because it is not looked for until the patient is symptomatic.

Majority of the Indian population is rural-based. According to the 2011 census, the total number of villages in India is 640,867. The major *population-based limitations* are ignorance about DR, illiteracy, and poor accessibility to healthcare facilities. Agricultural and harvesting seasons pose a major time constraint among the villagers, particularly for the spouses and elderly people. While community-based telemedicine is ideal for densely populated regions, mobile setups will be required in regions with sparse population. In urban areas too, busy office schedules pose a significant time constraint. In urban areas, there are healthcare facilities nearby, but the people may not like to spoil their productive working hours to participate in the screening. For them, unmanned kiosk for screening will be a better idea, which can run 24 h like the ATM machine. However, to make it successful, the interface should be robust and easy enough for a literate person to operate the screening setup using a fundus camera and computer. On the other hand, DR screening kiosk will require the least running cost compared to the screening teams running from mobile healthcare units and primary healthcare centers. In Figure 7.5, the overall flow of information for the DR screening is described.

The *physician-based constraints* include a relatively low number of ophthalmologists (about 16,000) in India. Of these, only about 2000 are trained for diagnosing and treating DR, and only a few hundred can treat diabetic macular edema, which is the main cause for causing moderate visual loss in patients with DR. The other limitations are posed by the *disease-based factors*. DR is an asymptomatic disease in the early stage. Patients become symptomatic in advanced stage. It is a truly preventable blindness by an early detection and intervention. Currently, there are no biomarkers for detecting early retinopathy. High prevalence and limited resources account for low treatable numbers of patients. The main goal of treating these patients is to preserve vision and prevent further deterioration of vision.

At present, screening in India is being undertaken in various ways such as eye camps, fundus evaluation of all diabetics attending eye care facilities for any ocular problem, and telemedicine where the digital retinal images are analyzed by remotely placed experts.

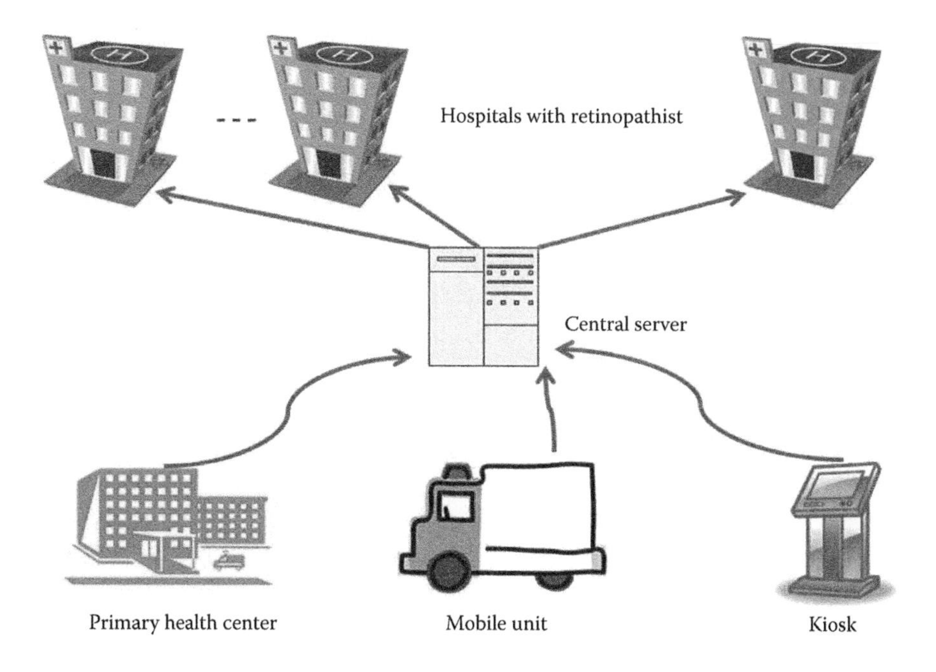

FIGURE 7.5
Block diagram of flow of information in DR screening.

The need of the hour is to develop an efficient imaging system that can be installed not only at a national level hospital, but also at the grassroot level primary healthcare units so as to be able to image a common man unaware of the problems related to diabetes and DR.

References

1. International Diabetes Federation. A summary of the figures and key findings. In *The IDF Diabetes Atlas*. 5th edn. Brussels, Belgium: International Diabetes Federation; 2011.
2. Shaw JE, Sicree RA, Zimmet PZ. Global estimates of the prevalence of diabetes for 2010 and 2030. *Diabetes Res Clin Practice* 2010;87:4–14.
3. Anjana RM, Pradeepa R, Deepa M et al. Prevalence of diabetes and prediabetes (impaired fasting glucose and/or impaired glucose tolerance) in urban and rural India: Phase I results of the Indian Council of Medical Research-INdia DIABetes (ICMR-INDIAB) study. *Diabetologia* 2011;54:3022–3027.
4. Klein R, Klein BE, Moss SE, Davis MD, DeMets DL. The Wisconsin Epidemiologic Study of Diabetic Retinopathy. II. Prevalence and risk of diabetic retinopathy when age at diagnosis is less than 30 years. *Arch Ophthalmol* 1984;102:520–526.
5. Klein R, Klein BEK, Moss SE, Davis MD, DeMets DL. The Wisconsin Epidemiologic Study of Diabetic Retinopathy. III. Prevalence and risk of diabetic retinopathy when age at diagnosis is 30 or more years. *Arch Ophthalmol* 1984;102:527–532.
6. Early Treatment Retinopathy Study Research Group. Grading diabetic retinopathy from stereoscopic colour fundus photographs—An extension of the modified Airlie House classification: ETDRS report number 10. *Ophthalmology* 1991;98(5 Suppl.):786–806.
7. Fong DS, Lloyd A, Gardner T et al. Retinopathy in diabetes. *Diabetes Care* 2004;27:S84–S87.
8. American Academy of Ophthalmology Retina Panel. Preferred Practice Pattern® Guidelines. Diabetic Retinopathy. San Francisco, CA: American Academy of Ophthalmology; 2008. Available at www.aao.org/ppp.
9. Ryder REJ, Vora JP, Atiea JA, Owens DR, Hayes TM, Young S. Possible new method to improve detection of diabetic retinopathy: Polaroid non-mydriatic retinal photography. *Br Med J* 1985;291:1256–1257.
10. Williams R, Nussey S, Humphry R, Thompson G. Assessment of non-mydriatic photography in detection of diabetic retinopathy. *Br Med J* 1986;293:1140–1142.
11. Dervan EWJ, O'Brien PD, Hobbs H, Acheson R, Flitcroft DI. Targeted mydriasis strategies for diabetic retinopathy screening clinics. *Eye* 2010;24:1207–1212.
12. Chan JC, Malik V, Jia W et al. Diabetes in Asia: Epidemiology, risk factors, and pathophysiology. *JAMA* 2009;301:2129–2140.

8

Application of Ocular Fundus Photography and Angiography

Caroline Ka Lin Chee, Patrick A. Santiago, Gopal Lingam, Mandeep S. Singh, Thet Naing, Aria E. Mangunkusumo, and Mohamed Naeem Naser

CONTENTS

8.1 Introduction

The fundus of eye is the back portion of the interior of the eyeball, visible through the pupil by use of the ophthalmoscope. In this chapter, imaging of the ocular fundus with color photography, photography with filters, and fluorescence angiography will be discussed.

8.1.1 Examination of the Fundus and Angiography

The most basic of examination of the retinal fundus can be achieved using the direct ophthalmoscope (Figure 8.1a). This portable handheld instrument produces an upright, virtual, monocular, and magnified view (15×) of the retina. It allows a quick view of the optic nerve and macula, as well as the surrounding vasculature. The limitations of the direct ophthalmoscope are the following: (1) it is a monocular instrument—the observer only uses one eye—thus cannot provide a 3D view required to detect pathology such as retinal edema; (2) the field of view is small, thus viewing of the peripheral retina is difficult; (3) it needs the examiner to position his/her head very close to the patient to be able to see the fundus; (4) high degrees of refractive errors can interfere with a good visualization; and (5) since illumination provided by the halogen lamp in the direct ophthalmoscope is limited, any medial opacity can severely impair one's ability to see the fundus. The major advantage of the monocular direct ophthalmoscope is its portability, ability to use by the bedside, and the ease with which it can be learnt—making it the instrument of choice for most nonophthalmologists who are mostly interested in visualizing just the optic disc.

The binocular indirect ophthalmoscope (*BIO*), which is used in combination with a handheld lens, provides a wide field of view, allowing a more rapid scanning of the entire retina, particularly the peripheral retina (Figure 8.1b). The disadvantages are that it has a lower magnification (2–3×) and produces an inverted real image. With scleral depression, this allows examination up to the ora. Although the BIO allows for a stereo view of the retina, its relatively low magnification limits the ability to detect small, subtle lesions in the fundus.

Slit-lamp biomicroscopy is favored by many ophthalmologists. This is performed with a handheld lens and a slit-lamp ophthalmoscope and provides a magnified, stereoscopic view (Figure 8.1c). Optically, it is similar to indirect ophthalmoscopy since it provides an inverted real image. However, the adjustable magnification allows detection of subtle posterior segment signs such as retinal edema, especially cystoid macular edema and glaucomatous optic nerve changes. While observation of the retina is possible with the various modalities, recording by the human observer using retina drawings is certainly not ideal, even if one is skilled and practiced. Retinal photography is essential for adequate and accurate recording of the appearance of the retina and following the changes over time.

8.1.2 Fundus Photography

The earliest recording of the appearance of the retina was made by hand drawing, just like old botanical and zoological specimens. Fundus photography revolutionized the ability to capture accurately the appearance of fundus and changes over time, allowing exponential advances in the study of the eye, patient care, training of health-care

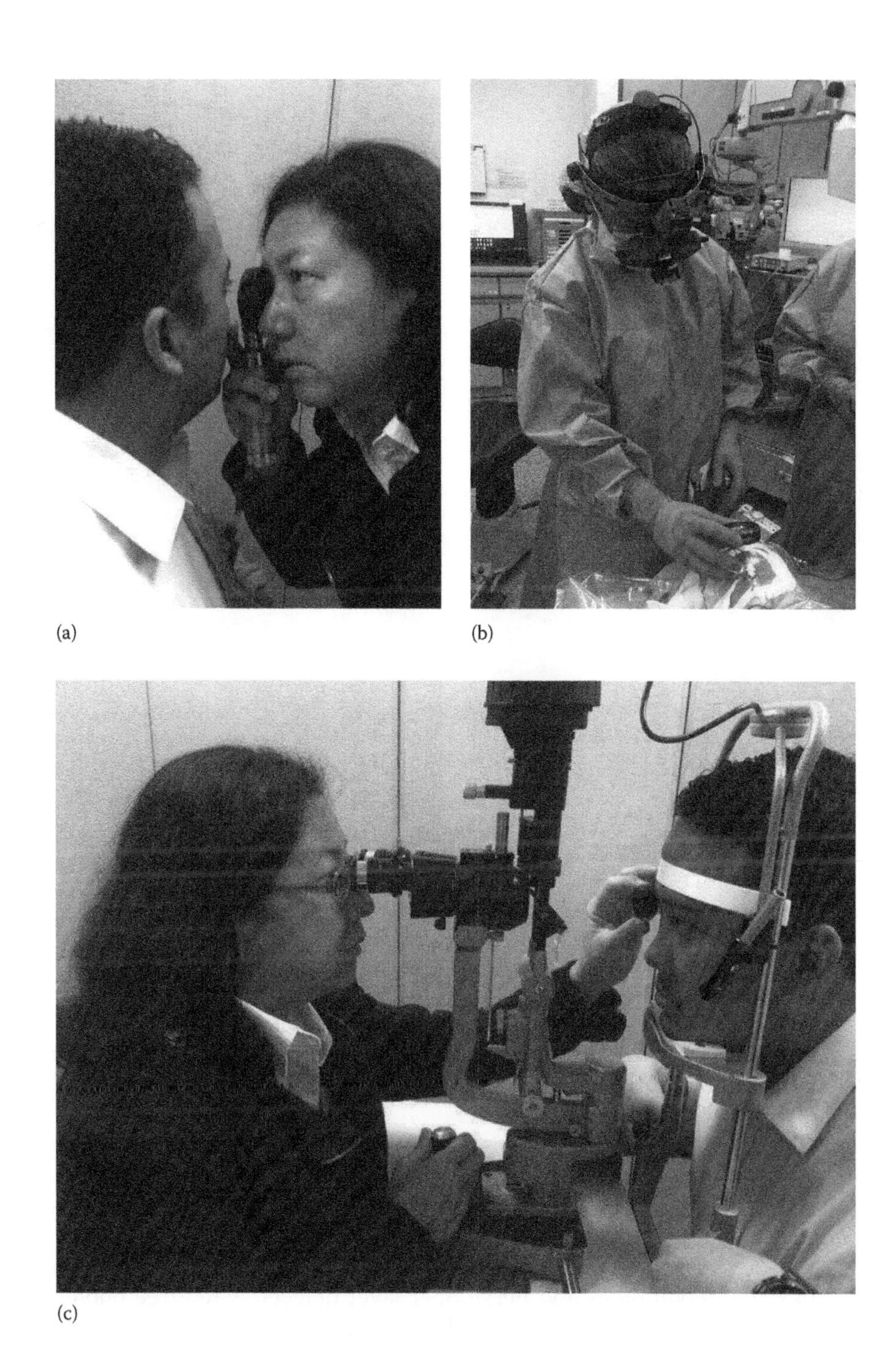

FIGURE 8.1
Instruments for viewing the fundus. (a) Using direct ophthalmoscope; (b) using the indirect ophthalmoscope, a head-mounted ophthalmoscope with a handheld lens, examining an eye in the operating theater; and (c) slit-lamp biomicroscopy, using a slit-lamp and a handheld lens.

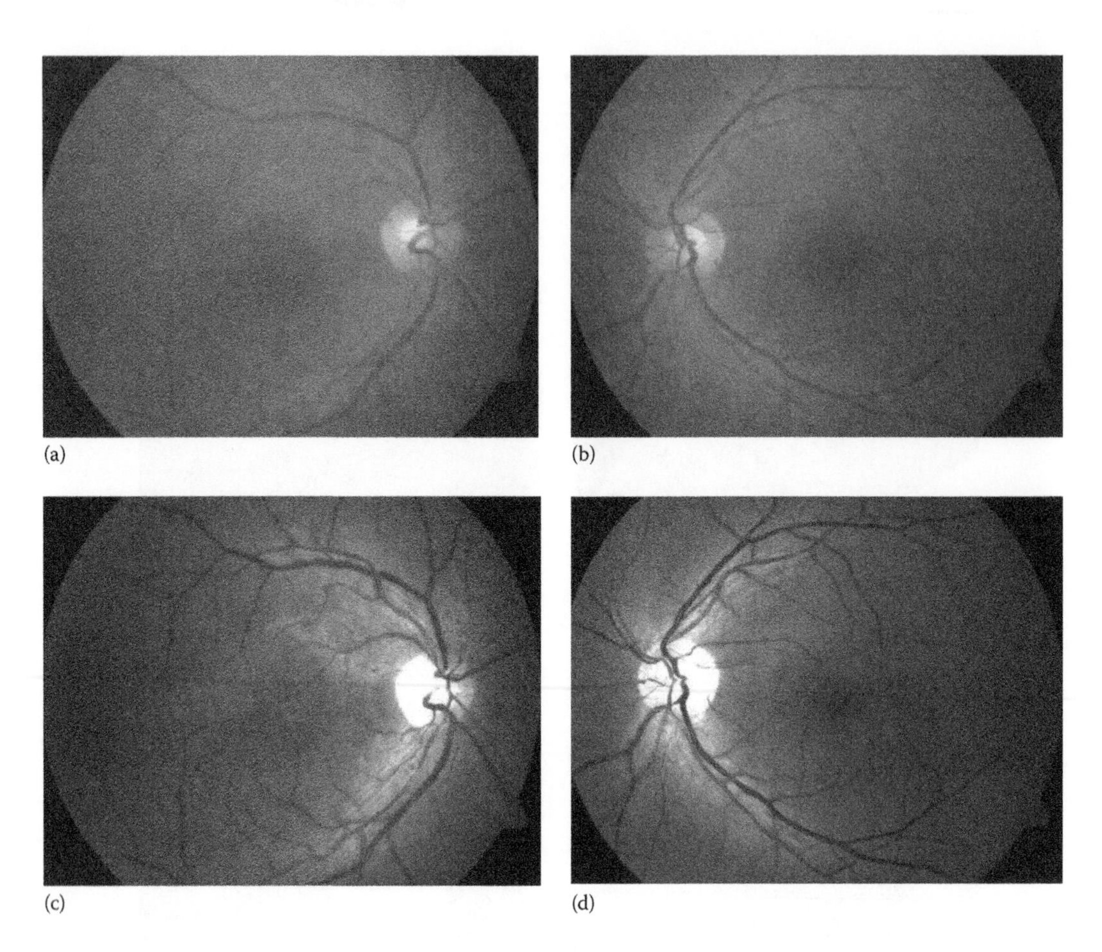

FIGURE 8.2
(See color insert.) Fundus photographs. (a, b) Color fundus photographs of the right and left eyes and (c, d) red-free fundus photographs of the right and left eyes using a green filter, about 540–570 nm.

professionals, and research. Color fundus photography (Figure 8.2a and b) is commonly used as a screening tool for diabetic retinopathy, a major cause of preventable blindness. It was also used for community-based surveys of eye diseases such as age-related macular degeneration (ARMD).

The use of filters in fundus photography enables certain features of the fundus to be accentuated. A red-free or green monochromatic photograph (Figure 8.2c and d) is obtained by using a green filter, about 540–570 nm, which blocks the red wavelengths. It highlights superficial retinal lesions well, such as retinal blood vessels and hemorrhages, as well as pale lesions such as drusen and exudates. It brings out contrast in conditions such as in epiretinal membranes and nerve fiber layer defects. A red-free photograph is usually taken as a baseline fundus photograph before angiography.

8.1.3 Fundus Angiography

Fundus angiography utilizes the fluorescent dyes fluorescein and indocyanine green (ICG) to image the blood vessels and other structures of the fundus. It revolutionized the understanding of physiology and pathology of the retina and many retinal and choroidal diseases and remains an essential investigation for diagnosis, treatment, and follow-up in the management of these diseases.

Fundus fluorescein angiography (FFA) was established many years before ICGA and is more useful for imaging retinal and retinal vascular disease such as cystoid macular edema (Figure 8.3a through f) and diabetic retinopathy (Figure 8.4b through d).

Indocyanine green angiography (ICGA) is more useful for imaging choroidal diseases (Figure 8.6c through f). ICGA cameras are not as commonly available in ophthalmology

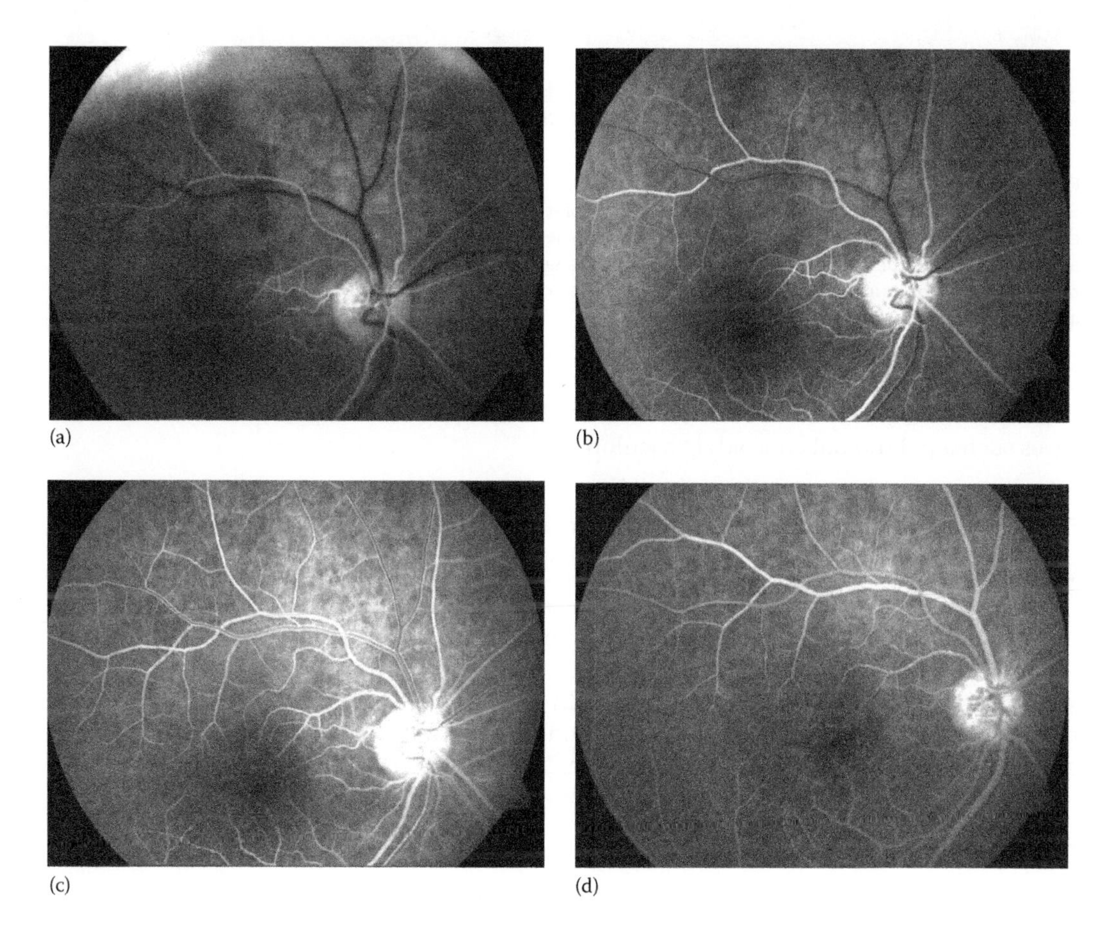

FIGURE 8.3
FFA of a right eye with cystoid macular edema. The color fundus photograph and red-free photograph of this eye are shown in Figure 8.2a and c. (a) Arterial phase: the background choroidal flush is present, and the arteries are filled with fluorescein dye. The veins are still unfilled and black against the background choroidal flush. (b) Early arteriovenous phase: there is laminar flow in the veins, where the fluorescein dye is prominent along the wall of the vein. The central macular area is dark because there are no vessels right in the center of the foveal avascular zone (FAZ), and increased density of xanthophyll pigment and taller RPE cells containing more melanin pigment in the area surrounding the FAZ, causing blocked fluorescence. (c) Mid arteriovenous or early venous phase: the arteries are filled, and the veins are nearly completely filled. Small spots of hyperfluorescence at the macula are beginning to appear and gradually increase over the next few frames. (d) Late arteriovenous or mid-venous phase: the veins are more prominent than the arteries.

(continued)

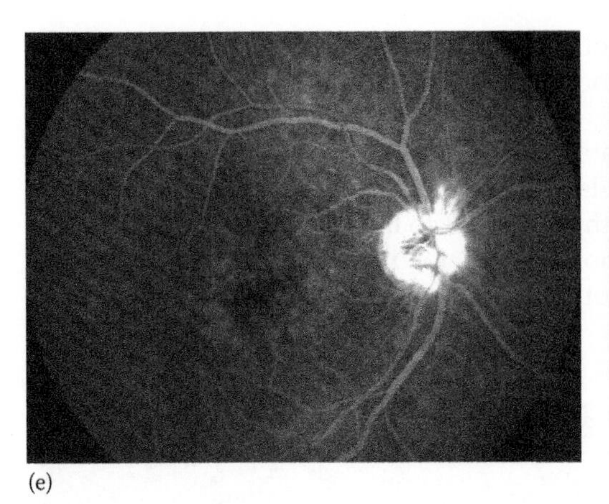
(e)

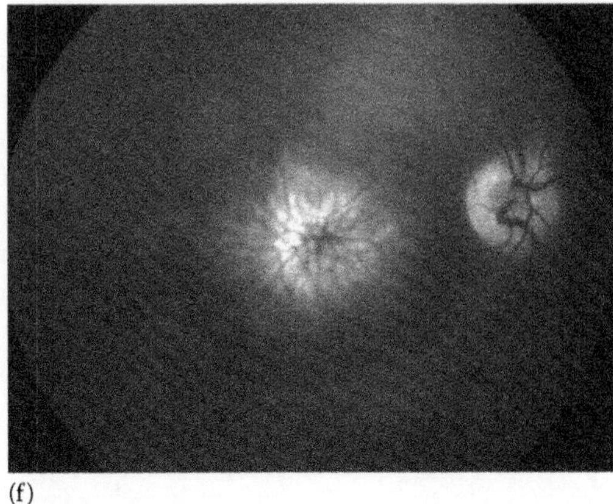
(f)

FIGURE 8.3 (continued)
FFA of a right eye with cystoid macular edema. The color fundus photograph and red-free photograph of this eye are shown in Figure 8.2a and c. (e) Late venous phase: the veins are much more prominent than the arteries. The macular hyperfluorescence is increasing and size and intensity. (f) Late phase: fluorescein has left the retinal vessels, but staining of the optic disc is present (normal). There is a petaloid pattern of hyperfluorescence at the macula demonstrating cystoid macular edema.

departments as FFA cameras. It is essential in the imaging and treatment of choroidal diseases such a polypoidal choroidal vasculopathy.

8.1.4 Fundus Reflectance and Autofluorescence

When a specific wavelength of light is projected on to the retina and reflected by the fundus structures, this is known as fundus reflectance. Filters are used to produce blue reflectance and near-infrared (NIR) reflectance in order to image the fundus (Figure 8.7a).

Autofluorescence (AF) imaging is done with excitatory and barrier filters in place. Blue-light AF uses the FFA filters (Figure 8.7b), and the fluorescence comes from fluorophores existing in the retina, for example, lipofuscin. NIR AF uses ICG filters.

8.1.5 Development of Fundus Imaging

The following chart traces the development of fundus imaging [1]:

1826	Niepce invents photography
1851	Helmholtz invents the modern ophthalmoscope
1854	Using the ophthalmoscope, Van Trigt publishes the first color fundus illustration
1871	Bayer synthesizes fluorescein
1881	Ehrlich examines aqueous flow with fluorescein in rabbits
1886	Refinement of in vivo photography of the retina
1899	Dimmer creates high-quality fundus photographs
1910	Examination of the retina and choroid using fluorescein
1926	Zeiss introduces the first commercially available fundus camera
1927	Dimmer and Pillat publish the first fundus photography atlas

1930	Application of filters to observe dyes better in the retina
1939	Fluorescein dye flow described in retinal blood vessels
1946	Edgerton introduces the electronic flash tube
1953	Electronic flash tube adapted to fundus photography
1954	Maumenee observes injected fluorescein in a patient with a retinal hemangioma
1959	Fluorescein photography with filters observed in cat retinas
1961	Novotny and Alvis described the modern fluorescein technique used today
1969	Kogure et al. performed the first ICG absorption angiography on an owl monkey
1972	Flower et al. produced first ICG fluorescence angiogram
1980	First commercial ICG fundus camera
1980s	Development of filters, infrared (IR)-sensitive videoangiography advances ICGA

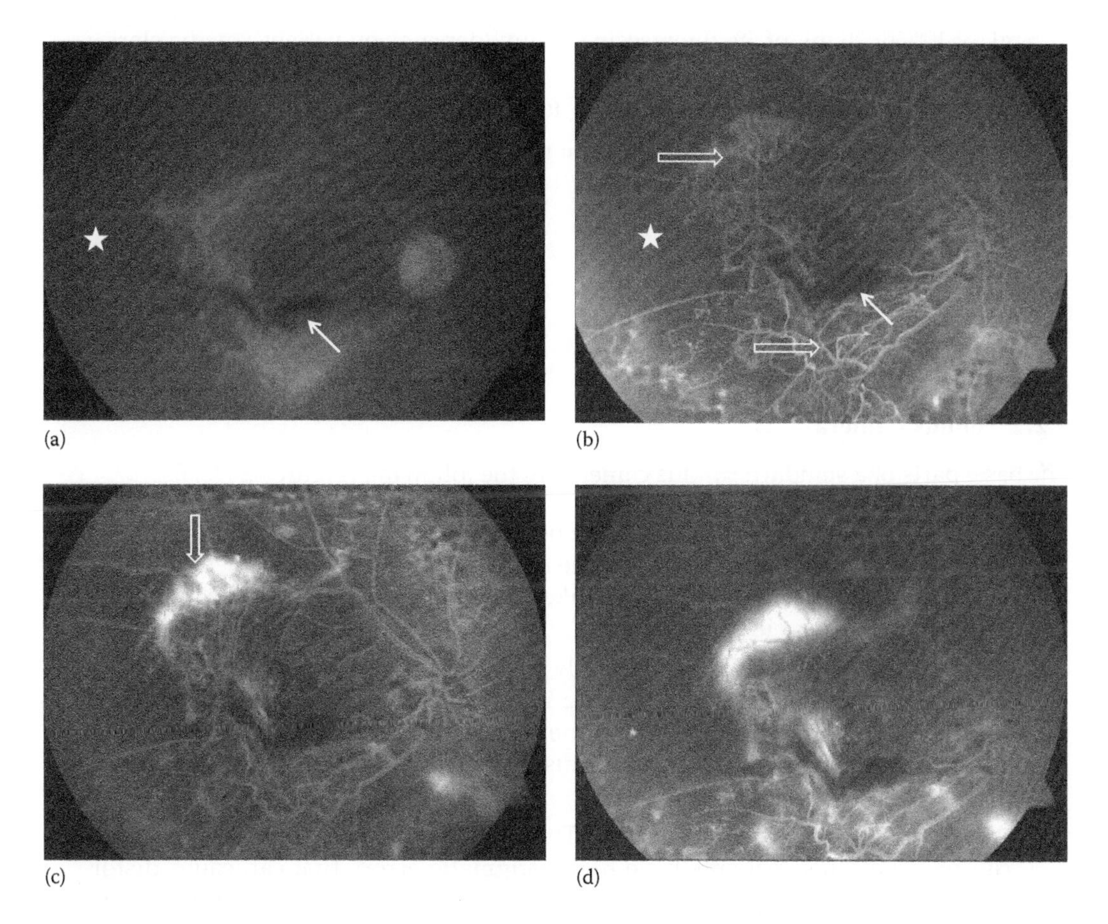

FIGURE 8.4
Fundus photograph and FFA of right eye with proliferative diabetic retinopathy. (a) There is extensive fibrosis (scar tissue) along the superior and inferior vascular arcades and preretinal hemorrhage (white arrow). The star marks the area corresponding to the nonperfusion demonstrated in (b). (b) The preretinal hemorrhage is outlined as an area of blocked fluorescence (white arrow). There is extensive neovascularization—growth of abnormal *new vessels* (two horizontal arrows pointing to the areas). There is an area of capillary nonperfusion temporal to the macula, marked by the star. (c) The vertical arrow shows the area of leakage from the new vessels (hyperfluorescence). (d) The hyperfluorescent leakage from the new vessels increases, and now there is a component of staining of the scar tissue as well.

8.2 Equipment and Procedure for Fundus Photography and Angiography

8.2.1 Equipment for Photography and Angiography

Fundus camera and accessories
Red-free or green-free filters
Matched barrier and excitation filters for FFA or ICGA
Computer software for digital photoprocessing and storage
Mydriatic (pupil-dilating) eyedrops
Intravenous cannula
5 mL syringe
5 mL of 10% or 10 mL of 5% fluorescein sodium (depends on patient's media clarity) for FFA
1 mL with 25 mg ICG or 2 mL with 50 mg ICG for ICGA
20 gauge needle to withdraw the dye from the fluorescein vial
Tourniquet
Alcohol swabs
Micropore tape
Consent for the procedure
Emergency equipment

8.2.2 Fundus Camera

The basic parts of a standard fundus camera are the following (Figure 8.5) [2,3]:

1. Angle selection lever: This changes the power of the lenses in the optical pathway. This can either increase or decrease the angle subtended by the camera. This can also modify the clarity of the image taken, depending on the glass quality of the lens built into each viewing angle.
2. Anterior segment lens: This essentially is a high-plus lens that brings the focus of the fundus camera nearer, allowing it to focus on the front part of the eye to take photographs of the anterior segment (cornea, iris, lens) of the eye. Turning the diopter compensation lens can also be done to do this in some camera models.
3. Astigmatism compensation control: This is an adjustable cylindrical lens that can be used when patients have high astigmatic errors that can cause distortions of the photograph being taken. This is also useful for photographs of the far retinal periphery as the tilt of the cornea can give astigmatic distortion of images.
4. Excitation and barrier filter slide: This is a replaceable filter slide positioned in front of either the film or the sensor of the camera.
5. Camera body/sensor: In the era of film fundus photography, this housed the camera body with its film. Modern fundus cameras have the sensor built into the body of the camera itself.

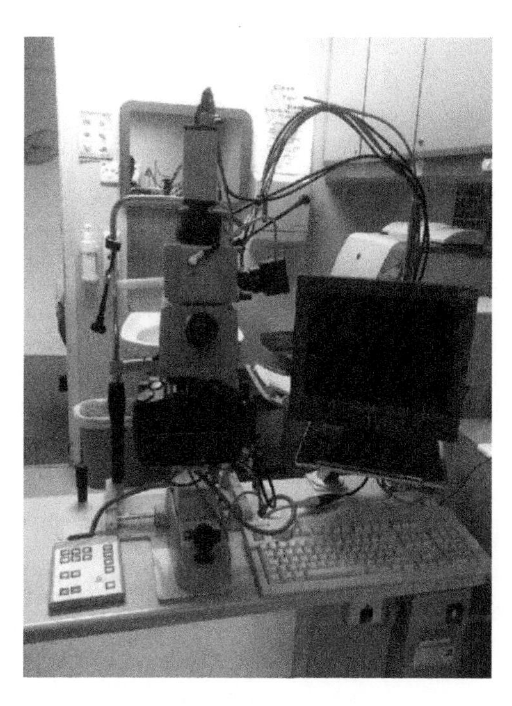

FIGURE 8.5
Imaging equipment: fundus and angiography camera.

6. Chin rest and forehead strap: Allows the patient to position his head for photography. These should be cleaned in between patients.
7. Diopter compensation lens: Places a positive or negative lens for unusually shorter or longer eyes, in order to refine the focus.
8. Eyepiece diopter adjustment: Allows sharp focusing of the reticle depending on the error of refraction of the photographer. This must be done prior to all photography session in order for the photographer to perceive a sharp image. There is no need for adjustment if the photographer wears the necessary corrective spectacles while operating the machine.
9. External fixation light: This allows the photographer to direct the patient's gaze with the fellow eye (the one not being photographed). They come in different colors and some models have lights that blink.
10. Filter slide and filter wheel: This allows different photographic techniques to be done (color, red-free, AF, etc.).
11. Flash intensity control: Allows adjustment of the amount of light emitted by the electronic flash. This must be adjusted by doing test shots prior to the injection of dye. Too little flash gives dark photographs, and too much flash gives overexposed photographs.
12. Focusing knob: Adjust the distance between the lens and the screen/sensor to maximize sharpness of images.
13. Internal fixation device: Different models have different fixation devices built into them. This fixation target is within the camera and is viewed by the patient while

the photograph is being taken. It is best to view this yourself in order to instruct patients better.

14. Joystick: Controls the forward–backward and the side to side movement of the optical head.
15. Objective lens: The front element of the fundus camera. This must be kept clean to avoid photographic artifacts.

Photograph orientation: Depending on the brand of fundus camera, photographs taken by it may be identified with the identification tab. This tab also helps orient the photographs with regards to whether it is the right or left eye. This is important especially in the era where images can easily be modified using the computer. Figures 8.2 through 8.6 are taken on the FF-450plus (Carl Zeiss Meditec) camera and has a tab protruding at 4 o'clock.

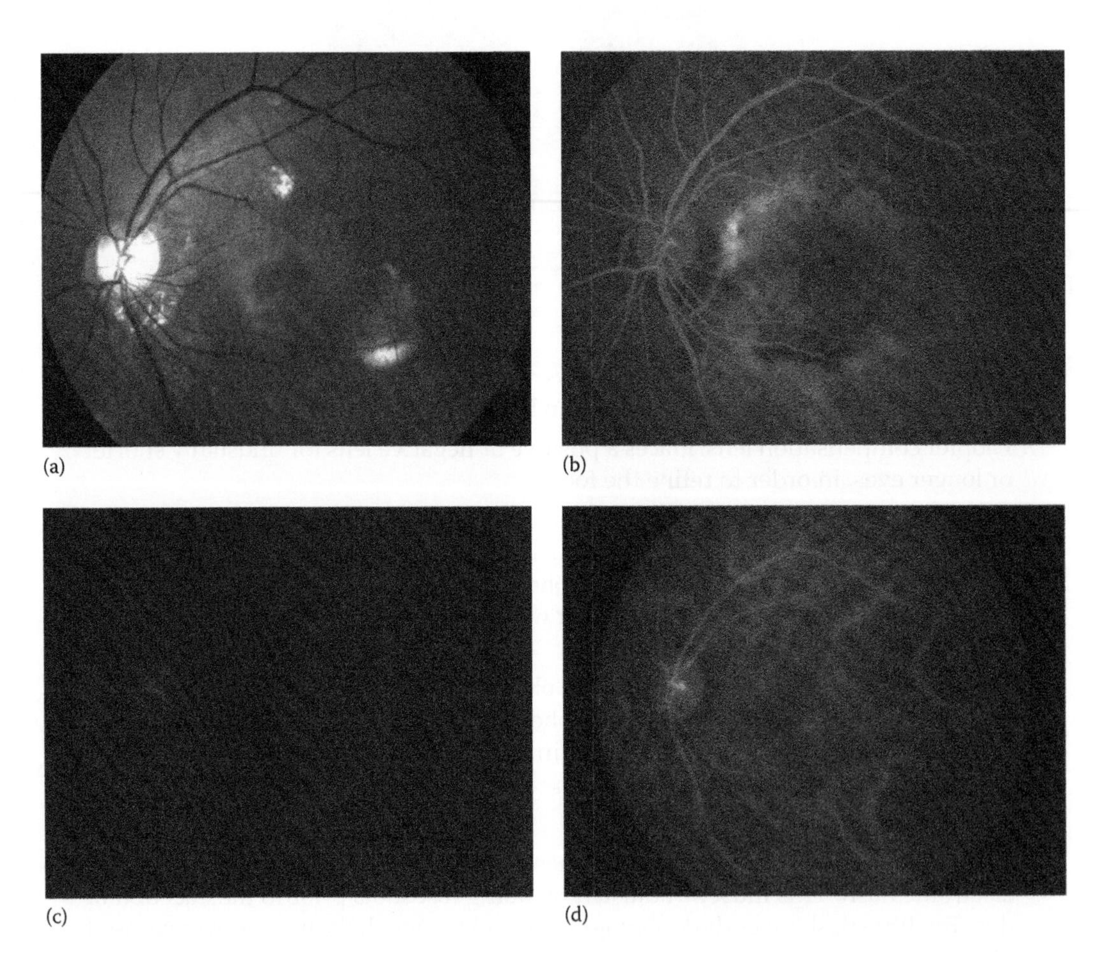

FIGURE 8.6
ICGA. (a) Red-free fundus photograph of a left eye. (b) A mid-phase FFA of the same eye shown for comparison. The retinal vessels are well demarcated, but the choroidal vessels are not visible. (c) Early phase shows ICG in the retinal vessels and the large choroidal vessels. (d) Early to mid phase shows retinal vessels and large and medium choroidal vessels.

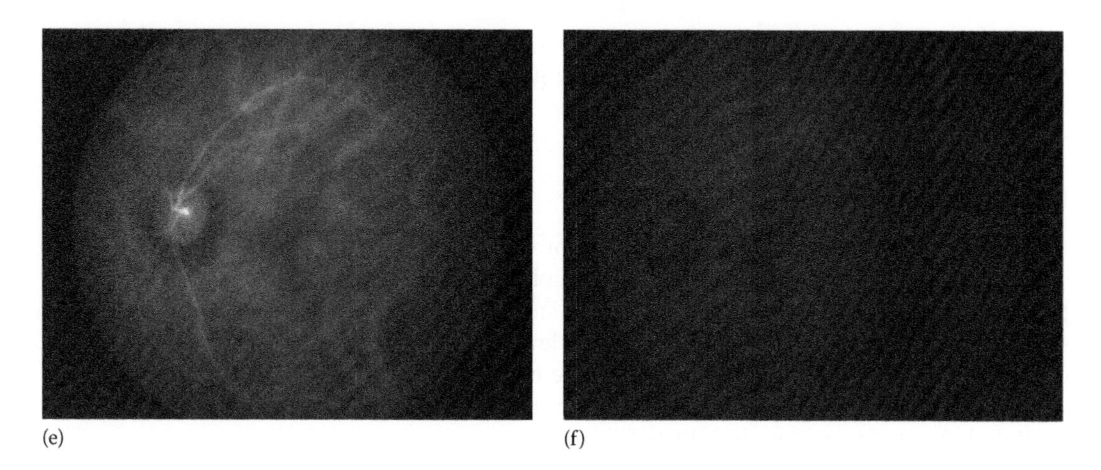

(e) (f)

FIGURE 8.6 (continued)
ICGA. (e) Midphase showing less distinct choroidal vessels and hazy background from dye leaking from the choroidal capillaries. (f) Late phase where the vessels are indistinct, and background haze and staining are seen. The optic disc is dark.

8.2.3 Types of Fundus Cameras Available

Fundus cameras are best described by the angle of view which they subtend the area of the retina. The most common angle used is around 30°. This essentially is used for the most common shot in retinal photography, the view of the optic nerve, and the macula (the area encircled by the two temporal retinal arcades). Larger angles of 45°–140° or more are taken by wide-angled fundus cameras, which provide a panoramic view of the retina up to its periphery, but gives less magnification. Views like this are good for general surveys of the retina for pathology such as retinopathy of prematurity and retinoblastoma. Smaller angles of 20° or less are best for photographing details in the lesions, the optic disc, and the macula, as they give a well-magnified view of the subject of interest.

Today, most fundus cameras have multiple modes for capturing images at different angles and magnifications. Furthermore, the higher pixel densities provided by newer fundus cameras allow us to overcome the problem of poor retinal details in wide-angle photographs. Computer software allows us to zoom in on details to a certain extent. This improvement is very important especially in examination of tumors.

Portable handheld fundus cameras are now available, which allows retinal photography outside the clinic, for example, in the ward or the operating room. These are specially useful for examination of children or bed-ridden patients and in animal studies. While these patients are under anesthesia, these cameras allow photographic documentation of lesions such as tumors, assisting clinicians in management decisions and documentation of lesion growth.

The Ret-Cam® is excellent for photography at the bedside or operating theater because of its portability and the ability to image the retina of patients in the supine position.

Fundus cameras also have mydriatic and nonmydriatic modes (dilated and undilated pupil modes). Mydriatic modes are the ones used for usual retinal photography and angiography, after the patient's pupils have been prepared with dilating eyedrops. The nonmydriatic mode is useful for screening (as in diabetic retinopathy) and for patients with poorly dilating pupils (like in uveitis) and patients who have contraindications to pupillary dilatation (e.g., untreated angle closure glaucoma, patients who will be driving in bright sunlight after photography).

8.2.4 Development of Digital Angiography

Before the advent of digital photography, fluorescein angiography was performed on film. This was a more meticulous process, as the color, red-free, and angiography shots had to be arranged in a certain sequence. Moreover, stereo images of the disc and retina had to be side by side when the film was cut, to allow viewing in 3D. This also had the disadvantage of limited shots per session as limited by the roll of film. Even though film photography gave superb resolution of images, because of its disadvantages, it was later surpassed by digital photography as the modality of choice.

An important development that came with digital photography was the development of ICGA. ICG fluorescence is much lower than that of fluorescein dye, and IR film sensitivity is too low to capture it. Improved illumination with continuous laser diodes, filter systems, video angiography, and digital imaging systems, which boost the ICG fluorescence, allowed ICGA to become commercially available.

Advantages of digital photography are the following:

1. An unlimited number of frames can be taken per session.
2. The computer software can be used to edit images digitally, for example, contrast and brightness, which can provide better resolution of the picture.
3. Computer software allows creation of a montage from several individual photographs, rapidly and seamlessly.
4. Accurate measurements of lesions using the caliper facility.
5. Images can be shared and transmitted easily.
6. Storage and retrieval of digital data is simplified.

8.3 Performing and Understanding Fundus Photography and Angiography

8.3.1 Preparation

8.3.1.1 Pupillary Dilation

Photography involves capturing light that reflects off the subject, in this case, the retina. Because the internal eye has no light source of its own, we need to shine a light or a flash in order to create a good photograph. But because of the eye's natural physiology of regulating light, closing the pupil when there is too much light and opening it when there is not enough, it makes taking photographs of the retina difficult in normal circumstances. This is the reason we use mydriatic agents that counteract the natural pupillary constriction when the eye encounters a bright light source, like the camera's flash. Mydriasis allows the pupil size to be larger than normal and permits adequate photography of the periphery.

Nonmydriatic cameras are available but are of limited use—more for photographing the posterior pole and not for angiography.

Mydriatic eyedrops

Generic Name	Actions	Maximal Effect (min)	Duration (h)
Tropicamide 1%	Mydriatic and cycloplegic (parasympatholytic)	20–30	Up to 4–6
Cyclopentolate 1%	Mydriatic and cycloplegic (parasympatholytic)	15–30	Up to 24
Phenylephrine 2.5% or 10%	Mydriatic (sympathomimetic)	20–40	Up to 3

8.3.1.2 Informed Consent

Before any procedure is done, written informed consent should be obtained from the patient. The patient should be informed of the indication for the procedure and its risks, which can range from mild urticaria or rhinitis to anaphylactic reaction and collapse (fortunately very rare) to the dye. The patient is also warned that the fluorescein is excreted in the urine, and therefore colors the urine bright orange.

Color fundus photographs and red-free photographs are obtained prior to fluorescein dye injection. An intravenous cannula is usually used to access the antecubital vein or a vein in the back of the hand. It is important to note where the venous access had been done as this makes a difference in the time it takes for the dye to travel from the hand or elbow, through the general circulation into the eye. The intravenous cannula is preferred to a butterfly needle as it is more reliable in the event of an emergency (anaphylaxis). It also important for staff to know how to perform emergency resuscitation procedures and where the emergency equipment is stored.

8.3.1.3 Fluorescein or ICG Dye Injection

Fluorescein sodium (500 mg) for injection is available in solutions of 10% of 5 mL or 5% of 10 mL. ICG is injected in 1–2 ml (25–50 mg).

The advantage of using a larger volume allows for a longer injection time while the smaller volume but higher concentration is useful for patients with media opacities. This allows for stronger fluorescence to pass through the hazy media.

Injection of fluorescein by a physician is coordinated with the photographer as he/she starts the timer. The photographer also takes one photograph at this time and is marked as zero time. Some photographers wait for the first sign of fluorescence before taking another photograph to show the time fluorescein first appears. It is recommended to take serial photographs continuously from time zero, so as not to miss out on important early shots. Digital photography allows unnecessary blank photographs to be deleted (unlike film photography), rather than missing out on essential early phase frames, which may not be immediately apparent.

Rapid injection of dye yields a higher concentration of dye in the circulation and creates sharper photographs. However, this may potentially cause more nausea and may lead to failure of the patient to be in position in order for photographs to be taken.

It is possible to perform simultaneous FFA and ICGA with some imaging systems. The problem with this is that ICGA requires more light than FFA; thus with the same flash settings, the ICGA may be underexposed and the FFA overexposed.

8.3.2 Basic Principles of Fundus Angiography

8.3.2.1 Functional Anatomy

Fluorescein or ICG dye is introduced intravenously through a vein at the elbow or the back of the hand. It reaches the ophthalmic artery and enters the ocular circulation, lighting up the spaces it occupies. There are two circulations in the eye: the retinal circulation supplied by the central retinal artery and the choroidal circulation supplied by the posterior ciliary arteries. As will be explained, fluorescein angiography delineates the retinal circulation better, and ICGA delineates the choroidal circulation better.

8.3.2.2 Physical Properties of Fluorescein and ICG

8.3.2.2.1 Some Technical Terms

Luminescence

- When light energy is absorbed into a luminescent material, free electrons are elevated into higher energy states. This energy is then reemitted by spontaneous decay of the electrons into their lower energy states.
- When this decay occurs in the visible spectrum, it is called luminescence.
- Luminescence therefore entails a shift from a shorter wavelength (higher energy) to a longer wavelength (lower energy).

Fluorescence

- Luminescence that is maintained only by continuous excitation.
- Excitation at one wavelength occurs and is emitted immediately at a longer wavelength.
- Once excitation stops, emission stops. It does not have an afterglow.

8.3.2.2.2 Properties of Sodium Fluorescein

Fluorescence

- Absorbs blue light, the excitation wavelength is 465–490 nm.
- Blue light is changed and emitted as a longer green-yellow emission wavelength of 520–530 nm.
- Therefore, if blue light is directed to unbound sodium fluorescein, it will emit green-yellow light.

Protein binding

About 70%–85% of fluorescein is bound to protein in the blood. Thus 15%–30% remains unbound as free fluorescein. In the retinal circulation, both bound and free fluorescein remain within the blood vessels and do not leak except in disease states. In the choriocapillaris (capillaries of the choroid), which contains fenestrations (or *windows*), only bound fluorescein remains within the vessel, and unbound fluorescein is free to move out into the extravascular space.

8.3.2.2.3 Properties of ICG

Fluorescence

- Green color.
- Peak absorption and emission is in IR, 800–850 nm.
- Maximal excitation: 790–805 nm (NIR).
- Maximal fluorescence: 835 nm (NIR).
- Fluorescence efficacy is much lower than sodium fluorescein.

Protein binding

ICG is about 98% protein bound, reducing its passage through the fenestrated choriocapillaris, thus allowing it to delineate the choroidal vessels more precisely.

8.3.2.2.4 Principles of the FA and ICGA Imaging Systems

FA: In the fundus camera, a white light source emits light that passes through blue excitation filters. This blue light stimulates the circulating fluorescein, which then emits a yellow-green light. A barrier filter now blocks all other reflected light except yellow green coming from the eye. This then is recorded onto a film or a digital camera sensor.

In ICGA, the use of continuous laser diodes as the excitatory light source allows a single wavelength to be used, which even the best excitation filters cannot match. A barrier filter is used, which can transmit shorter wavelengths.

8.3.2.3 Interpretation of Fundus Angiography

Anatomical considerations: There are two vascular circulations in the eye: the retinal circulation and the choroidal circulation. *The retinal circulation* is supplied by the central retinal artery and supplies the inner two-thirds of the neurosensory retina. The cells forming the retinal blood vessels have tight junctions, which do not allow plasma, fluorescein, or ICG to leak out. These tight junctions form the *inner blood retinal barrier. The choroidal circulation* is supplied by the posterior ciliary arteries and supplies the retinal pigment epithelium (RPE), which lies between the choroid and the neurosensory retina, and the outer one-third of the neurosensory retina (the photoreceptors and the outer nuclear layer).

The choroid has fenestrated blood vessels; this means there are tiny gaps between the cells forming the blood vessels, allowing fluid and fluorescein to leak through the choroidal vessels into the interstitial spaces of the choroid. Since fluorescein does not remain in the choroidal vessels, this is the first reason why it does not demonstrate the choroidal circulation well. ICG does not leak out of the choroidal vessels but remains within the choroidal vessels, outlining them. Therefore, ICGA delineates the choroidal circulation more clearly than fluorescein angiography and thus is more useful for demonstrating the anatomy and diseases of the choroidal circulation. *The outer blood retinal barrier* is formed by the tight junctions at the apices of the RPE; thus fluorescein and ICG do not leak into the neurosensory retina from the choroidal circulation.

The *RPE* lies between the neurosensory retina and the choroid. It is the supporting tissue for the highly metabolically active photoreceptors, controlling the supply of oxygen and nutrients and the removal of metabolic waste products from the choroidal circulation. The RPE is pigmented and masks the fluorescence from fluorescein in the choroidal circulation. This is the second reason why fluorescein angiography does not demonstrate the choroidal circulation well. ICGA relies on NIR wavelengths, which are able to pass through the pigment in the RPE. Thus the choroid is well demonstrated and not masked by the pigmented RPE in ICGA.

In diseased states, the inner and outer blood retinal barriers can break down, allowing leakage to occur and allowing angiography to detect the pathology. In ischemia (lack of blood supply) or inflammation of the retinal blood vessels, a breakdown of the inner blood–retinal barrier can occur, resulting in fluorescein leaking into the neurosensory retina, for example, macular edema. ICG generally does not leak out of the retinal vessels, even in these circumstances; thus fluorescein angiography is generally more useful than ICGA for diseases of the retinal circulation. In central serous chorioretinopathy, increased choroidal blood flow results in increased hydrostatic pressure in the choroid to the stage where the outer blood–retinal barrier can break down, resulting in leakage of fluid into the subretinal space, between the RPE and neurosensory retina.

8.3.2.4 Phases of the Fluorescein Angiogram

After the fluorescein passes from the brachiocephalic vein in the arm to the heart and then into the arterial circulation, it eventually goes into the ophthalmic artery to enter the eye. Fluorescein enters the choroidal circulation 1–2 s before the longer retinal circulation. Due to the pattern of blood circulation in the eye, the phases of the angiogram are as follows [3,4,6]:

1. Choroidal phase: This is also called the prearterial phase. Fluorescein fills the choroidal vessels. This usually takes 8–12 s from the time of injection of fluorescein. Choroidal fluorescence comes as a generalized flush that gradually increases in intensity. A portion of the choroidal fluorescence is decreased/blocked by the RPE layer. It is the length of time it takes for blood to travel up from the arm to the heart and into the eye. It takes a longer time as a person ages and also proportional to the arm length of the individual undergoing the test.
2. Arterial phase: This follows the choroidal phase about a second later and is marked by the first appearance of fluorescein in the retinal arteries (Figure 8.3a). Delays in this phase of the angiogram can be a sign of blockage further upstream in the blood circulation.
3. Arteriovenous phase: This is also known as the capillary phase. This is when fluorescein transitions from the arterial into the venous circulation (Figure 8.3b). This is marked by the completion of filling of the retinal arteries and lamellar flow into the veins. This is also the time when choroidal fluorescence is maximal, as free fluorescein saturates the extravascular space underneath the RPE. The arteriovenous phase overlaps with the venous phase.
4. Venous phase: This can be divided into early, mid, and late venous phases. Early venous is seen as the lamellar flow, as fluorescein adheres more to the walls of the vein compared to the center of the vessel (Figure 8.3c). Mid-venous is the complete filling of the veins (Figure 8.3d). And late is the complete filling of the veins with fluorescein dye with the fading of dye from the arteries (Figure 8.3e). Delays in the venous phase can be seen in diseases where there is obstruction to the outflow, such as in central and branch vein occlusions.
5. Late phase: This is also known as the elimination or recirculation phase. Fluorescein is absent in circulation but commonly shows the staining of the optic disc (Figure 8.3f).

8.3.2.5 Hyperfluorescence and Hypofluorescence

Descriptions of abnormal fluorescence in angiography are described in terms of hyperfluorescence, when there is greater fluorescence than normal, and hypofluorescence, when there is reduced fluorescence compared to normal [3,4,6].

8.3.2.5.1 Patterns of Hyperfluorescence

1. Window or transmission defects: These are caused by defects in the RPE layer. Since the RPE normally masks the choroidal fluorescence, when the RPE is atrophic and loses its pigment, the choroidal fluorescence shows through as hyperfluorescence called a window defect or transmission defect, the *window* being the area of defective RPE. This fluorescence appears early in the angiogram, in tandem with the choroidal circulation, remains the same size and shape, and then gradually fades toward the end of the angiogram.
2. Dye leakage: Dye leakage is fluorescence that increases in both size and intensity as the angiogram progresses. It may be due to leakage from breakdown of the inner blood retinal barrier (as in cystoid macular edema, Figure 8.3c through f), or abnormal new vessels (neovascularization) in the retinal or choroidal circulation (Figure 8.4b through d shows leakage from retinal neovascularization).
3. Pooling: This happens as fluorescein dye fills a defined space. It may be underneath the retina (subretinal) or underneath the RPE layer. Pooling in the subretinal space increases in size and intensity as the angiogram progresses, while pooling in the sub-RPE layer increases only in intensity but not in size. In the later phases of the angiogram, pooling of fluorescein usually allows us to outline the space that the dye has filled up.
4. Staining: Staining is hyperfluorescence due to the uptake of fluorescein dye by a tissue even after the dye has left the choroidal and retinal circulation. In general, staining occurs in tissues containing collagen, for example, sclera (if bared by RPE and choriocapillaris loss) and scar tissue (e.g., in trauma, advanced proliferative diabetic retinopathy, advanced exudative ARMD). (Figure 8.4d shows late staining of scar tissue in advanced proliferative diabetic retinopathy [3–6].)
5. Demonstration of abnormal vascular structures: Neovascularization, microaneurysms, collateral circulations, and other abnormal vascular structures are accentuated by fluorescein outlining their anatomy. Figure 8.4b through d shows neovascularization due to advanced proliferative diabetic retinopathy, a common cause of blindness.

8.3.2.5.2 Patterns of Hypofluorescence

1. Blocked fluorescence: Opaque structures (e.g., blood, pigment) anterior to normally fluorescent structures block the fluorescence. If they are in front of the retina, these lesions will block fluorescence from all deeper structures (e.g., preretinal blood indicated by white arrow in Figure 8.4a and b). If they are intraretinal or deeper, the lesion will only block fluorescence from either the capillaries or choroid, but not from the superficial large retinal vessels.
2. Filling defects: Filling defects are caused by either occlusions of vascular channels or absence of these channels themselves (e.g., Figure 8.4b shows hypofluorescence due to nonperfusion of capillaries in the area of the star).

8.3.2.5.3 Dark Foveal Appearance

The central fovea and the macula have a dark appearance throughout the angiogram (Figure 8.3b and c) because of the following:

1. Avascularity or absence of blood vessels at the fovea (foveal avascular zone [FAZ]).
2. Increased density of xanthophyll pigment in this area, blocking choroidal fluorescence.
3. RPE cells in this area are larger and contain more melanin, blocking choroidal fluorescence.

If there is leakage at the fovea, for example, macular edema or central serous chorioretinopathy, there is a characteristic hyperfluorescence pattern within the normally dark macular area [3–6].

8.3.2.6 Phases of ICGA

Unlike the blood–retinal barrier in the retinal circulation, endothelial cells in the choriocapillaris are connected by discontinuous zonular occludents, and there is a physiologic, slow leakage of ICG from the choriocapillaris in the mid to late phases. The choriocapillaris facing the RPE has large fenestrations too. Extravasation of ICG dye masks fluorescence of the underlying vessels and eventually blurs the ICG images. The choriocapillaris itself can only be appreciated as a faint haze in the early venous phase [2–4,6].

1. Early phase: Dye enters the large choroidal vessels within 1 min of injection (Figure 8.6c and d).
2. Mid phase: Between 5 and 15 min, the dye washes out, and the choroidal veins become less distinct, less fluorescent (Figure 8.6e). A diffuse, featureless choroidal hyperfluorescence is present as the dye leaks out into the interstitial spaces.
3. In the late phase, about 15 min after ICG injection, both the retinal and choroidal vasculature becomes indistinct (Figure 8.6f). The optic disc is dark (a sharp contrast to fluorescein angiography, where the optic disc shows *staining*), and the large choroidal vessels become hypofluorescent and may exhibit *silhouetting* against the hyperfluorescence of the interstitial spaces.

8.3.2.7 Interpretation of ICGA

ICGA is useful in ARMD, central serous chorioretinopathy, and choroidal hemangioma. The IR wavelength allows it to image lesions through mild to moderate hemorrhages, exudates, and lipofuscin, which fluorescein angiography cannot do [2–6].

In ARMD, hyperfluorescent lesions seen on ICGA, usually subretinal, may be described as either *hot spots* or *plaques*. Hot spots are also called focal choroidal neovascularisation (CNV) and are by definition smaller than 1 disc diameter in size and usually extrafoveal. They are believed to represent polypoidal lesions of idiopathic polypoidal choroidal vasculopathy most of the time. A faint hot spot is seen in Figure 8.6d and e. Plaques are by definition hyperfluorescent lesions, which are larger than 1 disc diameter in size, and involve the fovea; they usually represent occult choroidal neovascularization. Classic choroidal neovascularization may not leak ICG dye, and therefore may not light up with ICG dye.

In central serous chorioretinopathy, there is choroidal hyperfluorescence, representing choroidal hyperpermeability in addition to RPE detachments showing pooling and leaks into the subretinal space from the RPE detachments. This choroidal hyperfluorescence can be seen in areas separate from the RPE detachments, subretinal fluid, and in the apparently normal looking fellow eye.

Choroidal hemangioma is better delineated with ICGA due to the greater penetrance of the dye through the RPE.

8.4 Fundus Autofluorescence

8.4.1 Fundus Reflectance and Autofluorescence

While routine fundus photography became more of a tool for documentation, more hidden information can be unraveled without recourse to injecting contrasting dyes (sodium fluorescein, ICG) by the clever use of filters and choosing the right wavelength light to illuminate the retina.

Fundus reflectance is a term used when a particular wavelength light is projected on to the retina and the reflected light (image) is studied without any filtration of the reflected light. IR illumination using long wavelength (810–830 nm) penetrates subretinal tissues better than visible light. Fundus reflectance increases as illuminating wavelength increases. The combined quality of deeper penetration and increased reflectance produces finer detailed images of the RPE, RPE/Bruch's membrane complex, and choroidal pathology. Increased reflectance in IR imaging is seen in chorioretinal loss (geographical atrophy) (Figure 8.7a)

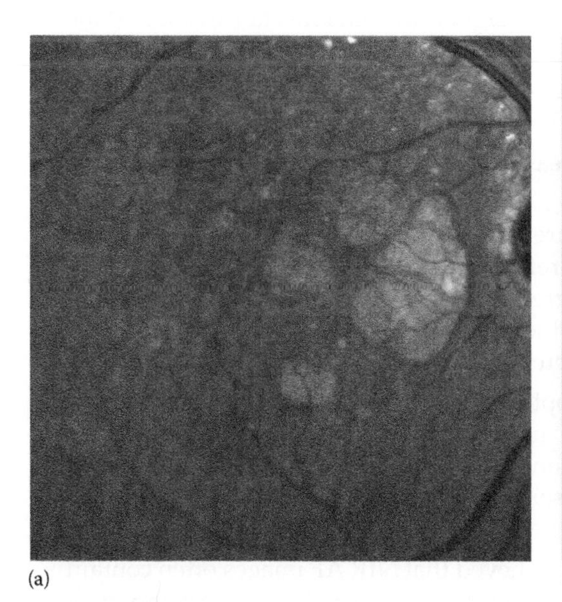
(a)

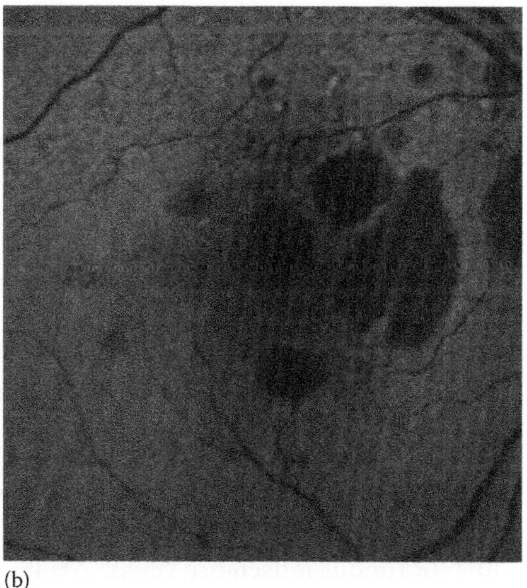
(b)

FIGURE 8.7
Fundus NIR reflectance and AF. (a) Fundus NIR reflectance of a right eye with ARMD showing RPE degeneration and atrophy. (b) The same eye showing AF. The area of RPE atrophy shows complete lack of AF indicating absence of any photoreceptor metabolism. There is background AF present.

and fibrin (scars). Decreased reflectance in IR imaging is seen in RPE hyperpigmentation, drusen, and presence of blood. Less light is required to take IR images; thus it is better tolerated than flash photography.

In contrast, in studies of AF, filters are used to help detect fluorescence caused by the incident light (change in wavelength caused by fluorophores existent in the retina).

1. Blue reflectance: With a 488 nm wavelength light, projected on the fundus, the image is captured. This represents the blue reflectance of the fundus.
2. NIR reflectance: With 820 nm wavelength light projected on the fundus, the image is captured and represents NIR fundus reflectance.
3. Blue-light AF (FAF): For AF studies using blue light, the fundus is excited with 488 nm wavelength light, and the emission spectrum is in the range of 500–700 nm.
4. NIR AF: The incident (excitation) light is of 790 nm wave length, and the emission is >810 nm.

The experience with the reflectance and AF is building up. Following are some of the observations made:

1. Signal to noise ratio is lower with NIR compared to blue light.
2. Lipofuscin in the RPE is the predominant fluorophore for blue light AF.
3. Melanin in RPE and choroid may be the source of the NIR AF signals.
4. Normal fovea is dark (hypo AF) on FAF surrounded by bright perifoveal area, while in NIR AF, there is progressive increase in signals toward the center of fovea.
5. In general, atrophic areas exhibit increased signals in both reflectance modes (blue and NIR) (Figure 8.7a).
6. In general, atrophic areas exhibit decreased signals in AF imaging with both blue and NIR light (Figure 8.7b).
7. The contrast with the nonatrophic areas is more marked with blue rather than with NIR AF.
8. Junctional zone around the atrophic area—FAF can show abnormalities that are not seen in fundus photos as well as reflectance images. NIR AF can also show abnormalities in this zone, but the degree and type of abnormalities between the two AFs (FAF and NIR) are mostly not identical. Occasionally, areas of increased NIR reflectance corresponded with increased NIR AF.
9. The increased blue AF around the atrophic areas has been attributed to increased collection of lipofuscin as a result of incomplete degradation of photoreceptor outer segments. However, accumulation of melanolipofuscin has also been suggested in this area. In addition, lipofuscin itself has been postulated to contain at least 10 different fluorophores.
10. NIR fundus reflectance versus AF: It is believed that NIR AF images often contain true AF as well as pseudofluorescence caused by leak from filters. This component of it is due to the reflectance.
11. Enhancing the NIR reflectance by manipulation of the image using denoising techniques improves the details further.

8.4.2 In Disease

1. Central serous retinopathy: Studies have shown four varieties of AF in these eyes—no focal AF, granular hypo AF, granular hyper AF, and mixed. Considering the AF generated by blue (FAF) and NIR, several combinations have been observed. In acute stage, the AF with both FAF and NIR shows reduction compared to background. Flecks with hyper AF appeared later in both blue and NIR images but not necessarily identical. Following resolution of subretinal fluid, the hyper AF spots reduced significantly in 8 weeks time. Several months after the event, the FAF showed some hyper AF specks, which were hypo AF in NIR images.
2. ARMD:
    a. Spots of increased AF on blue light imaging are the commonest finding, followed by spots of decreased AF and lines of increased AF. On NIR AF, spots of increased and reduced AF were seen equally frequently. Lines were less frequently made out on NIR. Serial imaging showed different variations in the level of AF on blue light (FAF) versus NIR.
    b. Geographic atrophy: Area of RPE loss is dark in both FAF and NIR AF (Figure 8.7b). The area of geographic atrophy was noted larger on NIR compared to blue light but never the other way around. Zone beyond the visible geographic atrophy showed increased intensity of AF on only FAF, only NIR, or both.
    c. Exudative AMD: Minimal or gross reduction in AF in both modalities is seen when significant blood or fluid was present. Areas of exudation tend to more often have increased AF on blue light compared to NIR AF.
3. Best's vitelliform dystrophy: In preclinical stage, no abnormalities have been found on imaging. In vitelliform stage, the margins of the lesion are well demarcated on FAF. The yellow material gives increased fluorescence on FAF. In pseudohypopyon stage, also the inferior yellow material shows hyper AF on FAF. NIR AF delineates the retinal elevation clearly.
4. Pseudoxanthoma elasticum: With NIR AF, angioid streaks appear as well-defined dark fissures against a bright background—far more than what can be detected on color imaging. Comets and comet tails have been described as bursts of hyper AF spots. These lesions are not well seen on color photography. The hyperpigmented borders of the lesions are seen uniformly as hypo AF lesions on both FAF and NIR AF.
5. Choroidal nevus: Both NIR reflectance and AF are increased while FAF does not show the nevus well.

8.5 Conclusion

Imaging the fundus with various wavelengths of light permits the appreciation of some details that are not otherwise seen. While contrast with injection of dyes such as sodium fluorescein and ICG gives good amount of information both of the retinal and choroidal vasculature, imaging with blue and NIR light gives additional information without recourse to injection of dyes. This is not to say that one can replace dye injection techniques with AF studies. Studies have shown that the lipofuscin—especially A2E—is responsible for the blue light autofluorescence (FAF), while melanin contributes mostly to the AF observed with NIR light. Diseases such as AMD and angioid streaks are more easily followed up with these AF imaging techniques since subtle changes are picked up easily. With more experience, there is a potential for greater role of these techniques of imaging in routine ophthalmic practice.

References

1. Duke-Elder S, *System of Ophthalmology*, Vol. X, London, U.K.: Henry Kimpton, 1961.
2. Yannuzzi LA, Flower RW, Slakter JS, *Indocyanine Green Angiography*, St. Louis: Mosby, 1997.
3. Sadda SR (ed.), *Retina*, Ryan SJ (Editor-in-Chief), *Part 1: Retinal Imaging and Diagnostics*, 5th edn, Vol. I, London: Saunders/Elsevier, 2013.
4. Saine P, Tyler M, *Ophthalmic Photography: Retinal Photography, Angiography, and Electronic Imaging*, 2nd edn, Boston, MA: Butterworth-Heinemann, 2002.
5. Kanski J, Milewski S, *Diseases of the Macula*, Edinburgh, U.K.: Mosby, 2002.
6. American Academy of Ophthalmology: Fundus Fluorescein Angiography and Indocyanine Green Choroidography, 1997.

9

Optic Nerve Analysis and Imaging in Relation to Glaucoma

Seng Chee Loon, Victor Koh, and Rosalynn Grace Siantar

CONTENTS

9.1 Introduction

Glaucoma is a major cause of blindness in the world and its prevalence is on the upward trend. Asia has one of the world's largest populations and an estimated half of the world's population with glaucoma is residing in Asia. We also have a higher rate of angle-closure glaucoma (ACG), especially among Asians of Chinese origin [1,2].

Imaging has become an essential component of the diagnosis and assessment of glaucoma. Ocular imaging tools of the posterior segment have the potential to provide quantifiable and reproducible measurements to complement clinical examination. Posterior imaging modalities such as the Heidelberg retinal tomography (HRT), optical coherence tomography (OCT), and GDx nerve fiber analyzer had proven to be good diagnostic and monitoring adjuncts in clinical practice. Posterior segment imaging involves primarily the optic nerve head and retinal nerve fiber layer (RNFL) measurements. Studies have convincingly shown that structural changes correlate well with functional tests [3] and structural changes preceded detectable visual field defects [4,5]. The diagnosis of glaucoma and monitoring its progression is challenging and difficult to the general ophthalmologist.

In a setting where there is lack of glaucoma expertise, instruments that quantify reproducible parameters and easy to interpret could improve diagnostic accuracy. However, each imaging modality has its strengths and weaknesses that resulted in accelerated modifications to improve its efficacy.

9.2 Posterior Segment Imaging

Posterior segment imaging focuses on the optic disc, RNFL, and macula. There are more tools to image the posterior segment and they have a longer duration of validation and level of maturity. The main disc parameters were rim volume, rim area, cup–disc ratio (CDR), and disc size. The main RNFL parameters were RNFL thickness and cross-sectional area. Both optic disc and RNFL parameters are presented as global and segmental values. There are different imaging modalities available and all had undergone modifications that addressed the limitations of their respective predecessors.

9.2.1 Stereo Disc Photographs

Arguably the oldest posterior imaging tool, this is a simple and easily available technology that continues to be useful even in our current technology-heavy practice. Stereoscopic disc photographs (Figure 9.1) are obtained simultaneously or sequentially with a fundus camera. Serial photos can track changes in the morphology of the disc. It is a highly reproducible technique, with studies reporting higher intraobserver than interobserver reproducibility [6]. However, the downsides are observer subjectivity and lack of specific quantitative measurements, and the trend analysis is less accurate than what HRT can

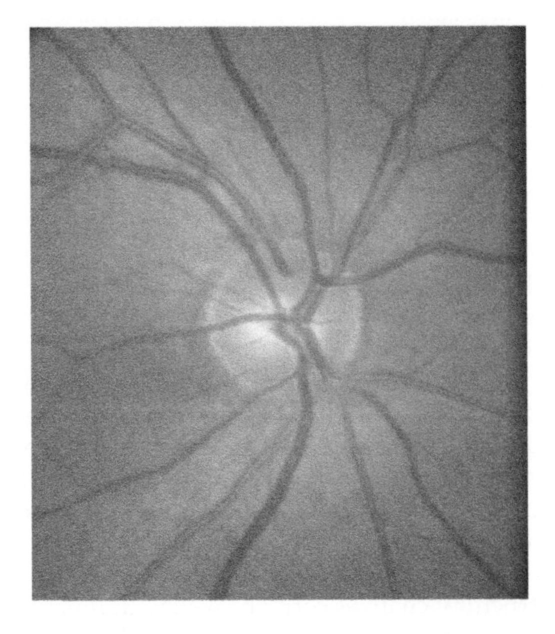

FIGURE 9.1
Photograph of normal optic disc.

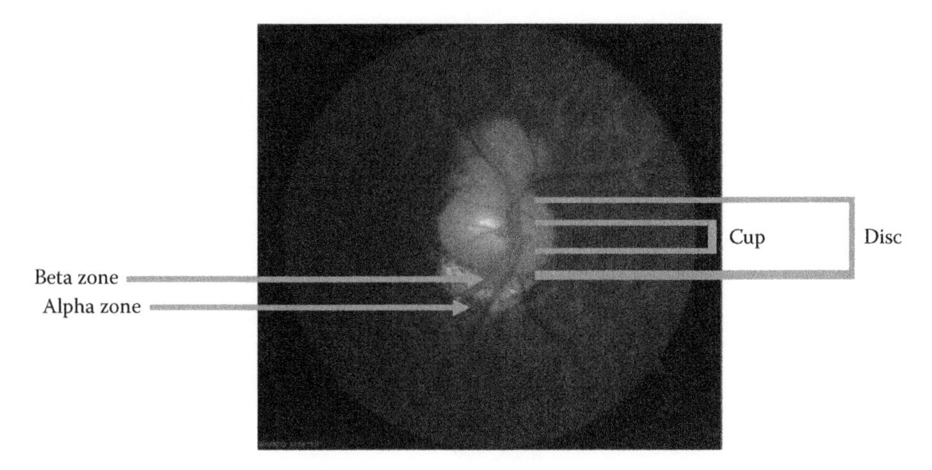

FIGURE 9.2
Optic disc with peripapillary atrophy showing alpha and beta zone.

offer. Nevertheless, in a clinical practice where technology is limited, stereo disc photographs can be an economical and effective tool in the diagnosis and monitoring of glaucomatous discs (Figure 9.2). It is also useful in documenting glaucomatous optic disc changes that cannot be easily captured with other imaging tools such as Drance disc hemorrhage, bayoneting of peripapillary blood vessels, and baring of circumlinear blood vessels.

9.2.2 Confocal Scanning Laser Ophthalmoscope

The confocal scanning laser ophthalmoscope (CLSO) has been used in clinical practice for around 15 years. The most widely available CLSO, HRT (Heidelberg Engineering, Heidelberg, Germany), is used primarily to measure optic nerve head parameters and provide peripapillary RNFL parameters. It utilizes a laser diode (wavelength 670 nm) and scans multiple cross sections of the retina resulting in 3D images. Topographic images of the optic nerve head are assimilated from 32 confocal images (Figure 9.3).

There have been a number of diagnostic algorithms that have been described to aid in analysis of the data captured by the HRT. Mikelberg et al. [7] used a stepwise discriminant analysis on a combination of stereometric parameters (cup shape measure, rim volume, and height variation contour) that yielded a sensitivity of 89% and specificity of 78% for the detection of early visual field loss. Bathija et al. also applied a discriminant analysis function based on cup shape measure, rim area, height variation contour, and RNFL thickness and yielded sensitivity of 78% and specificity of 88% [8].

The HRT is the single most reliable posterior segment imaging tool for the optic disc [9,10] despite newer Fourier domain OCTs. It is capable of measuring multiple area parameters, volumetric parameters, and ratios from the optic disc. It requires no patient interaction and is relatively small compared to the rest of posterior imaging tools. Image acquisition is also quite fast. One of its major strengths is that HRT has the most established normative database compared to the other tools such as the OCT or the GDx nerve fiber analyzer. However, it has its limitations including the observer-dependent step of optic disc contour drawing. This requires a trained observer who is familiar with the fundal anatomy and tools incorporated in the HRT software to accurately plot the disc margins (Figure 9.4).

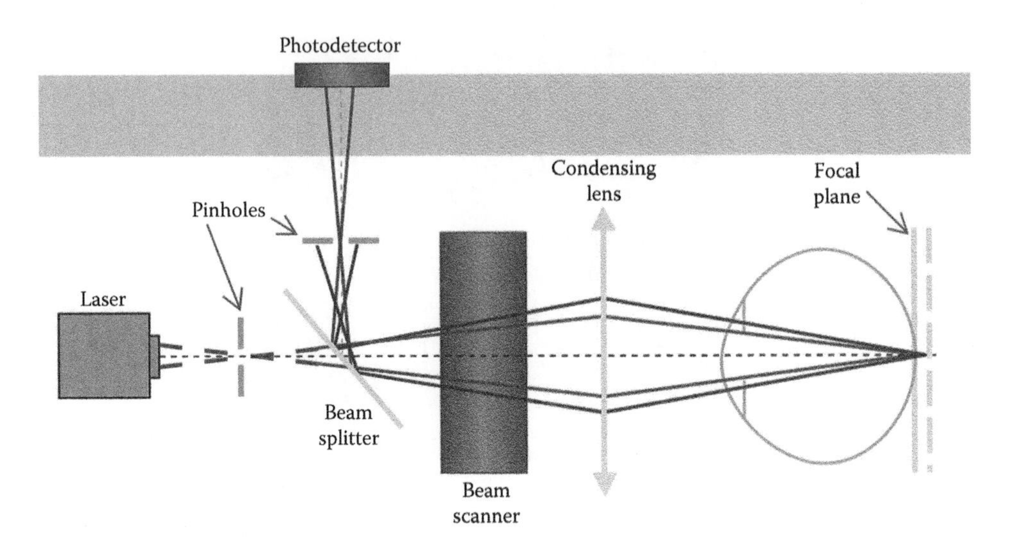

FIGURE 9.3
The confocal laser scanning system in HRT-2. (From http://www.heidelbergengineering.com/us/wp-content/uploads/chapter-1_principles-of-confocal-scanning-laser-ophthalmoscopy-for-the-clinician.pdf.)

One of the most difficult tasks that clinicians face is the longitudinal assessment of the optic disc to establish stability or progression of the disease. Comparing confocal scanning laser tomography (CSLT) to optic disc photography for the detection of progressive glaucomatous disc changes, results indicate that topographic change analysis (TCA) performs at least as well as either the individual or best combination of observer classifications of disc photographs [11]. Comparing HRT and conventional perimetry (using Humphrey Field Analyzer) in glaucoma patients, 40% showed progression with scanning laser tomography, while 4% progressed with conventional perimetry [12]. The HRT was also shown to be more sensitive than clinical assessment of stereoscopic optic disc photographs in distinguishing between healthy persons and patients with early glaucoma [13]. The HRT is also a better tool at detecting structural progression for monitoring purposes rather than diagnosis [14]. Other minor drawbacks include patient's movement during the scanning process resulting in degradation of image quality. The HRT is best used for optic nerve head imaging compared to the OCT, which should be preferably used to image the RNFL [15,16]. Comparing with optic nerve head analyzer measurements, there was lesser variability in HRT measurements [17]. It has been shown that optic disc morphology could also lead to a significant deviation of true optic disc parameters. This could pose a problem when used in Asian subjects, who are prone to refractive errors associated with optic disc tilting [18].

New statistical analyses have recently been developed to assess longitudinal changes of the optic disc by HRT, which greatly increases the specificity of detecting longitudinal optic disc changes. Comparative methods for longitudinal HRT follow-up of glaucoma such as direct comparison of baseline and subsequent follow-up stereometric parameters are readily available. They are easy to perform, allowing clinicians to work on mean topography images and standard parameters. While HRT provides highly reproducible measurement of optic disc stereometric parameters, the RNFL-related parameters should however be used with caution [19].

Good backward compatibility is another main strength of HRT. For HRT, each successive development of the analysis software is *backward compatible* with previous iterations.

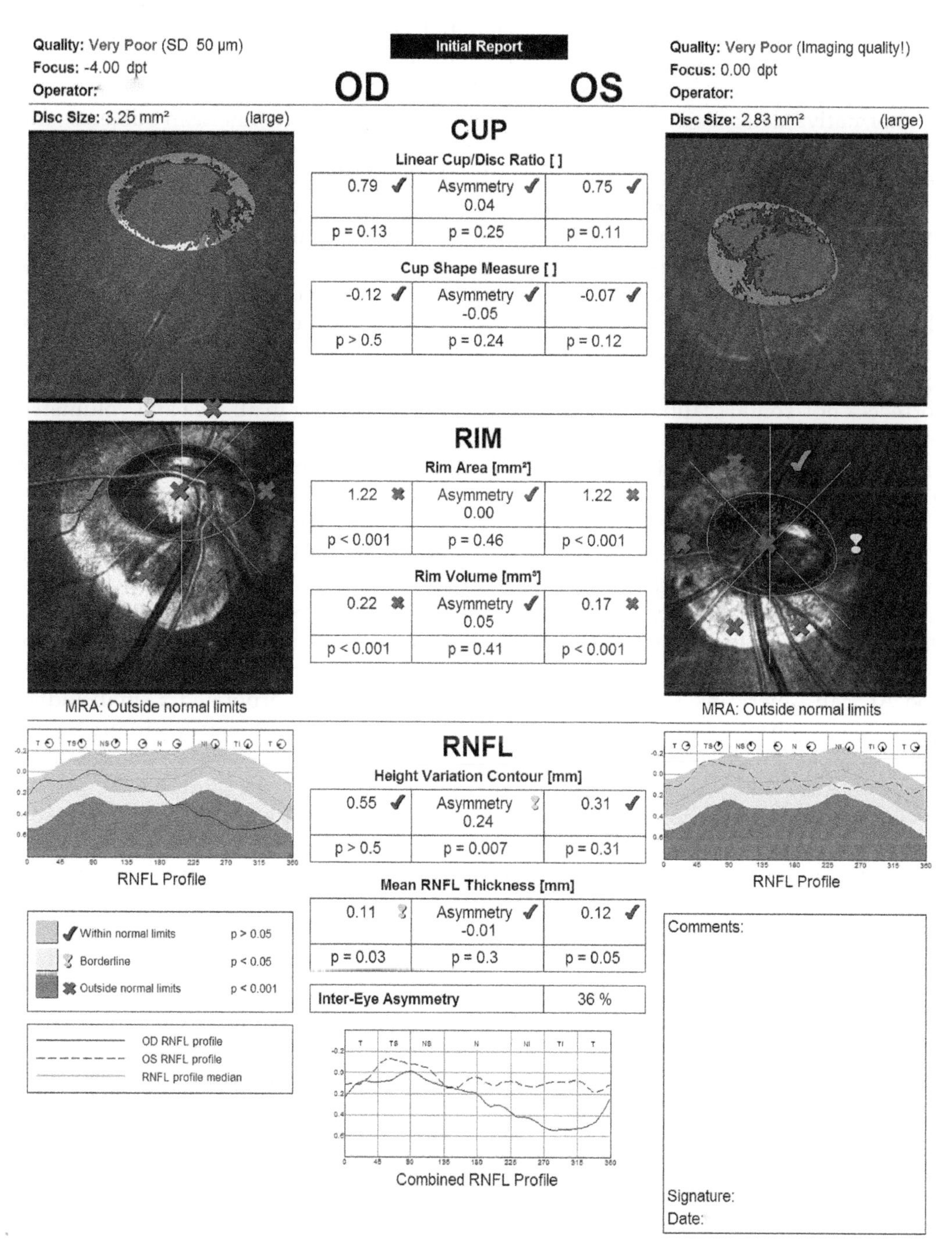

FIGURE 9.4
HRT-2 printout showing glaucomatous discs with large peripapillary atrophy.

This means that images acquired using the original device may be analyzed using the current software as part of a continuous time series. This is particularly valuable for monitoring glaucoma progression [20]. The HRT software has come a long way from HRT-1 to HRT-2 and more recently, HRT-3 has been introduced. The HRT-3 software has three main differences compared to HRT-2 [20,21]. Firstly, the HRT-3 has a bigger normative database comprising of 733 White, 215 African-American subjects, and other minor ethnic groups including Indians. This is in comparison to the relatively small group in HRT-2—349 White subjects. Secondly, the HRT-3 has a new operator-independent component known as the glaucoma probability score (GPS), which automatically *captures* the optic disc. The GPS automatically analyzes the profile of the disc to specify its outline and 3D shape and then, with comparison of data specific to ethnic groups, give an analysis of whether the disc is suspicious of glaucomatous changes. The GPS and the TCA are used for trend analysis in monitoring of glaucoma or glaucoma suspect patients. The HRT is capable of superimposing the baseline and follow-up images for automatic detection of glaucomatous changes. Lastly, the HRT-3 corrects a horizontal scaling error inherent in HRT-2 resulting in all area and volumetric parameters to be changed by 4%–6% from HRT-2 to HRT-3. Studies comparing HRT-2 and HRT-3 in Caucasians did not clearly show that one has better diagnostic ability for glaucoma [22–24].

One of the unique features of HRT is the glaucoma model introduced by Moorfields. The Moorfields regression analysis (MRA) compares the optic disc parameters with an ethnic-specific normative database to predict the risk of glaucoma and showed sensitivity of 96% and specificity of 84%. Although the HRT has been validated as a reliable diagnostic tool in the West, its diagnostic accuracy on Asian subjects are still controversial. The normative database used in HRT-2 is predominantly made up of Whites and African-Americans. Currently, the HRT-3 has already incorporated a small Indian normative database. However, there are well-documented ethnic-specific differences in the optic disc parameters and RNFL thickness [25–27]. Population studies involving the HRT-2 on Asian subjects such as the Malays in Singapore seem to suggest that the current HRT-2 algorithm seems to be inadequate as glaucoma screening tools. Despite unfavorable sensitivities and specificities of HRT-2, it is evidently a patient-friendly technique requiring a short time for processing. The HRT-2 images were successfully captured in 97.6% (3056/3131) of persons, a finding similar to that of Ohkubo et al.'s (99.0%) [14,28]. HRT-2 is also a much simpler and automated version of the original HRT, being small, light, and portable [17].

Using evidence-of-change analyses, although there was considerable overlap of eyes identified as having progressed by various tests, significant numbers of eyes were found to have progressed by only functional or structural criteria. These suggest that the separate sets of tests may represent independent indicators of progression. In a study using the same test procedures for detecting progression, Nicolela et al. [29] compared progression rates among different optic disc types. Across all four groups of different disc types (focal, myopic, senile sclerotic, and generalized), progression rates by HRT (44%–82%) were greater than those by standard automated perimetry (33%–57%), similar to earlier reported results [12], although Wollstein II [30] also reported higher rates of progression when a structural test was used (25%, OCT)—as compared with standard automated perimetry (12%), their population studied included glaucoma suspects and preperimetric glaucoma patients as well as patients with baseline visual field (VF) defects. It is not certain if this represents greater sensitivity for progression or hypersensitivity (false positives) of the structural test [31].

A statistical technique adopted by Chauhan et al. [32] aimed to estimate the amount of variability of small discrete areas for each eye using an empirical probabilistic approach. This allowed a higher frequency of progression detected by HRT as compared to visual field progression, suggesting higher sensitivity for longitudinal evaluation, although specificity is uncertain. Further studies are required to validate this novel technique in clinical situations.

9.2.3 Optical Coherence Tomography

The OCT uses low-coherence interferometry (820 nm wavelength) to produce a 2D image of optical scattering from internal tissue microstructures in a way that is analogous to ultrasonic pulse-echo imaging. It has a tissue resolution of up to 10–20 μm. The older time domain OCT (Figure 9.5) creates images of the retina by evaluating the pattern of interference created by the echo-time delays of backscattered light from both the retina and a moving reference mirror. The latest development is the spectral domain technology that made use of a spectrometer to detect multiple optical frequencies simultaneously from the diffracted spectrum. Using Fourier transformation, the relative retinal depths of each A-scan are derived. As such, the spectral domain OCT (Figure 9.6) is capable of much faster scan speed of around 0.04–0.05 s compared to 1.3 s for time domain OCT [33,34]. Typically, the optic disc cube is a glaucoma scan protocol extending over an area of 6×6 mm^2 covering the optic disc and the peripapillary retina. This area comprised of

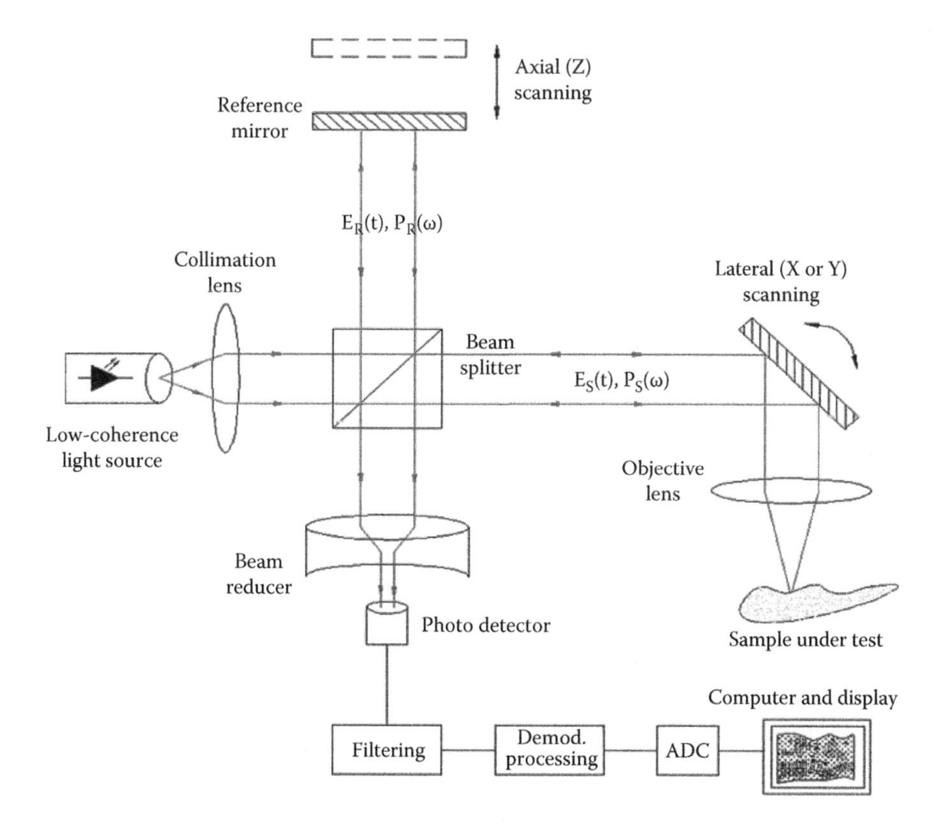

FIGURE 9.5
Schematic diagram of the time domain OCT.

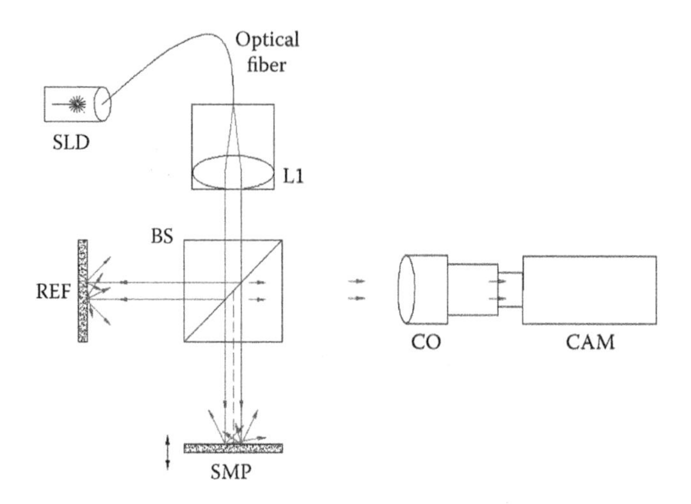

FIGURE 9.6
Schematic diagram of the spectral domain OCT.

40,000 (200 × 200) points compared to just 768 points for the time domain OCT. The OCT images were automatically centered on the optic disc with a scan circle of 3.46 mm in diameter consisting of 256 A-scans.

OCT is an imaging technique commonly used in assessments of disc cupping and peripapillary nerve fiber layer thickness to evaluate the optic nerve head. It is vital in diagnosing and managing both glaucoma and retinal diseases as well. It allows for the identification of macular holes, macular cysts, vitreomacular traction, subretinal fluid, pigment epithelial detachment, choroidal neovascularization, and macular edema. It can measure retinal thickness changes in response to therapy, which correlate well with visual acuity and leakage observed by fluorescein angiography. When used in combination with other optic nerve imaging techniques, it can be used to differentiate glaucomatous eyes from normal eyes [35] (Figure 9.7). As such, the OCT can play a dual function for patients who had concomitant both glaucoma and retinal diseases. In the ophthalmology clinic with limited resources or space, the OCT would be a good imaging tool of choice to provide both glaucoma and retinal service.

The OCT's main outcome measurement is its RNFL analysis. It performs circular scans around the optic nerve head to capture RNFL measurement of the peripapillary region. The software analyzes the RNFL thickness and provides comparison of measurements to a normative database with demonstration of asymmetry and serial analysis. The OCT also performs optic nerve head analysis with radial line scans through the optic disc creating cross-sectional and topographical data. The key analysis parameters include CDRs and horizontal integrated rim volume. OCT provides high-resolution cross-sectional images of the retina, allowing us to better identify, monitor, and quantitatively assess diseases of the macula and optic nerve head. The role of improved retina segmentation and macular ganglion cell layer imaging has provided any means of diagnosing and monitoring glaucoma. This would be discussed further in the following.

Wang et al. [36] analyzed the agreement and correlation of mean RNFL thickness between OCT and GDx in normal and glaucomatous subjects. Results showed high correlation despite a poor agreement. Leung et al. [37] arrived at a similar conclusion of high correlation of mean RNFL thickness between GDx-VCC and Stratus OCT measurements.

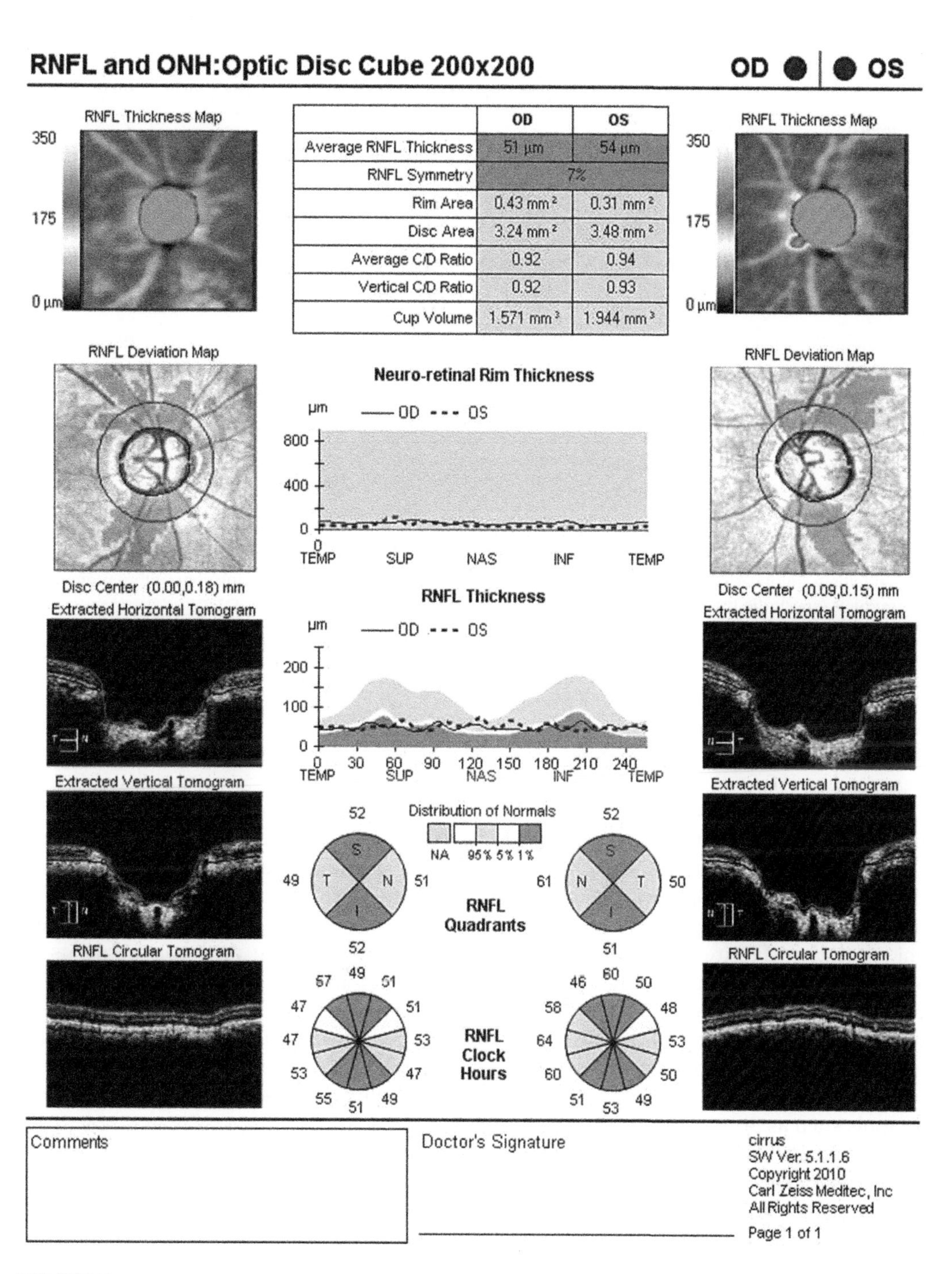

FIGURE 9.7
OCT printout showing glaucomatous optic discs.

TABLE 9.1

Comparison of Commercially Available OCT Instruments

	NIDEK RS-3000[a]	TOPCON 3D OCT[b]	Zeiss Cirrus OCT[c]	Heidelberg HRA-3[d]	Optovue RTVue-100[e]
Autofocus	✓		✓		✓
Acquisition time	53,000 scan/s	27,000 A-scan/s	27,000 A-scan/s	40,000 A-scan/s	26,000 A-scan/s
SLD wavelength (nm)	880	840	840	870	840
OCT resolution (μm)	Z: 4	Z: 6	Z: 5	Z: 7	Z: 5
	XY: 20	XY: 20	XY: 20	XY: 14	XY: 15
Minimal pupil size	Φ2.5 (ϕ3 recommended)	Φ4	Φ2.5 (ϕ3 recommended)	ϕ3	ϕ3
Field view of fundus imaging	SLO 785 nm	Fundus camera	SLO 750 nm	SLO 488/760/785	IR camera
	40° × 30°	45°	36° × 30°	30° × 30°	32° × 23°
Segmentation	6 layers	4 layers	4 layers	2 layers	4 layers

[a] NIDEK—advanced OCT/SLO system RS-3000.
[b] TOPCON Optical Coherence Tomography 3D OCT-1000. http://www.topcon.co.jp/en/eyecare/diag/oct/oct1000mark2.html.
[c] Cirrus™ HD-OCT for retina, glaucoma, and cornea by Carl Zeiss Meditec. http://www.meditec.zeiss.com/C125679E00525939/ContainerTitel/CirrusOCT/$File/products.html.
[d] Heidelberg Engineering—SPECTRALIS® HRA. http://www.heidelbergengineering.com/international/products/spectralis-hra/.
[e] RTVue overview—Optovue Inc. http://www.optovue.com/products/rtvue.

However, Naheedy et al. [38] found poor correlation for volumetric measurements between OCT and HRT. The macular volume measured by OCT was significantly greater than that measured by HRT.

The OCT has its strengths and limitations. Although machines from different manufacturers vary slightly in their algorithms, scan speed, and resolution (Table 9.1), they were based on similar principles. The OCT is a posterior segment imaging tool that provides highly reproducible objective measurements with multiple scanning regions. The OCT provides fast image acquisition speed and cross-sectional images of the retina with excellent resolution (Figure 9.8). With 3D OCT imaging, new imaging protocols allow us to better visualize and map retinal microstructures. OCT images of the retina with arbitrary orientations can be generated directly and cross-sectional OCT images and thickness maps with fundus features can be accurately mapped out, including thicknesses of the nerve fiber layer, photoreceptor layer, and other intraretinal layers. It is also possible to measure optic nerve head topography and disc parameters, similar to those of other imaging tools such as Stratus OCT, GDx, and HRT [39].

However, as the OCT is used mainly for RNFL imaging, compensation has to be made for the distortion caused by cornea birefringence. Image quality is dependent on operator technique and can be degraded in the presence of media opacity. Although change analysis software for glaucoma applications is still developing and there is a scarcity of age-, gender-, and race-specific normative data for comparison of eyes with retinal disease and glaucoma, the role of OCT as a method to diagnose and manage retinal disease and glaucoma will eventually be further defined, and many of the current limitations will be overcome [33]. OCT however is a useful imaging device for further qualitative and

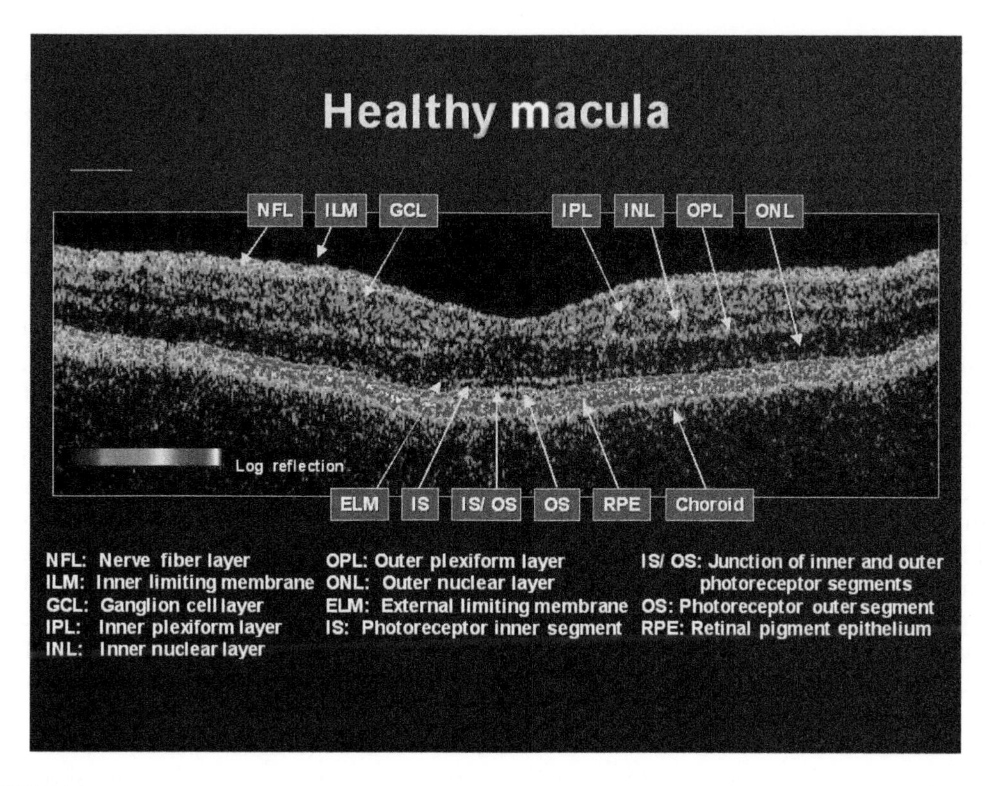

FIGURE 9.8
Spectral domain OCT scan of the macula showing various layers of the retina.

quantitative evaluation of injuries to the posterior segment and has potential in the diagnosis and follow-up of subtle key abnormalities [40].

9.2.4 Scanning Laser Polarimetry

The scanning laser polarimeter (SLP) is commercially available as the GDx nerve fiber analyzer (Laser Diagnostic Technologies Inc., San Diego, CA). Laser light double passes the RNFL and splits into two parallel rays by the birefringent fibers. The two rays travel at different speeds and this difference (called retardation) correlates to the thickness of the nerve fiber layer [41]. The GDx makes RNFL measurements in the peripapillary region and also uses a support vector machine learning classifier to calculate the nerve fiber indicator (NFI). It ranges from 0 to 100, and the higher the NFI, the greater the likelihood of glaucoma. Unfortunately, the birefringent property of the RNFL is also shared by the cornea and, to a lesser extent, the lens. Previous versions of the GDx had a fixed cornea fixator assuming that the cornea polarization axis and magnitude has the same values in all subjects. However, it was later reported that as high as 30% of the eyes had cornea polarization axis and magnitude that deviates significantly from the standardized values [42–44]. Thus, the variable cornea compensator (VCC) was introduced to adjust for different anterior segment birefringence [45]. There is good correlation between the RNFL measurements by GDx with histological measurement of RNFL thickness [13,46]. The GDx-VCC was also validated by clinical studies to have higher reproducibility than its original and higher diagnostic accuracy for glaucoma [47–50].

Morishita et al. compared GDx with VCC and enhanced corneal compensation (ECC) when applied to myopic glaucomatous eyes. ECC showed a better retardation pattern and structure–function relationship than VCC, and ECC appeared to be more suitable for RNFL assessment in glaucomatous eyes that are moderately to highly myopic [51]. However, it is unable to produce the quality cross-sectional images of RNFL and macula for diagnosis, which the OCT is able to [52].

The GDx provides quantitative RNFL measurements and analysis. It has its own normative database and with its unique guided progression analysis (GPA) helps to facilitate long-term monitoring of structural progression in glaucoma patients [44]. It works best on undilated pupils and could be used in eyes with significant cataracts, up to best corrected visual acuity of 20/60 (Snellen chart). However, GDx is limited by its range of imaging, only able to measure RNFL thickness, and lacks versatility of HRT and OCT. Unlike OCT, the GDx is capable of automatic optic nerve head registration. HRT also uses automatic optic nerve head registration for the follow-up exams. However, for the initial exam, the optic nerve head position has to be adjusted manually. Some studies that compared OCT with GDx provided areas under the receiver-operating characteristic (ROC) curve (AUCs) for diagnostic accuracy revealing relatively equivalent abilities to discriminate glaucoma from normal eyes [31]. Medeiros et al. [53] compared GDx-VCC, HRT-2, and Stratus OCT. At specificities of at least 95%, no statistically significant differences were found among parameters with the highest sensitivities from each instrument: GDx-VCC (sensitivity 61%), Stratus OCT (sensitivity 71%), and HRT-2 (sensitivity 59%). At specificities of at least 80%, there was a statistically significant difference between the parameter of HRT-2 (sensitivity 73%) and that of GDx-VCC (sensitivity 87%) and Stratus OCT (sensitivity 89%). No statistically significant difference was found between parameters with the highest sensitivities from the GDx-VCC and Stratus OCT. Regression analyses have found that OCT values in general had better correlation with visual function than GDx-VCC [54].

9.2.5 Comparison of HRT, OCT, and GDx

Table 9.2 summarizes the different features of HRT, OCT, and GDx. There are many studies investigating the diagnostic accuracy of each individual test or just two of the three instruments. To draw meaningful conclusions by direct comparison of instruments from these studies is hard as there were differences in the instrument versions/models, population characteristics, severity of glaucoma, methodology, definitions, and outcome measures. Thus, the best way to compare the three imaging modalities is to use all of them on the same sample of subjects and using a standardized outcome measure to determine diagnostic accuracy.

Badala et al. [15] compared HRT-3, Stratus OCT, and GDx-VCC for their ability to discriminate early glaucoma from normal eyes. The authors reported no significant difference among AUC for the best parameters of the three devices. This was consistent with other studies comparing the three instruments despite being of different versions [16,55–57]. Vessani et al. [58] compared Stratus OCT, HRT-3, and GDx with clinical evaluation of the optic nerve that showed no significant differences in performance between the automated imaging systems and experienced clinicians. Each of the quantitative imaging techniques was independently performed as well as, but not better than, evaluation of stereo-photographs by experienced clinicians. Clinical assessment of optic disc photos is influenced largely by the examiner's experience, and results may vary in different clinical settings.

OCT has the highest axial resolution out of the three, with the development of an ultrahigh-resolution system allowing the identification of otherwise unseen intermediate

TABLE 9.2

Comparison of HRT, OCT, and GDx

	HRT	OCT	GDx
Mechanism	A 670 nm diode laser provides 3D reconstruction of the optic disc.	Low-coherence near-infrared light and backscatter construct cross-sectional retinal image.	Phase shift of polarized laser passing the birefringent RNFL correlates with RNFL thickness.
Outcome measurements	Rim area, rim volume, cup shape measure, CDR, retinal height variation, and RNFL thickness.	RNFL thickness, CDR, rim volume, macular thickness.	RNFL thickness.
Analysis	MRA, GPS, TCA.	—	Guided progression analysis.
Strengths	Large ethnic-specific normative database, trend analysis, undilated pupils.	Fast scanning speed, excellent resolution of the retina cross section.	Undilated pupils, automatic optic nerve head registration.
Weaknesses	Operator-dependent disc contouring.	Pupil dilation, lack of ethnic-specific normative database, lack of progression analysis software.	Ocular comorbidities reduce accuracy of GDx; atypical birefringence patterns.

retinal layers [17]. HRT has greater usefulness in the evaluation of optic disc swelling and elevation, while OCT provides the most convenience and accuracy for determining and monitoring RNFL thickness. Some variables such as disease severity and optic disc size have an impact on the diagnostic accuracy of these three imaging techniques. Medeiros et al. [59] reported that the HRT-2, Stratus OCT, and GDx-VCC all had increased sensitivity when used in subjects with more severe glaucomatous disease and field loss. On the other hand, larger optic discs correlated with decreased sensitivity for the Stratus OCT and GDx-VCC but increased sensitivity for the HRT-2 and vice versa. DeLeon Ortega et al. [60] also showed that repeatability of these techniques are affected by the degree of glaucomatous damage with the HRT-2 and GDx-VCC showing better repeatability than the Stratus OCT. Test–retest variability of RNFL using GDx-VCC and OCT were consistent through all stages of disease severity, but repeatability results of GDx-VCC were better than those of OCT, except in severe cases. Test–retest variability of optic nerve head topography using HRT-2 and OCT increased with increasing disease severity for rim area, cup area, and CDR, but vertical CDR from HRT-2 and horizontal CDR from OCT showed stable variability through all stages. Regardless of disease severity, repeatability results of HRT-2 were superior to OCT.

Comorbidities in the eye may also affect the diagnostic accuracy of these imaging tools. Mild to moderate nonproliferative diabetic retinopathy was found to cause a quantitative discrepancy between RNFL measurements from GDx-VCC and Stratus OCT. Nevertheless, both tools were still able to effectively detect glaucomatous changes in eyes with diabetic retinopathy [61]. Zheng et al. reported that the presence of diabetes mellitus had no influence on both the sensitivities and specificity for all HRT algorithms. In the multivariate analyses adjusting for optic disc size, the presence of diabetic retinopathy was significantly associated with higher false-positive rates for the Burk and Bathija linear discriminant functions [62].

Eyes with large areas of age-related macular degeneration have optic disc structural alterations that mimic optic neuropathy and they were more likely to be classified as glaucomatous clinically as well as by HRT [63]. When Fourier domain OCT was used, age-related macular degeneration influenced the measurement of inner macular thickness parameters, and all ganglion cell complex parameters were significantly higher [64].

We suggest that structural imaging instruments should be used in combination of each other and as an adjunct to clinical examination of the optic nerve head and peripapillary RNFL. By combining the different posterior segment imaging techniques, we could harness the unique strengths of each machine to improve diagnostic reliability. This would give the ophthalmologist the confidence to detect glaucomatous changes early and start treatment earlier instead of adopting the wait-and-see approach for glaucoma suspect or preperimetric glaucoma. Similarly, by providing quantitative measurements, these machines provide an objective means of detecting structural progression due to glaucomatous damage. Progression could be detected earlier and modifications to treatment regimes can be instituted. However, it is important to remember that static automated perimetry is still the predominant functional method of monitoring the severity and progression of glaucoma. Perimetry depends on subjective input from the patient and takes a longer time to complete. In addition, patients require several practices over time to be able to perform the tests reliably. This may delay diagnosis of glaucoma, and patients with certain comorbidities such as dementia, arthritis involving the hands, and short attention span, may not be able to perform perimetry tests accurately. As such, structural imaging tools both complement and act as an alternative means for monitoring glaucoma in these patients. It should be emphasized that posterior imaging tools like the HRT, OCT, or GDx are best utilized in detecting progression rather than diagnosis [65]. Due to the long duration of experience and familiarity with HRT, it is used with much more regularity in glaucoma patients compared to OCT and GDx. Of the three machines, the GDx is used the most sparingly as it is relatively new compared to HRT and OCT. Most of the ophthalmology clinics would already be using either the HRT or OCT to monitor the glaucoma patients. Despite GDx being most economical, as these tools are not interchangeable, there are little clinical and economic indications to switch to GDx. Another advantage of the OCT is its ability to double up as an imaging tool for retinal diseases, which is a function that the GDx lacked. The popularity of these three imaging modalities for glaucoma imaging is also reflected in the number of publications available in the literature. A search on PubMed for HRT showed a total of 416 publications, with 179 of those being in the last 5 years. There were a total of 871 publications, including 631 in the last 5 years, on the use of OCT in glaucoma imaging. For the GDx, there were a total of 290 publications but only 114 in the last 5 years. Overall, posterior segment imaging can help prevent blindness and improve visual prognosis.

9.3 Looking Ahead

9.3.1 Automated Measurements of Disc Parameters

As the *silent thief of sight*, glaucoma causes significant irreversible visual field loss in asymptomatic patients. Clinically, glaucoma is diagnosed through slit lamp examination of the fundus looking for characteristic optic disc neuropathy and RNFL thinning. However, this is subjective and is prone to high inter- and intraobserver variability depending on experience level [66]. Similarly, most of the posterior segment imaging tools' algorithms are semiautomatic consisting of an operator-dependent step—identification of optic disc margins. This is a major obstacle in glaucoma screening of the general population as it is time consuming and requires trained manpower. Thus, there is a need for more automated measurements of optic nerve head and retinal parameters.

The *a*utomatic cup–disc *r*atio measurement system for *g*laucoma detection and *a*na*l*ys*i*s (ARGALI) is currently being developed to automatically measure the CDR to assess the risk of glaucoma [67,68]. ARGALI employs a unique algorithm to calculate the CDR using a level-set-based technique. The software detects the region of interest containing the optic disc from fundal photographs. After automatically recognizing disc and cup contours, an ellipse fitting step is used to smooth the contours and the CDR is calculated. In a study by Wong et al., 104 retinal photographs were tested with the ARGALI and gave a 96% confidence of obtaining results within a range of 0.2, comparable to the variability of manual grading of CDR [68].

9.3.2 Optic Disc Tilt

Optic disc morphology plays an important role in the diagnostic accuracy of semiautomatic posterior segment glaucoma imaging tool. The contours of the classic oval optic disc would be ideal to delineate and translates into high reproducibility of area and volumetric data.

However, in Asia where there is a high proportion of myopia and astigmatism, optic disc morphology is much more varied including large discs, tilted discs, torted discs, and peripapillary atrophy. As such, accurate identification of disc contours is harder and inconsistent. Studies have shown that tilted optic discs have significant impact on the subsequent area and volumetric data. Optic disc tilt is a 3D concept that was not accounted for by any current glaucoma imaging tools that were based on 2D images. Our preliminary results (unpublished) showed that we are able to make sure of mathematical models to adjust area and volumetric data according to the type and severity of optic disc tilt. Potentially, this may provide a means for further stratification and normality classification algorithms of glaucoma imaging tools to improve diagnostic accuracy.

9.3.3 3-T Diffusion Tensor Imaging

The 3-T diffusion tensor imaging (DTI) is a new technique recently evaluated to compare the axonal architecture of the optic nerve with morphological features of the optic nerve head and RNFL obtained with HRT-3, GDx-VCC, and OCT [69].

DTI is the MRI technique in which water molecule diffusivity is analyzed to develop a reconstruction of axonal density [70]. The internal structure of the axonal microtubules leads to linear water molecule movement in intact axons (high fractional anisotropy [FA] and limits mean diffusivity [MD]). Increases in MD and reductions in FA recorded in the central nervous system by DTI reflect the extent of axonal damage as shown by ultrastructural studies [71]. The MRI examinations were performed using a 3-T scanner (Achieva Intera 3T; Philips Healthcare, Best, the Netherlands). The imaging protocol included a T1-weighted 3D fast field echo sequence and a fluid-attenuated inversion-recovery T2-weighted sequence. Data were then processed on the magnetic resonance console (Achieva Intera 3T; Philips Healthcare) with an automatic customized script. Diffusion tensor trace images were created by averaging all 32 diffusion-weighted images, and MD and FA maps were automatically created. MD displayed the strongest correlation with linear cup/disc ratio (LCDR) from HRT-3, RNFL thickness from OCT, and NFI from GDx, whereas FA was strongly correlated with the LCDR.

The aforementioned study has introduced 3-T DTI as a plausible new adjunct in the diagnosis and monitoring of glaucoma. Nevertheless, larger-scale longitudinal studies would be required to ascertain its reliability as a routine imaging tool.

9.3.4 3D OCT

The introduction of 3D ultrahigh-resolution OCT is a relatively new tool capable of producing 3D quantification of ONH and RNFL parameters. This imaging modality was derived from enhanced depth imaging technique and was described elsewhere [72]. Briefly, the ONH was imaged with approximately 65 sections (30–34 μm apart), which were processed to construct a 3D optic disc image (Figure 9.9). Image is considered of good quality if the quality score is >15. Studies have showed that 3D OCT is capable of imaging the different isolated optic nerve head structures such as the lamina cribrosa, thought to be the site of primary injury in glaucoma, and the RNFL with good reproducibility and structure–function correlation [73–75]. However, further studies are required to validate its use for diagnosis and monitoring of glaucoma.

9.3.5 Macular Ganglion Cell Layer Imaging

High-definition OCT has allowed accurate segmentation of the different intraretinal layers possible. The retinal ganglion cell layer has been reported to be the first site of early glaucomatous damage and the macula comprised of the highest concentration of ganglion cells [76]. Thus, advanced imaging algorithms are targeted at imaging the macula ganglion cell layer. The Fourier domain RTVue OCT (Optovue Corporation, Fremont, CA) first introduced the macular ganglion cell complex (GCC—sum of RNFL, ganglion cell layer,

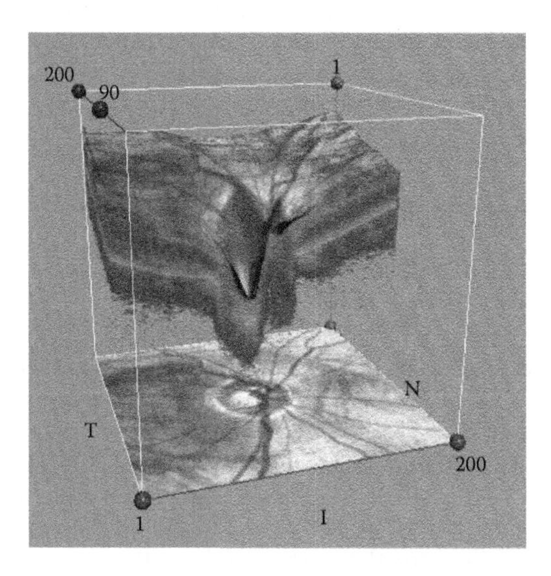

FIGURE 9.9
(See color insert.) 3D OCT scan of the optic disc.

and inner plexiform layers) thickness, which was further streamlined by Cirrus HD-OCT (Cirrus 6.0 software version, Carl Zeiss Meditec, Dublin, CA) to comprise of ganglion cell–inner plexiform layer (GC–IPL) while excluding the RNFL [77,78]. Studies have shown that GCC layer thickness has similar glaucoma discriminating performance compared with RNFL thickness [77], but further studies are required to study the diagnostic ability of GC–IPL thickness.

9.4 Summary and Conclusions

Ocular imaging has come a long way from experimental tools to its role as diagnostics and monitoring adjuncts. While clinical examination remains the mainstay, imaging tools are slowly gaining recognition as possible solutions for increased automation and quantification of ocular parameters pertinent to glaucoma.

Glaucoma imaging should always be an adjunct, rather than a replacement for a good clinical examination. The amount of investigation will vary according to the patient. We suggest a simple clinical pathway applicable to general ophthalmology practice. The first step would be clinical examination of both the anterior and posterior segment looking for signs of glaucoma such as shallow anterior chambers (usually via Van Herick sign), gonioscopic features of narrow anterior chamber angles, raised intraocular pressure, glaucomatous optic neuropathy, and RNFL defects.

If there are obvious signs of glaucoma, a comprehensive investigation of the patient will be needed. This will also apply if there are strong risk factors in the history taking, which include a family history of glaucoma, or a history of significant blood loss.

Posterior segment glaucoma imaging will be complemented by functional tests such as the standard automated perimetry. At this point, the ophthalmologist would have to assess the risk of glaucoma and progression. If deemed high risk, the ophthalmologist may choose to monitor the eyes at risk with increased frequency, or if there is low risk, then the patient can be reviewed with a longer duration. Ideally, the ophthalmologist should stick to the same imaging tool and version throughout the duration of the review as it had been shown that different tools give different results for the *same* measurements. This is the case illustrated by RNFL thickness measurements where the spectral domain OCT gave smaller values compared to time domain OCT [34,79]. As such, the results may not be interchangeable from each other.

Currently, there are many machines available commercially that it may be hard to decide which tools would be most appropriate to employ or, for new centers, to procure so as to maximize its clinical applications. In general, for a tertiary center to provide a competent glaucoma service, it would be good if there is an anterior segment imaging tool and a posterior imaging tool that provides optic nerve head measurements such as the HRT. For the general practice, it would be an advantage to procure a posterior imaging tool that also allows the macula to be imaged such as the OCT.

Ultimately, it is important to reiterate that imaging devices are meant to complement the clinical examination and visual field tests, and the ophthalmologist needs to retain his clinical acumen and use the images to assist his management of glaucoma. Imaging equipment is more useful as a tool for assessing progression and should be used together with other clinical data.

Acknowledgment

Special thanks to Carl Zeiss Meditec for Figures 9.5, 9.6, 9.8, and 9.9.

References

1. Quigley HA, Broman AT. The number of people with glaucoma worldwide in 2010 and 2020. *Br J Ophthalmol* 2006; **90**(3): 262–267.
2. He M, Foster PJ, Ge J et al. Prevalence and clinical characteristics of glaucoma in adult Chinese: A population-based study in Liwan District, Guangzhou. *Invest Ophthalmol Vis Sci* 2006; **47**(7): 2782–2788.
3. Bowd C, Zangwill LM, Medeiros FA et al. Structure–function relationships using confocal scanning laser ophthalmoscopy, optical coherence tomography, and scanning laser polarimetry. *Invest Ophthalmol Vis Sci* 2006; **47**(7): 2889–2895.
4. Quigley HA, Katz J, Derick RJ, Gilbert D, Sommer A. An evaluation of optic disc and nerve fiber layer examinations in monitoring progression of early glaucoma damage. *Ophthalmology* 1992; **99**(1): 19–28.
5. Sommer A, Katz J, Quigley HA et al. Clinically detectable nerve fiber atrophy precedes the onset of glaucomatous field loss. *Arch Ophthalmol* 1991; **109**(1): 77–83.
6. Zeyen T, Miglior S, Pfeiffer N, Cunha-Vaz J, Adamsons I, European Glaucoma Prevention Study Group. Reproducibility of evaluation of optic disc change for glaucoma with stereo optic disc photographs. *Ophthalmology* 2003; **110**(2): 340–344.
7. Mikelberg FS, Parfitt CM, Swindale NV, Graham SL, Drance SM, Gosine R. Ability of the Heidelberg retina tomograph to detect early glaucomatous visual field loss. *J Glaucoma* 1995; **4**(4): 242–247.
8. Bathija R, Zangwill L, Berry CC, Sample PA, Weinreb RN. Detection of early glaucomatous structural damage with confocal scanning laser tomography. *J Glaucoma* 1998; **7**(2): 121–127.
9. Miglior S, Guareschi M, Albe E, Gomarasca S, Vavassori M, Orzalesi N. Detection of glaucomatous visual field changes using the Moorfields regression analysis of the Heidelberg retina tomograph. *Am J Ophthalmol* 2003; **136**(1): 26–33.
10. Wollstein G, Garway-Heath DF, Fontana L, Hitchings RA. Identifying early glaucomatous changes. Comparison between expert clinical assessment of optic disc photographs and confocal scanning ophthalmoscopy. *Ophthalmology* 2000; **107**(12): 2272–2277.
11. Chauhan BC, Hutchison DM, Artes PH et al. Optic disc progression in glaucoma: Comparison of confocal scanning laser tomography to optic disc photographs in a prospective study. *Invest Ophthalmol Vis Sci* 2009; **50**(4): 1682–1691.
12. Chauhan BC, McCormick TA, Nicolela MT, LeBlanc RP. Optic disc and visual field changes in a prospective longitudinal study of patients with glaucoma: Comparison of scanning laser tomography with conventional perimetry and optic disc photography. *Arch Ophthalmol* 2001; **119**(10): 1492–1499.
13. Morgan JE, Waldock A. Scanning laser polarimetry of the normal human retinal nerve fiber layer: A quantitative analysis. *Am J Ophthalmol* 2000; **129**(1): 76–82.
14. Zheng Y, Wong TY, Lamoureux E et al. Diagnostic ability of Heidelberg retina tomography in detecting glaucoma in a population setting: The Singapore Malay Eye Study. *Ophthalmology* 2010; **117**(2): 290–297.
15. Badala F, Nouri-Mahdavi K, Raoof DA, Leeprechanon N, Law SK, Caprioli J. Optic disk and nerve fiber layer imaging to detect glaucoma. *Am J Ophthalmol* 2007; **144**(5): 724–732.

16. Deleon-Ortega JE, Arthur SN, McGwin G Jr, Xie A, Monheit BE, Girkin CA. Discrimination between glaucomatous and nonglaucomatous eyes using quantitative imaging devices and subjective optic nerve head assessment. *Invest Ophthalmol Vis Sci* 2006; **47**(8): 3374–3380.
17. Stein DM, Wollstein G, Schuman JS. Imaging in glaucoma. *Ophthalmol Clin North Am* 2004; **17**(1): 33–52.
18. Tong L, Chan YH, Gazzard G et al. Heidelberg retinal tomography of optic disc and nerve fiber layer in Singapore children: Variations with disc tilt and refractive error. *Invest Ophthalmol Vis Sci* 2007; **48**(11): 4939–4944.
19. Miglior S, Albe E, Guareschi M, Rossetti L, Orzalesi N. Intraobserver and interobserver reproducibility in the evaluation of optic disc stereometric parameters by Heidelberg retina tomograph. *Ophthalmology* 2002; **109**(6): 1072–1077.
20. Strouthidis NG, Garway-Heath DF. New developments in Heidelberg retina tomograph for glaucoma. *Curr Opin Ophthalmol* 2008; **19**(2): 141–148.
21. Gabriele ML, Wollstein G, Bilonick RA et al. Comparison of parameters from Heidelberg retina tomographs 2 and 3. *Ophthalmology* 2008; **115**(4): 673–677.
22. De Leon-Ortega JE, Sakata LM, Monheit BE, McGwin G Jr, Arthur SN, Girkin CA. Comparison of diagnostic accuracy of Heidelberg retina tomograph II and Heidelberg retina tomograph 3 to discriminate glaucomatous and nonglaucomatous eyes. *Am J Ophthalmol* 2007; **144**(4): 525–532.
23. Burgansky-Eliash Z, Wollstein G, Bilonick RA, Ishikawa H, Kagemann L, Schuman JS. Glaucoma detection with the Heidelberg retina tomograph 3. *Ophthalmology* 2007; **114**(3): 466–471.
24. Zelefsky JR, Harizman N, Mora R et al. Assessment of a race-specific normative HRT-III database to differentiate glaucomatous from normal eyes. *J Glaucoma* 2006; **15**(6): 548–551.
25. Samarawickrama C, Wang JJ, Huynh SC et al. Ethnic differences in optic nerve head and retinal nerve fibre layer thickness parameters in children. *Br J Ophthalmol* 2010; **94**(7): 871–876.
26. Tsai CS, Zangwill L, Gonzalez C et al. Ethnic differences in optic nerve head topography. *J Glaucoma* 1995; **4**(4): 248–257.
27. Girkin CA, McGwin G Jr, Long C, DeLeon-Ortega J, Graf CM, Everett AW. Subjective and objective optic nerve assessment in African Americans and whites. *Invest Ophthalmol Vis Sci* 2004; **45**(7): 2272–2278.
28. Ohkubo S, Takeda H, Higashide T. A pilot study to detect glaucoma with confocal scanning laser ophthalmoscopy compared with nonmydriatic stereoscopic photography in a community health screening. *J Glaucoma* 2007; **16**(6): 531–538.
29. Nicolela MT, McCormic TA, Drance SM, Ferrier SN, LeBlanc RP, Chauhan BC. Visual field and optic disc progression in patients with different types of optic disc damage. A longitudinal prospective study. *Ophthalmology* 2003; **110**(11): 2178–2184.
30. Wollstein G, Schuman JS, Price LL et al. Optical coherence tomography longitudinal evaluation of retinal nerve fiber layer thickness in glaucoma. *Arch Ophthalmol* 2005; **123**(4): 464–470.
31. Lin SC, Singh K, Jampel HD. Optic nerve head and retinal nerve fiber layer analysis. *Ophthalmology* 2007; **114**(10): 1937–1949.
32. Chauhan BC, Blanchard JW, Hamilton DC, LeBlanc RP. Technique for detecting serial topographic changes in the optic disc and peripapillary retina using scanning laser tomography. *Invest Ophthalmol Vis Sci* 2000; **41**(3): 775–782.
33. Chang RT, Knight OJ, Feuer WJ, Budenz DL. Sensitivity and specificity of time-domain versus spectral-domain optical coherence tomography in diagnosing early to moderate glaucoma. *Ophthalmology* 2009; **116**(12): 2294–2299.
34. Knight OJ, Chang RT, Feuer WJ, Budenz DL. Comparison of retinal nerve fiber layer measurements using time domain and spectral domain optical coherent tomography. *Ophthalmology* 2009; **116**(7): 1271–1277.
35. Jaffe G, Caprioli J. Optical coherence tomography to detect and manage retinal disease and glaucoma. *Am J Ophthalmol* 2004; **137**(1): 156–169.
36. Wang X, Li S, Fu J et al. Comparative study of retinal nerve fibre layer measurement by RTVue OCT and GDx VCC. *Br J Ophthalmol* 2011; **95**(4): 509–513.

37. Leung CK, Chan WM, Chong KK et al. Comparative study of retinal nerve fiber layer measurement by Stratus OCT and GDx VCC, I: Correlation analysis in glaucoma. *Invest Ophthalmol Vis Sci* 2005; **46**(9): 3214–3220.
38. Naheedy JH, Bartsch DU, Freeman WR. Comparison of retinal thickness and macular volume using three imaging techniques. *Invest Ophthalmol Vis Sci* 2004; **45**: 2407 (E-Abstract).
39. Wojtkowski M, Srinivasan V, Fujimoto JG et al. Three-dimensional retinal imaging with high-speed ultrahigh-resolution optical coherence tomography. *Ophthalmology* 2005; **112**(10): 1734–1746.
40. Rumelt S, Karatas M, Ophir A. Potential applications of optical coherence tomography in posterior segment trauma. *Ophthalmic Surg Lasers Imaging* 2005; **36**(4): 315–322.
41. Da Pozzo S, Marchesan R, Ravalico G. Scanning laser polarimetry—A review. *Clin Exp Ophthalmol* 2009; **37**(1): 68–80.
42. Greenfield DS, Knighton RW, Feuer WJ, Schiffman JC, Zangwill L, Weinreb RN. Correction for corneal polarization axis improves the discriminating power of scanning laser polarimetry. *Am J Ophthalmol* 2002; **134**(1): 27–33.
43. Garway-Heath DF, Greaney MJ, Caprioli J. Correction for the erroneous compensation of anterior segment birefringence with the scanning laser polarimeter for glaucoma diagnosis. *Invest Ophthalmol Vis Sci* 2002; **43**(5): 1465–1474.
44. Weinreb RN, Bowd C, Greenfield DS, Zangwill LM. Measurement of the magnitude and axis of corneal polarization with scanning laser polarimetry. *Arch Ophthalmol* 2002; **120**(7): 901–906.
45. Mai TA, Reus NJ, Lemij HG. Structure–function relationship is stronger with enhanced corneal compensation than with variable corneal compensation in scanning laser polarimetry. *Invest Ophthalmol Vis Sci* 2007; **48**(4): 1651–1658.
46. Weinreb RN, Dreher AW, Coleman W, Quigley H, Shaw B, Reiter K. Histopathologic validation of Fourier-ellipsometry measurements of retinal nerve fiber layer thickness. *Arch Ophthalmol* 1990; **108**(4): 557–560.
47. Bowd C, Zangwill LM, Weinreb RN. Association between scanning laser polarimetry measurements using variable corneal polarization compensation and visual field sensitivity in glaucomatous eyes. *Arch Ophthalmol* 2003; **121**(7): 961–966.
48. Medeiros FA, Bowd C, Zangwill LM, Patel C, Weinreb RN. Detection of glaucoma using scanning laser polarimetry with enhanced corneal compensation. *Invest Ophthalmol Vis Sci* 2007; **48**(7): 3146–3153.
49. Weinreb RN, Bowd C, Zangwill LM. Glaucoma detection using scanning laser polarimetry with variable corneal polarization compensation. *Arch Ophthalmol* 2003; **121**(2): 218–224.
50. Medeiros FA, Vizzeri G, Zangwill LM, Alencar LM, Sample PA, Weinreb RN. Comparison of retinal nerve fiber layer and optic disc imaging for diagnosing glaucoma in patients suspected of having the disease. *Ophthalmology* 2008; **115**: 1340–1346.
51. Morishita S, Tanabe T, Yu S et al. Retinal nerve fibre layer assessment in myopic glaucomatous eyes: Comparison of GDx VCC with GDx ECC. *Br J Ophthalmol* 2008 **92**(10): 1377–1381.
52. Trick GL, Calotti FY, Skarf B. Advances in imaging of the optic disc and retinal nerve fiber layer. *J Neuroophthalmol* 2006; **26**(4): 284–295.
53. Medeiros FA, Zangwill LM, Bowd C, Weinreb RN. Comparison of the GDx VCC scanning laser polarimeter, HRT II confocal scanning laser ophthalmoscope, and stratus OCT optical coherence tomograph for the detection of glaucoma. *Arch Ophthalmol* 2004; **122**(6): 827–837.
54. Leung CK, Chong KK, Chan WM. Comparative study of retinal nerve fiber layer measurement by Stratus OCT and GDx VCC, II: Structure/function regression analysis in glaucoma. *Invest Ophthalmol Vis Sci* 2005; **46**: 3702–3711.
55. Kanamori A, Nagai-Kusuhara A, Escano MF, Maeda H, Nakamura M, Negi A. Comparison of confocal scanning laser ophthalmoscopy, scanning laser polarimetry and optical coherence tomography to discriminate ocular hypertension and glaucoma at an early stage. *Graefes Arch Clin Exp Ophthalmol* 2006; **244**(1): 58–68.

56. Zangwill LM, Bowd C, Berry CC, Williams J. Discriminating between normal and glaucomatous eyes using the Heidelberg retina tomograph, GDx nerve fiber analyzer, and optical coherence tomograph. *Arch Ophthalmol* 2001; **119**(7): 985–993.
57. Medeiros FA, Zangwill LM, Bowd C, Weinreb RN. Comparison of the GDx VCC scanning laser polarimeter, HRT II confocal scanning laser ophthalmoscope, and stratus OCT optical coherence tomograph for the detection of glaucoma. *Arch Ophthalmol* 2004; **122**(6): 827–837.
58. Vessani RM, Moritz R, Batis L, Zagui RB, Bernardoni S, Susanna R. Comparison of quantitative imaging devices and subjective optic nerve head assessment by general ophthalmologists to differentiate normal from glaucomatous eyes. *J Glaucoma* 2009; **18**(3): 253–261.
59. Medeiros FA, Zangwill LM, Bowd C, Sample PA, Weinrev RN. Influence of disease severity and optic disc size on the diagnostic performance of imaging instruments in glaucoma. *Invest Ophthalmol Vis Sci* 2006; **47**(3): 1008–1015.
60. DeLeon Ortega JE, Sakata LM, Kakati B et al. Effect of glaucomatous damage on repeatability of confocal scanning laser ophthalmoscope, scanning laser polarimetry, and optical coherence tomography. *Invest Ophthalmol Vis Sci* 2007; **48**(3): 1156–1163.
61. Takahashi H, Chihara E. Impact of diabetic retinopathy on quantitative retinal nerve fibre layer measurement and glaucoma screening. *Invest Ophthalmol Vis Sci* 2008; **49**(2): 687–692.
62. Zheng Y, Wong TY, Cheung CY. Influence of diabetes and diabetic retinopathy on the performance of Heidelberg retina tomography II for diagnosis of glaucoma. *Invest Ophthalmol Vis Sci* 2010; **51**(11): 5519–5524.
63. Law SK, Sohn UH, Hoffman D, Smll K, Coleman AL, Caprioli J. Optic disk appearance in advanced age-related macular degeneration. *Am J Ophthalmol* 2004; **138**(1): 38–45.
64. Garas A, Papp A, Hollo G. Influence of age-related macular degeneration on macular thickness measurement made with Fourier-domain optical coherence tomography. *J Glaucoma* 2013; **22**(3):195–200.
65. Fayers T, Strouthidis NG, Garway-Heath DF. Monitoring glaucomatous progression using a novel Heidelberg retina tomograph event analysis. *Ophthalmology* 2007; **114**(11): 1973–1980.
66. Varma R, Spaeth GL, Steinmann WC, Katz LJ. Agreement between clinicians and an image analyzer in estimating cup-to-disc ratios. *Arch Ophthalmol* 1989; **107**(4): 526–529.
67. Wong DW, Liu J, Lim JH et al. Intelligent fusion of cup-to-disc ratio determination methods for glaucoma detection in ARGALI. *Conf Proc IEEE Eng Med Biol Soc* 2009, Minneapolis, MN, Vol. 2009, pp. 5777–5780.
68. Wong DK, Liu K, Lim JH et al. Level-set based automatic cup-to-disc ratio determination using retinal fundus images in ARGALI. *Conf Proc IEEE Eng Med Biol Soc* 2008, Vancouver, British Columbia, Columbia, Vol. 2008, pp. 2266–2269.
69. Nucci C, Mancino R, Martucci A et al. 3-T diffusion tensor imaging of the optic nerve in subjects with glaucoma: Correlation with GDx-VCC, HRT-III and stratus optical coherence tomography findings. *Br J Ophthalmol* 2012; **96**(7): 976–980.
70. Garaci FG, Cozzolino V, Nucci C et al. Advances in neuroimaging of the visual pathways and their use in glaucoma. *Prog Brain Res* 2008; **173**: 165–177.
71. Wheeler-Kingshott CA, Trip SA, Symms MR et al. In vivo diffusion tensor imaging of the human optic nerve: Pilot study in normal controls. *Magn Reson Med* 2006; **56**(2): 446–451.
72. Spaide RF, Koizumi H, Pozzoni MC. Enhanced depth imaging spectral-domain optical coherence tomography. *Am J Ophthalmol* 2008; **146**: 496–500.
73. Inoue R, Hangai M, Kotera Y et al. Three-dimensional high-speed optical coherence tomography imaging of lamina cribrosa in glaucoma. *Ophthalmology* 2009; **116**: 214–222.
74. Lee EJ, Kim TW, Weinreb RN et al. Three-dimensional evaluation of the lamina cribrosa using spectral-domain optical coherence tomography in glaucoma. *Invest Ophthalmol Vis Sci* 2012; **53**: 198–204.
75. Menke MN, Knecht P, Sturm V, Dabov S, Funk J. Reproducibility of nerve fiber layer thickness measurements using 3D Fourier-domain OCT. *Invest Ophthalmol Vis Sci* 2008; **49**: 5386–5391.

76. Desatnik H, Quigley HA, Glovinsky Y. Study of central retinal ganglion cell loss in experimental glaucoma in monkey eyes. *J Glaucoma* 1996; **5**(1): 46–53.
77. Tan O, Chopra V, Lu AT et al. Detection of macular ganglion cell loss in glaucoma by Fourier-domain optical coherence tomography. *Ophthalmology* 2009; **116**(12): 2305–2314, e1–e2.
78. Koh VT, Tham YC, Cheung CY et al. Determinants of ganglion cell-inner plexiform layer thickness measured by high-definition optical coherence tomography. *Invest Ophthalmol Vis Sci* 2012; **53**(9): 5853–5859.
79. Sung KR, Kim DY, Park SB, Kook MS. Comparison of retinal nerve fiber layer thickness measured by Cirrus HD and Stratus optical coherence tomography. *Ophthalmology* 2009; **116**(7): 1264–1270, 1270.e1.

10

Imaging of the Eye after Glaucoma Surgery

Mandeep S. Singh, Maria Cecilia D. Aquino, and Paul Tec Kuan Chew

CONTENTS

10.1 Introduction

10.1.1 Glaucoma: A Significant Disease

Glaucoma is an important human disease and so it has attracted much attention in research including its imaging aspects. In one study earlier this decade, it was estimated that 70 million people worldwide were affected by glaucoma, of which 6.7 million were blind in both eyes from this disease [1]. By the year 2020, these numbers are projected to be 79.6 million and 11.2 million, respectively [2]. Aside from the individual human burden and the loss of quality of life suffered by glaucoma patients [3], the global impact of this disease is significant.

10.1.2 Essential Clinical Background

In broad terms, glaucoma may be described as a chronic optic neuropathy. In other words, it is a disease in which the function and structure of the optic nerve is affected over time, due to insults to the neurons (known as the retinal ganglion cells) that make up this nerve [4]. The optic nerve normally functions to carry impulses from the retina to visual nuclei in the brain.

In glaucoma, the peripheral visual field is lost over time if disease progression is not controlled. In severe cases, the patient is left with only a small island of remaining vision at the center of the visual field. The main modifiable risk factor for glaucoma is the pressure inside the eye, or intraocular pressure (IOP). IOP-lowering treatment is the current mainstay of therapy for glaucoma. Medications or surgery can be employed to achieve a reduction in IOP.

10.1.3 Surgical Therapy for Glaucoma

It is critical to have a general understanding of glaucoma surgery in order to appreciate the relevance of imaging in this context.

Surgery is employed in cases where IOP is not lowered sufficiently by medications. Surgery for glaucoma aims to allow flow of fluid (termed the aqueous humor) out of the eye. There are a number of methods to do this, but it may be useful to understand trabeculectomy surgery as the main form of current surgical treatment.

In trabeculectomy, originally described in humans in 1968 [5], a small millimeter-scale opening (the keratotrabeculectomy ostium) is made in the eye wall to allow the outflow of aqueous. The opening is made under a partially thick flap of sclera. The flap is sutured and closed at the end of surgery as a form of protection from excessive early flow that would lead to dangerously low pressure, but it is intended that in the longer term, the flap does not heal back completely as that would shut off the newly created channel for flow.

The Tenon capsule and conjunctiva, the most superficial layers, are then draped over the flap and sutured to recreate the outer protective layer of the eyeball. Over time, the fluid flowing out of the eye though the ostium results in hydration of the Tenon capsule (also called episcleral tissue) and the conjunctiva, resulting in the expansion of these tissues like a wet sponge (Figure 10.1). The expanded portion is called a bleb and it is usually visible by magnified external observation. The fluid then collects into the vessels around the eye and is drained away.

In this surgery, complete healing of the scleral wound—unlike in other types of surgery—is not desired as an outcome, as it would seal off the outflow channel. If, however, the fibrotic response is excessive, the scleral flap, Tenon layer, or conjunctiva may seal up by fibrosis, and the IOP would begin to rise again.

10.1.4 Postoperative Course and Assessment

The flap is shut at the end of the operation to guard against too much outflow—which would deflate the eye too much and lead to other complications. However, after a few days or weeks, it would be safe to release some of these sutures to encourage gradually increasing flow in the later safe period. This technique is called laser suture lysis (LSL) [6]. LSL, if used, is considered a routine procedure of the postsurgical process.

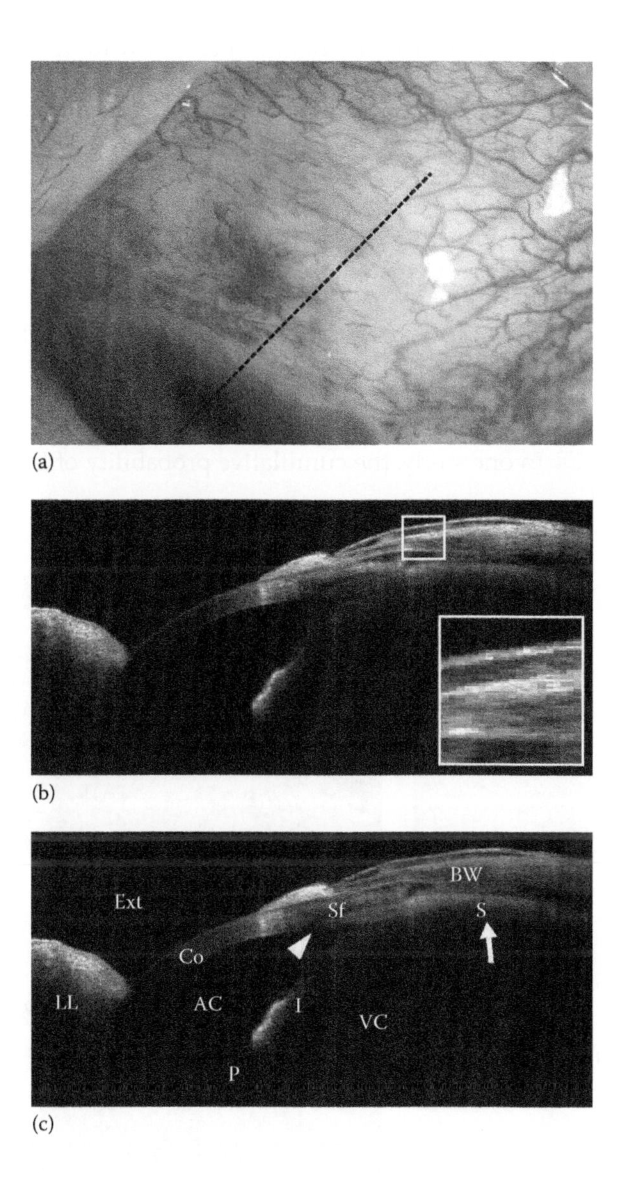

FIGURE 10.1
(See color insert.) Imaging and surgical anatomy of the bleb. (a) Photograph of a glaucoma surgery bleb; the dashed line indicates the approximate orientation of the ASOCT line scan shown in (b) and (c). The location of the bleb is indicated by the relatively opaque area of the conjunctiva. Deep features are not easily seen by direct observation. (b) ASOCT line scan shown without labels for clarity. The inset shows portion of the bleb wall to highlight stripes of differing reflectivity due to hydration of episcleral–conjunctival tissue. (c) The same optical section from (b), with labels added. The bleb wall is shaded blue, the scleral flap is shaded purple, and the sclera is shaded green. The arrowhead indicates the internal keratotrabeculectomy ostium. The deep boundary of the sclera (arrow) is indistinct. Ext, exterior of the eye; Co, cornea; AC, anterior chamber; LL, lower lid; P, pupil; I, iris; VC, vitreous cavity; BW, bleb wall; Sf, scleral flap; S, sclera.

If fluid flow remains poor over time and there is poor bleb formation, then other additional measures can be employed to encourage the outflow of fluid. A needle can be passed into the bleb to break up fibrotic strands that are presumed to be a cause of increased obstruction to flow. This intervention is called *needling* [7]. Needling can be combined with injection of an antifibrotic medication such 5-fluorouracil [8] or mitomycin C [9] near the bleb, to further reduce fibrosis.

Inflammation also must be adequately controlled. It is a normal reaction to any surgery; however, inflammation has to be suppressed with medications. If it occurs over a prolonged duration or to an excessive degree, inflammation can result in excessive scarring of the tissues, with more fibrosis and greater obstruction to fluid flow.

After the surgery, and the surgeon's best efforts to slowly and safely encourage the flow of fluid in the weeks and months after surgery, the bleb is then left to mature, and it is hoped that in the years ahead, this one operation would be successful in achieving a sustained low IOP for the remainder of the patient's life. A picture of a mature bleb is shown in Figure 10.2. However, trabeculectomy surgery unfortunately suffers from a rate of failure in the long term [10]. In one study, the cumulative probability of failure was estimated at 13.5% at 1 year [11].

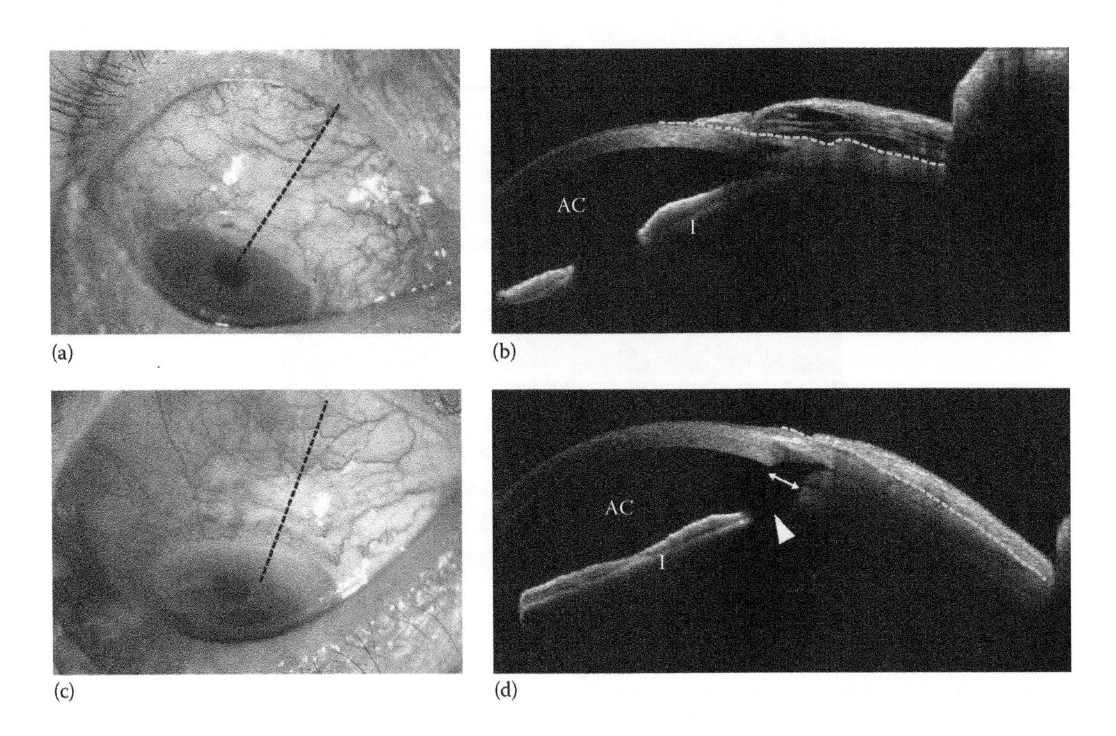

FIGURE 10.2
Imaging of a successful and a failed bleb. (a) Photograph of a successful bleb after trabeculectomy; dashed line indicates approximate orientation of the scan shown in (b). (b) ASOCT scan of the bleb in (a). Although not readily evident from the photograph in (a), expansion of the bleb (region above the dashed yellow line) is clearly seen in this image and is taken as an indicator of good flow of fluid outside of the eye. (c) Photograph of a failed bleb after trabeculectomy; dashed line indicates approximate orientation of the scan shown in (d). (d) ASOCT of the bleb in (c), showing a lack of hydration of the bleb wall above the yellow line. The internal ostium (double-headed arrow) is patent; however, the level of obstruction to flow is inferred to be higher than this, that is, between the flap and sclera or at the episcleral level. Arrowhead shows the peripheral iridectomy that is performed as part of the surgery. AC, anterior chamber; I, iris.

So, in the period immediately following surgery, the clinician examines the eye with a number of questions in mind. It is in the context of these questions that the role of imaging can be understood:

Is the aqueous humor flowing out though the ostium, under the flap, and out of the eye? Is there any evidence that the tissues outside the eye wall are now well hydrated?

Is the flow enough, to reduce IOP for this patient?

Is the degree of flow increasing, decreasing, or stable over time?

Is the keratotrabeculectomy ostium or sclerostomy blocked by tissue or other material?

Is the scleral flap scarring up excessively?

Is the Tenon capsule scarring up excessively?

Is the conjunctiva scarring up excessively?

Is inflammation adequately controlled?

In effect, the surgeon is asking this:

> Are there any clues now that this bleb will fail in the future? Should intervene at this stage, so that I can improve its long-term survival?

The intervention performed would ideally depend on the exact cause of the failure. At the deepest level, the internal ostium may be blocked by iris tissue. This can be detected by routine clinical visualization methods at the slit lamp. The next level of potential obstruction is at the level of the scleral flap. This level of obstruction is not readily diagnosed by direct clinical observation as the flap is underneath the visible outer layers of the eye. A third location of resistance is at the most superficial level, that is, at the subconjunctival plane. This occurs when the episclera–conjunctiva heals too tightly over the scleral flap due to aggressive fibrosis, in effect sealing over the surgical site like a cap. The latter two situations are often indistinguishable using routine examination and indeed may coexist in the same patient.

10.2 Role of Bleb Imaging: Surface versus Subsurface Assessment

10.2.1 Surface Assessment

Surface assessment of bleb morphology using routine clinical equipment (i.e., a slit-lamp ophthalmoscope, which provides a magnified and well-illuminated view) is the conventional method of bleb evaluation after glaucoma surgery [12].

Bleb elevation indicates whether or not there is any flow though the newly created outflow channel. The surface tissues, that is, episclera–conjunctiva, can be thought of as an expansible sponge. If there were no flow through them, they would appear *flat* as in a nonoperated eye. However, if there is flow, the increased hydration expands these tissues and results in an elevated appearance. This elevation can be subtle and may be difficult to appreciate using a slit-lamp ophthalmoscope.

The *surface extent of the elevated bleb* is another parameter for assessment. The elevated bleb may be localized to a small area over the scleral flap or be more spread out. The spread-out bleb is taken to represent a better outcome as it presumably indicates a good rate of fluid flow and at the same time avoids some of the complications associated with extremely elevated blebs.

Microcysts within the conjunctiva are a result of hydration and so are regarded as a favorable finding. Their absence may indicate low flow. These are tiny structures and are sometimes difficult to appreciate clinically.

The degree of conjunctival and episcleral *vascularity* is also assessed. The vessels can be so engorged and dilated such that they take on a *corkscrew* appearance. Increased vascularity is an unfavorable sign and is associated with failure.

Clinical assessment, being dependent on the observer's prior experience and personal interpretation, can yield variable results from observer to observer. In one study, only certain parameters were reproducibly assessed by different observers, whereas others showed poor interobserver agreement [13]. Some researchers have attempted to standardize the clinical assessment protocol for clinical and research purposes. Among the systems used are the Moorfields Bleb Grading System (MBGS) [14], the Indiana Bleb Assessment Grading Score (IBAGS) [15], and the Wuerzburg Bleb Grading System (WBGS) [16]. All systems aim to define a structured semiquantitative grading system to describe visible changes.

Ideally, the application of a structured grading system would be able to detect morphological features of impending failure. Applying the WBGS, one group found that there were no correlations between the early WBGS score and the late outcomes in terms of success or failure of surgery [17]. This could be taken as an indication that surface evaluation in isolation does not always yield information relevant to future bleb function.

These grading systems in their present forms rely on clinical criteria and do not include imaging data.

10.2.2 Subsurface Assessment

From the preceding explanation, it becomes clear that the surface signs are a proxy for the clinician to gather information about processes occurring deeper than the surface.

Potentially, these questions may be answered directly using imaging technology. If the bleb can be imaged, subsurface features can be observed and may directly inform management decisions. The ideal imaging system would have a number of attributes as summarized in Table 10.1. It should be able to assess the entire area of the surgical site and the surrounding ocular surface, that is, a region of interest spanning a few centimeters. Aside from width, it should also have sufficient penetration to be capable of depth imaging, that is, to reveal structural information including the ostium, the scleral flap and fistula (route beneath the flap), the subconjunctival tissues, and finally, the surface conjunctiva. The resultant images should be of adequate resolution to enable detailed anatomical assessment. Ideally, a bleb imaging system should be able to provide information about the entire bleb, as different parts of the bleb may be undergoing different structural responses. For example, an area of subconjunctival fibrosis may be localized to a small area in one corner of the bleb. For this, a 3D imaging system would be the ideal or, at the least, be able to acquire images of several locations in depth and breadth at once. Ideally, the system would allow for reproducible length and volume measurements to be made to quantify aspects of bleb morphology.

TABLE 10.1

Properties of an Ideal Bleb Imaging System

Characteristic	Rationale
Fast acquisition	To minimize patient discomfort To minimize movement artifacts
Deep penetration	To visualize entire bleb, scleral thickness, and underlying uvea beneath the bleb
Wide field of view	To capture data simultaneously from the entire bleb region, e.g., >5 × 5 mm^2 area
3D imaging	To capture volume data
High resolution	To reveal fine structures such as microcysts and fine vessels
Noncontact	To eliminate potential for injury or bleb distortion

Additionally, it would be best for there to be no contact with the eye during assessment, as the surgical site is prone to infection and may be injured by contact from the imaging device. These considerations are further explored in the following.

10.3 Variables in Imaging

10.3.1 Ultrasound versus Optical Coherence Tomography

Ultrasound biomicroscopy (UBM) is an imaging modality that has been applied to the structures in the anterior segment (front) of the eye [18,19], including trabeculectomy blebs [20] and blebs resulting from another related procedure, deep sclerectomy [21]. UBM imaging relies on echoes produced by high-frequency ultrasonic waves at 50–100 mHz. Indeed, ultrasound imaging has a track record of safe and effective human application, most notably in the imaging of the uterus in pregnancy. In general, UBM is able to provide images of the ocular anterior segment at 20–60 µm resolution.

UBM is advantageous in that it is able to perform subsurface imaging at relatively great depth of about 4 mm. This means that deep structures within and beneath the bleb—such as the scleral flap, subflap route, and internal ostium—are usually visible using this technique. However, its main disadvantage is the need for contact with the eye during imaging, either directly by the transducer or through a coupling medium such as methylcellulose or water contained in a bath placed over the eye surface during imaging. This is not ideal, as explained in Section 10.3.3.

Optical coherence tomography (OCT) is an imaging modality that relies on the differential optical scatter of incident light by different cell or tissue layers [22]. Its initial application in the eye was for retinal imaging [23], but it has now been adapted for use in the anterior segment [24,25] including trabeculectomy blebs [26–29]. Its resolution is far greater than UBM imaging—OCT provides images up to a resolution of a few micrometers in tissue. One of its main advantages over ultrasound is that it is a noncontact imaging modality. Examples of OCT-based systems in use are listed in Table 10.2.

OCT may employ time domain (TD) or Fourier domain protocols [30]. The latter includes spectral domain (SD) OCT and swept source OCT methods. Fourier domain OCT methods run at much higher acquisition speeds, enabling quicker acquisition and therefore have led to the development of 3D OCT imaging techniques for human application [31].

TABLE 10.2

Selected Instruments That Have Been Applied for Bleb Imaging

Category	Name	Detail	Manufacturer
Ultrasound biomicroscopy	UBM840	50 MHz ultrasound	Carl Zeiss
	UD-6010	40 MHz ultrasound	Tomey
Optical coherence tomography	Stratus OCT	820 nm light	Carl Zeiss
	ASOCT	1310 nm light	Heidelberg
	Visante OCT	1310 nm light	Carl Zeiss
	3D OCT	1310 nm light	Custom device
	Cirrus OCT	840 nm light	Carl Zeiss
	HRTII	670 nm light	Heidelberg
Thermography	Thermotracer TH1106		NEC San-Ei

It also features a higher signal-to-noise ratio and so yields more detailed images than TD OCT. Generally, however, OCT-based systems have a relatively low penetration depth and so are less able to image deep sclera and uvea than UBM.

10.3.2 Imaging Light Wavelength and Interferometry Approach

Broadly speaking, the wavelength of light used in imaging affects the resolution and depth of imaging.

In their landmark 1991 paper, David Huang and colleagues described the use of an OCT device using a fiber-optic Michelson interferometer, illuminated by low-coherence 830 nm light from a superluminescent diode, to image the human retina and optic nerve head [22]. Its advantages included <20 µm resolution and a high sensitivity with >100 dB dynamic range. Later, the same technology was applied to generate automated transpupillary measurements of the retina [23] and anterior segment structures such as cornea, anterior chamber angle, and lens [24].

As it became clear that 830 nm OCT could be useful not only for posterior segment imaging but also for the anterior segment, specific devices for the anterior segment were developed [32]. Imaging using a 1310 nm light source [33] showed less scattering in tissues such as cornea, and due to its lower transmittance in ocular media, higher optical power could be used safely. Coupled with high-speed Fourier domain optical depth scanning technology and a handheld probe, high-frame-rate imaging of the anterior segment in real time was achieved at even better resolution [34]. The 1310 nm imaging also allowed deeper penetration than 830 nm–based systems and so yielded better images of deep structures such as the ciliary body.

The 1310 nm wavelength enabled higher-resolution imaging of the glaucoma surgery bleb [26,28,35] than the ≈0.8 µm devices [36,37]. Anterior segment OCT (ASOCT) imaging was able to demonstrate features of the bleb and underlying structures in cross section, such as the ostium, the route under the scleral flap, and the subconjunctival tissues. In this way, the patency of a route for the flow of aqueous could be directly assessed.

OCT devices can rely on different methods to determine distance information. The TD approach relies on the mechanical movement of a reference arm, which limits the speed of acquisition. OCT with SD interferometry—a type of frequency domain imaging and also known as Fourier domain OCT—relies on a spectrometer to measure the cross-spectral density at the detector arm, therefore eliminating the need for mechanical scanning of a reference arm. This approach increased the speed of acquisition and improved both the signal-to-noise ratio [38,39] and the detection sensitivity [40]. One SDOCT system with an 840 nm light source has been applied to image trabeculectomy blebs and, while showing relatively low penetration, was able to show tiny structures such as microcysts at even higher resolution of about 5 μm in tissue [41]. The faster acquisition time also made it possible to perform 3D imaging as discussed in the following.

10.3.3 Contact versus Noncontact Imaging Modalities

As mentioned earlier, the issue of direct ocular contact with the imaging device or a probe is undesirable. Contact with the surgical site may result in infection due to inadvertent contamination from the imaging probe. Furthermore, any direct contact with the bleb may result in injury and may cause a leak and excessive fluid flow. Also, any contact device has the potential to alter the morphology of the target being investigated and so may yield erroneous information. For example, a contact probe may compress the subconjunctival tissues and falsely give the impression of a *compressed* layer that is, in actual fact, expanded in situ.

Of the imaging modalities reported, ultrasound and in vivo confocal microscopy (IVCM) [42,43] are those that feature contact-based devices. OCT devices obviate the need for contact and are therefore advantageous.

10.3.4 Resolution and Field of View

Another conflicting issue in imaging is the resolution of structures versus the field of view obtained. This aspect may be exemplified by comparing the use of IVCM and OCT in bleb imaging.

The IVCM device shows rather clear and detailed images of minute structures and among the first reports of its use in the eye related to the cornea [44,45]. For glaucoma surgery blebs, IVCM could show features such as microcysts and even individual inflammatory cells [46–48] due to its very high resolution of 2–4 μm or even 1–1.5 μm [49]. Strands of tissue, presumably collagen, could also be visualized as being organized in distinct stromal patterns [50] and so gave information about the *compactness* of the subconjunctival tissues. However, the field of view with IVCM using the Rostock cornea module coupled with the Heidelberg retina tomograph II is small (about 400 μm × 400 μm), and so information can be gathered from only a very small region in the bleb. Furthermore, each layer of interest at different depths would have to be imaged individually.

This concern is important as the bleb is not a homogenous structure, and so multiple scans would have to be acquired of each layer across different locations in the bleb. Only then can an overall impression be made. On the other hand, ASOCT is unable to discern cellular detail but can provide structural information about a large area of interest. Many layers can be imaged at once with the ASOCT.

With the current technologies, the assessor is forced to choose among the devices depending on the question at hand. If he or she were specifically interested to assess the extent of cellular infiltration or to determine the structure of stromal bands in a small, localized area of the glaucoma bleb, IVCM would have to be used. However, for a broader structural assessment, the ASOCT would be the tool of choice. The idealized bleb imaging system would combine both these capabilities.

10.3.5 Imaging in Two and Three Dimensions

The modalities mentioned so far—UBM, OCT, and IVCM—all provide mainly 2D images as the output. In other words, data are acquired and displayed from only one cross-sectional plane. Repeated imaging can be used to acquire images from other planes if they are of interest. As blebs are composed of different layers of tissue and span some distance across the surface of the eye—that is, the glaucoma surgery bleb is a heterogeneous 3D structure—a more desirable approach would be to use 3D imaging. One group has investigated 3D OCT in relation to bleb imaging, and striking images were shown by the authors of the overall shape of the bleb and its many regions in 3D [51,52].

The high acquisition speed achieved by using frequency domain OCT was a critical feature enabling the acquisition of the 3D 256 × 256 × 1024 voxel dataset in 3.3 s [52]. The volume imaged was also relatively large, that is, 16 mm × 16 mm wide and 6 mm deep, thus giving information covering the different regions in the bleb and superior to the 2D images provided by conventional OCT devices. The device used by the authors used a 1310 nm light source and gave an axial resolution of about 11 μm.

This capability may further reduce operator dependence for data acquisition. In the case of 2D imaging, the assessor must have the requisite skill to acquire data from the specific area of interest and focus the acquisition device accordingly. Thus, the assessor would need to critically assess the clinical question at hand and make decisions in real time in order to select the relevant 2D plane for assessment. 3D imaging, however, allows for simultaneous data capture from a broad lateral area and so lessens the need to target the imaging device precisely. So, a global picture of the bleb can be acquired by imaging personnel if the clinician is not available, and then the clinician may interpret the image remotely.

10.3.6 Thermography

In an interesting development, trabeculectomy blebs have also been imaged with thermography [53]. While this technique did not accurately delineate morphological features, it could discern temperature differences that suggested that well-functioning blebs were cooler than those with poor function. This difference may reflect higher flow and so higher turnover of aqueous humor in functional shunts. However, the method may potentially be influenced by other parameters such as vascularity, tear film status, and ambient temperature.

10.4 Correlation of Imaging Findings with Histology

Data to correlate OCT appearance with histology are scant, as understandably tissue is not routinely collected after bleb imaging in humans. A small number of exceptions to this have occurred, when human bleb tissue was available for analysis after imaging, as the bleb had to be removed because of complications.

Theelen and coworkers in their OCT study [54] identified a patient who required partial bleb excision due to presumed overfiltration and excessively low IOP. This portion of excised bleb tissue was analyzed histologically and showed conjunctival epithelium, lamina propria, Tenon capsule, and scleral layers that the authors correlated to stripes or bands seen in the OCT image. They were also able to identify nonendothelized fluid channels, which were the suggested anatomical correlate of the low-reflectivity cavities seen within the bleb. Taking their data as a whole, they proposed that the *striping* characteristic, where there were alternating hyper- and hyporeflective bands in the bleb, was due to the presence of fluid channels interposed between connective tissue septae. In support of this hypothesis, blebs with *striping* were, in general, well functioning.

In another report, Kim and colleagues used ASOCT imaging before surgery to repair a large overhanging bleb, as knowledge of the detailed structure of the different portions of the bleb was considered useful to plan a safe surgical approach [55]. The histological specimen obtained also showed multiloculated cystic structures that correlated to the cysts seen in OCT images.

10.5 Examples of Bleb Imaging in Clinical and Research Applications

10.5.1 Imaging Findings in Successful and Failed Blebs

Qualitative correlation. The earliest studies of bleb imaging with UBM began to yield correlations between bleb morphology and function (as indicated by IOP). Blebs with low internal reflectivity were found to have good function [56,57], and this confirmed the generally accepted clinical impression that flowing shunts showed hydrated and expanded episclera–conjunctiva. Additionally, the early studies demonstrated the utility of depth imaging—by carefully assessing the patency of the route beneath the scleral flap by UBM, reports showed that patent routes favored good function not only concurrently [56,58] but also in the long term [59]. Although intuitive, this finding showed how imaging could complement clinical assessment, as the subflap route cannot normally be seen using routine clinical examination techniques. Indeed, if the subflap route is obstructed, specific interventions may be performed to lift the flap and reestablish a route for flow.

Moving forward to the application if 1310 nm OCT, once again, similar qualitative characteristics were found to correlate with function and so confirmed the earlier UBM data. OCT imaging, yielding greater detail than UBM, showed the broadly similar result that blebs with loose internal structure and a low intrableb signal were those that functioned well [35]. Owing to the higher resolution, layers could be seen within the bleb itself, and in at least one study, the presence of high and low reflecting layers or stripes indicated good IOP control [54]. TD OCT images were of high enough resolution to show microcysts in the wall, and these were found mostly in well-functioning blebs [35]. Microcysts in successful blebs were also demonstrated using SDOCT [41], which as mentioned earlier could easily discern the presence of these structures owing to even better resolution than TD OCT.

Poor IOP control was in general associated with compact, uniformly high-reflecting blebs with no small cysts. These findings were in general agreement with the IVCM data [42,43,46,47].

Semiquantitative correlation: To approach the question in a more quantitative way, our group used 1310 nm ASOCT images to classify blebs according to cross-sectional height into low, moderate, and high blebs. We found that high blebs were mostly successful, and low blebs were associated with failure [26]. We found ASOCT assessment to be useful in failed cases, where it was able to show the level of obstruction as being in the ostium, the subflap route, or at the episcleral level and so could potentially contribute additional information to inform the management plan [60].

An example each of a well-expanded bleb and a poorly expanded bleb are shown in Figure 10.2.

Quantitative correlation: Going one step further to 3D imaging, with its capability to image almost the entire bleb at once [51], the potential lay that accurate measurements of the bleb parts in their entire volume—rather than in just one 2D slice that may not be representative—could yield data regarding quantitative features that would correlate with function. Indeed, in a study of 38 blebs in 31 patients, Kawana et al. from the University of Tsukuba, Japan, demonstrated using 1.3 µm frequency domain 3D OCT that the actual dimensions of the fluid cavity, bleb wall thickness, bleb height, the number of microcysts, and the volume of hyporeflective areas all correlated with pressure reduction and so were indicators of good IOP control [52]. The linear dimensions of the fluid-filled cavity and the bleb height were those indices that showed the strongest correlation with IOP. This was arguably the most comprehensive study of quantitative bleb measurements in relation to concurrent IOP control.

It should be emphasized, however, that the data discussed in this section relate to the structure–function correlation at the same time point, as a one-time snapshot, and for this reason does not yield much additional useful information in the clinic. A clinician would know at once if a bleb was functioning well by simply measuring the IOP. However, contemporaneous structure–function correlation data were a useful starting point as it provided clues on which early imaging features would indicate future success or failure. In other words, these data may pave the way toward the ultimate goal in OCT imaging of blebs—to prognosticate.

10.5.2 Predictive Value of Early Imaging on Final Outcome

Ultimately, for the clinician, the main value of bleb imaging lies in its potential ability to predict which blebs will fail and which will succeed, so that the failing filters may be targeted with interventions. Many of the imaging studies to date have examined structure in relation to contemporaneous function, and data are just becoming available on the prospective ability of bleb imaging to provide clues about future function.

Nakano and colleagues examined blebs just 2 weeks after surgery using ASOCT and found imaging data that were of prognostic value—blebs at 2 weeks that showed *multiform walls*, that is, containing hypo- and hyperreflective areas within the bleb, were more likely to function well at 6 months. This is contrasted with blebs with more uniform internal reflectivity, 67% of which had poor function at 6 months. The histological correlation of these different appearances are not conclusively known—for example, they could be attributed to differences in inflammatory cell infiltrate or the nature and quantity of fluid within the bleb tissues. Interestingly, they also found that microcysts discovered at 2 weeks by ASOCT imaging were lost over time in the eyes that eventually functioned poorly but remained detectable only in eyes with good flow. Bleb microcysts have traditionally been viewed as a sign of good function; however, these data indicate that this may only be true in mature and not early blebs, as they can be lost over time. Their work could lead the way for the development of a protocol for functional prognostication based on imaging young blebs.

10.5.3 Role in Postoperative Management

In terms of relevance to patient management, ASOCT imaging has the potential to provide information that directly affects patient management. One study demonstrated the potential role of imaging in clinical decisions after glaucoma surgery [60]. As imaging could reveal features not visible clinically, cases of a blocked ostium or a tight scleral flap could be distinguished from conjunctival fibrosis and specific interventions performed depending on the findings. ASOCT was also able to demonstrate changes in these structures after LSL [61], a common postoperative maneuver used to release the scleral flap in order to increase the rate of fluid flow.

10.5.4 Assessment of the Effects of Novel Surgical Approaches

Techniques to further optimize shunt function after trabeculectomy are continually being developed, in an effort to increase long-term surgical success. Therefore, imaging may also be useful in evaluating the effects of these novel surgical approaches, three of which are illustrated here.

Implants: The Ologen biodegradable porcine collagen matrix implant was proposed as a method to decrease scarring and promote the development of an organized, moderately elevated bleb consisting of regularly arranged fibrous tissue after the absorption of the implant. ASOCT imaging was applied by one group to assess the morphological sequelae, and the authors found that about one third of the implants were still visible on imaging at 90 days, whereas these were less readily visible on the slit lamp [62]. Hence, if only clinical examination was relied upon, an erroneous impression could be made of a rapid biodegradation time; however, using imaging more accurate data can be obtained about subsurface implants.

Superficial modification: The additional use of amniotic membrane transplantation (AMT) over the scleral flap area is thought to provide a scaffold for organized epithelialization and additionally leads to reduced scarring by growth factor suppression. Using 40 MHz UBM, one group found that AMT-augmented blebs were more likely to have a larger fluid-filled episcleral space and were less likely to be highly reflective than those without AMT.

Deep modification: Chihara and colleagues reported their results from a procedure they termed *D-lectomy*, which was a modified deep sclerectomy technique. Their aim in using UBM imaging was to examine the presence of the lake of aqueous as this anatomical feature was invisible by clinical examination methods. In selected cases, the window and lake were examined UBM and OCT, to provide data on the morphological effects of this surgical approach.

10.6 Conclusions and Future Directions

Imaging of the trabeculectomy bleb has developed briskly since the late 1990s since ultrasound was first applied for this purpose. The advent of newer imaging technologies has enabled more detailed and comprehensive imaging than previously possible. Data are gradually emerging on how morphological data provided by bleb imaging may assist in the clinical management of glaucoma patients after filtration surgery. In addition, bleb imaging may have a role in investigating novel surgical approaches and adjuncts in development. In the future, the development of a complete bleb characterization system, which may include clinical as well as imaging data, may potentially enable predictions of the future course of glaucoma control in patients after trabeculectomy.

References

1. Quigley, H. A. Number of people with glaucoma worldwide. *Br. J. Ophthalmol.* **80**, 389–393 (1996).
2. Quigley, H. and Broman, A. T. The number of people with glaucoma worldwide in 2010 and 2020. *Br. J. Ophthalmol.* **90**, 262–267, doi:10.1136/bjo.2005.081224 (2006).
3. Gutienez, P. et al. Influence of glaucomatous visual field loss on health-related quality of life. *Arch. Ophthalmol.* **115**, 777–784 (1997).
4. Quigley, H. A. et al. Retinal ganglion cell death in experimental glaucoma and after axotomy occurs by apoptosis. *Invest. Ophthalmol. Vis. Sci.* **36**, 774–786 (1995).
5. Cairns, J. E. Trabeculectomy. Preliminary report of a new method. *Am. J. Ophthalmol.* **66**, 673–679 (1968).
6. Savage, J. A., Condon, G. P., Lytle, R. A., and Simmons, R. J. Laser suture lysis after trabeculectomy. *Ophthalmology* **95**, 1631–1638 (1988).
7. Pederson, J. E. and Smith, S. G. Surgical management of encapsulated filtering blebs. *Ophthalmology* **92**, 955–958 (1985).
8. Broadway, D. C., Bloom, P. A., Bunce, C., Thiagarajan, M., and Khaw, P. T. Needle revision of failing and failed trabeculectomy blebs with adjunctive 5-fluorouracil: Survival analysis. *Ophthalmology* **111**, 665–673, doi:10.1016/j.ophtha.2003.07.009 (2004).
9. Greenfield, D. S., Miller, M. P., Suner, I. J., and Palmberg, P. F. Needle elevation of the scleral flap for failing filtration blebs after trabeculectomy with mitomycin C. *Am. J. Ophthalmol.* **122**, 195–204 (1996).
10. Scott, I. U. et al. Outcomes of primary trabeculectomy with the use of adjunctive mitomycin. *Arch. Ophthalmol.* **116**, 286–291 (1998).
11. Gedde, S. J. et al. Treatment outcomes in the tube versus trabeculectomy study after one year of follow-up. *Am. J. Ophthalmol.* **143**, 9–22, doi:10.1016/j.ajo.2006.07.020 (2007).
12. Picht, G. and Grehn, F. Classification of filtering blebs in trabeculectomy: Biomicroscopy and functionality. *Curr. Opin. Ophthalmol.* **9**, 2–8 (1998).
13. Crowston, J. G., Kirwan, J. F., Wells, A., Kennedy, C., and Murdoch, I. E. Evaluating clinical signs in trabeculectomized eyes. *Eye* **18**, 299–303, doi:10.1038/sj.eye.6700638 (2004).
14. Wells, A. P. et al. A pilot study of a system for grading of drainage blebs after glaucoma surgery. *J. Glaucoma* **13**, 454–460, doi:10.1097/00061198-200412000-00005 (2004).
15. Cantor, L. B., Mantravadi, A., WuDunn, D., Swamynathan, K., and Cortes, A. Morphologic classification of filtering blebs after glaucoma filtration surgery: The Indiana Bleb Appearance Grading Scale. *J. Glaucoma* **12**, 266–271, doi:10.1097/00061198-200306000-00015 (2003).
16. Furrer, S., Menke, M. N., Funk, J., and Töteberg-Harms, M. Evaluation of filtering blebs using the Wuerzburg bleb classification score compared to clinical findings. *BMC Ophthalmol.* **12**, 24, doi:10.1186/1471-2415-12-24 (2012).
17. Klink, T. et al. The prognostic value of the Wuerzburg bleb classification score for the outcome of trabeculectomy. *Ophthalmologica* **225**, 55–60, doi:10.1159/000314717 (2011).
18. Pavlin, C. J., Harasiewicz, K., Sherar, M. D., and Foster, F. S. Clinical use of ultrasound biomicroscopy. *Ophthalmology* **98**, 287–295 (1991).
19. Pavlin, C. J., Harasiewicz, K., and Foster, F. S. Ultrasound biomicroscopy of anterior segment structures in normal and glaucomatous eyes. *Am. J. Ophthalmol.* **113**, 381–389 (1992).
20. Yamamoto, T., Sakuma, T., and Kitazawa, Y. An ultrasound biomicroscopic study of filtering blebs after mitomycin C trabeculectomy. *Ophthalmology* **102**, 1770–1776 (1995).
21. Chiou, A. G. Y., Mermoud, A., Underdahl, J. P., and Schnyder, C. C. An ultrasound biomicroscopic study of eyes after deep sclerectomy with collagen implant. *Ophthalmology* **105**, 746–750, doi:10.1016/s0161-6420(98)94033-7 (1998).
22. Huang, D. et al. Optical coherence tomography. *Science* **254**, 1178–1181 (1991).
23. Swanson, E. A. et al. In vivo retinal imaging by optical coherence tomography. *Opt. Lett.* **18**, 1864–1869 (1993).

24. Izatt, J. A. et al. Micrometer-scale resolution imaging of the anterior eye in vivo with optical coherence tomography. *Arch. Ophthalmol.* **112**, 1584–1589 (1994).
25. Akiyama, H. et al. Observation of the anterior ocular segment by optical coherence tomography. *Jpn. J. Clin. Ophthalmol.* **52**, 829–832 (1998).
26. Singh, M. et al. Imaging of trabeculectomy blebs using anterior segment optical coherence tomography. *Ophthalmology* **114**, 47–53, doi:10.1016/j.ophtha.2006.05.078 (2007).
27. Akiyama, H. and Kimura, Y. Optical coherence tomographic findings of the anterior ocular segment following filtering surgery for glaucoma. *Jpn. J. Clin. Ophthalmol.* **52**, 1574–1575 (1998).
28. Leung, C. K. S. et al. Analysis of bleb morphology after trabeculectomy with Visante anterior segment optical coherence tomography. *Br. J. Ophthalmol.* **91**, 340–344, doi:10.1136/bjo.2006.100321 (2007).
29. Singh, M. et al. Anterior segment optical coherence tomography imaging of trabeculectomy blebs before and after laser suture lysis. *Am. J. Ophthalmol.* **143**, 873–875, doi:10.1016/j.ajo.2006.12.001 (2007).
30. Leitgeb, R., Hitzenberger, C. K., and Fercher, A. F. Performance of Fourier domain vs. time domain optical coherence tomography. *Opt. Exp.* **11**, 889–894 (2003).
31. Wojtkowski, M. et al. Three-dimensional retinal imaging with high-speed ultrahigh-resolution optical coherence tomography. *Ophthalmology* **112**, 1734–1746, doi:10.1016/j.ophtha.2005.05.023 (2005).
32. Hoerauf, H. et al. Slit-lamp-adapted optical coherence tomography of the anterior segment. *Graefes Arch. Clin. Exp. Ophthalmol.* **238**, 8–18 (2000).
33. Hoerauf, H. et al. First experiences with a slit-lamp-adapted optical coherence tomography (OCT) system in the anterior and posterior segment of the eye. *Proc. SPIE—Int. Soc. Opt. Eng.* **3564**, 158–162 (1999).
34. Radhakrishnan, S. et al. Real-time optical coherence tomography of the anterior segment at 1310 nm. *Arch. Ophthalmol.* **119**, 1179–1185 (2001).
35. Müller, M. et al. Filtering bleb evaluation with slit-lamp-adapted 1310-nm optical coherence tomography. *Curr. Eye Res.* **31**, 909–915, doi:10.1080/02713680600910528 (2006).
36. Savini, G., Zanini, M., and Barboni, P. Filtering blebs imaging by optical coherence tomography. *Clin. Exp. Ophthalmol.* **33**, 483–489, doi:10.1111/j.1442-9071.2005.01066.x (2005).
37. Babighian, S., Rapizzi, E., and Galan, A. Stratus OCT of filtering bleb after trabeculectomy [4]. *Acta Ophthalmol. Scand.* **84**, 270, doi:10.1111/j.1600-0420.2006.00616.x (2006).
38. De Boer, J. F. et al. Improved signal-to-noise ratio in spectral-domain compared with time-domain optical coherence tomography. *Opt. Lett.* **28**, 2067–2069 (2003).
39. Yun, S. H., Tearney, G. J., Bouma, B. E., Park, B. H., and De Boer, J. F. High-speed spectral-domain optical coherence tomography at 1.3 μm wavelength. *Opt. Exp.* **11**, 3598–3604 (2003).
40. Nassif, N. et al. In vivo human retinal imaging by ultrahigh-speed spectral domain optical coherence tomography. *Opt. Lett.* **29**, 480–482, doi:10.1364/ol.29.000480 (2004).
41. Singh, M., See, J. L. S., Aquino, M. C., Thean, L. S. Y., and Chew, P. T. K. High-definition imaging of trabeculectomy blebs using spectral domain optical coherence tomography adapted for the anterior segment. *Clin. Exp. Ophthalmol.* **37**, 345–351, doi:10.1111/j.1442-9071.2009.02066.x (2009).
42. Labbé, A., Dupas, B., Hamard, P., and Baudouin, C. In vivo confocal microscopy study of blebs after filtering surgery. *Ophthalmology* **112**, 1979.e1971–1979.e1979, doi:10.1016/j.ophtha.2005.05.021 (2005).
43. Messmer, E. M., Zapp, D. M., Mackert, M. J., Thiel, M., and Kampik, A. In vivo confocal microscopy of filtering blebs after trabeculectomy. *Arch. Ophthalmol.* **124**, 1095–1103, doi:10.1001/archopht.124.8.1095 (2006).
44. Petrolll, W. M., Cavanagh, H. D., and Jester, J. V. Three-dimensional imaging of corneal cells using in vivo confocal microscopy. *J. Microsc.* **170**, 213–219 (1993).
45. Cavanagh, H. D. et al. Clinical and diagnostic use of in vivo confocal microscopy in patients with corneal disease. *Ophthalmology* **100**, 1444–1454 (1993).

46. Amar, N., Labbé, A., Hamard, P., Dupas, B., and Baudouin, C. Filtering blebs and aqueous pathway. An immunocytological and in vivo Confocal Microscopy Study. *Ophthalmology* **115**, 1154.e4–1161.e4, doi:10.1016/j.ophtha.2007.10.024 (2008).
47. Sbeity, Z., Palmiero, P. M., Tello, C., Liebmann, J. M., and Ritch, R. Noncontact in vivo scanning laser microscopy of filtering blebs. *J. Glaucoma* **18**, 479–483, doi:10.1097/IJG.0b013e31818d38bf (2009).
48. Ciancaglini, M. et al. Filtering bleb functionality: A clinical, anterior segment optical coherence tomography and in vivo confocal microscopy study. *J. Glaucoma* **17**, 308–317, doi:10.1097/IJG.0b013e31815c3a19 (2008).
49. Wells, A. P., Wakely, L., and Birchall, W. In vivo fluorescence mode confocal microscopy of subepithelial tissues in glaucoma filtering blebs. *Ophthalmic Surg. Lasers Imaging* **41**, 78–82, doi:10.3928/15428877-20091230-14 (2010).
50. Guthoff, R., Klink, T., Schlunck, G., and Grehn, F. In vivo confocal microscopy of failing and functioning filtering blebs: Results and clinical correlations. *J. Glaucoma* **15**, 552–558, doi:10.1097/01.ijg.0000212295.39034.10 (2006).
51. Miura, M. et al. Three-dimensional anterior segment optical coherence tomography of filtering blebs after trabeculectomy. *J. Glaucoma* **17**, 193–196, doi:10.1097/IJG.0b013e31815a34cd (2008).
52. Kawana, K., Kiuchi, T., Yasuno, Y., and Oshika, T. Evaluation of trabeculectomy blebs using 3-dimensional cornea and anterior segment optical coherence tomography. *Ophthalmology* **116**, 848–855, doi:10.1016/j.ophtha.2008.11.019 (2009).
53. Kawasaki, S. et al. Evaluation of filtering bleb function by thermography. *Br. J. Ophthalmol.* **93**, 1331–1336, doi:10.1136/bjo.2008.152066 (2009).
54. Theelen, T., Wesseling, P., Keunen, J. E. E., and Klevering, B. J. A pilot study on slit lamp-adapted optical coherence tomography imaging of trabeculectomy filtering blebs. *Graefes Arch. Clin. Exp. Ophthalmol.* **245**, 877–882, doi:10.1007/s00417-006-0476-2 (2007).
55. Kim, W. K., Seong, G. J., Lee, C. S., Kim, Y. G., and Kim, C. Y. Anterior segment optical coherence tomography imaging and histopathologic findings of an overhanging filtering bleb. *Eye* **22**, 1520–1521, doi:10.1038/eye.2008.166 (2008).
56. Avitabile, T. et al. Ultrasound-biomicroscopic evaluation of filtering blebs after laser suture lysis trabeculectomy. *Ophthalmologica* **212**, 17–21, doi:10.1159/000055414 (1998).
57. Wang, X., Zhang, H., Li, S., and Wang, N. The effects of phacoemulsification on intraocular pressure and ultrasound biomicroscopic image of filtering bleb in eyes with cataract and functioning filtering blebs. *Eye* **23**, 112–116, doi:10.1038/sj.eye.6702981 (2009).
58. Jinza, K., Saika, S., Kin, K., and Ohnishi, Y. Relationship between formation of a filtering bleb and an intrascleral aqueous drainage route after trabeculectomy: Evaluation using ultrasound biomicroscopy. *Ophthalmic Res.* **32**, 240–243 (2000).
59. Kaushik, S., Tiwari, A., Pandav, S. S., Ichhpujani, P., and Gupta, A. Use of ultrasound biomicroscopy to predict long-term outcome of sub-Tenon needle revision of failed trabeculectomy blebs: A pilot study. *Eur. J. Ophthalmol.* **21**, 700–707, doi:10.5301/ejo.2011.6468 (2011).
60. Singh, M., Aung, T., Aquino, M. C., and Chew, P. T. K. Utility of bleb imaging with anterior segment optical coherence tomography in clinical decision-making after trabeculectomy. *J. Glaucoma* **18**, 492–495, doi:10.1097/IJG.0b013e31818d38ab (2009).
61. Sng, C. C. A. et al. Quantitative assessment of changes in trabeculectomy blebs after laser suture lysis using anterior segment coherence tomography. *J. Glaucoma* **21**, 313–317, doi:10.1097/IJG.0b013e31820e2d23 (2012).
62. Boey, P. Y. et al. Imaging of blebs after phacotrabeculectomy with Ologen collagen matrix implants. *Br. J. Ophthalmol.* **95**, 340–344, doi:10.1136/bjo.2009.177758 (2011).

11

Confocal Microscopy of Cornea

Manotosh Ray, Anna W.T. Tan, Aria E. Mangunkusumo, and Dawn K.A. Lim

CONTENTS

Microscopic evaluation of the ocular structures has always been a challenge for ophthalmic clinicians and researchers. Ocular diagnostic imaging techniques have evolved rapidly over the past decades. The clinical diagnostic capability of detecting corneal diseases has grown exponentially in accord with technological innovation. Confocal microscopy, one such most advanced imaging technology, offers several advantages over conventional wide-field optical microscopy. It has the ability to control the depth of field and eliminate or reduce the background information away from the focal plane and the capability to collect serial optical sections from thick specimens. The basic key to the confocal approach is the use of spatial filtering techniques to eliminate out-of-focus light or glare. There has been a tremendous interest in confocal microscopy in recent years, due in part to the relative ease with which extremely high-quality images can be obtained. Confocal microscopy has enhanced the ability to image the cornea in vivo. The application of this technology permits the acquisition of images of high spatial resolution and contrast as compared to conventional microscopy.

The major limiting factor of conventional light microscopy is that the reflected light from the structures surrounding the point of interest obscures the image. The fringing effect produced by this reflection reduces the image contrast. Therefore, the useful magnification in slit-lamp biomicroscope and other related ophthalmic instruments is limited to approximately 40×. Further magnification compromises the image quality and produces significant image blur. Confocal microscope, on the other hand, utilizes a principle where both illumination and observation system are focused on a single point. Thus, the resolution is improved dramatically and the system allows a magnification up to 600×.

Confocal microscope employs an oscillating slit aperture in an ophthalmic microscope configuration, especially suitable for the analysis of cell layers of cornea. It can focus through the entire range of a normal cornea from epithelium to endothelium. A series of scan shows (a) epithelium, (b) corneal nerves, (c) keratocytes, (d) endothelium, and (e) a computer generated slice of cornea. There are distinct advantages of confocal microscope over the regular microscope. When focused on a transparent tissue like cornea with regular microscope, the unfocused layers affect the visibility of the focused layer. Confocal microscope, on the other hand, can focus on different layers distinctly without affecting the quality of the image.

11.1 Optics

The principle of confocal microscopy was first described by Minsky in 1957 [1]. He postulated that both the illumination and observation systems be focused on a single point, hence proposed the name *confocal* microscopy. A halogen light source passes through movable slits (Nipkow disk). A condenser lens (front lens) projects the light to the cornea. Only a small area inside the cornea is illuminated to minimize the light scattering. The reflected light passes through the front lens again and is directed to another slit of the same size via a beam splitter. Finally, the image is projected onto a highly sensitive camera and displayed on a computer monitor (Figure 11.1).

The confocal microscope utilizes a transparent viscous sterile gel that is interposed between front lens and cornea to eliminate the optical interface with two different refractive indices. The front lens works on *distance immersion principle.* The working distance (distance between front lens and the cornea) is 1.92 mm. The back and forth movement of the front lens enables scanning of the entire cornea starting from anterior chamber and corneal endothelium to most superficial corneal epithelium. The use of standard ×40 immersion lens gives magnified cellular detail and an image field of 440 × 330 μm. Other lenses (e.g., ×20) delivers wide field but less distinct cell morphology. Newer model (Confoscan 2.0) captures 350 images per examination at a rate of 25 fps. Thickness of the captured layers varies from 3 to 5 μm depending on scanning slit characteristics.

In addition, every recorded image is characterized by its position on the *Z*-axis of the cornea. Every time a confocal scan is performed, a graphic shows the depth coordinate on the *Z*-axis and the level of reflectivity on the *Y*-axis. The graphic also displays the distance between two images along the anteroposterior line. This simultaneous graphic recording is called *Z*-scan graphic. The reflectivity on *Z*-scan is entirely dependent on the tissue being scanned. A transparent tissue displays low reflectivity, whereas a

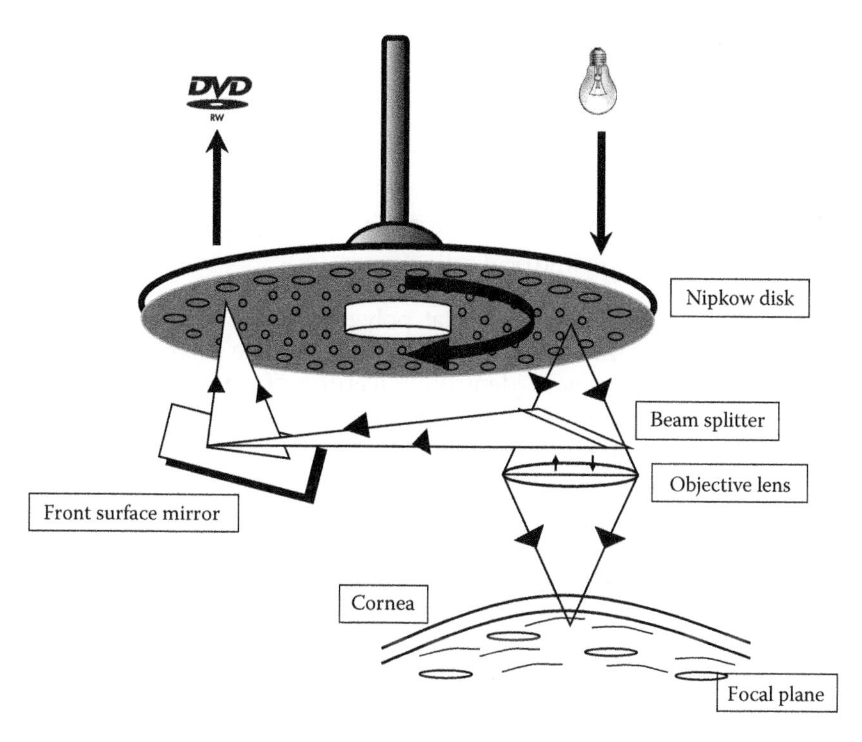

FIGURE 11.1
Optics of the confocal microscope. (Reproduced with permission © 2013 E. A. Mangunkusumo, Dawn K.A. Lim.)

higher reflectivity is obtained from an opaque layer. Therefore, different corneal layers would display different reflectivities on Z-scan. The corneal endothelium displays the maximum reflectivity while stroma is the lowest. An intermediate reflectivity is obtained from epithelial layers. A typical Z-scan of the entire normal cornea shows high endothelial reflection curves followed by low stromal reflection and then late intermediate reflectivity from superficial corneal epithelium. Thus, confocal microscopy enables to perform corneal pachymetry or even can measure the distance between two corneal layers.

11.2 Confocal Microscopy of Normal Cornea

This is a noninvasive technique of imaging of corneal layers that provides excellent resolution with sufficient contrast. A well-executed scan can visualize the corneal endothelium, stroma, subepithelial nerve plexus, and epithelial layers distinctly. The limitations are nonvisualization of normal Bowman's layer and Descemet's membrane since these structures are transparent to this microscope. However, it is possible to view these structures when they are pathologically involved. Eyes with corneal opacity or edema can also be successfully scanned [2]. The quality of image depends on (a) centration of the light beam, (b) stability of the eye, and (c) optimum brightness of the illumination.

11.2.1 Epithelium

Corneal epithelium has five to six layers. Three different types of cellular component are recognized in the epithelium:

- Superficial (two to three layers): flat cells
- Intermediate wing cells (two to three layers): polygonal cells
- Basal cells (single layer): cylindrical cells

The superficial epithelial cells appear as flat polygonal cells with well-defined border, prominent nuclei, and uniform density of cytoplasm. They are 40–50 μm in diameter and approximately 5 μm thick. The main identifying features of superficial epithelial cells are nuclei, which are brighter than the surrounding cytoplasm and usually associated with perinuclear hypodense ring (Figure 11.2). Superficial cells often display a large variation in cytoplasmic reflectivity representing various stages of progression toward cell death. The intermediate epithelial cells, also known as wing cells, are similar polygonal cells as superficial layers but the nuclei are not evident. They are typically 30–45 μm in size and are characterized by bright cell borders. Basal cell layers are smaller in size (10–15 μm) and appear denser than other two layers (Figure 11.3). They display a uniformly bright cell border with a dark cytoplasmic mass. The nucleus is not evident in basal layers also.

11.2.2 Subepithelial Nerve Plexus

Corneal nerves originate from long ciliary nerve, a branch of ophthalmic division of trigeminal nerve. Nerve fibers from long ciliary nerve form a circular plexus at the limbus. Radial nerve fibers originate from this circular plexus and run deep into the stroma to

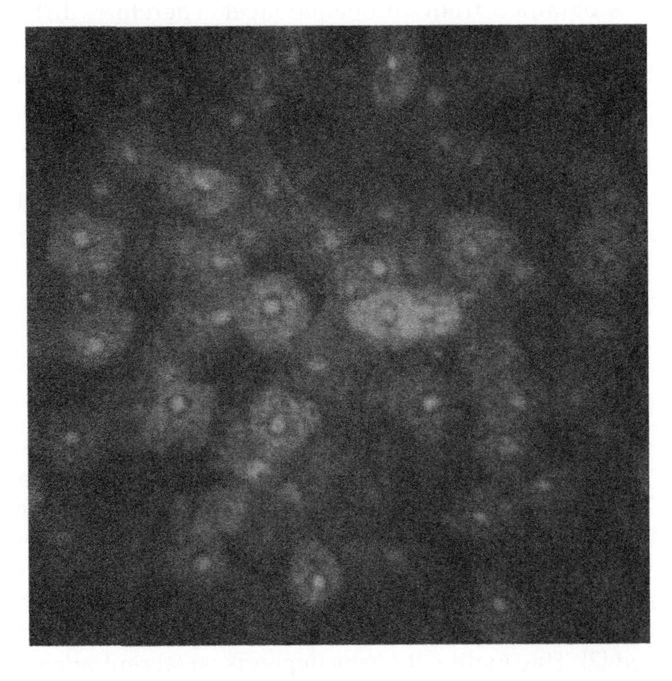

FIGURE 11.2
Superficial epithelial cells with prominent nuclei.

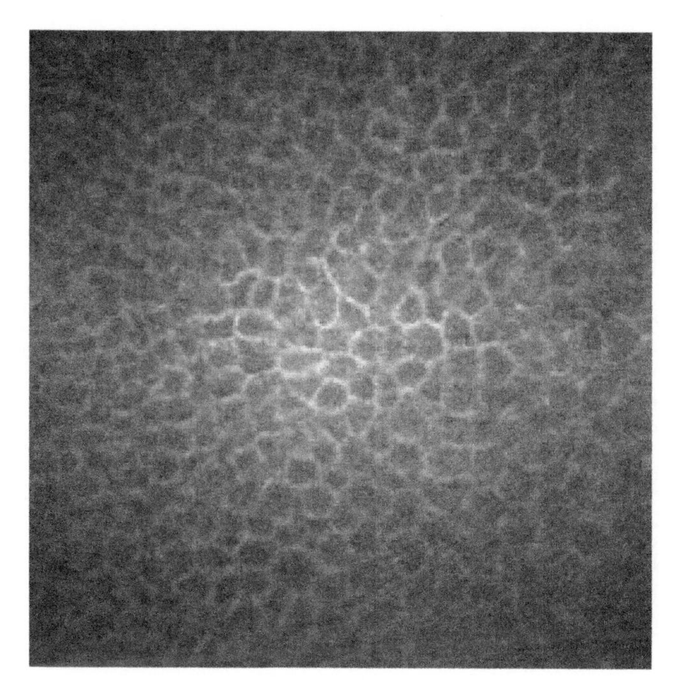

FIGURE 11.3
Basal epithelial cells. High-density cells with well-demarcated cell borders.

form deep corneal plexus. Now deep vertical fibers derive from deep corneal plexus to run anteriorly to form subbasal and subepithelial nerve plexus. Small nerve fibers from subbasal plexus terminate at the superficial epithelium.

This complex anatomy was not possible to visualize in vivo until the advent of corneal confocal microscope. Generally, the nerve fibers appear bright and well contrasted against a dark background (Figure 11.4). Confocal microscopy can visualize the orientation, tortuosity, width, branching pattern, and any abnormality of the corneal nerves [3]. The unmyelinated subbasal nerve plexus is visible on confocal microscopy images at the level of the acellular Bowman's layer. Single nerve fibers are beyond the resolution limit of confocal microscopy and only beaded nerve bundles can be observed. In the anterior corneal stroma, larger nerve fiber bundles are easily observed and signs of apparent keratocyte–nerve interactions are occasionally noted in the central cornea.

11.2.3 Stroma

Corneal stroma accounts for 90% of total corneal thickness. It has three components:

1. Cellular stroma: Composed of keratocytes and constitutes 5% of entire stroma.
2. Acellular stroma: Represents the major component (90%–95%) of stroma. The main component is regular collagen tissue (type I, III, IV) and interstitial substances.
3. Neurosensory stroma: Represented by stromal nerve plexus and nerve fibers originating from it.

The keratocyte concentration is much higher in the anterior stroma and progressively decreases toward the deep stroma. Generally, the keratocyte count is approximately

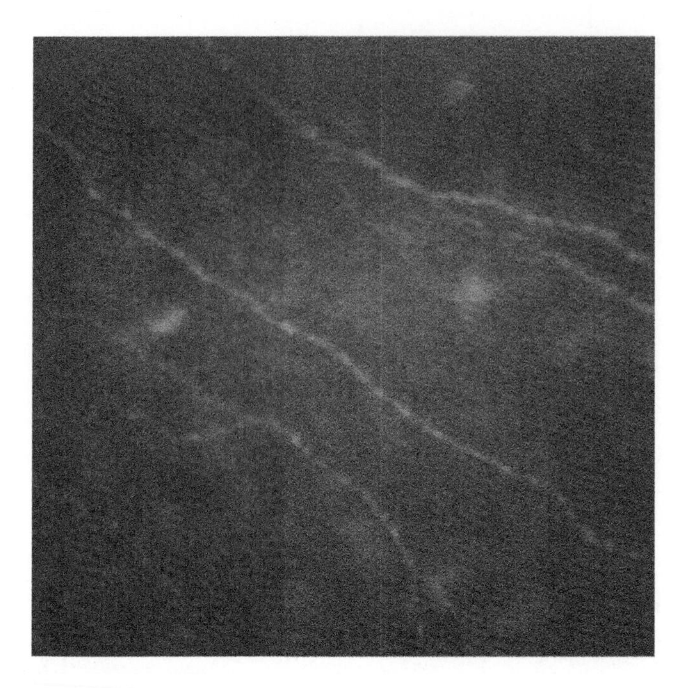

FIGURE 11.4
(See color insert.) Subepithelial nerve fibers.

1000 cells/mm^2 in the anterior stroma, while the average value drops to 700 cells/mm^2 in the posterior stroma. Confocal image of stroma shows multiple irregularly oval-, round-, or bean-shaped bright structures that represent keratocyte nuclei. These nuclei are well contrasted against dark acellular matrix (Figure 11.5). Anterior stromal keratocyte nuclei assume rounded bean-shaped morphology, while the same in rear stroma are more often irregularly oval. A bright highly reflective keratocyte represents a metabolically activated keratocyte of a healthy cornea. In a normal healthy cornea, collagen fibers and interstitial substances appear transparent to confocal microscope and impossible to visualize. It is possible to identify stromal nerve fibers in the anterior and mid stroma. These nerve fibers belong to deep corneal plexus and appear as linear bright thick lines. The stromal nerve fiber thickness is greater than epithelial nerves. Occasionally, nerve bifurcations are also clearly visible.

11.2.4 Descemet's Membrane

Descemet's membrane appears as generalized hazy layer and no cellular structure can be identified. The normal Descemet's membrane is not visible in young subjects but becomes more apparent with increasing age.

11.2.5 Endothelium

Corneal endothelium is comprised of a single layer of cells that are 4–6 μm thick and approximately 20 μm in diameter. This is a noninnervated single layer of cells at the most posterior part of the cornea. Endothelial cell density is maximal at birth and progressively declines with age. Normal endothelial cell count varies from 1600 to 3000 cells/mm^2

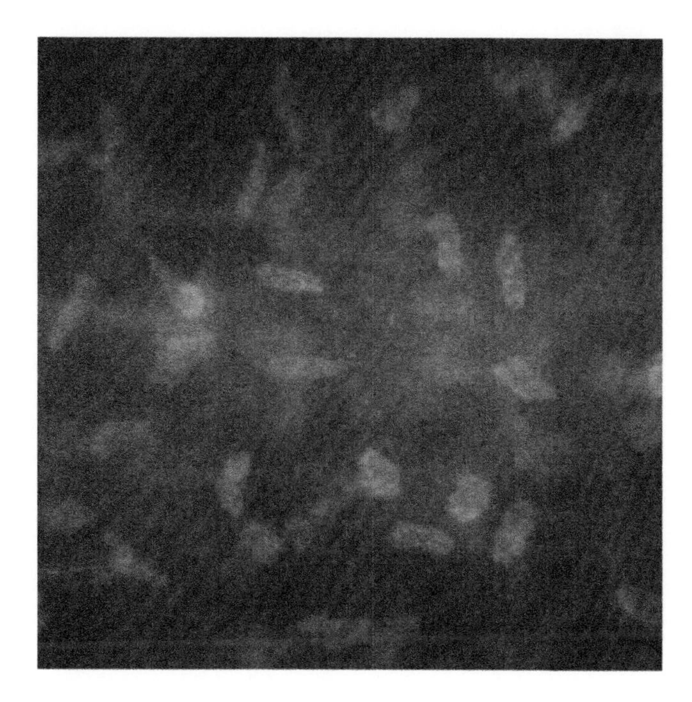

FIGURE 11.5
Stromal keratocytes with bright oval nucleus.

(average 2700 cells/mm^2) in a normal healthy adult [3–5]. However, the cornea can still maintain the integrity till the cell count declines below 300–500 cells/mm^2.

Homogeneous hexagonal cells with uniform size and shape represent healthy endothelial cells. Increasing age and endothelial assault cause pleomorphism and polymegathism. Confocal microscopy easily identifies endothelial cells. These cells appear as bright hexagonal and polygonal cells with unrecognizable nucleus. The cell borders are represented by a thin, nonreflective dark line (Figure 11.6). A ×20 objective lens provides wide field with less magnification. It is possible to perform cell count and study the minute details of cellular morphology.

11.2.6 Corneal Thickness Measurement

Confocal microscopes can be used to measure corneal thickness. This function is called confocal microscopy through focusing (CMTF). This technique is considered as one of the major advances in confocal imaging. As all the points of the CMTF curve correlate directly with high-resolution images, the exact position in the Z-axis of a corneal structure such as the epithelium, the subepithelial nerve plexus, and the endothelium can be used to calculate precisely the distance between the different corneal layers. Specialized software allows interactive viewing of the image corresponding to the cursor location on the Z-curve and measurement of the distance between any two points on the curve. Because different layers of the cornea reflect light at different intensities, the depth-intensity profile allows for the determination of corneal sublayer location. Thus, corneal confocal microscope may provide not only the total corneal thickness but also the epithelial thickness, Bowman's layer thickness, and, following laser in situ keratomileusis (LASIK) surgery, flap thickness also.

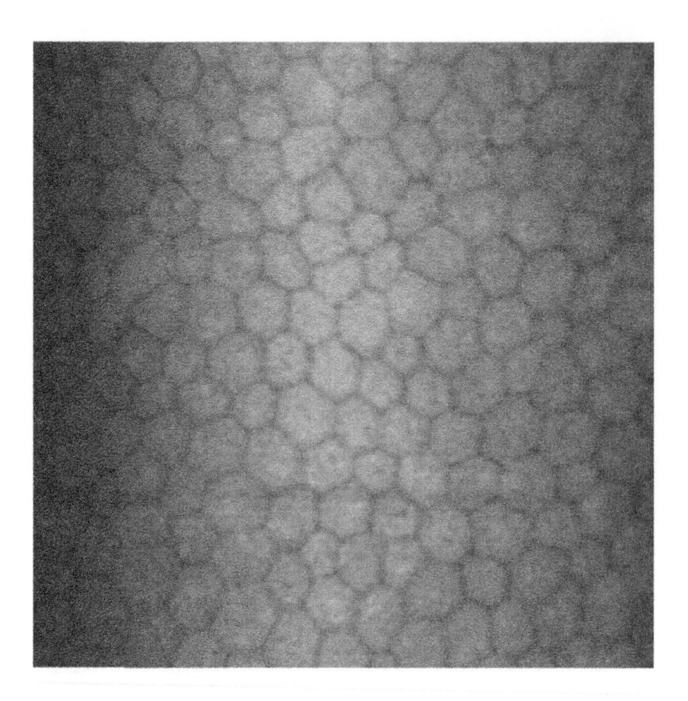

FIGURE 11.6
Hexagonal endothelial cells.

11.3 Confocal Microscopy in Corneal Pathologies

11.3.1 Keratoconus

Keratoconus is a progressive, noninflammatory, bilateral (but usually asymmetrical) ectatic corneal disease, characterized by paraxial stromal thinning and weakening that leads to corneal surface distortion. The thinning is most apparent at the apex of the cornea. The steep conical protrusion of the corneal apex causes high myopia with severe irregular astigmatism. Other features of keratoconus include an iron ring, known as Fleischer's ring that partially or completely encircles the cone [5,6]. The cone appears as *oil drop* reflex on distant direct ophthalmoscopy due to internal reflection of light. Deep vertical folds oriented parallel to the steeper axis of the cornea at the level of deep stroma and Descemet's membrane are known as *Vogt's striae.* An acute corneal hydrops appears when there is a break in the Descemet's membrane. The corneal edema usually subsides after few months leaving behind scar and flattening the cornea. The corneal nerves become more readily visible due to thinning of the cornea. High irregular astigmatism precludes adequate spectacle correction. Visual loss occurs primarily from irregular astigmatism and myopia, and secondarily from corneal scarring. In the early stages, the use of contact lenses may improve the visual acuity. However, contact lens fitting can be extremely difficult, and in advanced cases, it ceases to improve visual acuity, optimally forcing the patient to rely on the only option left, corneal transplantation.

The most effective way to identify early cases of keratoconus is computerized corneal topography that has become a gold standard for diagnosis and follow-up of the disease

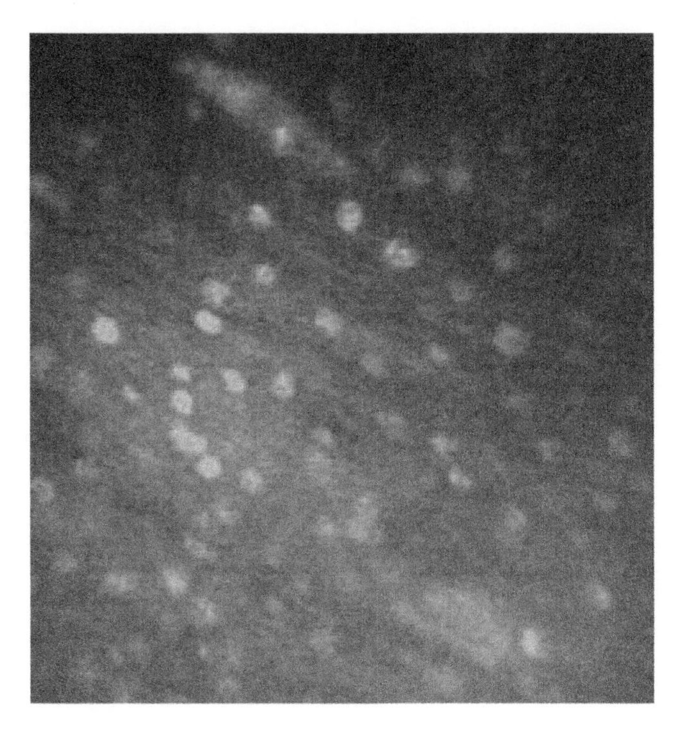

FIGURE 11.7
Superficial epithelium with obliquely elongated cells in keratoconus.

in recent years [7,8]. Confocal microscopy is a relatively newer investigative modality to assess the keratoconic cornea. Quantitative and qualitative structural changes are observed in all corneal layers in eyes with keratoconus by using slit-scanning confocal microscopy. Morphological changes in keratoconus are mostly confined to the corneal apex and depend on the severity of the disease. The rest of the cornea may appear normal. The typical polygonal shape of superficial epithelial cells is lost. They appear distorted and elongated in an oblique direction with highly reflective nuclei (Figure 11.7). Cell borders are not distinguishable. There may be areas of basal epithelial loss as evident by a linear dark nonreflective patch in confocal microscopy. The subepithelial nerve plexus generally appear normal. However, the subbasal nerve fibers are curved and take the course of stretched overlying epithelium. Corneal stroma is also affected by keratoconus. The confocal images of stroma are highly specific. The characteristic stromal changes are multiple *striae* represented by thin hyporeflective lines oriented vertically, horizontally, or obliquely (Figure 11.8). These are confocal representation of Vogt's striae [8,9]. In advanced stages of keratoconus, the keratocyte concentration is reduced in anterior stroma. The shape of the keratocytes is also altered. Occasionally, highly reflective bodies with tapering ends are visible in anterior stroma near the apex. The nature of these abnormal bodies is not yet known but it may be due to altered keratocytes. The corneal endothelial changes vary from none to occasional pleomorphism and polymegathism.

11.3.2 Corneal Dystrophies

Corneal dystrophies are inherited abnormalities that affect one or more layers of cornea. Usually both eyes are affected but not necessarily symmetrically. They may present at

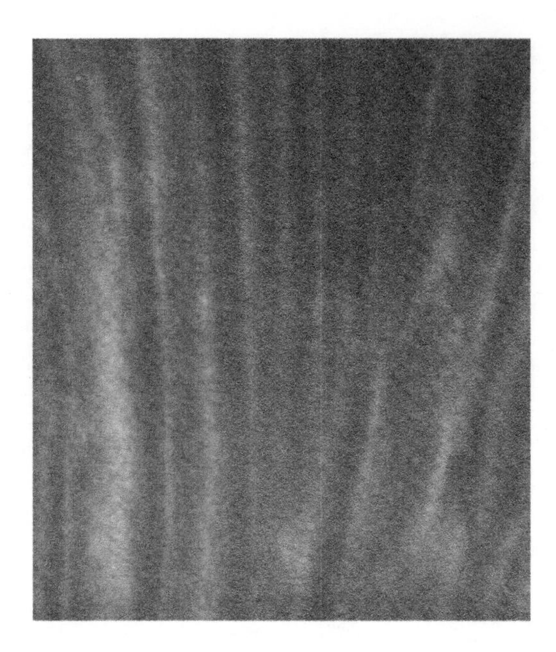

FIGURE 11.8
Vertical striae in the stroma in advanced keratoconus.

birth but more frequently develop during adolescence and progress gradually throughout life. Some forms are mild, others severe.

11.3.3 Granular Dystrophy

Granular dystrophy is an autosomal dominant, bilateral, noninflammatory condition that results in deposition of opacities in the cornea by adulthood. It specifically affects the corneal stroma and eventually can cause decreased vision and eye discomfort. The eye condition results from deposition of eosinophilic hyaline deposits in the corneal stroma [10]. It specifically affects the central cornea and eventually can cause decreased vision and eye discomfort. Initially, the lesions are confined to superficial stroma, but with the progression of the disease, they can involve the posterior stroma as well. Severe cases of granular dystrophy can be treated with either excimer laser ablation or by replacing cornea (corneal transplant).

Confocal microscopy reveals highly reflective, bright, dense structures in the anterior and mid-stroma. Keratocytes are not involved. Depth of stromal involvement may be ascertained by using Z-scan function. This is an added advantage over other contemporary investigations that enables the surgeon to plan for surgical modalities. Confocal microscopy is also useful in differential diagnosis and follow-up of the disease.

11.3.4 Posterior Polymorphous Dystrophy

This uncommon form of corneal dystrophy may present at birth or later during life and is characterized by lesions affecting the endothelium. Majority of patients are asymptomatic. The condition is bilateral but asymmetric and slowly progressive. In severe cases, individuals with posterior polymorphous dystrophy (PPMD) may develop corneal edema, photophobia, decreased vision, and foreign body sensation in the eye. In rare cases, intraocular pressure may increase. The characteristic endothelial changes are small vesicles or areas of geographic lesions. In fact, endothelial cell lining of the posterior surface of the cornea has epithelial-like features [11,12]. These cells can also cover the trabecular meshwork, leading to glaucoma in some patients. Most severe cases may develop corneal edema due to compromised pump function of the endothelial cells.

Confocal microscopy shows multiple round vesicles at the level of Descemet's membrane and endothelium [13]. PPMD usually distorts the normal flat profile of the endothelial cells and present large dark cystic impressions on confocal scan. The endothelial cells surrounding the lesion appear large and distorted.

11.3.5 Fuchs Endothelial Dystrophy

Fuchs endothelial dystrophy is a chronic bilateral hereditary (variable autosomal dominant or sporadic) disorder of corneal endothelium. It typically presents after the age of 50 and more common in females. There is a loss of endothelial cells that results in deposition of collagen materials in Descemet's membrane (guttata). Corneal guttata is the hallmark of this disease. The integrity of corneal endothelium is essential to maintain the metabolic and osmotic function of the entire cornea. Corneal edema in Fuchs dystrophy initially involves the posterior and mid-stroma. As the disease advances, the edema progresses to involve the anterior cornea; resulting in formation of bullous keratopathy.

Confocal microscopy is useful to visualize the corneal guttata. This technique has a distinct advantage over conventional specular microscopy that fails to visualize the endothelium when there is significant corneal edema [14]. The corneal guttata appears dark with bright central reflex [15] (Figure 11.9). In advanced stage, the endothelial morphology is altered completely but it is still possible to identify the distorted cell borders [15].

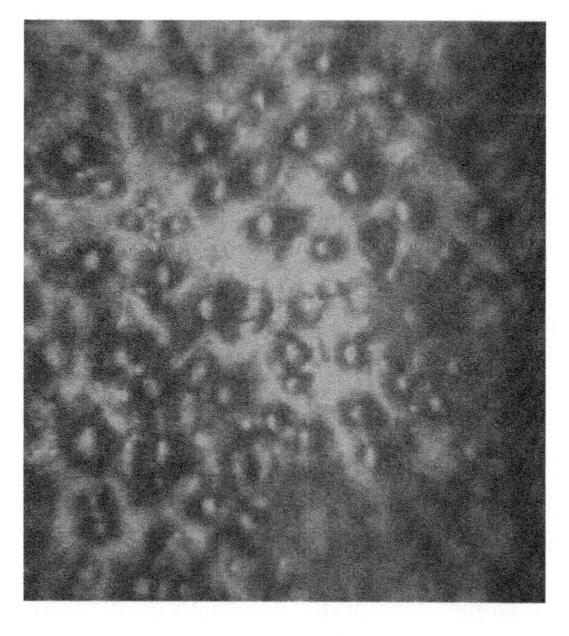

FIGURE 11.9
Distorted endothelium in Fuch's endothelial dystrophy.

In the early stages of bullous keratopathy, intraepithelial edema is seen as distorted cellular morphology with increased reflectivity. It can also identify the bullae in the basal epithelial layer.

11.3.6 Laser In Situ Keratomileusis

LASIK is one of the latest techniques of excimer laser refractive surgery that is currently being successfully used by refractive surgeons for the correction of various types of refractive errors. LASIK has become the technique of choice to correct myopia and hyperopia with or without astigmatism [16]. LASIK is a modification of photorefractive keratectomy (PRK) where excimer laser is used to ablate superficial corneal stroma after the epithelium has been removed. LASIK involves the use of microkeratome to prepare a hinged corneal flap of uniform thickness. The excimer laser is subsequently used to ablate the midcorneal stromal bed, and thereafter, the flap is reposited to its original position without applying any suture. After LASIK, the healing of corneal tissue occurs quickly since there is minimal damage to the corneal epithelium and Bowman's membrane.

Traditionally, the cornea is evaluated with slit-lamp biomicroscopy and computerized corneal topography both pre- and postoperatively. Confocal microscopy adds newer dimensions to the commonly employed investigations. Functional outcome of LASIK depends on many factors including the biomechanics, healing process, and the inflammatory response of the flap interface that is created between the epithelial flap and stromal bed. Confocal scan is useful in the evaluation of the following parameters:

- Corneal flap thickness
- Interface study
- Healing process
- Inflammatory response
- Abnormal deposits
- Corneal nerve fiber regeneration
- Residual stromal thickness

A well-designed flap is the key to successful outcome of LASIK. Thinner flaps are more at risk from flap complications. A few studies with confocal microscopy had suggested that actual flap thickness after LASIK is consistently lower than predicted thickness [17]. The reasons are not yet known. However, corneal edema that may be caused by microkeratome cut and suction may play an important role. Postoperative scarring and tissue retraction could be other possible factors. Using a Z-scan, it is possible to identify the interface that corresponds to a very low level of reflectivity. The flap thickness is obtained by measuring the distance between high reflective spike from the front surface of the cornea and the low reflective interface (Figure 11.10).

The interface usually appears as a hyporeflective space in between relatively hyperreflective cellular stroma. Interface can easily be imaged by confocal microscope. Typically, the keratocyte concentration is lower than normal in the interface. Bright particles and microstriae are consistently visible in the interface. These bright particles most probably originate from microkeratome blade and represented by highly reflective white bodies (Figure 11.11). Microstriae are present at Bowman's layer. Excessive interface microstriae and bright particles may lead to astigmatism and eventually poor outcome after LASIK.

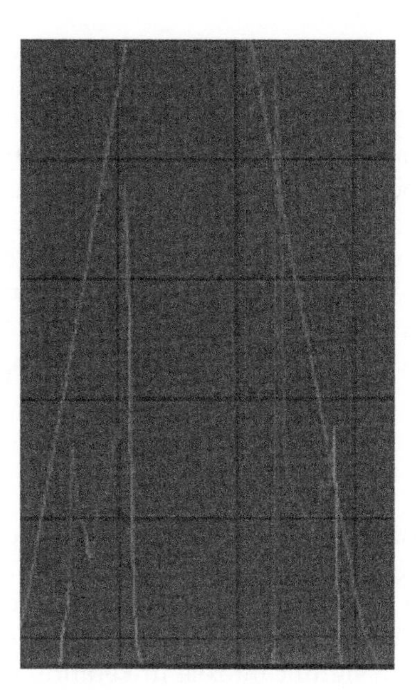

FIGURE 11.10
Flap thickness measurement in LASIK.

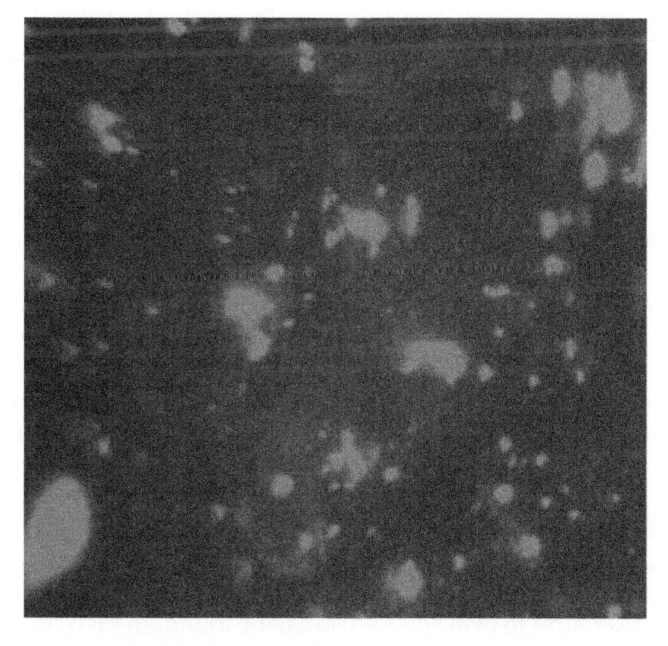

FIGURE 11.11
Highly reflective particles in the interface after LASIK.

These microstriae can be imaged with confocal microscope even when the slit-lamp examination is unremarkable.

Diffuse lamellar keratitis (DLK), also known as *sands of Sahara syndrome*, is a noninfectious inflammation of the interface. The etiology is not known but it is assumed to be toxic or allergic in nature. In confocal scan, DLK appears as diffuse and multiple infiltrates in the interface with no anterior or posterior extension.

Subepithelial nerve fibers are affected by LASIK. No nerve is visible in the immediate postoperative period. However, the regenerating nerve fibers appear as thin irregularly branching line when confocal scan is performed 5–7 days after surgery. The residual stromal thickness can also be measured using Z-scan technique as described while evaluating the epithelial flap.

11.3.7 Infectious Keratitis

Accurate and prompt diagnosis of sight threatening infectious keratitis is one of the major challenges in ophthalmic practice today. Delay in diagnosis and inappropriate treatment can adversely affect the visual outcome. Current microbiological diagnostic techniques can identify most of the offending organisms if the tests are carried out meticulously. However, confocal microscopy can play a significant role in keratitis with prolonged course, polymicrobial keratitis, and in the scenario when conventional techniques are unable to identify any organism. The usefulness of confocal microscopy was demonstrated in eyes with *Acanthamoeba* [18] and fungal keratitis [19,20].

It is frequently difficult to identify *Acanthamoeba* on the ocular surface since the presentation can mimic herpetic keratitis and several forms of bacterial keratitis. This diagnostic confusion has often led to delays in making the diagnosis and subsequently affecting the visual outcome significantly. Most cases of Acanthamoeba keratitis are diagnosed by tissue culture, corneal biopsy, and histological analysis [21–23]. Confocal microscope offers a useful noninvasive technique to diagnose Acanthamoeba keratitis. Although confocal microscopy lacks sufficient resolution to be the only method of diagnosis, it can be used in screening patients suspected of having Acanthamoeba keratitis [24,25]. Sometimes internal structures of *Acanthamoeba* along with vacuoles are also visible. On confocal microscopy, *Acanthamoeba* are visualized typically as round or ovoid highly reflective structures ranging in size from 10 to 25 μm, which is larger than leukocytes (Figure 11.12). Sometimes double-walled cystic forms of the parasite are also well visualized (Figure 11.13). *Acanthamoeba* are smaller and much more iridescent than corneal parenchymal cells such as epithelial cells and keratocyte nuclei.

Mycotic keratitis is common in many countries in tropical latitudes. Filamentous fungi are the most common cause of mycotic keratitis [26]. It is important to establish a specific diagnosis as early as possible to ensure prompt institution of antifungal therapy. Although confocal microscopic examination may help in to reach a rapid presumptive diagnosis, the in vivo confocal microscopic characteristic of fungal keratitis continues to confuse ophthalmologists over the years. However, clear understanding of confocal characteristics of fungal hyphae and spores may play an important role to establish a rapid diagnosis. Identification of fungal organisms by confocal microscopy is important, not only for rapidly diagnosing fungal keratitis but also to monitor the antifungal therapy. On confocal microscopy, the mycotic organisms appear as thin, extensively branching, beaded filaments and sometimes round to oval spores also can be found. In vivo confocal microscopy offers either of the four morphologic features of mycotic keratitis such as (a) the branching

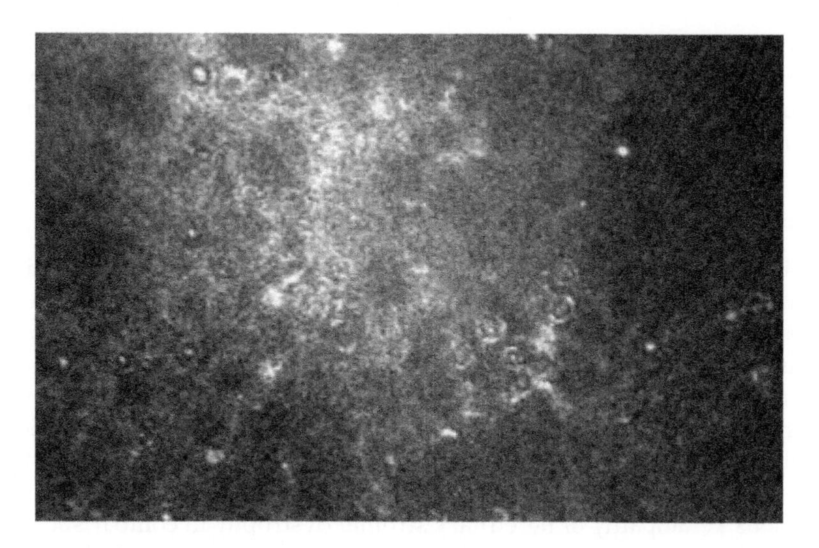

FIGURE 11.12
In vivo confocal microscopy demonstrating active *Acanthamoeba* represented by bright refractile bodies. Few trophozoites are also visible.

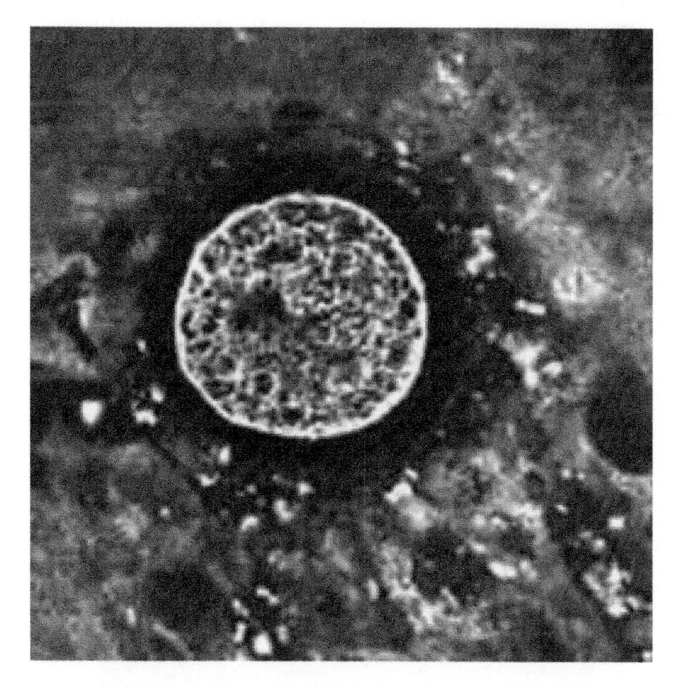

FIGURE 11.13
In vivo confocal microscopy showing typical double-walled cystic form of *Acanthamoeba*.

hyperreflective structures, (b) the long line hyperreflective structures, (c) the short rod hyperreflective structures, and (d) the round to oval structures (spores). The hyphae must not be confused with corneal nerves, which appear regular, elongated, and uniform with sharp margins.

11.3.8 Corneal Grafts

Confocal microscope is a useful tool to follow up the corneal grafts and to diagnose the abnormal changes that may occur postoperatively. It provides images at the cellular level to identify any pathological changes even before it becomes clinically evident. It can also be used to assess the donor cornea.

Corneal graft survival is entirely dependent on optimum number of healthy endothelial cells. Endothelial cell loss occurs rapidly after corneal transplantation [27]. Majority of cell loss takes place during the first 2 postoperative years [28]. Several studies had suggested that endothelial cell loss is much higher after corneal grafting when the primary indications are bullous keratopathy or hereditary stromal dystrophy in comparison to keratoconus and corneal leukomas [29,30]. Another interesting fact is that endothelial cell loss is greater when corneal transplantation is performed on phakic eyes than on aphakics [31].

Confocal microscopy scores over conventional specular microscopy while evaluating endothelial cell characteristics especially in eyes with stromal edema. Endothelial morphology in confocal scan has been described earlier. In the immediate postoperative period, the endothelium looks normal and healthy. However, as time progresses, endothelial cell density decreases as evidenced by pleomorphism and polymegathism. Occasionally, bright preendothelial deposits appear, the significance of which is not yet known (Figure 11.14).

Reinnervation after grafting is another issue well addressed by confocal microscopy. The first sign of innervation that starts a few months after keratoplasty is visible at the

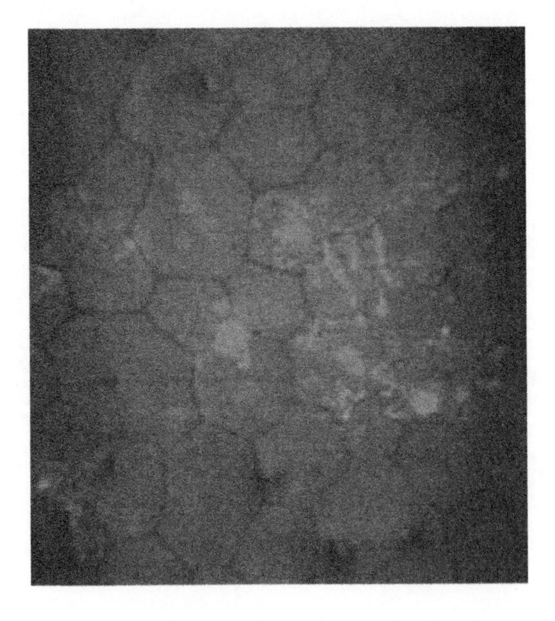

FIGURE 11.14
Pleomorphism, polymegathism, and preendothelial deposits in a corneal graft.

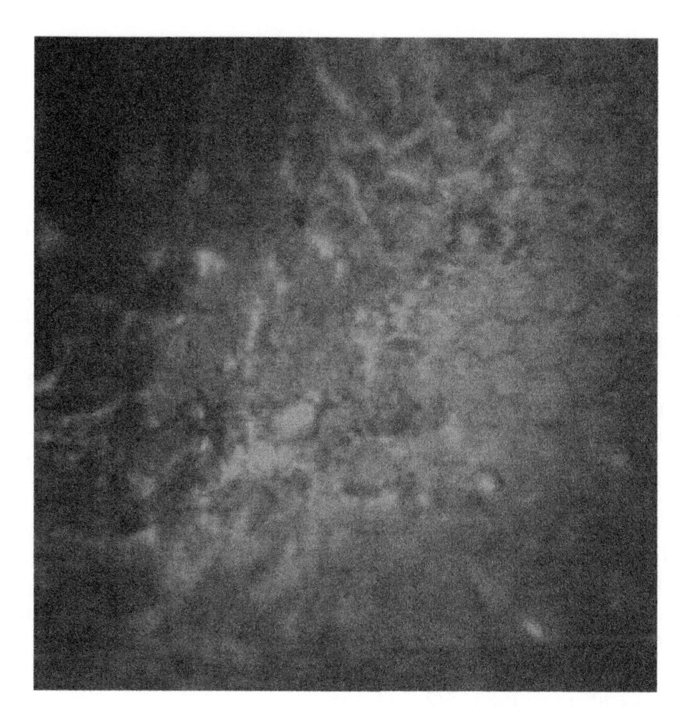

FIGURE 11.15
Coexistence of degenerated and normal endothelial cells in early endothelial allograft rejection.

periphery of the graft stroma. However, complete innervation may take many years to develop. Regenerated nerve fibers look similar to that found in a normal cornea. Occasionally, they may take a tortuous and convoluted course depending on age (e.g., older patients) and primary indications of keratoplasty (e.g., bullous keratopathy, corneal dystrophies).

It is well known that allograft rejection is one of the most common causes of graft failure. Graft rejection can be classified as epithelial, subepithelial, and endothelial rejection, of which the endothelial rejection is the worst. Confocal features of epithelial rejection are distorted basal epithelial cells with altered subepithelial reflectivity. Subepithelial rejection is identified by discrete opacities underneath the epithelial layer [32]. Endothelial rejection, on the other hand, is characterized by coexistence of normal-looking and degenerated endothelial cells, focal endothelial cell lesions, and bright highly reflective microprecipitates [33] (Figure 11.15).

11.4 Conclusion

Ophthalmic investigations and instrumentations have come a long way over the past decades. Confocal microscope is one of those wonderful innovations in recent times. It is becoming more popular everyday and its indications are expanding. Confocal microscopy is truly an exciting tool that can be useful for the clinical diagnosis, follow-up, and analysis of many corneal lesions.

References

1. Minsky M. Memoir on inventing the confocal scanning microscope. *Scanning* 1988;10:128–138.
2. Weigand W, Thaer AA, Kroll P et al. Optical sectioning of the cornea with a new confocal in vivo slit-scanning videomicroscope. *Ophthalmology* 1995;102(4):485–492.
3. Oliveira-Soto L, Efron N. Morphology of corneal nerves using confocal microscopy. *Cornea* 2001;20(4):374–384.
4. Tuft SJ, Coster DJ. The corneal endothelium. *Eye* 1990;4:389.
5. Nucci P, Brancato R, Mets MB et al. Normal endothelial cell density range in childhood. *Arch Ophthalmol* 1990;108:247.
6. Gass JD. The iron lines of the superficial cornea: Hudson-Stahli line, Stocker's line, and Fleischer's ring. *Arch Ophthalmol* 1964;71:348–358.
7. Maguire LJ, Bourne WM. Corneal topography in early keratoconus. *Am J Ophthalmol* 1989;108:107.
8. Maguire LJ, Lowry J. Identifying progression of subclinical keratoconus by serial topography analysis. *Am J Ophthalmol* 1991;112:41.
9. Somodi S, Hahnel C, Slowik C et al. Confocal in vivo microscopy and confocal laser-scanning fluorescence microscopy in keratoconus. *Ger J Ophthalmol* 1996;5(6):518–525.
10. Werner LP, Werner L, Dighiero P et al. Confocal microscopy in Bowman's and stromal corneal dystrophies. *Ophthalmology* 1999;106(9):1697–1704.
11. Hirst LW, Waring GO. Clinical specular microscopy of posterior polymorphous endothelial dystrophy. *Am J Ophthalmol* 1983;95(2):143–155.
12. Mashima Y, Hida T, Akiya S et al. Specular microscopy of posterior polymorphous endothelial dystrophy. *Ophthalmic Paediatr Genet* 1986;7(2):101–107.
13. Chiou AG, Kaufman SC, Beuerman RW et al. Confocal microscopy of posterior polymorphous endothelial dystrophy. *Ophthalmologica* 1999;213(4):211–213.
14. Chiou AG, Kaufman SC, Beuerman RW et al. Confocal microscopy in cornea guttata and Fuch's endothelial dystrophy. *Br J Ophthalmol* 1999;83(2):185–189.
15. Rosenblum P, Stark WJ, Maumenee IH et al. Hereditary Fuch's dystrophy. *Am J Ophthalmol* 1980;90:455.
16. Reviglio VE, Bossana EL, Luna JD et al. Laser in situ keratomileusis for the correction of hyperopia from +0.50 to +11.50 diopters with Keracor 117C laser. *J Refract Surg* 2000;16(6):716–723.
17. Durairaj VD, Balentine J, Kouyoumdjian G et al. The predictability of corneal flap thickness and tissue laser ablation in laser in situ keratomileusis. *Ophthalmology* 2000;107(12):2140–2143.
18. Cavanagh HD, Petrol WM, Alizadeh H et al. Clinical and diagnostic use of in vivo confocal microscopy in patients with corneal disease. *Ophthalmology* 1993;100:1444–1454.
19. Winchester K, Mathers WD, Sutphin JE. Diagnosis of aspergillus keratitis in vivo with confocal microscopy. *Cornea* 1997;16:27–31.
20. Florakis GJ, Moazami G, Schubert H et al. Scanning slit confocal microscopy of fungal keratitis. *Arch Ophthalmol* 1997;115:1461–1463.
21. Mathers WD, Sutphin JE, Folberg R et al. Outbreak of keratitis presumed to be caused by *Acanthamoeba*. *Am J Ophthalmol* 1996;121:129–142.
22. Auran JD, Starr MB, Jakobiec FA. Acanthamoeba keratitis: A review of the literature. *Cornea* 1987;6:2–26.
23. D'Aversa G, Stern GA, Driebe WT. Diagnosis and successful medical treatment of Acanthamoeba keratitis. *Arch Ophthalmol* 1995;113:1120–1123.
24. Winchester K, Mathers WD, Sutphin JE. Diagnosis of Acanthamoeba keratitis in vivo with confocal microscopy. *Cornea* 1995;14:10–17.
25. Chew SJ, Beuerman RW, Assouline M et al. Early diagnosis of infectious keratitis with in vivo real time confocal microscopy. *CLAO J* 1992;18:197–201.

26. Wang L, Zhang J, Sun S et al. In vivo confocal microscopic characteristics of fungal keratitis. *Life Sci J* 2008;5(1):51–54.
27. Harper CL, Boulton ML, Marcyniuk B et al. Endothelial viability of organ cultured corneas following penetrating keratoplasty. *Eye* 1998;12(5):834–838.
28. Vasara K, Setala K, Ruusuvaara P. Follow up study of corneal endothelial cells, photographed in vivo before enucleation and 20 years later in graft. *Acta Ophthalmol Scand* 1999;77(3):273–276.
29. Obata H, Ishida K, Murao M et al. Corneal endothelial cell damage in penetrating keratoplasty. *Jpn J Ophthalmol* 1991;35(4):411–416.
30. Abott RL, Fine M, Guillet E. Long-term changes in corneal endothelium following penetrating keratoplasty. A specular microscopic study. *Ophthalmology* 1983;90(6):676–685.
31. Ing JJ, Ing HH, Nelson LR et al. Ten-year postoperative results of penetrating keratoplasty. *Ophthalmology* 1998;105(10):1855–1865.
32. Cohen RA, Chew SJ, Gebhardt BM et al. Confocal microscopy of corneal graft rejection. *Cornea* 1995;14(5):467–472.
33. Cho BJ, Gross SJ, Pfister DR et al. In vivo confocal microscopic analysis of corneal allograft rejection in rabbits. *Cornea* 1998;17(4):417–422.

12

Corneal Topography and Tomography: The Orbscan II

Anna W.T. Tan, Manotosh Ray, and Dawn K.A. Lim

CONTENTS

The cornea accounts for approximately two-thirds of the eye's total optical power, making it the most important refractive element in the human eye. The emphasis on quantitative assessment of the cornea dates back to the 1600s [1], and its importance cannot be overemphasized in this current era of rapid advances in refractive surgery with an unprecedented demand to achieve optically perfect results. Cornea surface analysis has become indispensable for the current-day practice, where other important applications include diagnosis of forme-fruste keratoconus, monitoring of ectatic noninflammatory diseases, and complicated contact lens fitting in advance keratoconus. Technologies in corneal mapping have evolved from Placido-based (reflective technique) computerized videokeratography systems to slit-scanning (projective technique) topography methods to a hybrid of both technologies, revolutionizing the capabilities and precision of measuring corneal surfaces.

12.1 Orbscan

Topography gives a 2D representation of the anterior corneal surface, where *topos* in Greek refers to *place* and *tomos* in Greek to *a section*; hence, tomography describes a 3D representation (or section) of the cornea.

The Orbscan II (Bausch & Lomb) incorporates [2] both 2D anterior corneal topography and 3D corneal and anterior segment tomography data acquisition capabilities. This involves a slit-scanning technique using white light and Placido disk technology [3]. The Orbscan II acquires over 9000 data points in 1.5 s to meticulously map the entire corneal surface.

12.2 From Data Acquisition to Map Construction

The Placido disk is illuminated and the reflection of its mires (concentric illuminated rings) from the anterior stromal surface is stored and digitally analyzed to reconstruct a 3D corneal shape. Closely spaced mires indicate higher corneal powers and widely spaced rings, the reverse. The size and distortion of ring patterns serve as the basis for calculation. The scanning slit-section technique of imaging the cornea involves 40 slit sections of the cornea during 2 scans, from which the anterior and posterior corneal height profiles are reconstructed using 3D ray tracing.

Several algorithms are used for reconstructing the corneal shape from the mire positions; the arc-step being the most accurate. Using various methods, the dioptric power of the cornea can be derived from the local radii of curvature. The detailed discussion of these calculations is beyond the scope of this chapter.

12.3 Color-Coded Maps and Quantitative Indices

The color-coded map (Figure 12.1) is a qualitative display of the data, which is designed for ease of pattern recognition, which aids intuitive interpretation through the association of power with color and recognition of pathology with patterns given by the map contours. Depending on the corneal topographer used, each has its standard color scale and the actual power values, intervals, and colors used differ. In general, warm colors, for example, red and orange, denote relatively higher powers (steeper curvature), whereas cool colors, for example, blue, represents relatively lower powers, hence flatter curvatures.

The standard *quad map* presentation on a printout comprises of two elevation maps presented in the form of a contour map representing height deviations from the best-fit sphere, that is, anterior and posterior elevation, the keratometric map, and the pachymetry map.

Quantitative indices are derived through various mathematical formulae; these include the simulated keratometry (Sim K) reading.

12.4 Applications

12.4.1 Forme-Fruste Keratoconus and Keratoconus

Keratoconus (Figure 12.2) is a progressive noninflammatory ectatic disease of the cornea, characterized by apical thinning, localized conical protrusion, and irregular astigmatism.

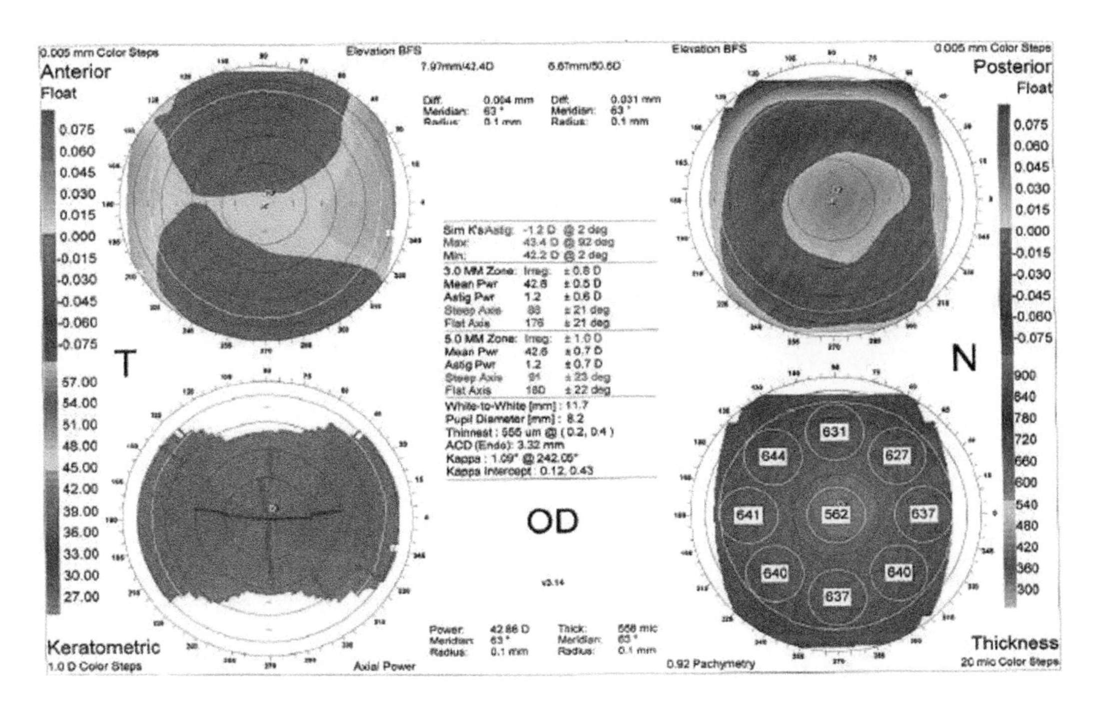

FIGURE 12.1
(See color insert.) Typical display of data from information acquired via the Orbscan II. This printout demonstrates the anterior elevation, posterior elevation, and keratometric and pachymetry maps.

Clinical features include Fleischer ring, Vogt striae, and anterior corneal stromal scar from previous hydrops.

The incidence of keratoconus [4,5] varies between countries with most estimates being between 50 and 230 per 100,000 in the general population—approximately 1 per 2,000 to 1 per 500.

Preclinical keratoconus or forme-fruste keratoconus is important to recognize as refractive surgery is contraindicated in these patients. Forme-fruste keratoconus is not easy to diagnose as these eyes frequently have normal clinical findings, hence the importance of a thorough and tedious assessment of the patient's corneal status through the use of corneal topography, to detect these eyes in the preoperative assessment before refractive surgery.

Before the advent of Orbscan, the Rabinowitz, Smolek/Klyce, and Klyce/Maeda criteria on videokeratography have been applied to identify subclinical cases. Several features on corneal topography have been described to aid the refractive surgeon in the diagnosis of forme-fruste keratoconus [6–9] with the advent of Orbscan:

- An area of central, inferior, or superior steepening
- Oblique cylinder >1.5 diopters
- Steep keratometric curvature greater than 47 D
- Central corneal thickness less than 500 µm
- Asymmetric bow tie
- Posterior float elevation greater than 40 µm

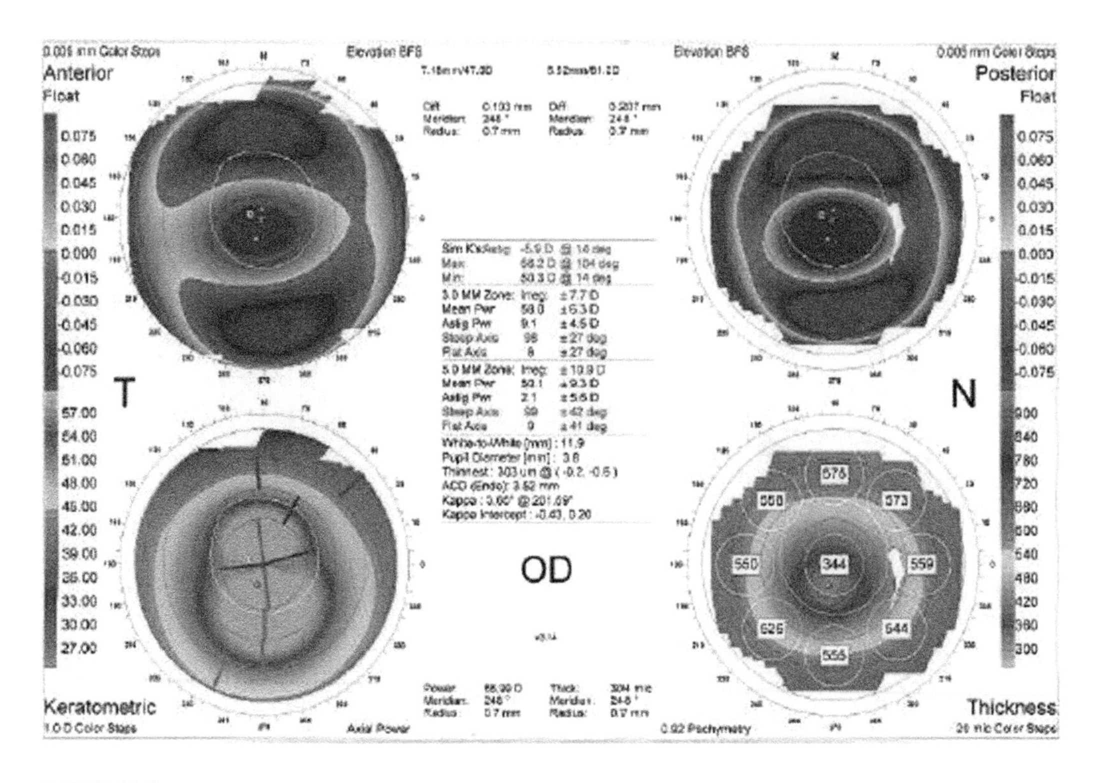

FIGURE 12.2
(See color insert.) Orbscan II topography in an eye with keratoconus. Note the irregular astigmatism in the keratometric map. The high Sim K and increased irregularity in the 3 and 5 mm zones.

- Anterior float elevation greater than 25 μm
- Skewed superior axis >21°
- Inferior–superior dioptric asymmetry (I–S value) >1.2
- Sim K > 2 D
- Irregularity indices
- At 3 mm zone: > ±1.5 D
- At 5 mm zone: > ±2.0 D

To date, no single index has been found to be expert in detecting forme-fruste keratoconus, hence the need for the use of a combination of indices and topographic features to aid the detection of subclinical keratoconus, hence reducing the incidence of the dreaded complication of corneal ectasia following laser in situ keratomileusis (LASIK).

12.4.2 Pachymetry in Pre-LASIK Assessment

Noncontact technology with the evolution of Orbscan has enabled the measurement of corneal thickness with much ease as opposed to traditional methods of ultrasound pachymetry that requires direct contact of the probe with the patient's cornea.

This enables pre-LASIK assessment of the patient's cornea thickness, as it has been recommended that a residual stromal bed thickness of at least 250–300 μm be maintained to prevent corneal ectasia after myopic keratomileusis [10,11]. A central corneal thickness of less than 500 μm is a contraindication to LASIK [11].

12.4.3 Contact Lens Fitting

As keratoconus progresses, irregular astigmatism increases. This irregular astigmatism is nonorthogonal; hence, achieving an accurate refraction, subjective, and objective is difficult. Spectacle correction will, therefore, not be able to correct the constant blur that the patient experiences. Hence, rigid gas permeable contact lens is one of the conservative measures employed to improve the best-corrected visual acuity in this group of patients.

The corneal topography with inbuilt gridlines allows the measurement of the size, position, and area of the cone to aid the estimation of the back optic zone diameter (BOZD) and also the determination of the lens diameter (TD) during the contact lens fitting process, from which the back optic zone radius (BOZR) is derived.

12.5 Limitations

Problems cited [1,2,12,13] in the use of corneal topography include its sensitivity to alignment and focusing errors, which can produce artefactual information.

Tear film break up can contribute to artefactual results if prolonged fixed gaze is requested by the operator. This results in poor tracking with missing data and a map with the appearance of irregular astigmatism.

The accuracy if the measurement of the posterior surface elevation on Orbscan cannot be validated against any other gold standard.

Compared to Scheimpflug imaging technology such as that used in the Pentacam (Oculus Inc., Germany), the scanning slit topography tends to overestimate central corneal thickness in eyes with corneas greater than 500 μm and an underestimation is observed in eyes with thinner corneas below 500 μm [14].

The Pentacam (Oculus Inc., Germany), a tomographer, which came on the scene much later, appears to be able to overcome the limitations of the Orbscan and also allow for validation of the measurements obtained via Orbscan [2]. It has been reported that the tear film does not affect measurements obtained. And it overcomes the issue of alignment and focusing errors, as minute eye movements are captured by a camera that rotates around a common axis while taking 3D image slices of the anterior segment, which automatically realigns the measurement process with the corneal apex, compensating for saccadic eye movements.

These factors have to be considered in the analysis of any data generated via the Orbscan.

12.6 Conclusion

Corneal analysis has evolved with recent-day software technologies since the advent of the Placido disk. This overview describes in brief how advancing technologies have evolved patient care to its current stage where corneal topography is part of the standard care in the current-day practice of the cornea and refractive surgeon.

References

1. Cairns G and McGhee CN. Orbscan computerized topography: Attributes, applications, and limitations. *J Cataract Refract Surg*. 2005 Jan;31(1):205–220.
2. Wheeldon CE and McGhee CNJ. Corneal tomography and anterior chamber imaging. In Brightbill FS and McDonnell PJ (eds), *Corneal Surgery: Theory, Technique and Tissue*, 4th edn. St Louis, MO: Mosby Elsevier, 2008, Chapter 10, pp. 83–88.
3. Klyce SD. Computer-assisted corneal topography. High-resolution graphic presentation and analysis of keratoscopy. *Invest Ophthalmol Vis Sci*. 1984 Dec;25(12):1426–1435.
4. Ertan A and Muftuoglu O. Keratoconus clinical findings according to different age and gender groups. *Cornea*. 2008;27:1109–1113.
5. Edmund C. Corneal topography and elasticity in normal and keratoconic eyes. A methodological study concerning the pathogenesis of keratoconus. *Acta Ophthalmol Suppl*. 1989;193:1–36.
6. Rao SN, Raviv T, Majmudar PA, and Epstein RJ. Role of Orbscan II in screening keratoconus suspects before refractive corneal surgery. *Ophthalmology*. 2002 Sept;109(9):1642–1646.
7. Lim L, Wei RH, Chan WK, and Tan DT. Evaluation of keratoconus in Asians: Role of Orbscan II and Tomey TMS-2 corneal topography. *Am J Ophthalmol*. 2007 Mar;143(3):390–400.
8. Rabinowitz YS. Keratoconus. *Surv Ophthalmol*. 1998;42:297–319.
9. Randleman JB, Russell B, Ward MA, Thompson KP, and Stulting RD. Risk factors and prognosis for corneal ectasia after LASIK. *Ophthalmology*. 2003 Feb;110(2):267–275.
10. Barraquer JI. Keratomileusis for myopia and aphakia. *Ophthalmology*. 1981 Aug;88(8):701–708.
11. Salz JJ and Binder PS. Is there a "magic number" to reduce the risk of ectasia after laser in situ keratomileusis and photorefractive keratectomy? *Am J Ophthalmol*. 2007 Aug;144(2):284–285.
12. Wang JY, Rice DA, and Klyce SD. Analysis of the effects of astigmatism and misalignment on corneal surface reconstruction from photokeratoscopic data. *Refract Corneal Surg*. 1991 Mar–Apr;7(2):129–140.
13. Hubbe RE and Foulks GN. The effect of poor fixation on computer-assisted topographic corneal analysis. Pseudokeratoconus. *Ophthalmology*. 1994 Oct;101(10):1745–1748.
14. Leung DY, Lam DK, Yeung BY, and Lam DS. Comparison between central corneal thickness measurements by ultrasound pachymetry and optical coherence tomography. *Clin Exp Ophthalmol*. 2006 Nov;34(8):751–754.

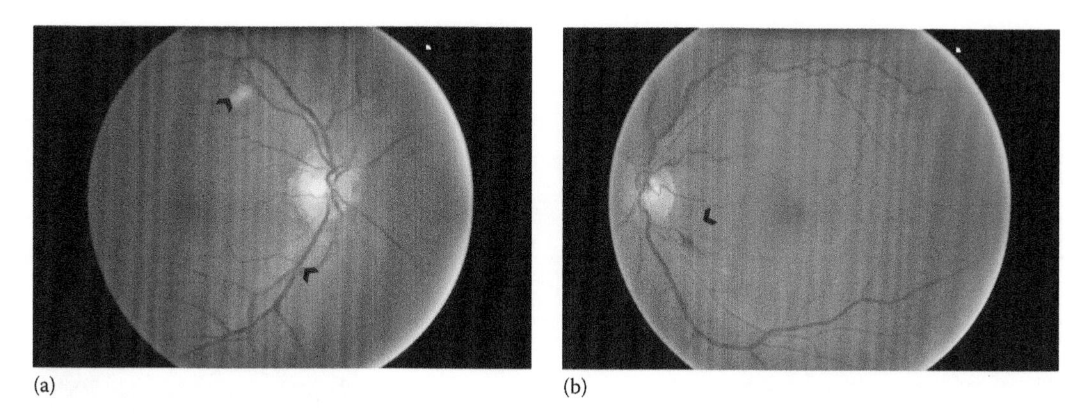

FIGURE 1.1
Retinal photograph showing examples of retinal microvascular signs: (a) including cotton-wool spots (arrow head pointing to a bright spot) and arteriovenous nicking (arrow head pointing to a crossing of arteriole and venule) and (b) hemorrhage (arrow head pointing to a dark spot).

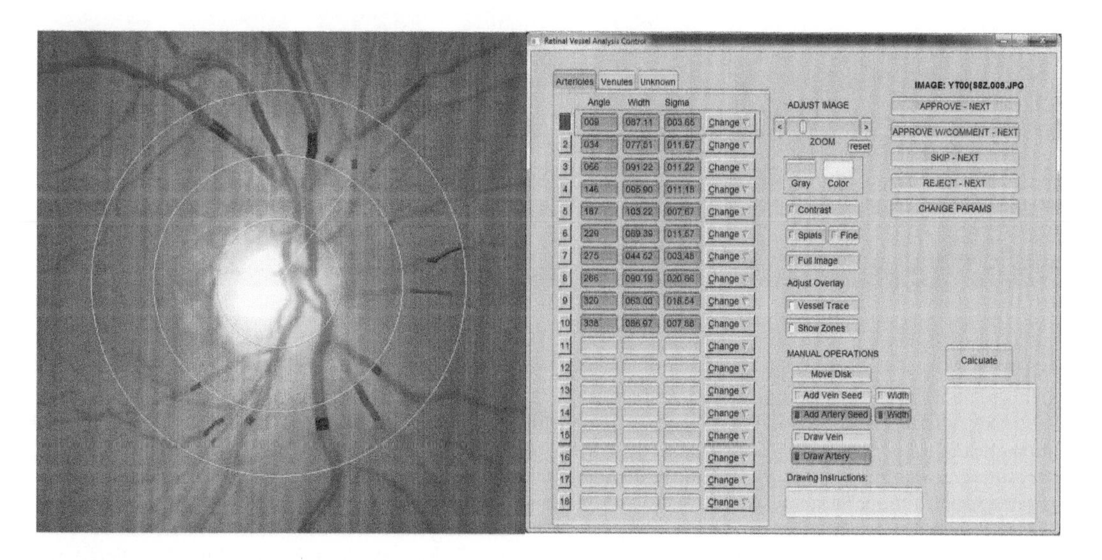

FIGURE 1.2
Retinal fundus photograph assessed quantitatively by the Interactive Vessel Analysis software. The measured area of retinal vascular parameters was standardized as the region from 0.5 to 1.0 disc diameters away from the disc margin. Retinal arteriolar and venular calibers were summarized as CRAE and the CRVE, respectively, from retinal fundus photograph. CRAE and CRVE were defined based on the revised Knudtson–Parr–Hubbard formula.

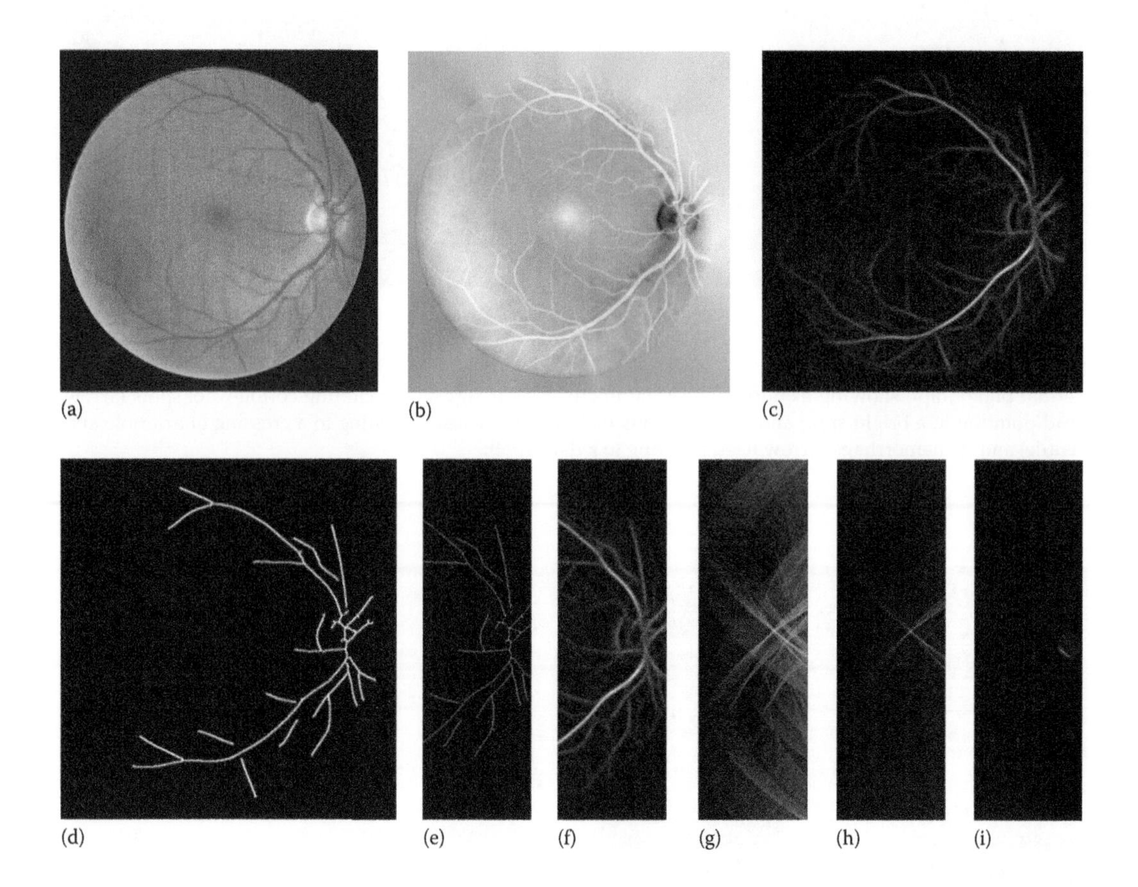

FIGURE 2.4
(a) Image 24 of the DRIVE database (584 × 565 pixels). (b) The inverted and preprocessed grayscale image. (c) The Gabor-magnitude response. (d) The skeletonized and filtered image obtained from the result in (c). (e) The automatically limited skeleton image used in the GHT procedure (584 × 180 pixels). (f) The automatically limited Gabor-magnitude image used to update the Hough space. (g) The Hough space for $a = -64$ using the unity-updated GHT without vertex restriction. (h) The Hough space for $a = -66$ using the Gabor-magnitude-updated GHT without vertex restriction. (i) The Hough space for $a = -75$ using the Gabor-magnitude-updated GHT with vertex restriction. (Reproduced with permission from Oloumi, F., Rangayyan, R.M., and Ells, A.L., Parabolic modeling of the major temporal arcade in retinal fundus images, *IEEE Trans. Instrum. Meas.*, 61(7), 1825–1838, © July 2012 IEEE.)

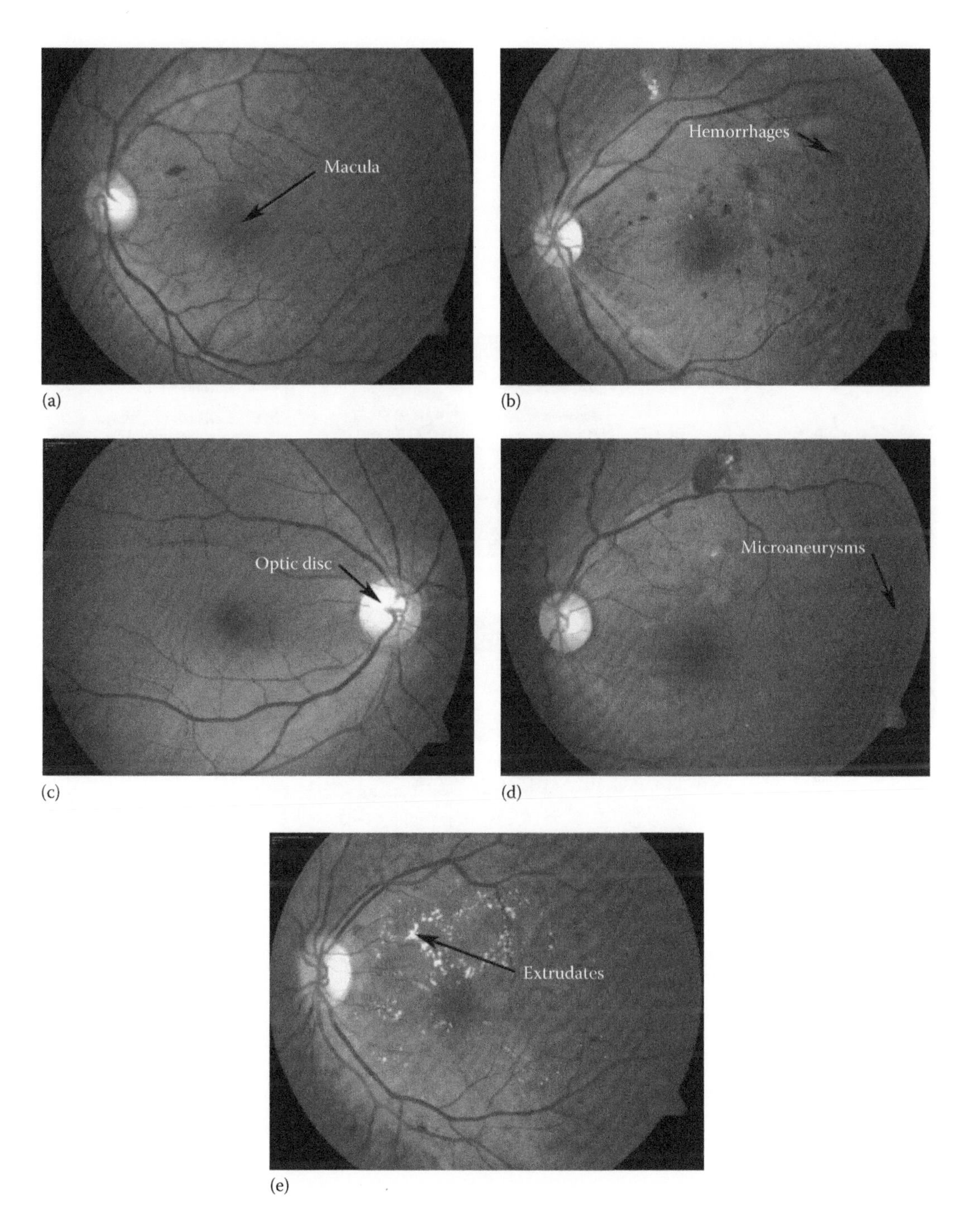

FIGURE 3.2
Sample retinal images of (a) normal, (b) mild NPDR, (c) moderate NPDR, (d) severe NPDR, and (e) PDR.

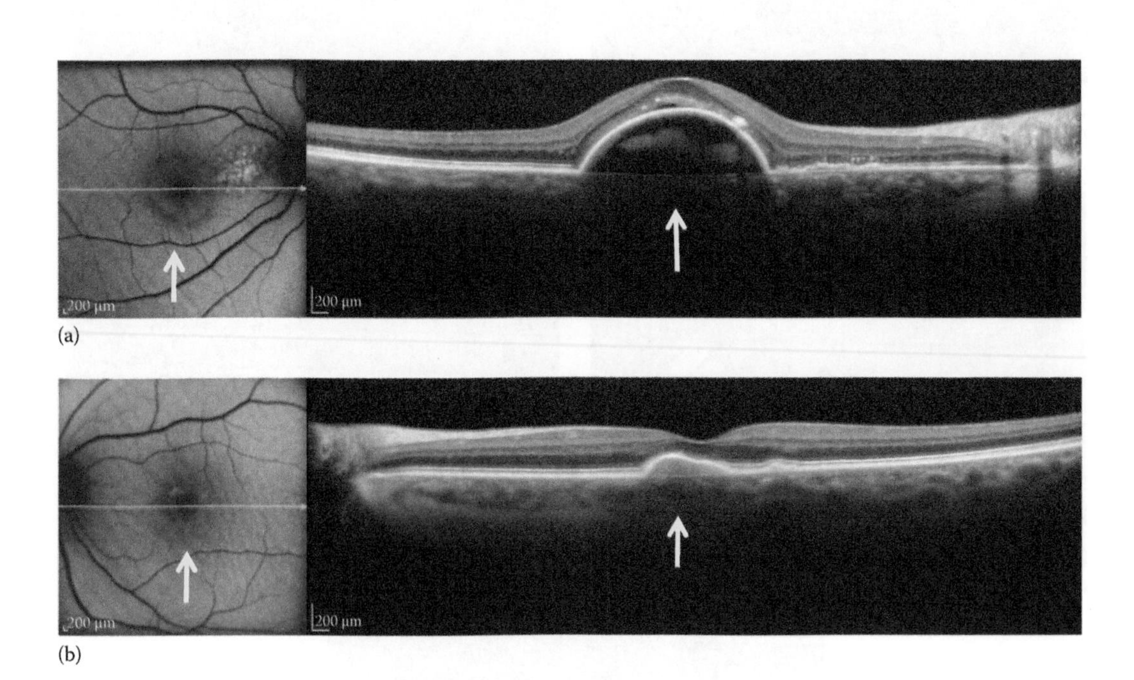

FIGURE 6.5
Neovascular AMD, right eye (a) with more advanced disease compared to left eye (b). Fovea surrounded by a band of hypoautofluorescence corresponding to the site of neovascularization shown by OCT. Both arrows in (a) and (b) are pointing towards the disease process surrounding the fovea.

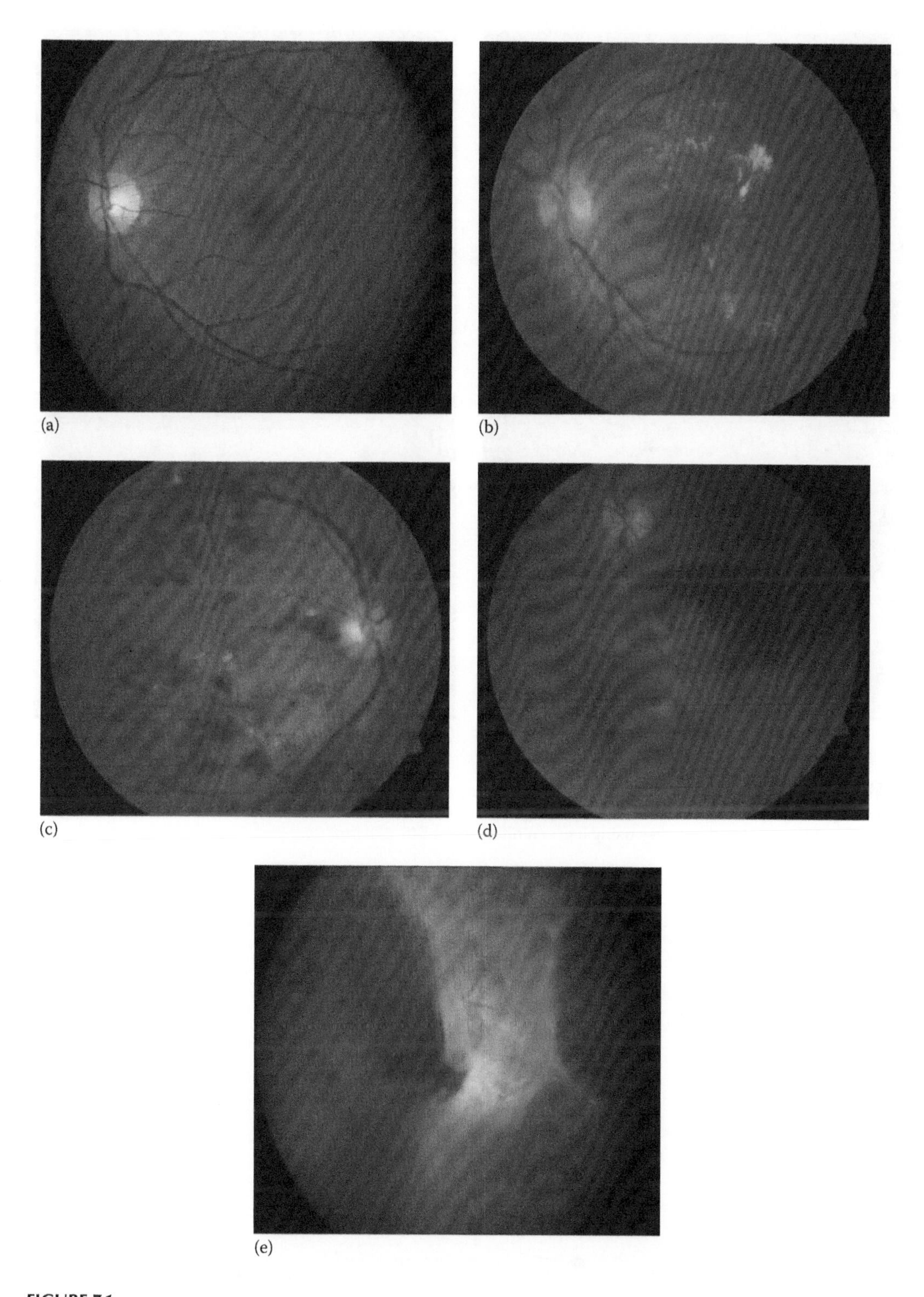

FIGURE 7.1
Different stages of DR: (a) early NPDR, (b) moderate NPDR, (c) severe NPDR, (d) PDR with vitreous and subhyaloid hemorrhage, and (e) PDR with tractional retinal detachment.

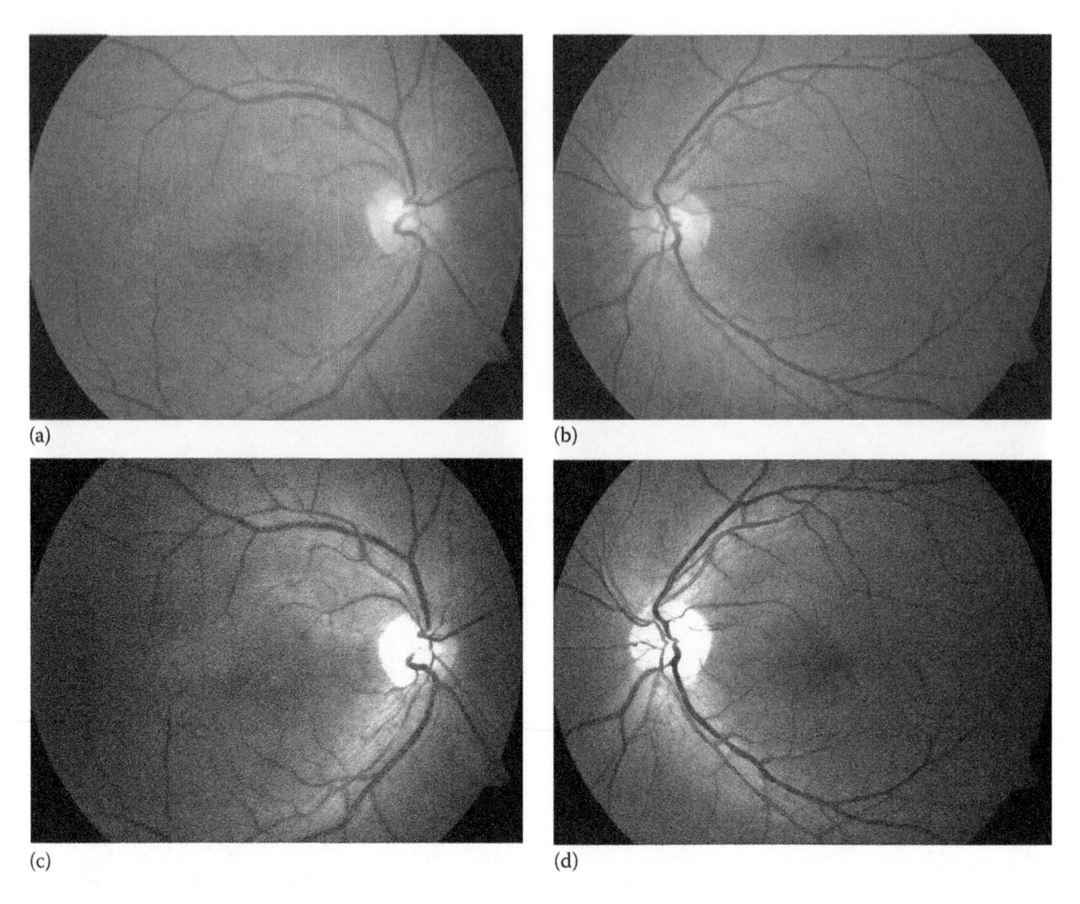

FIGURE 8.2
Fundus photographs. (a, b) Color fundus photographs of the right and left eyes and (c, d) red-free fundus photographs of the right and left eyes using a green filter, about 540–570 nm.

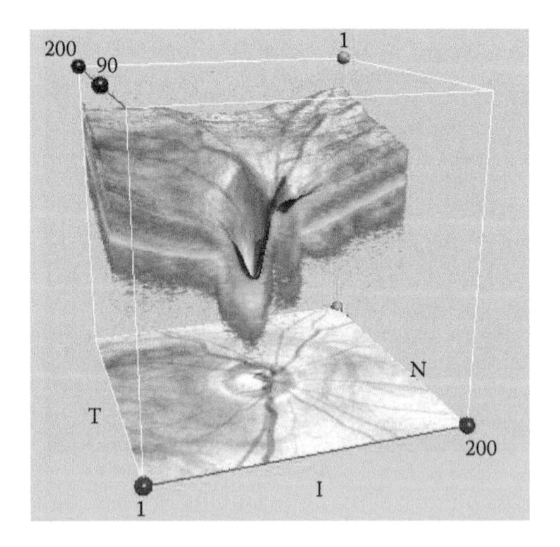

FIGURE 9.9
3D OCT scan of the optic disc.

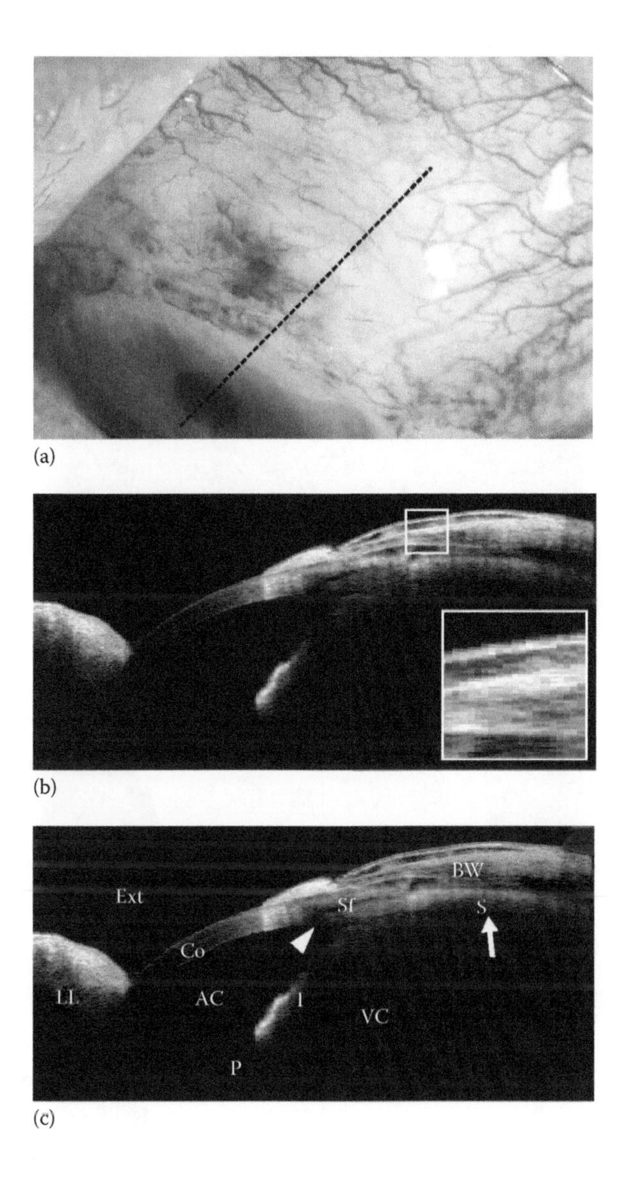

FIGURE 10.1
Imaging and surgical anatomy of the bleb. (a) Photograph of a glaucoma surgery bleb; the dashed line indicates the approximate orientation of the ASOCT line scan shown in (b) and (c). The location of the bleb is indicated by the relatively opaque area of the conjunctiva. Deep features are not easily seen by direct observation. (b) ASOCT line scan shown without labels for clarity. The inset shows portion of the bleb wall to highlight stripes of differing reflectivity due to hydration of episcleral–conjunctival tissue. (c) The same optical section from (b), with labels added. The bleb wall is shaded blue, the scleral flap is shaded purple, and the sclera is shaded green. The arrowhead indicates the internal keratotrabeculectomy ostium. The deep boundary of the sclera (arrow) is indistinct. Ext, exterior of the eye; Co, cornea; AC, anterior chamber; LL, lower lid; P, pupil; I, iris; VC, vitreous cavity; BW, bleb wall; Sf, scleral flap; S, sclera.

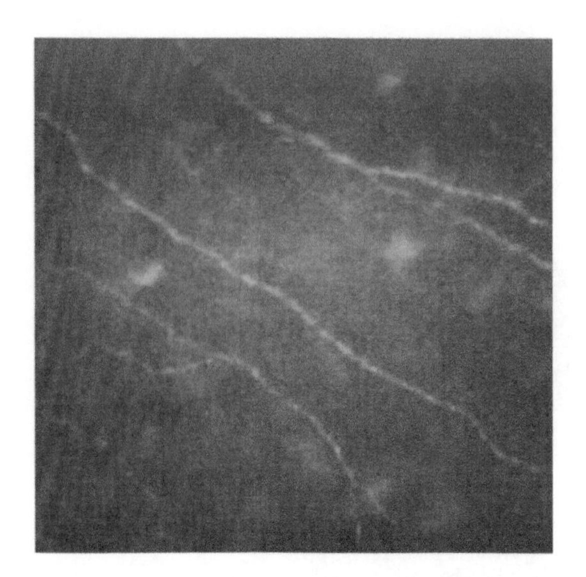

FIGURE 11.4
Subepithelial nerve fibers.

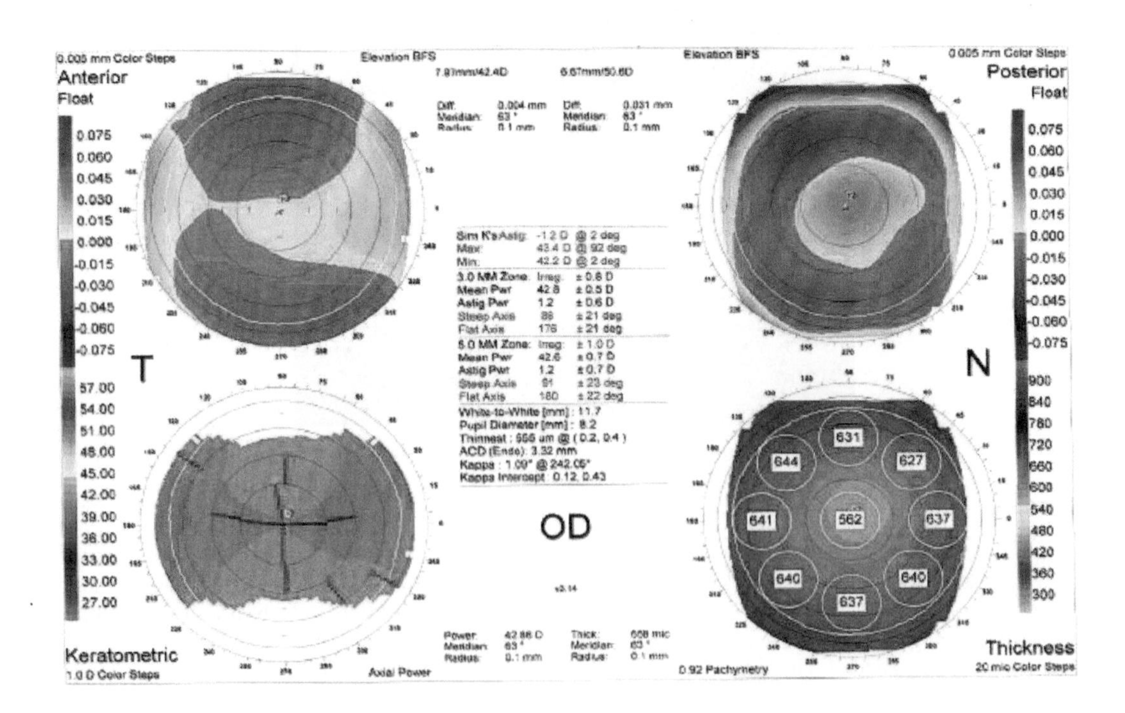

FIGURE 12.1
Typical display of data from information acquired via the Orbscan II. This printout demonstrates the anterior elevation, posterior elevation, and keratometric and pachymetry maps.

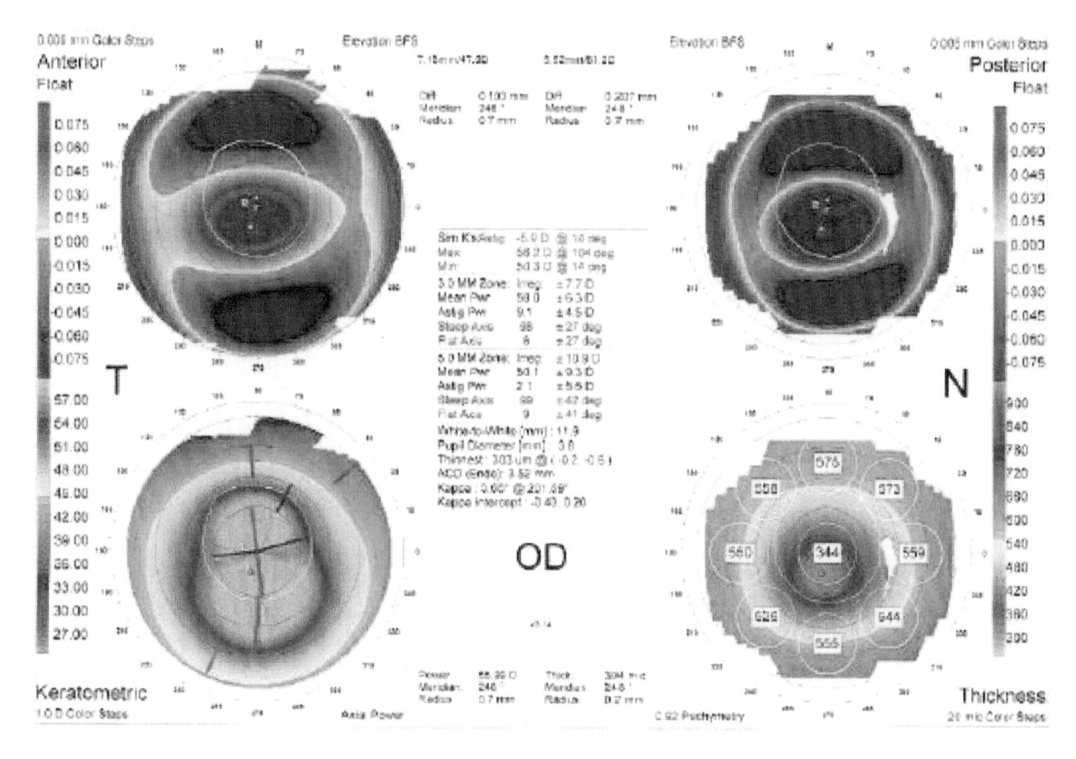

FIGURE 12.2
Orbscan II topography in an eye with keratoconus. Note the irregular astigmatism in the keratometric map. The high Sim K and increased irregularity in the 3 and 5 mm zones.

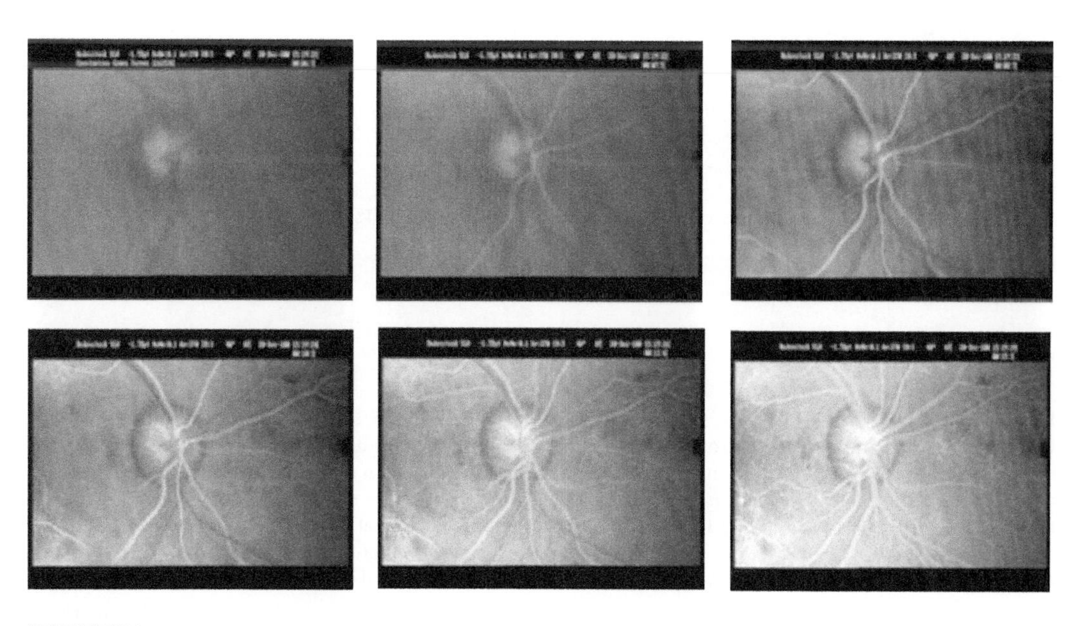

FIGURE 13.1
Frames from an SLO sequence. Note the increase in brightness as the sequence progresses because of the fluorescence dye.

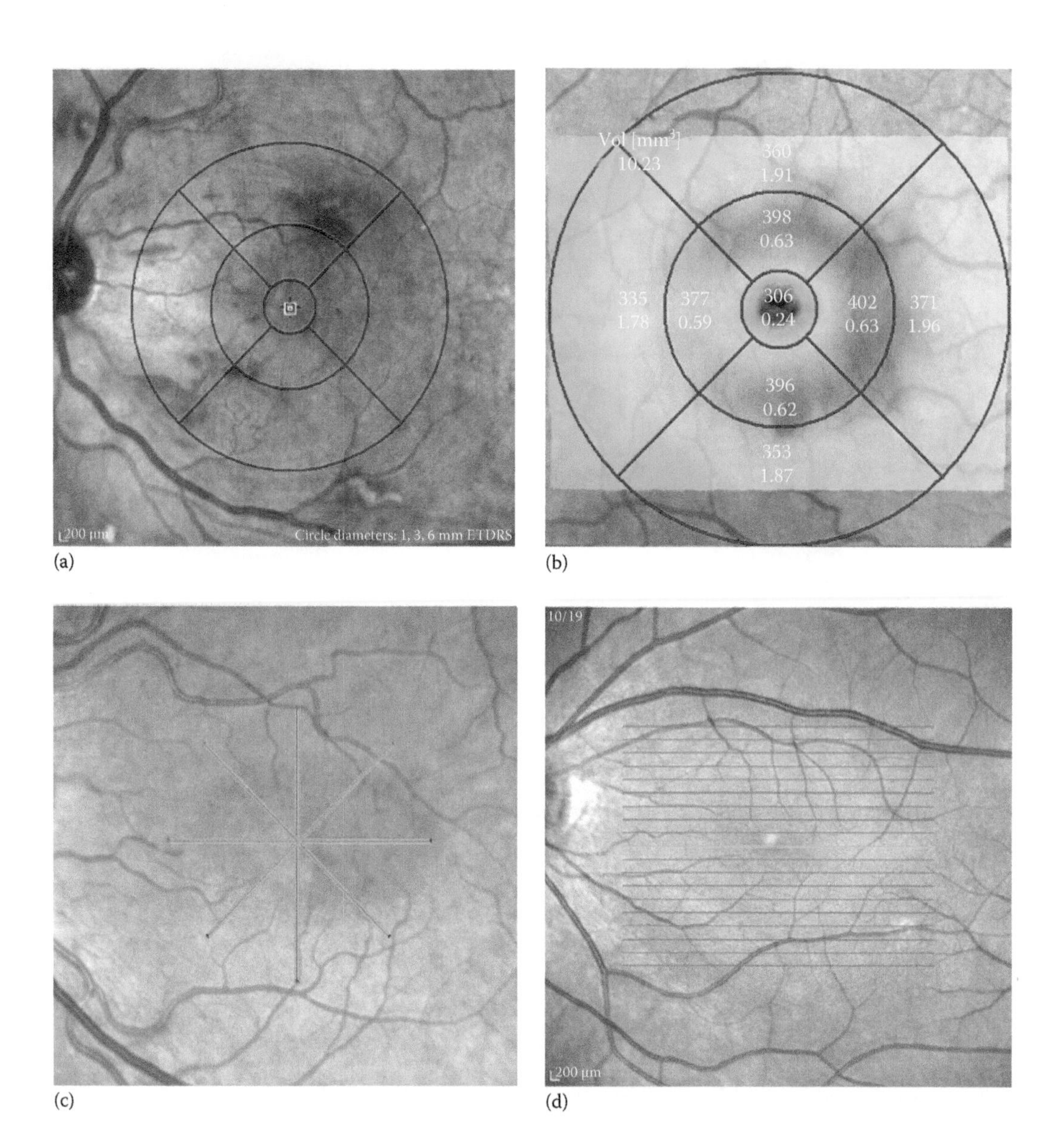

FIGURE 14.15
Quantitative scan patterns to measure macular thickness. The circles of the early treatment diabetic retinopathy study (ETDRS) grid (a) are 1, 3, and 6 mm in diameter. Thickness map within the central 6 mm of the retina is calculated from the absolute values measured and is presented in a false color scale (b). To calculate the thickness map, TD-OCT uses a scan pattern made of six radial scan lines intersecting at the center of the fovea (c). The average thickness of the areas in between is interpolated from the measurements of the six lines. SD-OCT devices adopted different approach with a scan pattern made of series of horizontal or vertical raster line scans (d).

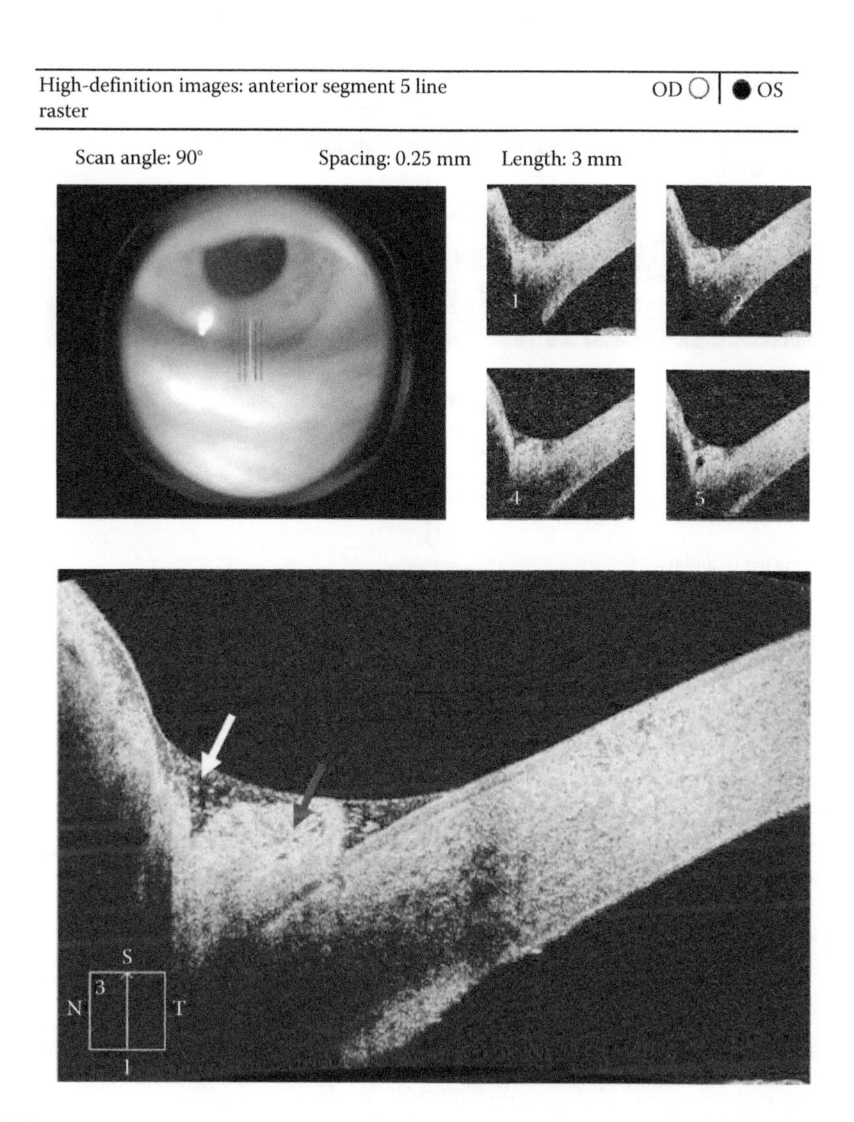

FIGURE 15.15
Conjunctivochalasis taken by a Cirrus OCT. A high-definition colored scan taken by a Cirrus OCT shows the cross-sectional view of the conjunctivochalasis (red arrow) surrounded by the tear meniscus (white arrow). The tear meniscus height and volume appear to be greater than they are with the conjunctivochalasis. Surrounding are the lower lid (to the left) and the cornea (to the right).

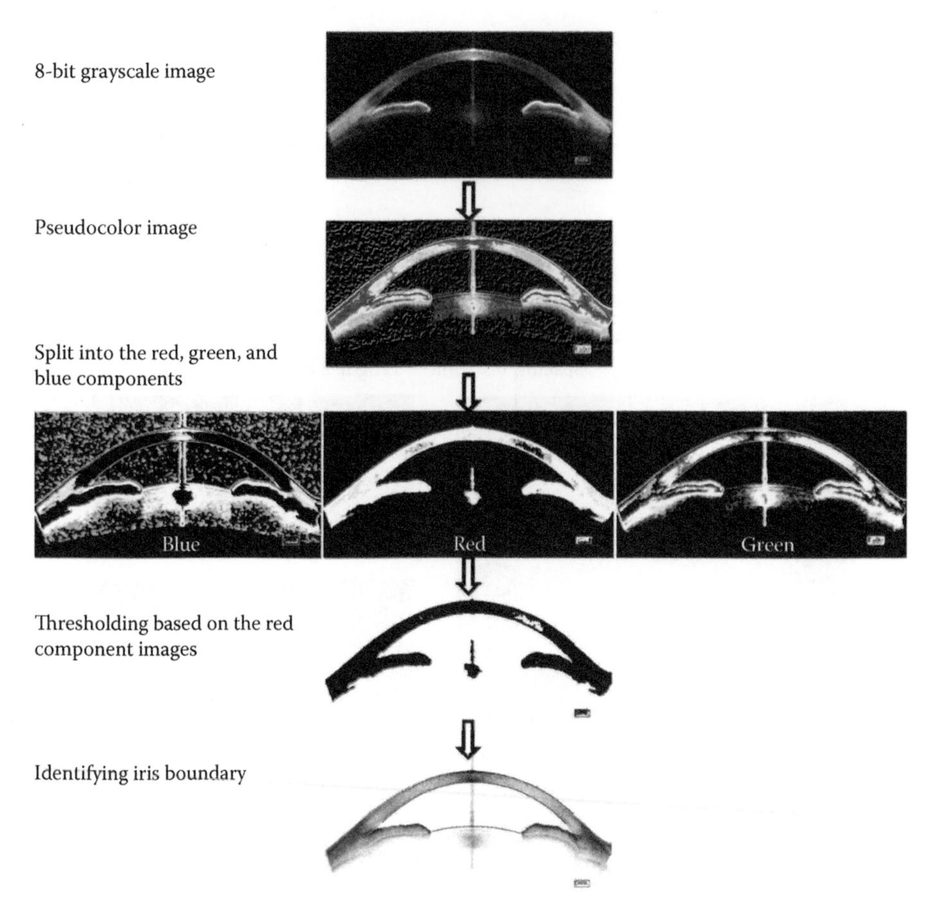

FIGURE 16.9
Flowchart of the segmentation algorithm for identifying the iris boundary.

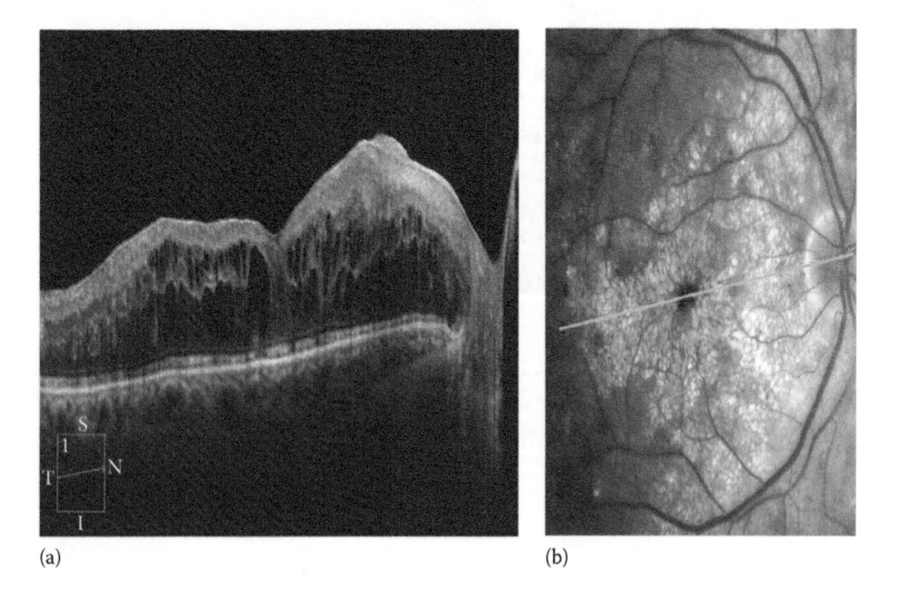

FIGURE 17.4
(a) Cystoid macular edema (CME) on a OCT image. (b) Fluorescein angiography, where petaloid placement of the cysts is appreciable, as well as other vascular disorders that provide information for more accurate diagnosis.

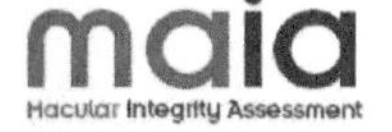

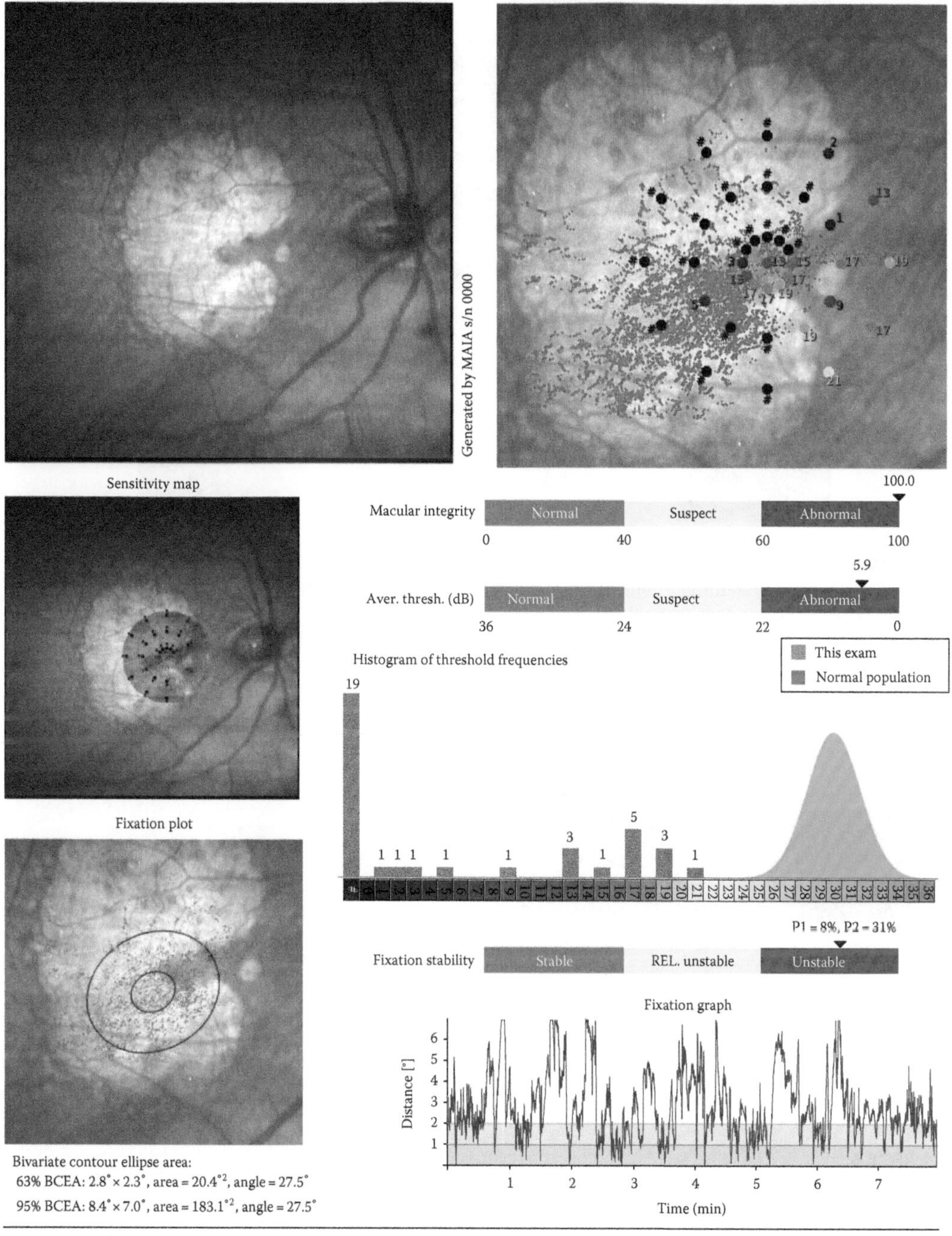

FIGURE 18.7
MAIA perimetry report. (Courtesy of Marco Morales, CenterVue Inc., Padova, Italy, 2013.)

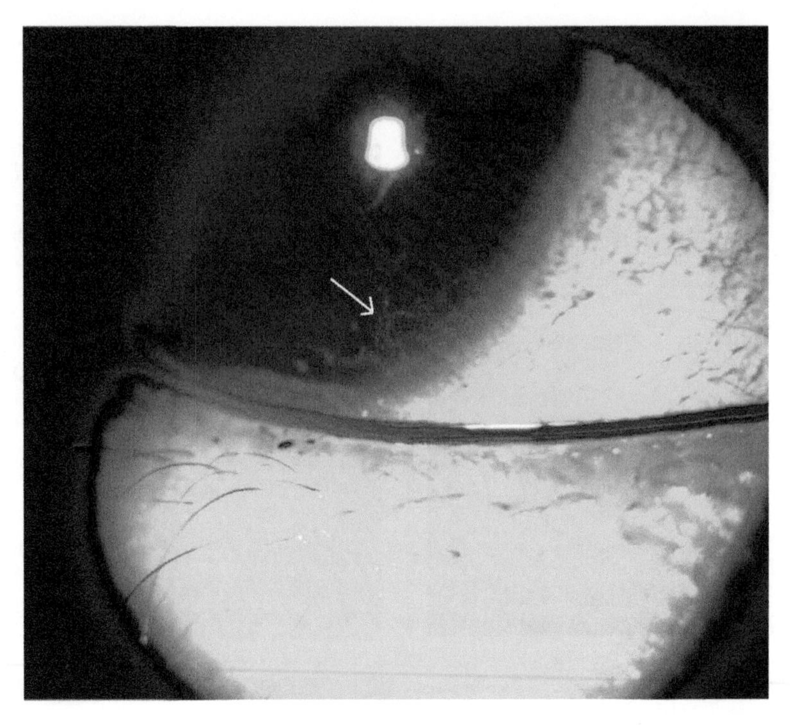

FIGURE 19.16
Corneal fluorescein dye staining. A slit-lamp photo of corneal fluorescein dye staining that would show up as flourescent green in the cornea (arrow).

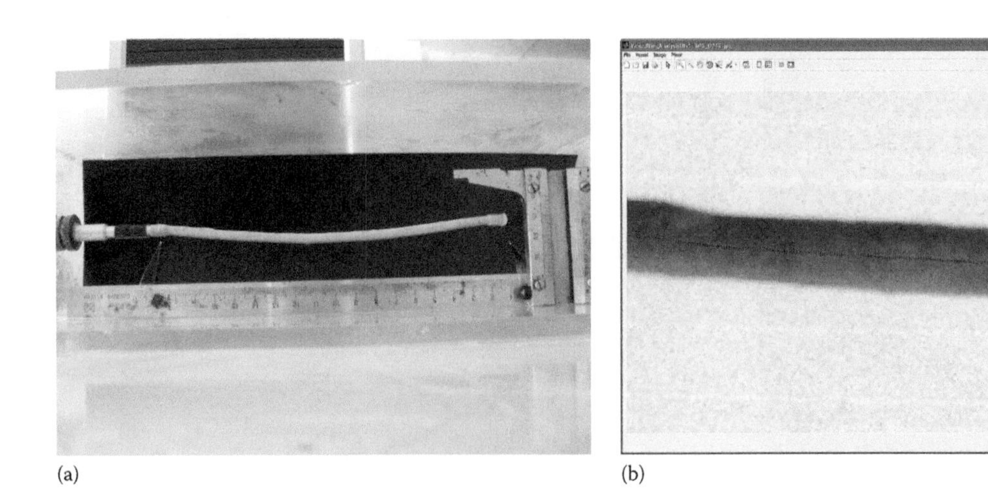

FIGURE 20.6
A sample picture of the latex tube (a) and finding the limits of the tube (b). (From Patašius, M. et al., Preliminary validation of FEM based blood vessel model, *Biomedicininė inžinerija = Biomedical engineering: tarptautinės konferencijos pranešimų medžiaga, 2008 m. spalio 23–24 d, Kaunas/Kauno technologijos universitetas*, Technologija, Kaunas, Lithuania, 2008, pp. 70–73.)

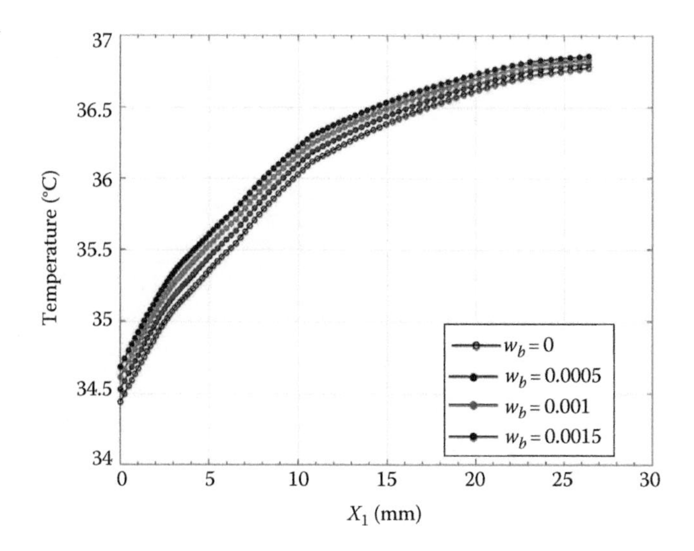

FIGURE 21.7
Temperature distribution along the papillary axis of eyeball for various blood perfusion rates.

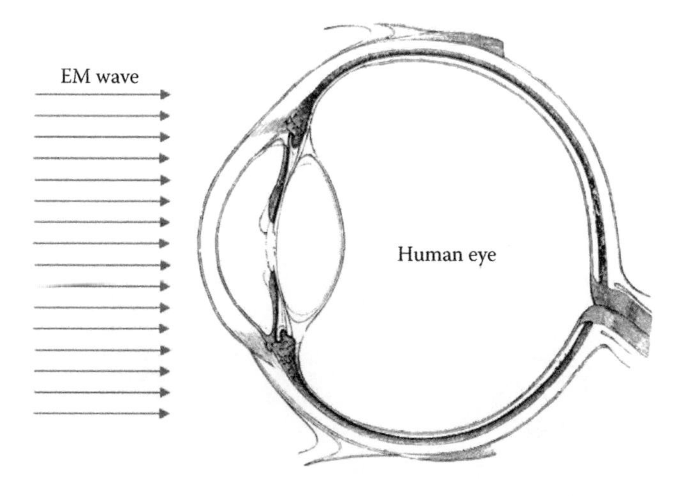

FIGURE 22.1
EM fields from an EM radiation device.

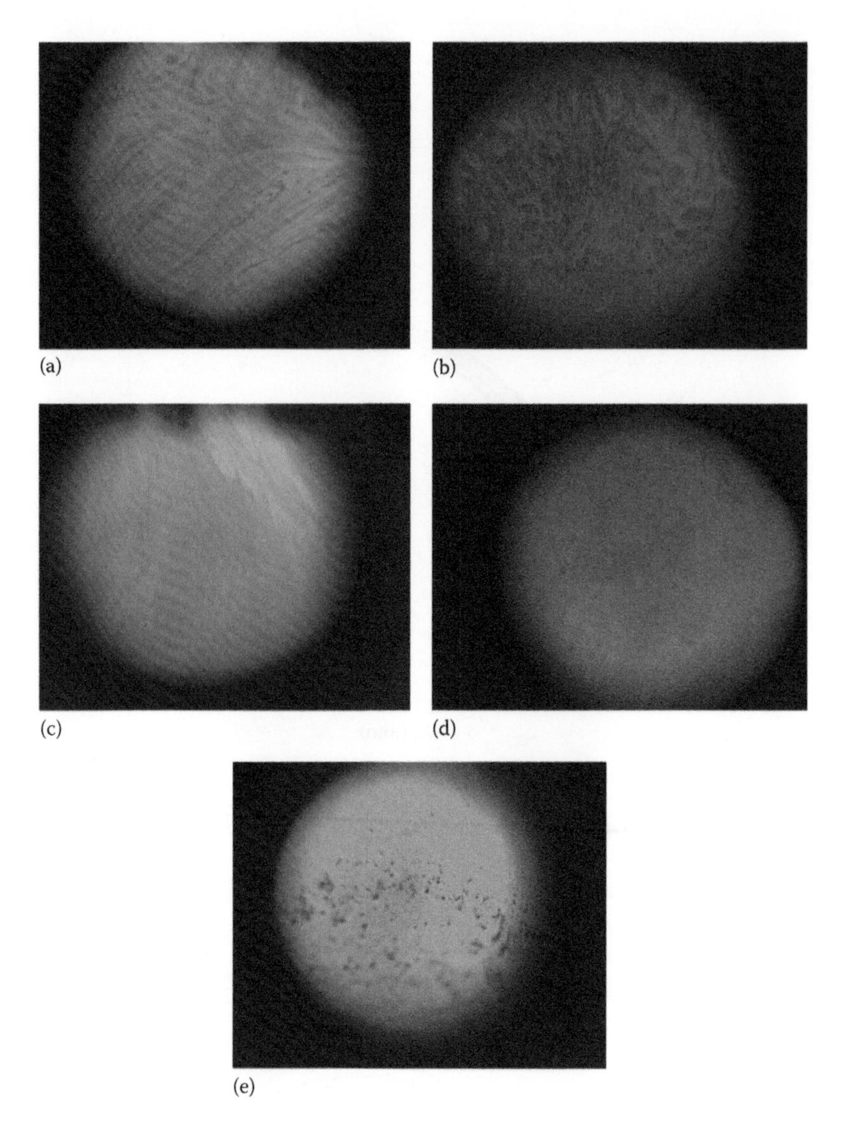

FIGURE 23.8
Lipid layer interference patterns observed with the Doane's interferometer. (a) Strong fringes, (b) coalescing strong fringes, (c) fine fringes, (d) coalescing fine fringes, and (e) debris.

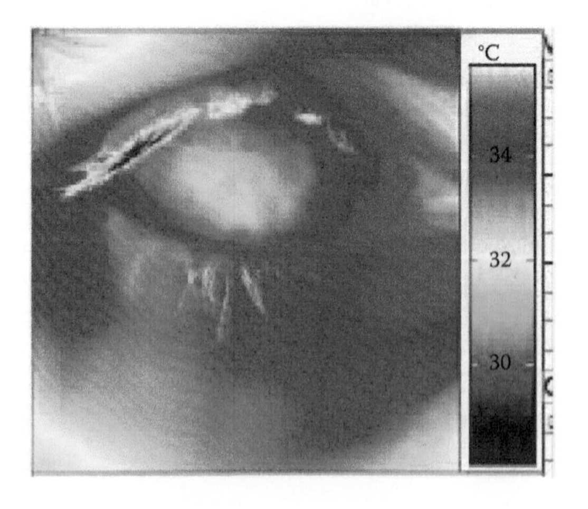

FIGURE 24.2
A normal ocular thermogram in color-coded display.

13

Automatic Analysis of Scanning Laser Ophthalmoscope Sequences for Arteriovenous Passage Time Measurement

C. Marino, Marcos Ortega, J. Novo, Beatriz Remeseiro, Alba Fernandez, and F. Gomez-Ulla

CONTENTS

Retinal microcirculation can vary with associated retinopathies. One of the most widely used techniques for analyzing these variations is fluorescein angiography. Scanning laser ophthalmoscope (SLO) sequences are obtained from a patient who was injected with a fluorescent dye. These SLO techniques are useful for measuring biomedical metrics such as the arteriovenous (AV) passage time. As the acquisition of the whole sequence takes a lot of time, the patient's eye will move during the process; hence an alignment procedure must take place afterward. This work discusses an automatic methodology for the alignment of large SLO sequences for AV passage time measurement. This methodology is a combination of two different approaches for registration: mutual information (MI) and landmark. The first one will be used for registration in dark frames where the dye is not yet present in the vessels. This is so because of its ability to work without any prior processing or structure segmentation. The second one will use the vessels as landmarks for registration. Although the methodology considers rigid transforms only, it has been proven to work well in the presence of alterations in the perspective of the eye. The results obtained in the experiments were validated by expert ophthalmologists.

13.1 Introduction

Diabetic retinopathy could lead to partial or total loss of vision. It is one of the most prominent causes in active population [1]. Among the population in Spain, diabetes has a prevalence of 4% [2]. Diabetes can be classified as two types: type I (insulin dependent) and type II (non-insulin dependent). In Spain, 98% of type I patients and 78% of type II are affected by retinopathy during the initial 15 years after diabetes is diagnosed. During the initial 20 years, more than 10% will suffer blindness. When the retinopathy is present, retinal microcirculation may present some abnormal deviations even before the neovascularization. Therefore, measurement of these deviations is crucial to prevent further development of the disease.

The aforementioned deviations cannot be correctly visualized by means of traditional retinography; thus, an alternative technique such as the fluorescein angiography must be used. In videos acquired using this technique, sodium fluorescein is injected intravenously before the sequence acquisition. As the blood stream transports the dye, vasculature and possible leakage into the tissue around it can be clearly visualized.

SLO is an imaging acquisition technique suitable for the study and quantitative evaluation of circulation in the retina. For the study setup presented here, the ophthalmoscope projects a laser beam (helium neon, HeNe 632.8 nm) and an infrared diode laser, 780 nm both simultaneously on the eye fundus with a 33 × 21 degree image size. The helium neon laser is modulated by means of an acoustic optic modulator. The retinal image is obtained by illuminating a group of almost confocal apertures by the infrared light.

SLO presents advantages over traditional fundus photography [3,4]. First, the speed of acquisition is higher in SLO with rates of up to 25 Hz. In addition, the light intensity needed for correct illumination of the retina using SLO is much lower than when using traditional cameras with consequent increase in patient comfort and risk prevention for retinal damages. The illumination is also more homogeneous in the SLO mainly because of the narrowness of the laser beam width and the optical geometry. However, as the acquisition process takes some time and because of exposure to the laser, the patient will tend to move the eye during the process, making typically fast movements with a maximum rotation rate of around 600°/s [5]. As a result of these movements, the consecutive frames of the sequence will not be aligned and will need a registration before any quantitative assessment of the retinal microcirculation can be done.

Image registration is an extensively discussed field in image processing literature [6,7]. Nevertheless, registration of large video sequences entails additional difficulties such as the large distortions between consecutive frames because of rapid eye movements, and there is a need for a more efficient approach to process the whole sequence and for the appropriate selection of reference pictures from among the video frames. This last issue must be taken into account to adjust the varying contrast of the frames, which go from darker to brighter and darker again, along the sequence as the dye passes through the vessels.

Among the different registration approaches, we can distinguish two big classes: intensity- and feature-based registration. In the feature-based registration method, some reference structures or landmarks are obtained from the images, then the geometric transform that more precisely matches landmarks from both images is calculated. In general, feature extraction must be very precise to get good results. In retinal images, extraction of landmarks (such as vessels or optic disc) may be too computation heavy as in [8] to be used for registration of a whole SLO sequence close to real-time.

In the group of techniques based on intensity, the need for precision is avoided as the whole image is transformed and compared to the referenced one on the basis of some similarity measurement. Wade and Fitzke [9] presented a fast methodology using a variation of normalized cross correlation by adding a hierarchical search approach to reduce computation time. The drawback in this was that their method only considered translations as a possible distortion from the reference image, ignoring rotations. Noack and Sutton [10] introduced a method focused on SLO registration that again ignored rotations. Xu et al. [11] presented a method for tracking the motion in the retina by analyzing intensity on SLO video sequences.

SLO sequences we worked with showed large intensity changes with some features that were visible or indistinguishable depending on the particular frame we were analyzing as the presence of the dye is not constant along the sequence (see Figure 13.1, where some frames of a standard sequence are depicted). For those frames where relevant features (vessels) are distinguishable, a landmark-based registration method can be used as in [8,12,13]. However, for those frames belonging to sections of the sequence where the dye has not yet arrived or has already been dissolved, an intensity-based method must be used. In our case, we used an alignment process based on MI [14–18]. So the methodology presented here combines both the approaches of registration by automatically selecting the most appropriate based on frame properties.

The goal of this work is to apply and validate the registration approach by automatically estimating dye-dilution curves and computing AV passage time in fundus images. This chapter consists of the following: Section 13.2 where the methodology for registration of the sequences is presented. This section is divided into Section 13.2.1, where registration based on creaseness (feature) is introduced; Section 13.2.2 where the registration using MI is described; and Section 13.2.3 where a combination of both methods is proposed. Afterward, in Section 13.3, experiments performed and the results obtained are presented, whereas in Section 13.4, some conclusions are discussed.

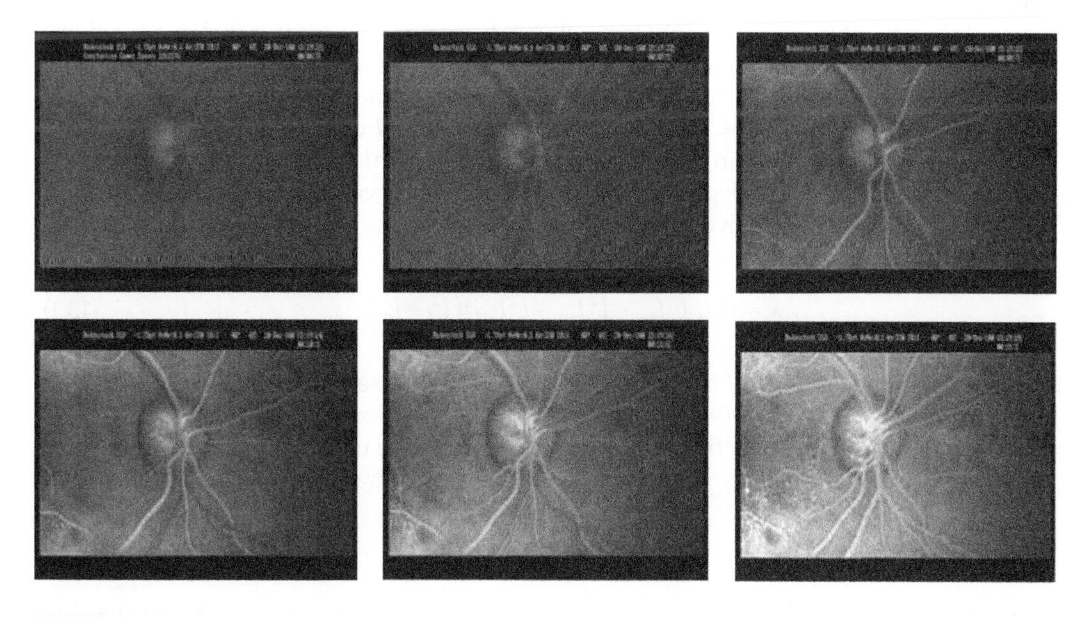

FIGURE 13.1
(See color insert.) Frames from an SLO sequence. Note the increase in brightness as the sequence progresses because of the fluorescence dye.

13.2 SLO Image Alignment

The classical approach clinicians used to analyze SLO sequences is based on manual alignment of the frames from the sequence. A point is selected and marked in all the frames in order to compute the evolution of its intensity along the sequence depicting a curve, usually known as a dye-dilution curve.

Our method consists in aligning frames by means of two different methods: First, a fast method based on crease alignment is used; if it performs adequately in a particular frame, it is considered as already registered. As there are frames where most vessel segments cannot be properly distinguished, an MI-based approach is used, as it does not require any landmark in the image. This allows all frames along the sequence to be registered.

13.2.1 Crease-Based Registration

This method, like most feature-based approaches, is similar to the way humans perform the image matching task, that is, finding common structures in both frames. In this case, the structures are the vessels in the retina so we propose the use of the vessel tree as the landmark for alignment. To avoid difficulties derived from the quality of the acquisition, we do not propose to rely, in this particular case, on the bifurcation points only, as the loss of a substantial amount of them could lead to misregistrations. Instead, the use of the whole vessel tree could help to improve the quality of registration although it will increase computation time.

The methodology consists of two stages: first, extraction of the vessels and, second, alignment of these vessels. As accurate vessel segmentation is not needed and some precision errors could appear derived from it, we propose the use of the centerlines estimation of the vessels for their alignment. This ensures the stability of the structure along frames, which is crucial to satisfactorily identify common structures between images. For this computation, we take advantage of the fact that vessels can be considered creases (valleys or ridges) if the image is thought of as a landscape where the height of each point comes from its own intensity. By means of level-set extrinsic curvature (LSEC), image creases can be extracted.

Given a function L, $\mathbb{R}^d \rightarrow \mathbb{R}$, the level set for a constant l consists of the set of points $\{x \mid L(x) = l\}$. For 2D images, L can be considered as a topographic relief or landscape and the level sets as its level curves. Negative minima of the level curve, curvature κ, level by level, form valley curves, and positive maxima form ridge curves:

$$\kappa = \left(2L_xL_yL_{xy} - L_y^2L_{xx} - L_x^2L_{yy}\right)\left(L_x^2 + L_y^2\right)^{-\frac{3}{2}}. \tag{13.1}$$

Typical discretization of LSEC is not well defined in some cases, giving rise to unexpected discontinuities at the center of elongated objects. As a result of this, the MLSEC-ST operator [19] for 3D landmark extraction of CT and MRI volumes is used. This alternative definition is based on the divergence (div) of the normalized vector field $\bar{\mathbf{w}}$:

$$\kappa = -\text{div}\left(\bar{\mathbf{w}}\right). \tag{13.2}$$

Although Equations 13.1 and 13.2 are equivalent in the continuous domain, in the discrete domain, when the derivatives are approximated by finite centered differences of the Gaussian-smoothed image, Equation 13.2 provides much better results. The creaseness measure κ is improved by prefiltering the image gradient vector field using a Gaussian function.

When crease lines are obtained for both images, their alignment takes place. The most straightforward approach is to iteratively optimize the transformation parameters to one image compared to the reference image. Correlation computation gives a valid measure of the similarity of the reference image compared to the transformed one:

$$\text{Corr}_{\mathcal{T}} = \sum_{x \in f} f(x) \cdot g(\mathcal{T}(x))$$

where
f and g are the creaseness images
$\mathcal{T}$ represents the transformation whose parameters we are testing

As most pixels are irrelevant as background pixels in the image, an important optimization in this process, is to avoid applying the transformation to pixels with an intensity below a given threshold. This step reduces computation time to 5% of the time originally employed.

The function $\text{Corr}_{\mathcal{T}}$ along with the transformation parameters (x and y translation and rotation and x and y scale) defines a search space difficult to optimize for several reasons: First, the function is nonmonotonic, that is, it possesses many local maxima. Second, the similarity metric $\text{Corr}_{\mathcal{T}}$ is not efficient to calculate as it requires the transformation of a whole 2D large image. Finally, parameters for translation and rotation cannot be separated in different searches to decrease dimensionality of the search space.

To avoid the first two issues, we propose an approach to explore the search space at multiple resolutions. This is performed by having two pyramids [20], where crease images are at the bottom and each upper level is a version of the previous one at a reduced resolution (typically halved). This is built up to a level where images have a minimum resolution. In our case, our final image size is 64 × 64.

The process of parameter searching starts at the top level of the pyramid (minimum size) where a complete exploration of the images is possible given their reduced size. As the best result in a given level cannot lead to the best final result because of false maxima, we carry many of the best results at one level to the lower one. In each step, we reduce by half the number of seeds carried to the next level until in the final one, we only have one, which is considered our optimal solution.

In each level, the correlation function needs to be computed as seen earlier. As this is the most expensive computation for this approach, we propose the use of downhill simplex iterative method [21]. As the seeds enter a new level from the previous one, the search in that particular level stops when the difference between the maximum and minimum values is below a given threshold in that zone. This threshold and the seed number of first level determine the performance in terms of precision and computation time.

Figure 13.2 shows the three sections the sequences are divided into. Frames in the middle of each section are selected as reference frames, since a representative frame must be selected for each section to get a good registration of floating frames.

Figure 13.3 shows frame samples for existing sections in the video sequence. In section 1, the level of fluorescein is not high enough, and so there is not enough feature information that can be used to align the frames in this section. For this reason, we consider an intensity-based registration method more suitable for section 1, which is presented next.

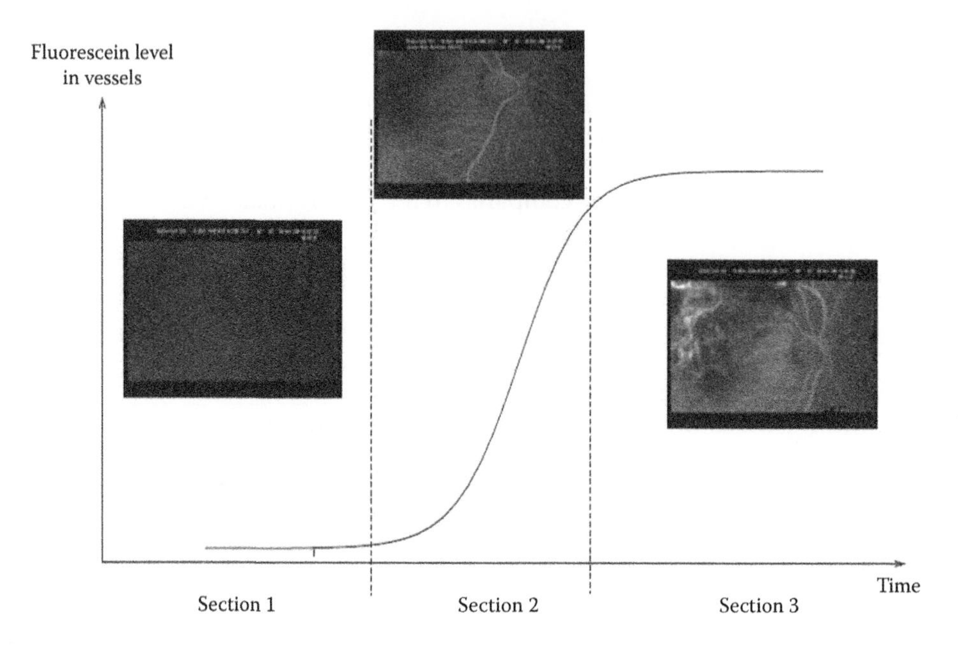

FIGURE 13.2
SLO sequences are separated into three sections, characterized by the fluorescein level in the vessels.

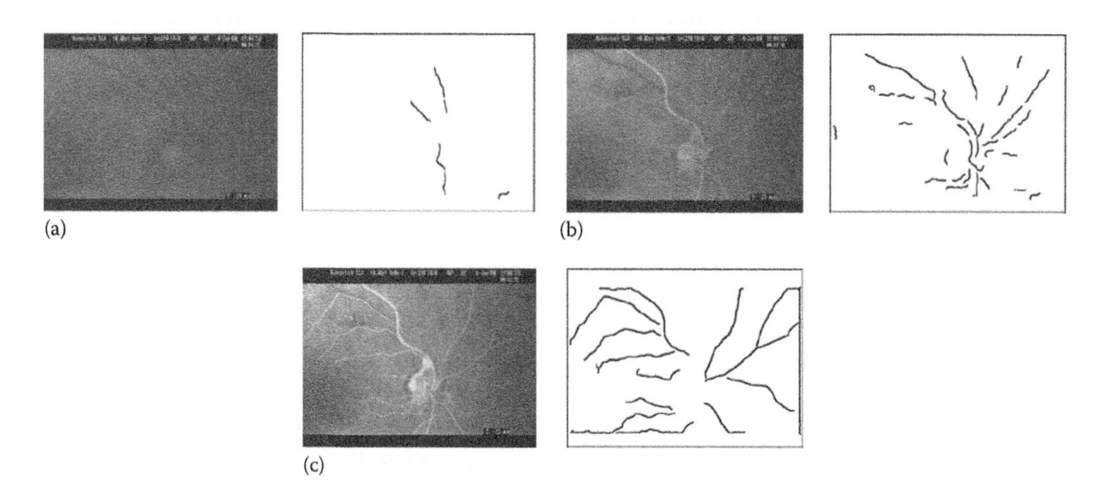

FIGURE 13.3
Examples of representative frames for each section in Figure 13.2 (left) and creases extracted from them (right): (a) frame #30 of 1459 is representative of section 1, (b) frame #640 of 1459 is representative of section 2, and (c) frame #989 of 1459 is representative of section 3. Here, we can see how creaseness measurement is available for sections 2 and 3, but not necessarily for the first section.

13.2.2 MI-Based Registration Method

The MI is a classical concept from information theory. MI measures the amount of information that one variable contains about the other or the reduction in the uncertainty of one variable owing to the knowledge of the other [22].

Given two random variables A and B with a joint probability $p(A,B)$ and marginal probabilities $p(A)$ and $p(B)$, the mutual information $\mathrm{MI}(A,B)$ is the relative entropy between the joint distribution and the product distribution $p(A)p(B)$:

$$\mathrm{MI}(A,B)=\sum_{a\in A}\sum_{b\in B}p(A,B)\log\frac{p(a,b)}{p(a)p(b)}. \tag{13.3}$$

MI can be obtained by calculating the entropy:

$$\mathrm{MI}(A,B)=H(A)+H(B)-H(A,B) \tag{13.4}$$

with $H(A),H(B)$ being, respectively, the entropy of A and B and $H(A,B)$ their joint entropy.

Several methods to compute the probabilities have been proposed. Wells et al. [18] proposed the use of the Parzen window, which is a method for nonparametric estimation of the density, generally defined as

$$P^*(x,a)=\frac{1}{N_a}\sum_{x_a\in a}R(x-x_a) \tag{13.5}$$

where
- a is a sample
- R is a valid density function

There is one Gaussian centered at each sample for smoothing. When applied to SLO sequences, this method proved to be computationally inefficient as it needed a large number of samples for a reasonably good estimation of the density. Maes et al. [14] propose an estimation of probabilities by means of the distribution of gray-level pixel pairs and pixel values across the common region for both images:

$$p(a)=\frac{h(a)}{N},\quad p(b)=\frac{h(b)}{N},\quad p(a,b)=\frac{h(a,b)}{N} \tag{13.6}$$

where
- $h(\,)$ is the value of the histogram ($h(a,b)$ is the joint histogram)
- N is the size of the common region in the sample space

After the MI is computed, parameters of the transformation maximizing MI are calculated by a simulated annealing minimization (minimizing $-\mathrm{MI}(A,B)$ is equivalent to maximizing $\mathrm{MI}(A,B)$), implemented as a variation of the downhill simplex method [21]. The objective function is the MI, the system state is the applied transformation that derived the value of the MI, and the control parameter T, which logically represents the temperature of the system, is progressively decreased from 0.001.

At this point, the only transformations that are searched are the rigid ones as the scaling term would greatly increase computation time, whereas the results obtained without it are precise enough as the results section will show.

Regardless of the optimization we propose, this method is still more time demanding than the crease-based approach; the computation time is approximately doubled. Because of this, this approach will be only used in frames where the other one fails. Keeping this in mind, the next section discusses how these methods are combined in our proposal.

13.2.3 Combination of Crease- and MI-Based Registration

As the need for two different alignment methodologies has been settled in the previous sections, we describe here how these can be combined to perform a whole alignment of the sequence.

As a first stage of the registration process, an expert selects two frames of the sequence (F_1 and F_2 in Figure 13.4a). These frames will act as reference frames in the sequence. The first frame will be a reference for those frames that belong to the initial part of the sequence (corresponding to lower levels of fluorescein). The second frame will be the reference for those frames with a higher level of fluorescein, corresponding to brightest section in the video sequence. This selection of multiple reference frames is because the variation in brightness along the sequence is very high, making it impossible to get a unique representative frame valid for each frame in the sequence.

Once the reference frames have been selected, the alignment process starts. Interval of frames starting with the first frame until the frame number $(F_2 - F_1)/2$ are aligned using F_1 as a reference, whereas the rest of frames are aligned using frame F_2 as the reference frame.

Because of the differences between F_1 and F_2, it is required to adjust the transforms calculated for the frames located between them, as in Figure 13.4b where the gray-level evolution in a selected pixel is shown. In Figure 13.4c, the final result after adjusting those values can be seen.

Let I_1, F_1, I_2, F_2 be four points requiring alignment, using F_1 as a reference for I_1 and F_2 as a reference for I_2. Let T be the transformation that aligns F_2 with F_1, defined by the transformation matrix M_t. By the affine transformation composition properties [23], the transformation that aligns I_2 with F_1, let it be T_f, will be

$$T\left(T_2\left(I_2\right)\right) = \left(TT_2\right)\left(I_2\right) = T_f\left(I_2\right) \tag{13.7}$$

where the matrix transformation of T_f will be

$$M_f = M_2 M_t. \tag{13.8}$$

The final transformation matrix, resulting from the composition of T_2 and T, will be obtained by multiplying transformation matrices M_2 and M_t.

In our particular domain, by aligning F_i against its representative frame, we can calculate the associated transformation. This transformation has a homogeneous coordinate matrix T_i. In this case, the readjustment is a registration between both reference frames, thus allowing the combination of the obtained transformation matrix T_t with T_i for each frame i between both reference frames. This combination helps in the correction of the misregistration that causes the gap in Figure 13.4b:

$$T_i^* = T_i \circ T_t, \quad F_1 < F_i < F_2. \tag{13.9}$$

By superimposing frames of the sequence, it is possible to visually explore and evaluate the alignment procedure. In Figure 13.5, a sample of such visualizations is shown. To build images of that kind, we need to intersect a 3D cube, defined by the composition of

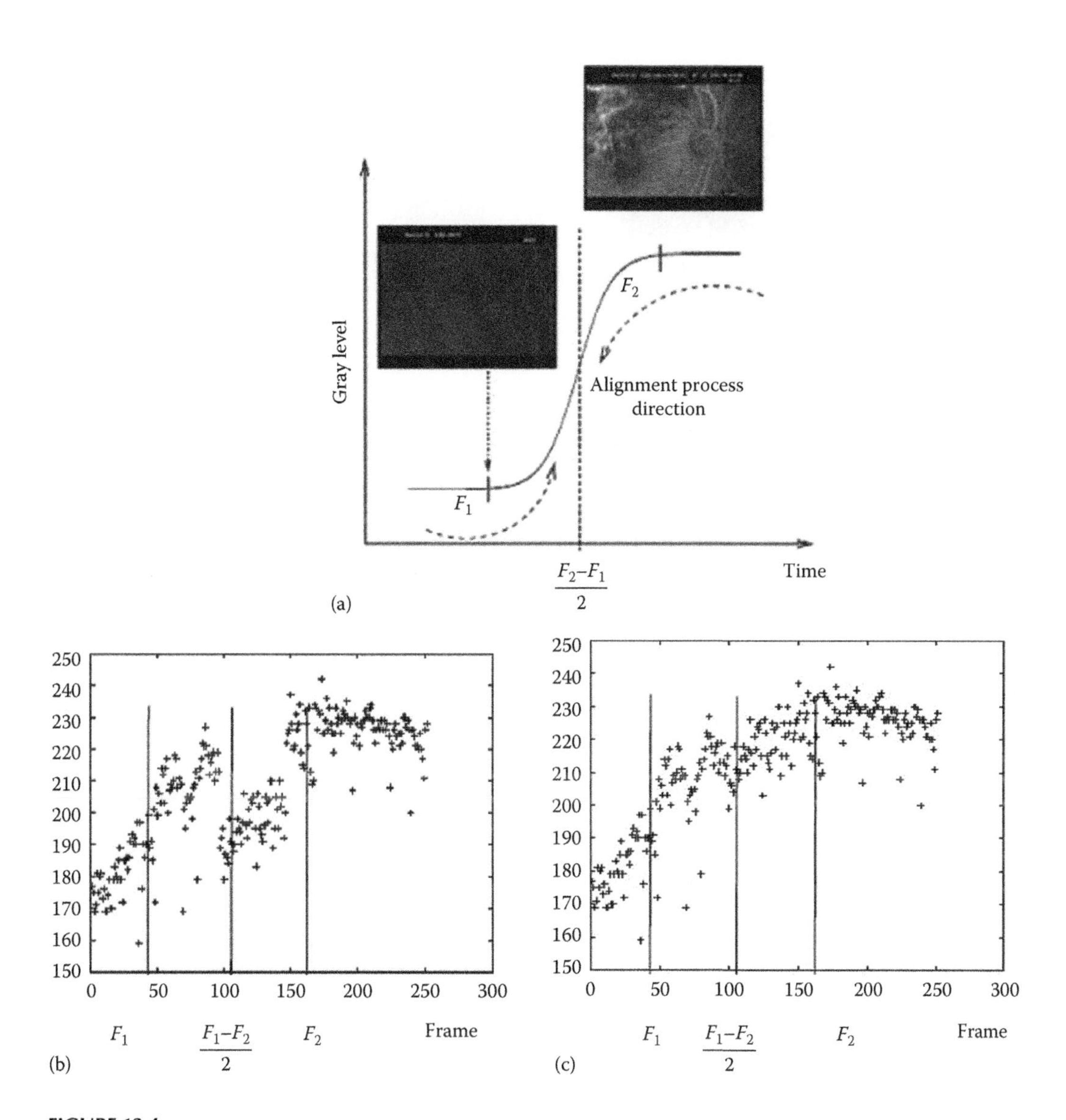

FIGURE 13.4
(a) A diagram of reference frames employed to register the SLO sequence. The frames from the beginning of the sequence are registered against the first reference frame (F_1), and the registration process goes forward from the first frame, but the last frames are registered against the second reference frame (F_2) from the last frame of the sequence backward. Evolution of the gray level in a selected point obtained after registration. (b) If the readjustment process is not performed, a gap between both areas of the registration appears. (c) This gap is removed if the readjustment is performed, and thus, curves are similar to that obtained manually by the expert clinicians. (From Lloret, D. et al., Landmark-based registration of full SLO video sequences, in *Proceedings of the IX Spanish Symposium on Pattern Recognition and Image Analysis*, Castellón, Spain, vol. I, pp. 189–194, 2001.)

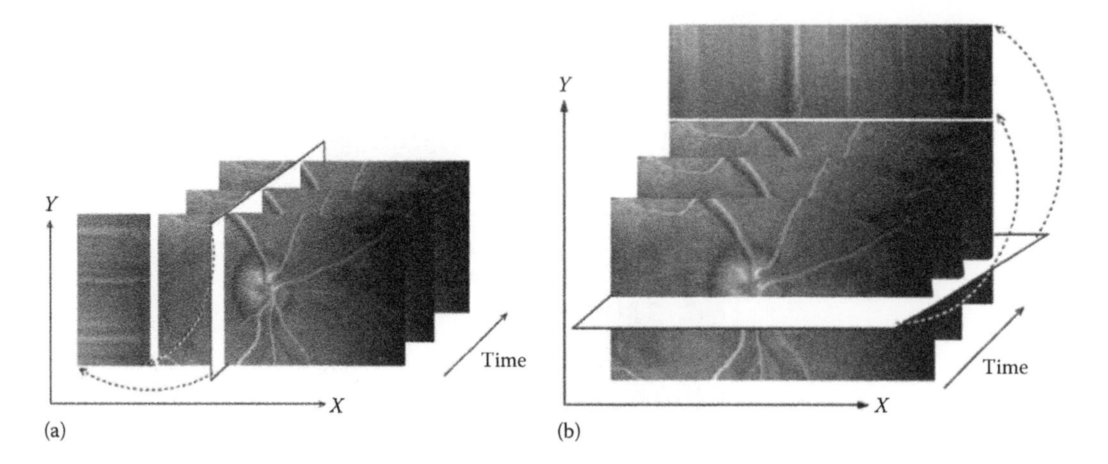

FIGURE 13.5
Image constructed by stacking the frames of the sequence. A 3D cube composed by the superposition in a stack of the frames of the SLO sequence is intersected by vertical and horizontal plane. (a) Shows the intersection process for vertical plane and (b) for horizontal plane.

all the frames in the sequence, by a horizontal and a vertical plane. Figure 13.5a and b illustrates the intersections and their results.

13.3 Experimental Validation and Results

The usual protocol at the ophthalmologic service in the Complejo Hospitalario Universitario de Santiago de Compostela (CHUS) for the acquisition of SLO sequences begins by injecting into the patient 3 mL of fluorescein sodium. After that, the ophthalmoscope laser begins to capture the frames. In this case, the device is a SLO-101 Rodenstock with argon laser. After digitalisation by a frame grabber at a normal 25 fps rate, a sequence is obtained with a resolution of 720 × 576 pixels. After the whole process of obtaining the sequence, a clinician corrects its alignment manually, calculates the dye-dilution curves, and obtains, from the sequence, the artery–vein time (AVT).

13.3.1 Artery–Vein Time

AVT can be described as the total time taken by the dye to go through the path between two particular points, one on the artery and the other point on its corresponding vein. If both points are set into the slope of a line, we can define the contrast arrival time to artery/vein as the moment when the line obtains half the maximum lighting for each vessel. The difference between contrast arrival time in both vessels is a measurement for AVT.

Assuming we have the frames aligned by the processes described in the previous sections, dye-dilution curves can be obtained and, from them, all the circulation variables. These curves express the changes in the intensity in a selected point along the frames in a sequence. As this sequence starts when the dye is still not present in the retinal vessels, curve shapes are expected to be very similar to the one depicted in Figure 13.6a, where we can establish three different zones depending on the presence or absence of the dye:

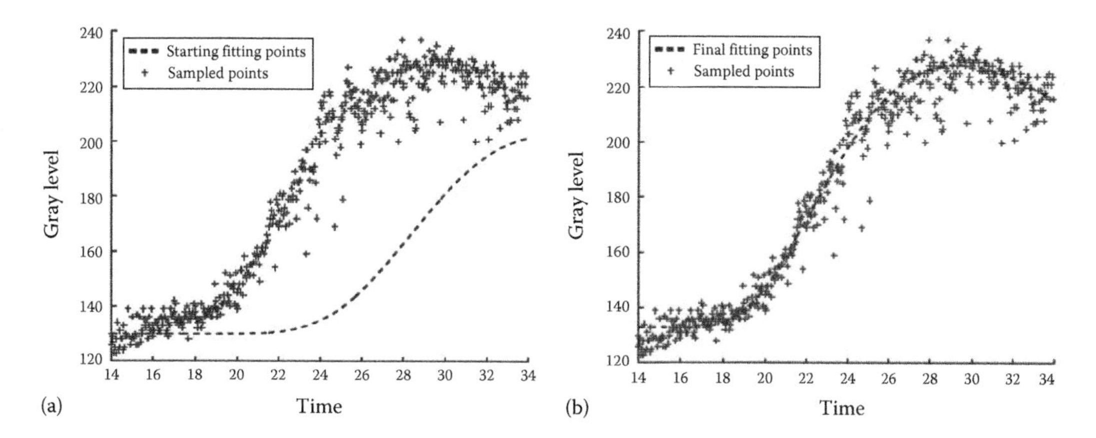

FIGURE 13.6
Results obtained with the developed fitting method. (a) Shows the initial set of points and the starting point of the theoretical curve of Equation 13.10, and (b) shows the final fitted curve and the removed points.

initially a zone where the dye has not arrived the vessels yet, a second zone where the dye is starting to reach the vessels, and a third zone where the dye is present in a great amount.

With the set of selected points, curves for dye dilution are calculated using the approach presented by Koyama et al. [24], where the intensity is represented as a function of time, and applying a regression of the data to adjust all points to a curve by using the formula in the following equation:

$$I_i' = I_0 + I_{max} \cdot e^{-A \ln^2 \frac{n-n_0}{n_{max}-n_0}}. \tag{13.10}$$

For our particular domain, I_0 is the intensity value in the first frame of the sequence, I_{max} is the maximum value for intensity, A is the parameter for shape, n_0 is defined by the number of the first frame in the computation, and n_{max} is the number of frame with the maximum intensity value.

In the original work of Koyama, the approach to calculate the fitting curve was a least-squares approach, but in our case, this solution is not enough given the presence of outliers associated with problems during the acquisition stage because of the blinking of the patient, for instance. When one of these frames appears in the sequence, neither of the alignment methods can perform well as both intensity values and landmarks are artificially altered. For the expert the usefulness of these frames is zero because of their lack of information, and hence, they are removed. We use simulated annealing [21] as it has been proved to be a good enough method for curve fitting. Also, the parameters from Equation 13.10 are the dimensions in our search space and we define the cost function as

$$C = \sum_i \left| I_i - I_i' \right| \tag{13.11}$$

where

i is the point picked by the expert in the sequence
I_i is the intensity in i
I_i' is the estimated intensity value computed using Equation 13.10

As the curve for dye dilution is obtained, we can remove outliers as mentioned earlier. A given point i is considered as an outlier if $I_i > 3\sigma_{i'}$, where $\sigma_{i'}$ is the standard deviation calculated from the sampled points.

We perform the fitting procedure up to three times as it is the minimum number needed for a satisfactory adjustment of the curve. Figure 13.6 shows a simulation of sampled data with the initial adjustment of the curve (a) and the final result obtained after three iterations with our approach (b).

13.3.2 Clinical Validation

To validate the methodology, an experiment was performed where the dilution measurements obtained by our system were compared to the manual results from three experts obtained by the usual process described earlier (see Figure 13.7). Intensity is depicted as a function of time enabling the observance of how the gray level evolves in a particular selected point over time. Figure 13.7b illustrates the results obtained by manual procedure, whereas Figure 13.7c shows the results using our method.

After the computation of the curves, parameters derived from the blood circulation analysis can be calculated. As mentioned earlier, we focus on the AVT [25]. It is important to note that AVT is not usually employed by expert clinicians in a very precise way but typically as an indicator of how a patient is responding to a particular treatment. In a patient

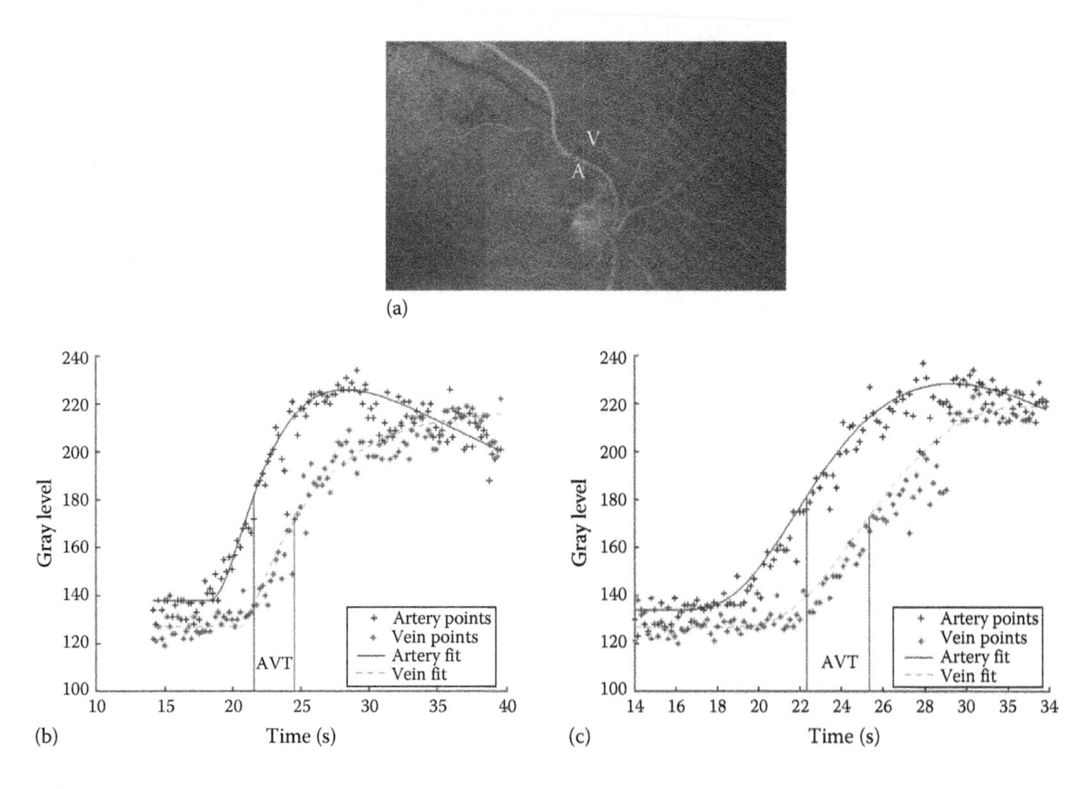

FIGURE 13.7
Graphs derived from the registered frames of the sequence: (a) depicts the points chosen by the clinician, which corresponds to an artery (A) and vein (V). (b) and (c) show the results obtained manually and with our method, respectively, as well as the lines estimating slopes. AVT is computed by measuring difference between both midpoints of the corresponding ascendant slope lines.

TABLE 13.1

AVTs (in Seconds) Obtained through the Manual (Second and Third Columns, Corresponding to Two Different Clinicians) and Automatic (Fourth Column) Registration Methods for the Five Analyzed SLO Sequences

	Clinician 1 Manual AVT (avt_{m1})	Clinician 2 Manual AVT (avt_{m2})	Automatic AVT (avt_a)	$\lvert avt_m - avt_a \rvert$
A	4098	3987	5208	0985
B	2728	2922	1685	1140
C	1923	1903	1226	0687
D	3505	3945	3430	0295
E	2168	2568	2935	0567

Note: The first column represents the SLO sequence and the fifth column represents the absolute difference between the average manual AVT and the automatic AVT.

presenting an initially abnormal AVT, any variation due to the treatment can be detected in future acquisitions.

Table 13.1 presents AVT for five SLO sequences (named A–E) with results by two different clinicians and by our automatic system. Results are expressed in seconds. We have also included a calculation of the deviation between the automatic and manual measurements.

Figure 13.8 shows the curves obtained for three of the sequences. In the left column, the curves from the manual process are shown, whereas the right column shows the curves from our automatic procedure.

Although there are deviations between manual and automatic calculations, it has been determined by the experts that these are derived from the intrinsic variability of the manual processes mainly from the alignment stage. Automatic measurements have been validated by clinicians confirming the coherence in the results. It is also important to note that this variability also appears in other works of the literature. In Bursell et al. [26], the obtained values are in a range of 3.1 ± 0.7 s for patients with no diabetes, whereas for patients presenting with diabetes, AVTs fall in the interval 5.1 ± 1.8 s. In Clermont et al. [27], these values were 3.5 ± 0.9 s and 4.9 ± 1.3 s, respectively.

13.4 Discussion and Conclusions

In this work, a novel registration algorithm has been presented. By combining two aligning techniques, the registration of whole SLO sequences is performed in a successful way. Moreover, computation times obtained in the registration process of the whole SLO sequence allow for the employment of the method in clinical environments as a fundamental tool in the evaluation and monitoring processes of eye diseases.

We described here how our technique can be used to assess the AVT. However, other hemodynamic features of the retinochoroidal vasculature could also be assessed. For instance, the time course of the front wave of the choroidal blood perfusion could be determined by performing some sort of calculation between consecutive frames. The clinical application of this procedure could help to detect hypoperfused areas that may be present in some ocular systemic diseases. Additionally, some dynamic features of vascular anomalies that may cause focal leaking could be better detected by, for instance, stabilizing the leaking point in the picture.

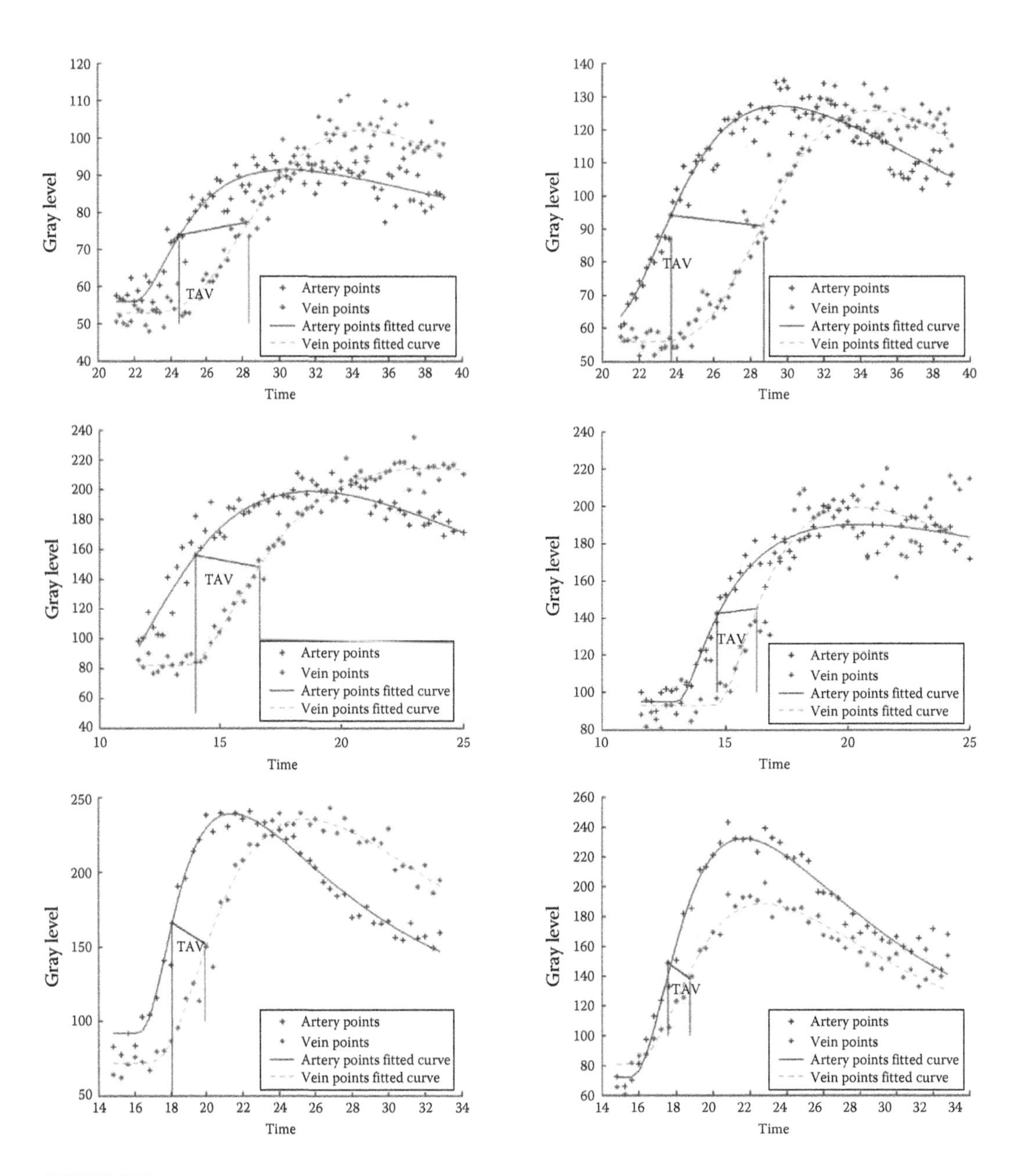

FIGURE 13.8
Dye-dilution curves and AVTs for three different SLO video sequences. Left column: manual results. Right column: automatic results. AVT from figures are included in Table 13.1.

Acknowledgments

This chapter has been partly funded by the Ministerio de Ciencia y Tecnología through the grant contract TIN2011-25476 and Xunta de Galicia through the grant contract 10TIC009CT.

References

1. R. Klein, B.E.K. Klein, and S.E. Moss. Visual impairment in diabetes. *Ophthalmology*, 91(1):1–9, 1984.
2. S. Bonafonte and C.A. García. Epidemiología de la retinopatía diabética. Harcourt Brace, Madrid, Spain, 1996.
3. F. Holz, R. Spaide, A.C. Bird, and S. Schmitz-Valckenberg (eds.). Fundus autofluorescence imaging with the confocal scanning laser ophthalmoscope. In *Atlas of Fundus Autofluorescence Imaging*, pp. 31–36. Springer-Verlag, Berlin, Germany, 2007.
4. Y. Zhang, P. Tiruveedhula, L. Sincich, J. Horton, and A. Roorda. Adaptive optics scanning laser ophthalmoscope (AOSLO) for precise visual stimulus presentation. *Journal of Vision*, 7(15):116, 2007.
5. M.S. Markov, H.G. Rylander, and A.J. Welch. Real-time algorithm for retinal tracking. *IEEE Transactions on Biomedical Engineering*, 40(12):1269–1281, 1993.
6. L.G. Brown. A survey of image registration techniques. *ACM Computer Surveys*, 24(4):325–376, 1992.
7. J.B.A. Maintz and M.A. Viergever. A survey of medical image registration. *Medical Image Analysis*, 2(1):1–36, 1998.
8. A. Pinz, S. Bernögger, P. Datlinger, and A. Kruger. Mapping the human retina. *IEEE Transactions on Medical Imaging*, 17(4):606–619, 1998.
9. A.R. Wade and F.W. Fitzke. A fast, robust pattern recognition system for low level image registration and its application to retinal imaging. *Optics Express*, 5(3):190–197, 1998.
10. J. Noack and D. Sutton. An algorithm for the fast registration of image sequences obtained with a scanning laser ophthalmoscope. *Physics in Medicine and Biology*, 59(5):907–915, 1994.
11. Z. Xu, R. Schuchard, D. Ross, and P. Benkeser. Tracking retinal motion with a scanning laser ophthalmoscope. *Journal of Rehabilitation Research and Development*, 42(3):373–380, 2005.
12. D. Lloret, C. Mariño, J. Serrat, A.M. López, and J.J. Villanueva. Landmark-based registration of full SLO video sequences. In *Proceedings of the IX Spanish Symposium on Pattern Recognition and Image Analysis*, Castellón, Spain, vol. I, pp. 189–194, 2001.
13. F. Zana and J.C. Klein. A multimodal registration algorithm of eye fundus images using vessels detection and Hough transform. *IEEE Transactions on Medical Imaging*, 18(5):419–428, 1999.
14. F. Maes, A. Collignon, D. Vandermeulen, G. Marchal, and P. Suetens. Multimodality image registration by maximization of mutual information. *IEEE Transactions on Medical Imaging*, 16(2):187–198, 1997.
15. F. Pardo, V. Leborán, C. Mariño, M.G. Penedo, M.J. Carreira, A. Mosquera, D. Cabello, F. GómezUlla, and F. González. Retinal angiography image registration applied to hemodynamic variable measurement. In *Proceedings of the IX Spanish Symposium on Pattern Recognition and Image Analysis*, Castellón, Spain, vol. II, pp. 139–144, 2001.
16. N. Ritter, R. Owens, and J. Cooper. Registration of stereo and temporal images of the retina. *IEEE Transactions on Medical Imaging*, 18(5):404–418, 1999.
17. C. Studholme, D.L.G. Hill, and D.J. Hawkes. Automated 3-D registration of MR and CT images of the head. *Medical Image Analysis*, 1(2):163–175, 1996.
18. W.M. Wells, P. Viola, H. Atsumi, S. Nakajima, and R. Kikinis. Multimodal volume registration by maximization mutual information. *Medical Image Analysis*, 1(1):35–51, 1996.
19. A. López Peña, F. Lumbreras, J. Serrat, and J.J. Villanueva. Evaluation of methods for ridge and valley detection. *IEEE Transactions on Pattern Analysis and Machine Intelligence*, 21(4):327–335, 1999.
20. P.A. Van den Elsen, J.B. Antoine Maintz, E.-J.D. Pol, and M.A. Viergever. Automatic registration of CT and MR brain images using correlation of geometrical features. *IEEE Transactions on Medical Imaging*, 14(2):384–396, 1995.
21. W. Press, S. Teukolsky, W. Vetterling, and B. Flannery. *Numerical Recipes in C*, 2nd edn. Cambridge University Press, Cambridge, U.K., 1992.

22. I. Vajda. *Theory of Statistical Inference and Information*. Kluwer Academic Publishers, Dordrecht, the Netherlands, 1989.
23. F.S. Hill Jr. *Computer Graphics Using OpenGL*, 2nd edn. Prentice Hall, Upper Saddle River, NJ, 2001.
24. T. Koyama, N. Matsuo, K. Shimizu, M. Mihara, Y. Tsuchida, S. Wolf, and M. Reim. Retinal circulation times in quantitative fluorescein angiography. *Graefe's Archive of Clinical and Experimental Ophthalmology*, 228:442–446, 1990.
25. S. Wolf, F. Jung, H. Kiesewetter, N. Körber, and M. Reim. Video fluorescein angiography: Method and clinical application. *Graefe's Archive of Clinical and Experimental Ophthalmology*, 227:145–151, 1989.
26. S.E. Bursell, A.C. Clermont, B.T. Kinsley, D.C. Simonson, L.M. Aiello, and H.A. Wolpert. Retinal blood changes in patients with insulin dependent diabetes mellitus and no diabetic retinopathy. *Investigative Ophthalmology and Visual Science*, 37(5):886–897, 1996.
27. A.C. Clermont, L.P. Aiello, F. Mori, L.M. Aiello, and S.E. Bursell. Vascular endothelial growth factor and severity of nonproliferative diabetic retinopathy mediate retinal hemodynamics in vivo: A potential role for vascular endothelial growth factor in the progression of nonproliferative diabetic retinopathy. *American Journal of Ophthalmology*, 124(4):433–446, 1997.

14

Optical Coherence Tomography

Mohamed A. Ibrahim, Yasir J. Sepah, Millena G. Bittencourt, Hongting Liu, Mostafa Hanout, Daniel Araújo Ferraz, Diana V. Do, and Quan Dong Nguyen

CONTENTS

14.1 Objectives

Optical coherence tomography (OCT) is widely used in imaging of biological tissues such as eye, skin, and most recently blood vessels. In this chapter, we will give a brief history of OCT and its development, especially during the most recent years. We will also discuss about the physical principles underlying the technology. The spectrum of

OCT applications is expanding quickly to include new medical and industrial disciplines. However, in this chapter, we will focus on the applications of OCT in the ophthalmological field, more specifically, in retina. Lastly, we will briefly discuss newer developments in OCT technologies with focus on research topics and future directions of use in ocular diseases.

14.2 Overview

Optical coherence tomography (OCT) is an optical imaging technique that employs light interferometry principles to capture 3D representations of optically scattering and reflective biological tissues. Real-time images of biological tissue can be obtained *in vivo* with an axial resolution of 1–15 μm [15,16]. Ideally, light within infrared wavelength is used, which allows deeper penetration of biological tissue. In ophthalmology, however, infrared waves are largely absorbed by aqueous and vitreous humor. For that reason, near infrared light is commonly employed for ophthalmological applications. The axial resolution of OCT is proportional to the width of the light source spectrum. Light sources such as superluminescent diodes, ultrashort pulsed lasers, and supercontinuum have been used and with spectrum width of over 100 nm.

In-depth imaging of ocular structures were traditionally acquired through techniques that employed the principles of ultrasonography, where the intensity of backscattered sound waves are measured and the in-depth reflectivity profile of the ocular structures is obtained through measurement of the echo delay. Ultrasonography has the advantages of being a quick noninvasive technique that yields cross-sectional images of the ocular and orbital structures even through opacified ocular media [41]. Compared to ultrasonography, OCT cannot penetrate through opacified media and does not have the same ability to image deeper structures. However, OCT provides unprecedented superior axial resolution about 10× that of ultrasound, hence the nickname *in vivo* biopsy.

While superb axial resolutions can be obtained in OCT through manipulating the light source, as we will explain later in this chapter, transverse resolution is usually limited by the optical properties of the eye, especially pupillary diffraction, to no less than 10 μm [23].

Superluminescent diode (SLD) has been traditionally employed as the light source in various OCT settings. Using SLD, axial resolutions of 10–15 μm were obtained. However, the axial resolution can be dramatically improved through using the ultrahigh-resolution OCT systems. Using ultrahigh-resolution OCT that employed ultrashort pulse laser source with broad-bandwidth femtosecond technology, Drexler et al. were able to obtain an *in vivo* longitudinal resolution of 1 μm and transverse resolution of 3 μm when scanning an African frog tadpole [8]. When applied in ophthalmology, the previous method yielded an *in vivo* axial resolution of 2–3 μm, whereas the transverse resolution was still limited to ~15 μm [7]. Ocular optics, in particular pupillary diffraction, is the limiting factor of the transverse resolution. Transverse resolution can even be degraded while scanning deeper layers of structures like the human retina due to the increase of the spot size by scatterings form the deeper retinal structures such as retinal pigment epithelium (RPE) and choroid [54]. Higher transverse resolutions, however, can be achieved using different imaging schemes such as en face (full-field) OCT technique, which will be discussed later. In addition, research in adaptive optics can help with improvement of transverse resolution.

Axial resolution in OCT is predominantly determined by the coherence length of the light source, that is, the smaller the coherence length, the higher the axial resolution. As we will see later in this chapter, coherence length is inversely proportional to the bandwidth of the light source. As a result, to acquire OCT images with high axial resolution, infrared light sources with wide bandwidth are ideally recommended. On the other hand, wavelengths longer than 1000 nm are greatly absorbed by aqueous and vitreous humor because of their high water content. For that reason, broadband light sources with central wavelength ~800 nm are commonly used in ophthalmological applications. The change from the infrared spectrum to a shorter wavelength comes with another trade-off as wavelengths around 800 nm suffer more scattering by the ocular media and retina, especially RPE, which limits to great extent the imaging of deeper intraocular structures such as the choroid.

The presence of intraocular structures that express birefringence, such as the nerve fiber layer (NFL), has encouraged the use of polarized light sources and the use of polarimetry techniques in combination with OCT to help retrieve depth-correlated information.

14.3 History and Development of OCT

OCT was first developed in industry as a mean for measuring the thickness of thin films that are otherwise too thin to be measured by other techniques using beta ray and x-ray scales. The use of optical interferometry to measure the thickness of micron-thick specimens was not exactly a new idea. However, the traditional settings used monochromatic light source and the sensitivity of the tool relied on the ability to compute accurately the absolute fringe shift, which was not easily done. Furthermore, the technique requires near-perfect stabilization of the traditional interferometer in order to limit its movement to fractions of a wavelength, which is almost impossible. Flournoy et al. were the first to use white light source, which is naturally broadband, instead of monochromatic light to measure film thickness using the principles of low-coherence interferometry [13].

Because of its low intensity and great scattering by ocular media, white light, however, is not suitable for ophthalmic applications. Fujimoto et al. employed the optical interferometry principles and used a light source of SLD to measure the axial length of the eye [11]. The first use of OCT technology to acquire cross-sectional data of internal ocular structures, such as the retina, came in 1991, when Huang et al. used a low-coherence light with a central wavelength of 830 nm to obtain *in vitro* cross-sectional images from the peripapillary region of a human retina. The device setup included a SLD light source and traditional Michelson interferometer. To acquire a 2D image, a series of axial (longitudinal) scans were performed with the optical beam position translated laterally along the x-axis between the axial scans. The obtained images demonstrated high accuracy when they were compared to a histologic section that was prepared from the same specimen. In 1991, Huang et al. reported an in-air longitudinal resolution of their system of 17 μm [25]. Two years later, the same group reported the first *in vivo* cross-sectional image of the human retina using SLD light source with central wavelength of 843 nm and 175 μW of power incident on the eye; the system reportedly had a sensitivity as small as 50 fW and a depth resolution of ~14 μm [53]. Correlations of the retinal images obtained using this method to the known histology of the human retina was established in 1995 [21].

Cross-sectional images of the retina are 2D images along the lateral (x) and axial (z) axes of the eye. They are also termed B-scans. The term *B-scan* was borrowed from ultrasound imaging along with other terms such as A-scan, which refers to axial or longitudinal scans, and C-scan, which refers to 3D images. Other terms, however, were borrowed from other imaging modalities. T-scan, for instance, was borrowed from confocal microscopy and refers to 2D images from the fundus along the x- and y-axes. Not only the term T-scan was borrowed from confocal microscopy but the scanning technique itself was also emulated to obtain 3D representations of the human retina. The first 3D representation using this technique was reported by Podoleanu et al. in 2000. In that report, a 3D representation of a 3 mm × 3 mm × 1.1 mm cube of the peripapillary region was compiled from 100 transverse frames that were collected in 56 seconds [44]. With such long acquisition time, motion artifacts are more than likely to happen, resulting in reduction of both the imaging quality as well as reproducibility. However, in 2003, Hitzenberger et al. have acquired 3D scans ($256(x) \times 128(y) \times 64(z)$ voxels) of the human retina in just 1.2 seconds. The research group achieved such speed through combining the scanning approach of confocal microscopy to the depth scanning advantage of OCT [22]. Such scanning technique is coined the name en face or *full-field OCT* imaging. Despite the impressive improvement in the speed and quality of 3D imaging using this technique, the new development of spectral domain OCT (SD-OCT) has provided an effective alternative while avoiding the confocal microscopy scanning approach.

Prior to SD-OCT, all OCT techniques relied on time domain principles (TD-OCT), where the presence of a moving mirror at the reference arm of the interferometer was essential to ensure that the reference wave will have the same optical pathlength as that of the sample arm. As a result to that principle, the optical path difference between the reference and the sample arms is always zero at any given scattering point along the axial axis, yielding the same sensitivity at all scanned points. However, relying on a moving mirror has limited the speed of A-scans and hence hindered the chances of getting a reliable 3D representation of the fundus. In contrast to TD-OCT, the reference mirror in SD-OCT is fixed. In SD-OCT, the depth information is acquired by analyzing the data obtained in a single A-scan all at once in Fourier domain, also called spectral or frequency domain. Analysis of data in the spectral domain is achieved through either replacing the photodetector at the receiving end of the traditional TD-OCT with a spectrometer and a high-pixel linear camera or by replacing the light source of the traditional TD-OCT with a tunable light source that would switch the frequency range of the emitted light at high speed. The first method is known as the spectral-based OCT (SB-OCT), whereas the second one is named swept-source OCT (SS-OCT).

As the case with TD-OCT, the first setups of SD-OCT were used to acquire a 1D reflectivity profile of the human eye and was based on the SB-OCT principles [10]. The concept of SS-OCT was introduced in 1997 [4]. In the same year, 1D profiles were obtained in high resolution in a model eye by slow tuning of a swept source over a wide wavelength range. In lower resolution, simultaneous *in vivo* measurements of the anterior segment length, vitreous chamber depth, and axial eye length in human eyes were possible with data-acquisition times in the millisecond range [38]. Another improvement in the SS-OCT speed came the same year when Golubovic et al. used a tunable laser with frequency range of 1200–1275 nm, which allowed an acquisition of 1D profiles of an axial resolution of 15 μm in less than half the time of previous SS-OCT methods [17].

Despite the early development and application of SD-OCT in ophthalmology in 1995, the first 2D scan of the human retina using SD-OCT came 7 years later [60], and the first 3D representation came after an additional 3 years [48]. The performance of both TD- and SD-OCT in ophthalmology has been an active area of research ever since with the SD-OCT being an obvious winner.

14.4 Theory and Physical Principle

The physical principles of OCT are similar in many ways to the principles of ultrasound imaging. In ultrasound, the sound signals are emitted and the intensity of echoes received is measured to detect the density of the imaged structures, with the in-depth information detected through measuring of the echo delays. In OCT, light waves are used instead of sound waves, and the intensity of the backscattered light is measured to detect the reflectivity profiles of the imaged structures. Contrary to ultrasound, however, the in-depth information in OCT cannot be accurately and directly obtained through measuring the flight time of backscattered light owing in part to the lack of hardware that can accurately do that and in part to the small scale (micron scale) at which biological tissues is required to be measured. To overcome the problem, the in-depth information in OCT is obtained indirectly using the low-coherence and interferometry principles.

14.4.1 Optical Interferometry

Interferometry is an optical phenomenon that occurs when two light beams of the same wavelength share one path direction (Figure 14.1). If the peaks and troughs of both waves are coinciding with one another, the wave beams are said to be in phase, and when they interfere, the result is a single wave with higher intensity (amplitude) than either parent beam (constructive interference). On the other hand, if the beams are out of phase so that peaks are largely coinciding with troughs, the resultant beam will have a lower intensity and will completely vanish if the peaks and troughs are exactly superimposed (destructive). The interference pattern of any two beams of the same wavelength (monochromatic) will therefore be composed of alternating zones of dark and bright gratings or fringes, with the dark zones representing areas of destructive interference and the bright zones representing constructive interference.

To obtain two light beams that are exactly in phase, a beam splitter is usually employed. If such split beams were to mix after traveling for some distances, the interference pattern of the mixed waves will depend on the phase at which the split beams are when interference happened. The phase of the split beams, on the other hand, depends on the optical pathlength (optical pathlength is the product of geometric length the light travels in a medium and the index of refraction of such medium) that each beam has traveled after the split until the interference. If the optical pathlength of one of the beams is known (reference beam), then analysis of the interference pattern should yield the optical pathlength of the other beam.

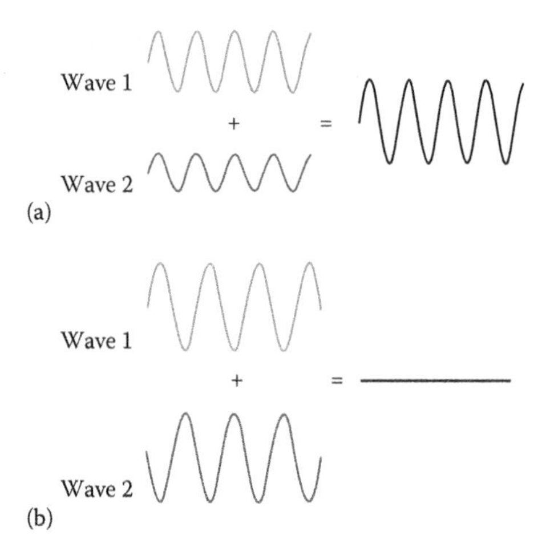

FIGURE 14.1
Optical interference. Constructive interference (a) occurs when two waves of the same wavelength (waves 1 and 2) and the same optical path are in the same phase of the wave cycle. The child wave of constructive interference will have higher amplitude than either parent wave but will have the same wavelength. Destructive interference (b) occurs when the two waves sharing one optical path are of the same wavelength but out of phase. If the waves are out of phase by half wavelength (waves 1 and 2) so that peaks of one wave coincide with troughs of the other, both parent wave will annihilate and no child wave is produced.

14.4.2 Interferometry in OCT

The principles of interferometry are employed in OCT in such way that the difference in the optical pathlengths of the reference and sample beams reveals the in-depth location of various backscattered light intensities. Monochromatic light, however, is highly coherent in nature in a way that deterioration of the fringes' contrast by the variations in the optical pathlength occurs very slowly, which limit largely the axial resolution of images obtained using this technique. Broad bandwidth light, in contrast, has low coherence and the deterioration of the interferometric fringes occurs rapidly. With low-coherence light, the fringe pattern deteriorates rapidly in such a way that the slightest change in the optical pathlength is easily detectable by current interferometry analyzers. In fact, the axial resolution of a traditional OCT system is nearly half the coherence length [56] and since the coherence length is given by the following formula:

$$l_C = \frac{4 \ln 2}{\pi} \frac{\bar{\lambda}^2}{\Delta\lambda}$$

where

l_C is the coherence length
$\bar{\lambda}$ is the central wavelength
$\Delta\lambda$ is the spectral width

It follows that if the bandwidth $\Delta\lambda$ is higher and the mean wavelength $\bar{\lambda}$ is lower, a higher axial resolution of a micron scale can be obtained.

For example, an OCT device with a source light that has a bandwidth $\Delta\lambda = 20$ nm and center wavelength $\bar{\lambda} = 840$ nm (both settings are common for the SLD light sources) will have a coherence length of 31,136 nm and hence an axial resolution of 15.5 µm. In contrast, a light source with a bandwidth of 60 nm and center wavelength of 810 nm will yield an axial resolution of 4.8 µm. Drexler et al. have used a light source of Ti:Al_2O_3 laser that generated pulses as short as 5.4 fs, which corresponds to bandwidths of up to 350 nm centered at 800 nm, which have produced an axial resolution of 2–3 µm. In theory, however, such settings should have yielded an axial resolution less than 1 µm [7].

14.5 OCT Setups and Types

In a typical OCT setup (Figure 14.2), an incident broadband light is split by a beam splitter into two arms, one travels to a reference mirror with a known distance from the splitter (reference arm) and the other beam travels to the specimen (sample arm). The backscattered light from both arms is then allowed to interfere and the interference pattern is measured by an interferometric analyzer. Variations in the light source, position of the reference mirror, and nature of the analyzer have yielded the various modalities

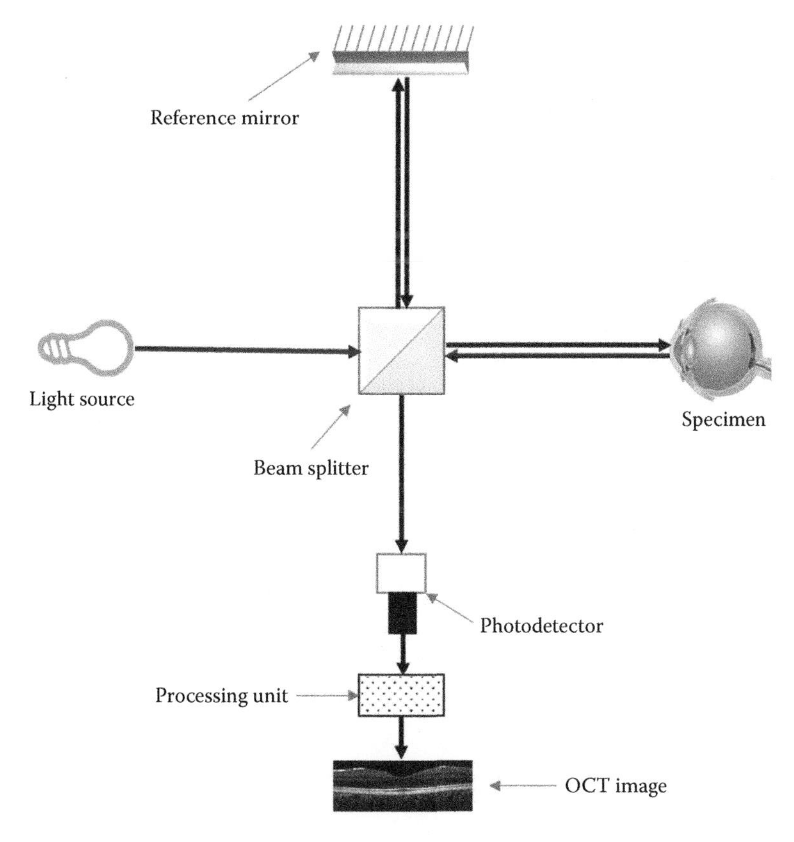

FIGURE 14.2
Typical OCT device setup.

of OCT imaging including the time domain versus SD-OCT on one hand and the swept source versus spectral broadband on the other.

14.5.1 Time Domain OCT

14.5.1.1 Device Setup

TD-OCT has the typical setup (Figure 14.3) of OCT with broadband light source, usually SLD; an interferometer, similar to Michelson interferometer; and a processing unit, usually a photodetector. The reference mirror, however, is movable and the continuous adjustment of the reference mirror during the scan provides variations in the optical pathlength of the reference arm to match the variations in the pathlength of the sample arm. Such movement ensures that at any scanned sample point, a reference beam with a matching optical pathlength, is available to interfere with the beam returned by the scanned point. In such case, the sample pathlength and the reference pathlength are equal with an optical path difference (OPD) = 0.

In a specimen that is composed of different layers at different distances (depths) from the beam splitter, each layer will backscatter a wavetrain of the incident beam with a phase delay correspondent to the depth of the layer. The maximum interference pattern from each layer will occur only at OPD = 0. By scanning the reference pathlength through moving the reference mirror, the layer satisfying the coherence gate condition, OPD = 0 can be selected.

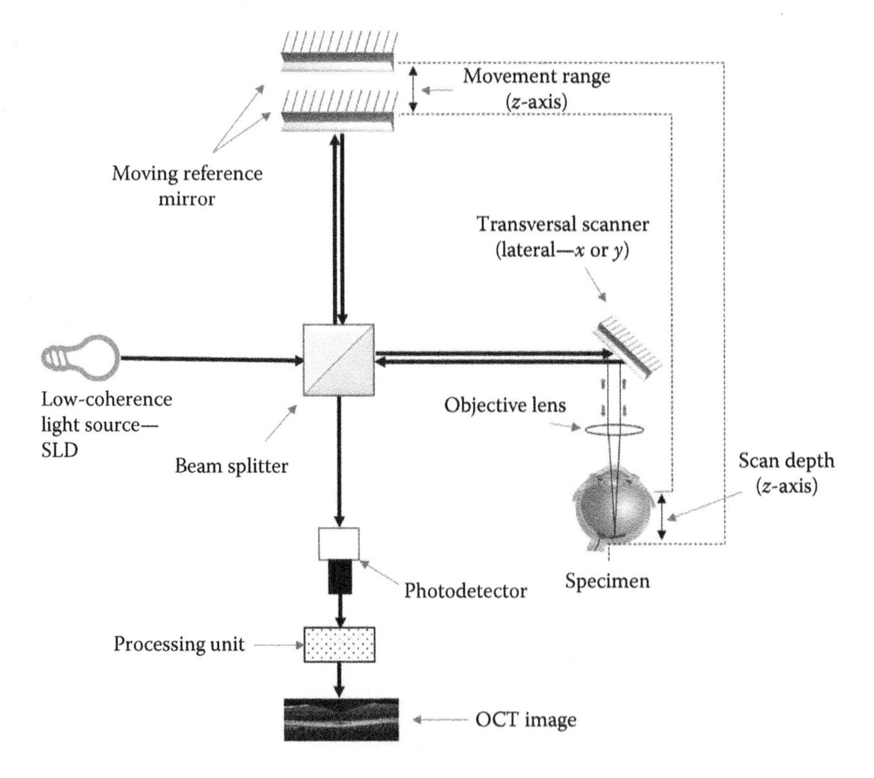

FIGURE 14.3
TD-OCT setup. The setup in the graph applies to both axial TD-OCT and the flying-spot en face TD-OCT, with the main differences lying within the scanning protocol.

14.5.1.2 Formats of TD-OCT

14.5.1.2.1 Longitudinal (Axial) TD-OCT (Figure 14.3)

The information returned from each layer through a single incident beam is then translated in time to output in-depth reflectivity profile, termed an A-scan. Another mirror (transversal scanner [25]) then deflects the incident beam form the light source to adjacent location of the specimen along the *x* (transverse)- or the *y* (vertical)-axis of the specimen, which enable the acquisition of another A-scan (Figure 14.4). Through compilation of a series of adjacent A-scans taken along either the *x* or *y* coordinates, cross-sectional image of the specimen, termed B-scan, is obtained. Such technique is the traditional method of scanning with TD-OCT devices in ophthalmology and is known as longitudinal (or axial) TD-OCT, and it is akin to the technique used in ultrasonography.

It is worth mentioning here that axial resolution and lateral (transverse) resolution of OCT are not related to each other. While axial resolution in TD-OCT is determined by

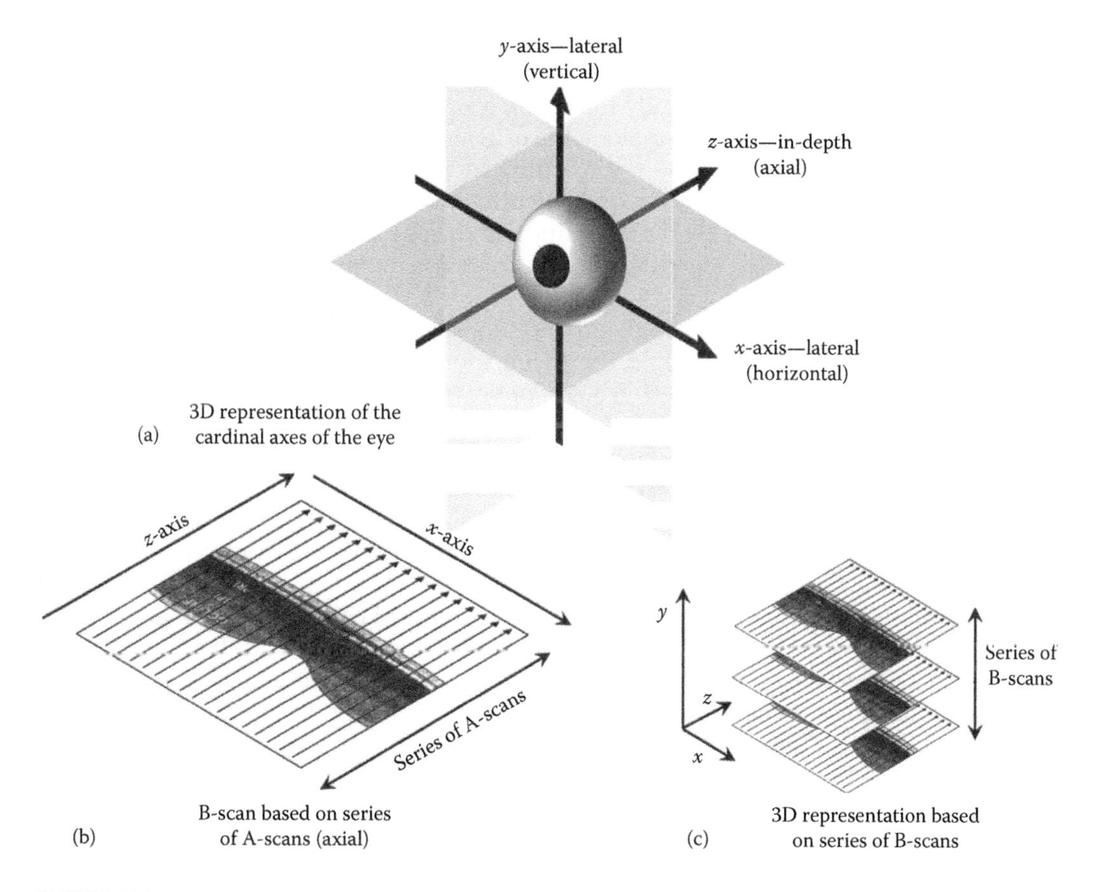

FIGURE 14.4
Types and conventional naming of OCT scans in ophthalmology with 3D representation of the cardinal axes of the eye (a). A single B-scan in this conventional scanning protocol is a 2D cross sectional representation along the *z*-axis (axial) and either one of *x* (horizontal)- or *y* (vertical)-axes. In this particular graph, the B-scan (b) is made of series of A scans along the *x*-axis. Most of commercially available OCT devices adopt this specific scanning protocol where 3D representations of the retina are made of series of B-scans (c).

the bandwidth and the center wavelength of the light source and hence the length of coherence, the lateral resolution is largely determined by the optics, spot size in particular, of the system. While very high lateral resolution is possible *in vivo*, the lateral resolution of retinal OCT is usually limited to 10–14 μm.

14.5.1.2.2 En Face OCT

The scanning speed of the traditional axial TD-OCT is limited by the speed of the reference mirror in a way that obtaining a 3D representation of a specimen requires relatively long time. Therefore, *in vivo* 3D representations of biological structures are greatly affected by motion artifacts, and with a particularly fast moving structure like the eye, accurate 3D representations are almost impossible. En face OCT is another type of OCT devices that uses similar hardware setup to that of axial TD-OCT with the exception of perhaps the processing unit in certain implementations. The main difference between both types of OCT lies, however, in the scanning technique rather than the device setup. While axial TD-OCT borrows its scanning technique from ultrasonography, the en face OCT borrows its scanning technique from confocal microscopy scanning.

In en face scanning, the reference mirror is initially fixed while the transversal scanner deflects the incident beam laterally to acquire a single line called T-scan (Figure 14.5). A series of T-scans are then acquired along the orthogonal coordinate. Compilation of the T-scans yields a 2D image along the x–y coordinates, which is termed C-scan. A series of C-scans is then acquired along the z-axis (in depth) of the specimen through moving the reference mirror to produce a 3D representation of the specimen. In other words, the en face OCT allows scanning fast laterally, since the reference mirror is fixed, and slow axially using the reference mirror.

The T-scans can be obtained through either flying-spot (Figure 14.3) or full-field implementations (FF OCT) (Figure 14.6). In the flying-spot implantation, galvoscanners, resonant scanners, piezoelements, and acousto-optic modulators are used to deflect the beam over the specimen, pixel by pixel. In contrast, the full-field implementations use a linear photodetector array or a 2D array, a charged couple (CCD) or complementary metal–oxide–semiconductor (CMOS), to capture the whole T-scan at single exposure to thermal lamp light [56]. In other words, instead of acquiring information from an axial direction, as both axial TD- and SD-OCT do, or acquiring point-by-point lateral information through deflecting the incident beam transversely, as in the flying-spot OCT, FF-OCT acquires backscattering data from the same (optical path) depth simultaneously. Therefore, though one needs the reference mirror to be moved for in-depth scanning, one does not need to move the incident light source in lateral directions over the sample. Using FF-OCT, submicron axial and lateral resolution with an image acquisition time of 1 second were possible *in vitro* [9].

14.5.2 Spectral-Domain (Fourier-Domain) Optical Coherence Tomography

14.5.2.1 Device Setup

Similar to TD-OCT, a broadband optical source is used. However, the main difference from TD-OCT is the use of fixed reference mirror (Figures 14.7 and 14.8). The identification of OPD through the mechanically moving reference mirror is replaced by the use of a processing unit that employs a spectrometer, usually built using a prism or a diffraction

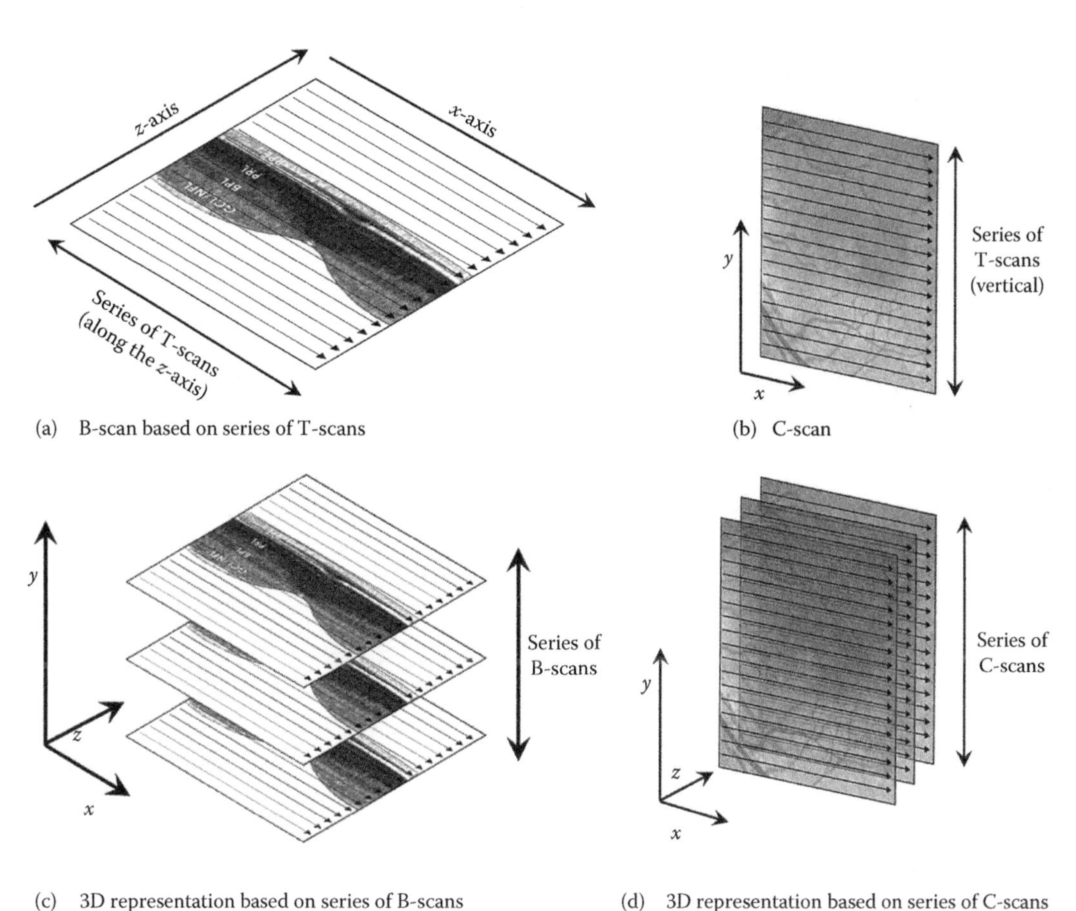

(a) B-scan based on series of T-scans

(b) C-scan

(c) 3D representation based on series of B-scans

(d) 3D representation based on series of C-scans

FIGURE 14.5
Demonstration of scanning protocols adapted from confocal microscopy. T-scans are series of single 1D scans made along either one of the orthogonal axes (x or y). A series of T-scans along the z-axis can produces a B-scan (a) and if made along the x- or y-axes, it can produce a two-dimensional image (x, y) termed C-scan (b). 3D representations using this imaging protocol can be made through series of B-scans (c) or a series of C-scans (d).

grating and a linear photodetector array, using a CCD or a CMOS linear camera. The depth information can be immediately obtained by a Fourier transform from the acquired spectra, without moving the reference arm. This feature improves imaging speed dramatically, while the reduced losses during a single scan improves the signal to noise proportional to the number of detection elements. The parallel detection at multiple wavelength ranges limits the scanning range, while the full spectral bandwidth sets the axial resolution. Such setups that employ spectrometers in the processing unit are termed spectral-based SD-OCT (SB-OCT).

Alternative method of the identification of OPD was achieved through replacing the light source with tunable laser source and the use of a processing unit that employs a photodetector. Such setups that employ tunable lasers as light source are termed swept-source SD-OCT (SS-OCT).

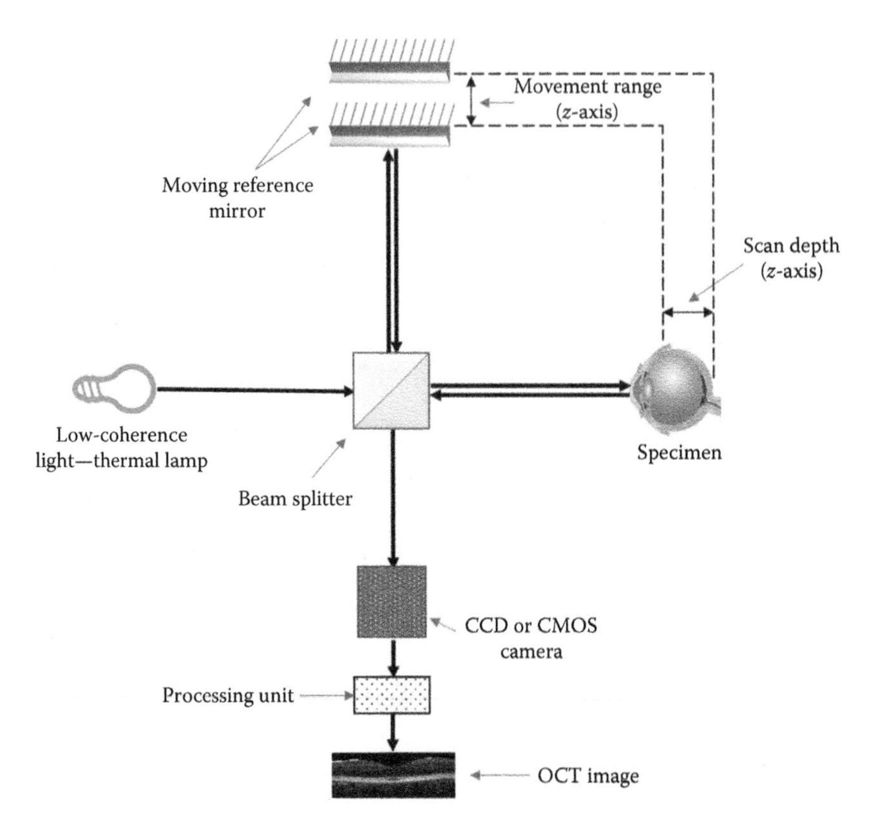

FIGURE 14.6
Setup of full-field en face TD-OCT (FF TD-OCT). Please note, the digital signal processor is made of CCD or CMOS camera to allow multipixel recording of the full-field image all at once instead of single registration with the photodetector as is the case with axial TD-OCT and flying-spot TD-OCT.

14.5.2.2 Formats of SD-OCT

14.5.2.2.1 Spectral-Based OCT

SB-OCT uses a spectrometer that is built of disperser, usually a prism or a diffraction grating, and a linear camera array to output a spectrum that is read in time in a Fourier transform to resolve the in-depth information (Figure 14.7). In such system, the number of cycles in the channeled spectrum, after passing through the disperser, is given approximately by the OPD/cl, where the coherence length, cl, is approximately given by cl $\approx \lambda^2/\Delta\lambda$. Consequently, the longer the OPD, the higher the number of cycles in the channeled spectrum and hence, the smaller the linewidth ($\delta\lambda$). It follows then that the linear camera must have a sufficient number of pixels to detect such small $\delta\lambda$, which is one of the determinant factors of the axial resolution of such system, in addition to the bandwidth of the source light and the center wavelength. In other words, the smaller the pixel sizes in the linear camera of the spectrometer, the higher the resolution of the system. Due to its sensitivity advantage and availability of fast digital linear cameras with high pixel density, the SB-OCT became the method of choice in current OCT investigations of the retina.

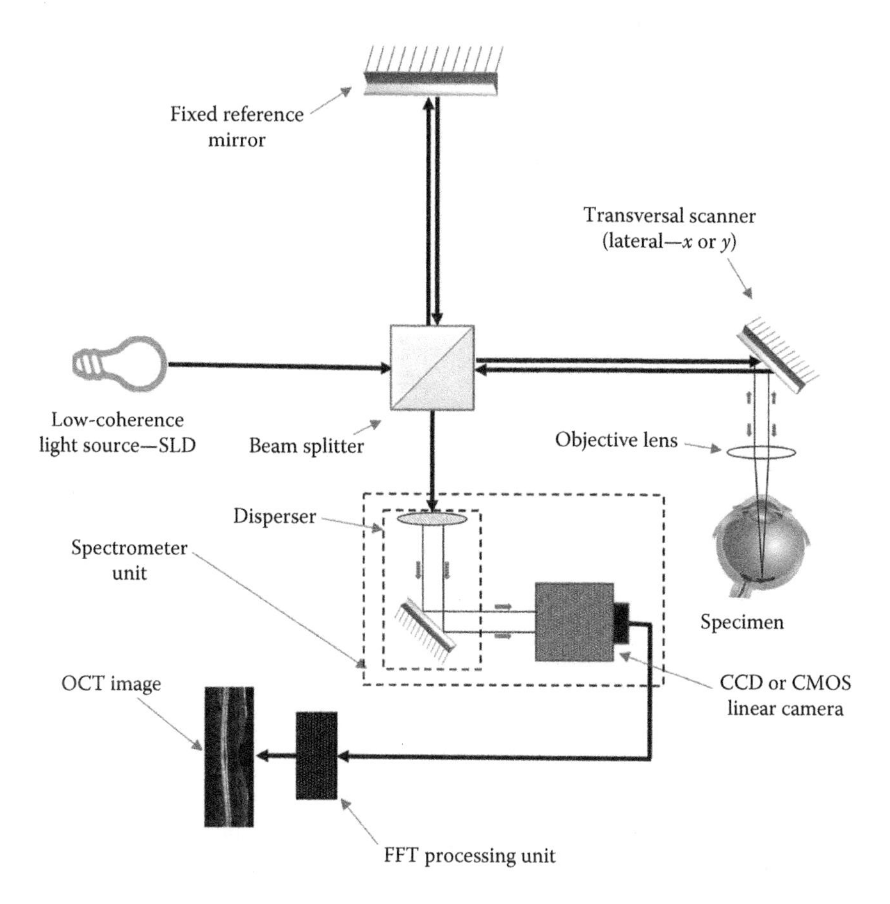

FIGURE 14.7
Setup of SB-OCT. The fixed reference mirror and the fast Fourier transform processing unit are characteristic for all spectral (Fourier) frequency (SD-) OCT devices. SB-OCT utilizes a disperser, usually a prism or diffraction grating, to channel the spectrum to a linear camera (CCD or CMOS). The disperser and the camera form the spectrometer unit.

14.5.2.2.2 Swept-Source OCT

In SS-OCT, a light source of tunable laser is used, which sweeps across the bandwidth (frequency range) in rapid succession in a process called frequency tuning (Figure 14.8). The frequency range of interest is swept through equally spaced frequency values, which is necessary to allow the use of fast Fourier transform. Because of the frequency tuning, by the time the initial wavetrain from the SS reaches the deeper layer of the specimen, the frequency of the next wavetrains changes and reaches the top of the specimen. Such continuous tuning of frequency gives a Doppler-like pulsations or beating signals resulting from the interference of the sample and reference light beams at the photodetector. As a result, the in-depth information of the axially scanned layers is encoded on the frequency of the pulsating light source. Needless to say, the faster the light source is tuning, the higher the frequency of the beating signal and hence the higher the axial resolution [17,38,46]. Tuning speeds in excess of 5 MHz [59] makes the

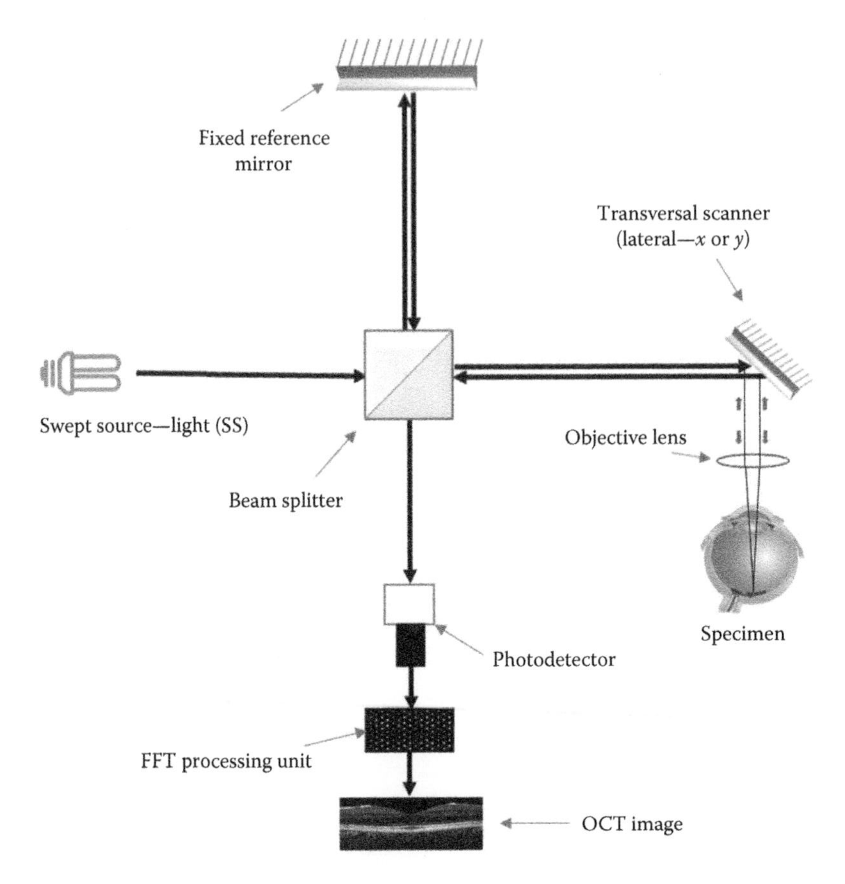

FIGURE 14.8
Setup of SS-OCT. As in all spectral (Fourier) frequency OCT devices, the unit has fixed reference mirror. However, the system is unique for having a fast tuning laser (swept-source) light source. Contrary to SB-OCT, the system utilizes a photodetector instead of a spectrometer as a digital signal processor.

SS-OCT the fastest scanning OCT method that has led to sufficient quality of *in vivo* images acquired from tissue to date [33].

The main advantage of SS-OCT over SD-OCT is the minimal signal drop-off with depth that arises from using the same beam for all frequencies, as is the case in SD-OCT.

14.6 Comparison of TD-OCT and SD-OCT

14.6.1 Imaging Resolution

Commercially available TD-OCT devices provide *in vivo* axial resolution of 14 μm and lateral resolution of 10–14 μm. Certain implementations of SD-OCT techniques allow submicron axial resolution with the commercially available solutions providing an axial resolution in the range of 4–8 μm. Such higher resolution is of critical importance while examining very small tissues with micron level layers such as the retina.

14.6.2 Acquisition Speed

In TD-OCT, the acquisition time is limited by the speed of mechanical movement of the reference mirror. Since SD-OCT does not have moving mechanical parts, great acquisition speeds of more than 100 MHz are possible. However, acquisition speeds in excess of 100 MHz do not allow enough exposure of individual pixels to the backscattered light resulting in significant falloff of signal noise ratio. The number of pixels in the linear camera along with the rate in which it discharges governs the acquisition speeds of the commercially available SB-OCT devices. The speed of tunability of the light source on the other hand governs the acquisition speeds of the SS-OCT devices.

14.6.3 Scan Depth Range and Spatial Extension

In TD-OCT, the scan depth range (Figures 14.3 and 14.6) is governed by the location and the range of movement of the reference mirror. In SD-OCT, however, the maximum depth range is given by the equation

$$z_{max} = \frac{N}{4n_s}\frac{\bar{\lambda}^2}{\Delta\lambda},$$

where
- N is the number of data points along the A-scan
- n_s is the reflective index of the medium
- $\bar{\lambda}$ and $\Delta\lambda$ are the center wavelength and the bandwidth of the light source, respectively

In an aqueous medium like the vitreous and aqueous humor, the $n_s = 1.33$ and in a typical SD-OCT setting, $\bar{\lambda} = 810$ nm, $\Delta\lambda = 60$ nm, and $N = 1024$, and hence, the maximum depth of scan is about 2.1 mm [50]. Since scanning larger depths requires higher center wavelength and narrower bandwidth, which is quite the opposite to the requirements of higher axial resolution, a trade-off between the desired axial resolution and scan depth range is usually thought of while designing OCT devices for specific biological applications.

A major drawback of SB-OCT is the decrease of signal level, and therefore of sensitivity, with sample depth. This is a consequence of the convolution between the point-spread function for each wavelength, whose width increases along the detector plan, toward its edge, due to optical aberrations, and the corresponding detector pixel, whose width is finite and fixed [24].

As an example, a specimen is made of layers (Figure 14.9) that are separated from each other by a distance δz, and with the distance between the top and bottom layers of the specimen equal Δz, the OPD axial extension of the specimen is $2\Delta z$, assuming for simplicity the index of refraction as 1. In TD-OCT, the coherence length, cl, of the optical source needs to be smaller than δz to be able to separate the layers in depth in the object. Because TD-OCT operates around OPD = 0 at every scanned point along the axial axis, the maximum of sensitivity is moved from one layer to the next. Therefore, all layers can be interrogated by the same sensitivity.

The system is different, however, in SD-OCT where the reference mirror is fixed. As an example, the reference mirror is adjusted for OPD = 0 to match the top of the specimen. In the case of SB-OCT, the total overlap of interfering wavetrains, from specimen and reference, will occur at the top of the specimen only where OPD = 0. For the deepest layer,

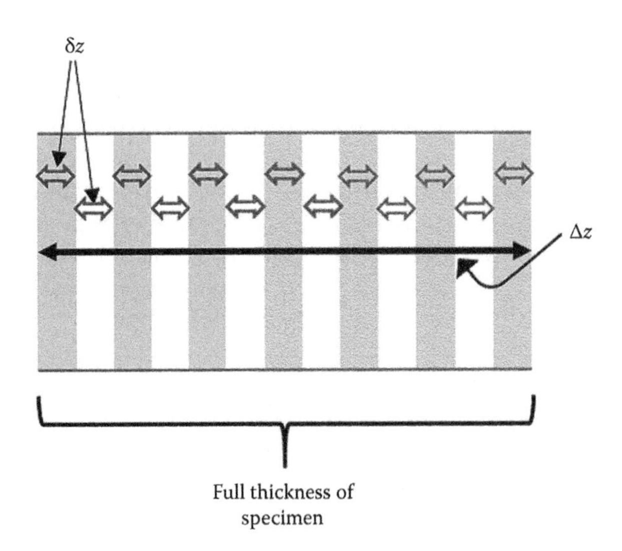

FIGURE 14.9
Scan depth range and spatial extension.

however, specimen and reference waves are superposed toward the tails of the waves only, which yields a lesser amount of overlap of interfering waves. Since the sensitivity depends on the amount of overlap of the two interfering wavetrains, the sensitivity in SD-OCT decays with depth [45].

At the same time, to ensure interference of the waves coming from the reference mirror with the waves coming from the top as well as the bottom of the specimen, the spatial extension of the waves coming from the top and bottom of the specimen, CL, needs to exceed the OPD axial range $2\Delta z$, in other words, $CL > 2\Delta z$. Such requirement for CL to be larger than $2\Delta z$ limits the axial range of SD-OCT.

The spatial extension, CL, in the SB is given by the extension of the specimen and reference wavetrains after suffering dispersion in the spectrometer. Whereas, in the SS-OCT case, the CL of the wavetrains emitted by the swept source is inversely proportional to the linewidth, $\delta\lambda$, of the spectrum [45].

14.6.4 Sensitivity

Choma and coworkers have demonstrated the superior sensitivity of SS- and SB-OCT techniques over the conventional TD-OCT approach. They also showed that SS- and SB-OCT have equivalent expressions for system signal-to-noise ratio, which results in a typical sensitivity advantage of 20–30 dB over TD-OCT [5].

14.7 Applications in Ophthalmology

Since its first introduction in the early 1990s, OCT has revolutionized the field of ophthalmic imaging. For many years, TD-OCT has been the gold standard for evaluation of the structural integrity of internal ocular structures. However, in the recent years and since the introduction of SD-OCT, TD-OCT has been rapidly phasing out. In the next section of this chapter, we will discuss some of the important aspects of the application of OCT, with a focus on SD-OCT, in the field of ophthalmic imaging, most specifically structural assessment of the retina in health and disease.

14.7.1 Retina

Retina is the photosensitive structure that lines the innermost surface of the eye. Composed mainly of neurons, retina is considered part of the central nervous system (CNS). It is the only part of the CNS that can be visualized noninvasively using methods such as slit-lamp biomicroscopy and indirect ophthalmoscopy. Being the innermost part of the eye with clear optical media in front of it (cornea, lens, and aqueous and vitreous humor) and being transparent itself, the retina represents a unique opportunity to noninvasively assess the integrity of certain aspects of the CNS and help diagnosing and monitoring various systemic diseases. Along with clinical examination, several imaging modalities have been developed to help assess the structural integrity of the retina, starting with color fundus photography, fluorescein angiography, and ending with OCT.

The retina itself is a transparent structure of 200–300 μm in thickness, which is composed of 10 layers with the internal limiting membrane (ILM) representing the innermost layer and the RPE representing the outermost layer. The only neurons that are directly sensitive to light are the photoreceptor (PR) cells whose outer segments are next to the RPE comprising the second outermost layer of the retina, which is named the PR layer (PRL). Photoreceptors are mainly of two types: rods and cones. Rods function mainly in dim light and provide black-and-white vision, while cones support daytime vision and the perception of color. The architecture of the retina is preserved by cytoskeletal cells unique to the retina called the Muller cells. Muller cells span the retinal thickness with their footplates fusing together to form the ILM and the outer limiting membrane (OLM), which represents the third outermost layer. The cell bodies of the PRs are located within the fourth outermost layer and termed the outer nuclear layer (ONL). The cell bodies of the bipolar cells, amacrine cell, and horizontal cells are located within the bipolar cells layer (BPL), which represents the sixth outermost layer, with the fifth layer composed of the synapses between the PRs cells and cells of the BPL and therefore termed the outer plexiform layer (OPL). The synapses between the cells of BPL and the dendrites from the ganglion cells form the seventh layer, which is termed the inner plexiform layer (IPL). The cells bodies of the ganglion cells are located in the eighth layer, the ganglion cell layer (GCL). The ninth layer is composed of the axons of the GCL and is called the NFL. The axons of the NFL span around the macula and converge toward the optic nerve head where they exit the eye and form the optic nerve, which travels to the brain.

The macula is the central region of the retina and occupies the entire posterior pole of the eye. In the center of the macular region lies the fovea.

Neural signals from the rods and cones undergo processing by intermediate neurons within the retina, mostly the cells of the BPL before the signals are synapsed to the ganglion cells whose axons carry the signals to the brain through the optic nerve.

14.7.2 Qualitative Assessment of Retina

OCT technology, SD-OCT in particular, has provided unprecedented ultrahigh-resolution images of the retinal structure *in vivo* (Figure 14.10). Such high resolution combined with quickness and noninvasiveness nature of the test itself has made OCT scanning of the

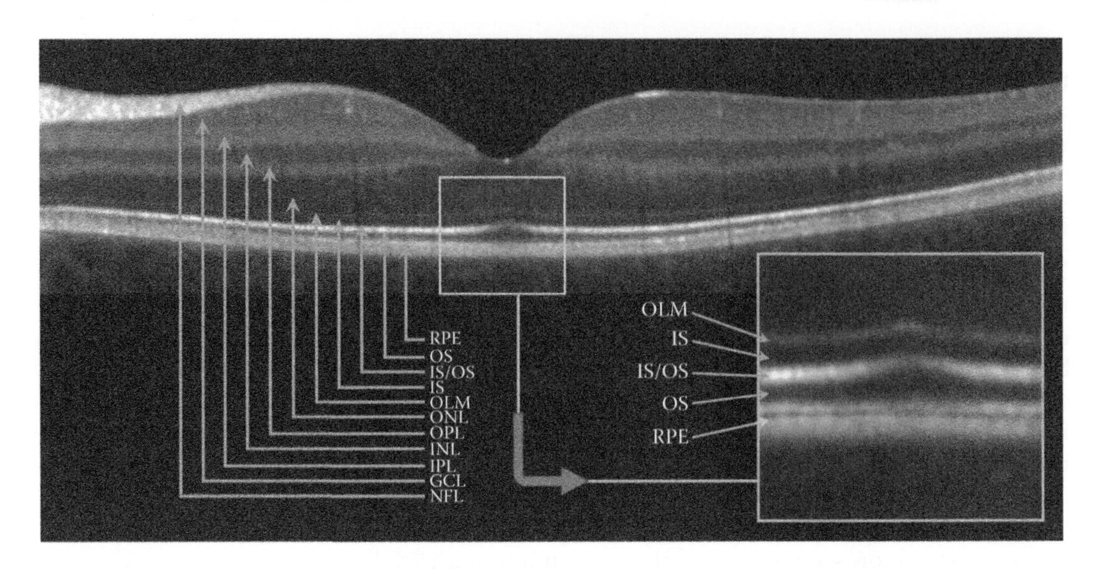

FIGURE 14.10
B-scan of SD-OCT displaying normal retinal structure. The scan represents a 6 mm horizontal section of the left retina with the line centered on the fovea. The magnified part of the retina demonstrates the ultrahigh resolution that is possible with the SD-OCT devices available today. RPE, retinal pigment epithelium; OS, outer segments of PRs; IS/OS, junction between inner and outer segments of PRs; IS, inner segments of PRs; OLM, outer limiting membrane; ONL, outer nuclear layer; OPL, outer plexiform layer; INL, inner nuclear layer; IPL, inner plexiform layer; GCL, ganglion cell layer; and NFL, nerve fiber layer.

retina a very popular tool in very much all retina clinics today. Examination of cross-sectional B-scans and 3D representations of the retinal structure can provide invaluable information that help clinicians in managing the most difficult retinal diseases with great accuracy and efficiency.

OCT can provide highly detailed images of the vitreomacular interface (Figure 14.11) that can affect the clinical decision on whether to treat conservatively or to perform vitreomacular surgery. Several studies have assessed the extent of inner retinal abnormalities and have described minute changes in early stages of chloroquine retinopathy [30], retinoschisis [18,68], and ocular albinism [40,49], among others. In their study of 84 eyes from 73 patients to detect the impact of OCT on clinical decision, Do et al. have demonstrated that an epiretinal membrane (ERM) was identified in 66 (78.6%) eyes with clinical examination alone compared with 72 (85.7%) when OCT was added; vitreomacular traction (VMT) was identified in 5 (6%) prior to OCT compared with 18 (21.4%) after the OCT was used; and macular edema was identified in 57 (67.9%) using clinical examination alone compared with 70 (83.3%) using OCT. Surgical intervention was recommended in 19 cases (57.6%) before reviewing the OCT images. Reviewing the OCT images has resulted in consideration of surgery in additional 14 cases (42.2%) [6].

In addition to the vitreomacular interface assessment, SD-OCT can provide detailed structural images of the most posterior retinal layers, which can be used in assessment and follow-up of diseases that can affect RPE. Punctate inner choroidopathy (PIC) is an ocular inflammatory disease that can serve as a perfect example of such diseases. In a retrospective case series, lesions form PIC not associated with choroidal neovascularization (CNV) were reviewed and characterized on macular SD-OCT scans [2]. Channa et al. have reported the presence of many lesions of RPE elevations (Figure 14.12), which have fluctuated with disease activity. Bruch's membrane (BM) and the choroid, on the other

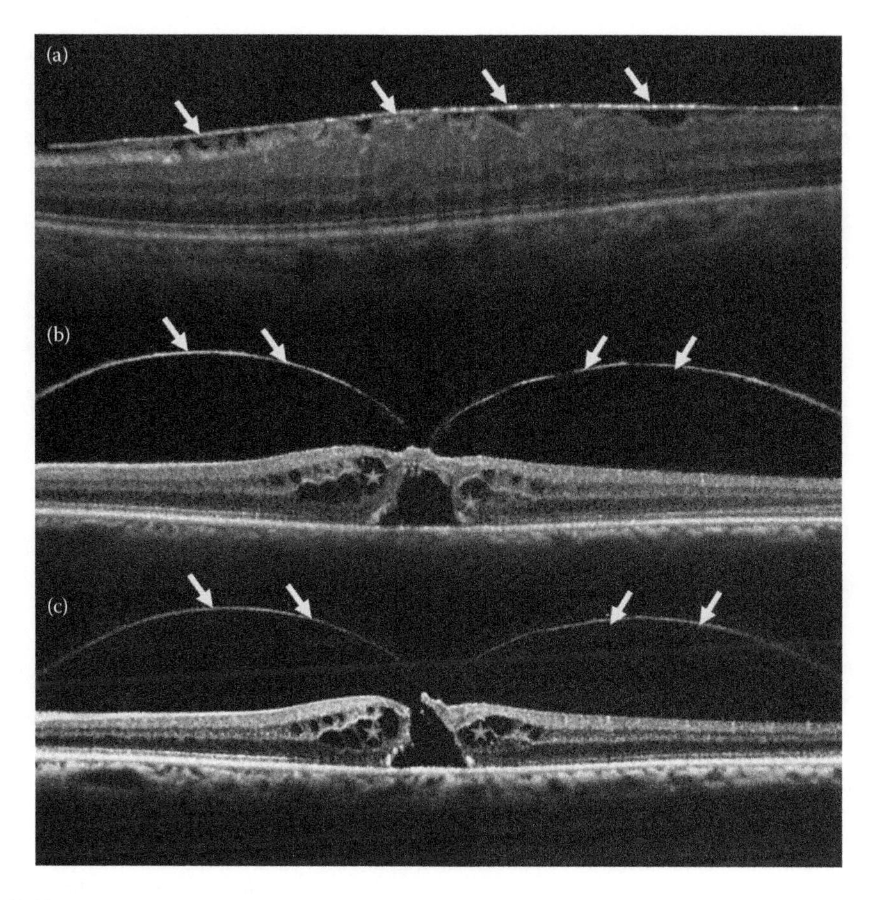

FIGURE 14.11
Ultrahigh-resolution SD-OCT images of the retina showing changes at the level of the vitreomacular interface. Conditions such as the presence of epiretinal membrane (ERM) (a) can be accurately confirmed with SD-OCT. The changes of the retina pertinent to the presence of the ERM (arrows) may alter the treatment decision significantly. Other abnormal structures that may cause vitreo-macular traction (VMT) (arrows in b and c) can also be visualized with high details with SD-OCT. The VMT in (b) is causing the accumulation of intraretinal fluid (edema; stars in b and c). The high speed of SD-OCT has enabled the acquisition of highly dense scans with duration within reasonable limits. Such scan density enables the detection of pathologies that may go otherwise undetected. For example, the scan in (b) shows just the VMT; however, the adjacent scan in the same patient (30 μm away) shows that a part of the macula has already broke with the formation of a full thickness macular hole (c). Such finding could easily be missed had fewer OCT scans were available as the case with TD-OCT.

hand, appeared to be intact, which is a finding contrary to what was previously suggested in many previous studies, where the disease was thought to be of choroidal inflammatory origin, hence the nomenclature. The study has also reported the presence of PR-associated bands on SD-OCT that appear compressed during clinically active stages of the disease but return to normal visibility with the disease is stabilized [2].

RPE morphology can also be affected in early stages of age-related macular degeneration (AMD), where sub-REP deposits, known as drusen (Figure 14.13), result in the distortion of the REP contour and in many cases result in significant focal elevation of REP. Yi et al. has been able to develop an automated algorithm to quantify drusen area and volume from SD-OCT images in patients with AMD [65]. In addition, alterations of the outer retinal layers imaged with SD-OCT have been demonstrated in various retinal diseases such as

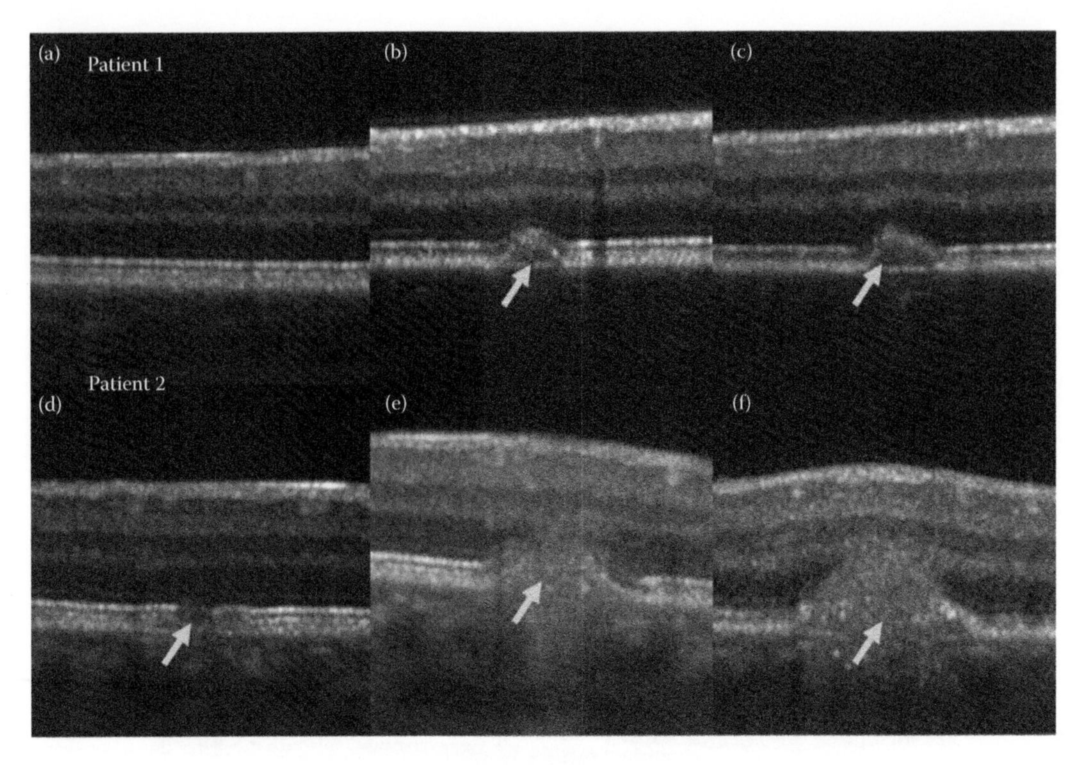

FIGURE 14.12
Magnified B-scans of SD-OCT from retina of two patients with punctate inner choroidopathy (PIC). (a) and (d) show almost normal retinal layers configuration with the exception of few irregularities at the level of retinal pigment epithelium (RPE) in (d) (arrow). The patients showed disease activity at the visit when (b) and (e) were imaged. (b) and (e) show sub-RPE deposits with RPE elevation (arrows); the inner segment–outer segment (IS/OS) is preserved in (b) and almost disappeared in (e). (c) and (f) were taken 2 months later and show further progression of the disease with increased elevation of RPE and near disappearance of IS/OS junction overlying the lesions. The lesions measure 50 μm in with (b) and 120 μm (e).

in vitelliform macular dystrophy [12,64], acute zonal occult outer retinopathy [57], occult macular dystrophy [1], in type 2 idiopathic perifoveal telangiectasia [34], and acute-stage Vogt–Koyanagi–Harada disease [29].

Qualitative assessment of high-resolution OCT images can also help evaluate the integrity of very minute retinal structures such as the PR inner segment/outer segment (IS/OS) junction. Yohannan et al. have evaluated the relationship between retinal sensitivity and the integrity of the IS/OS junction in patients with DME. The authors have performed point-by-point analysis of the IS/OS junction integrity at the 1036 individual points where retinal sensitivity could be assessed using fundus microperimetry (MP). IS/OS junction was found to be intact in 76.5% of the tested points and compromised in 23.5%. The study has revealed that the absence of the IS/OS junction was significantly associated with a 3.28 dB decrease in retinal point sensitivity ($P < 0.001$) [66].

Macular hole (Figure 14.14) represents another retinal disease in which SD-OCT has proved to be of utmost usefulness. The ultrahigh-resolution images of the anteroposterior and tangential VMTs, which are involved in the pathogenesis of idiopathic macular holes, help early identification of impending holes in a way early surgery can be a sight saving. In addition, changes associated with macular holes such as cystoid macular edema and

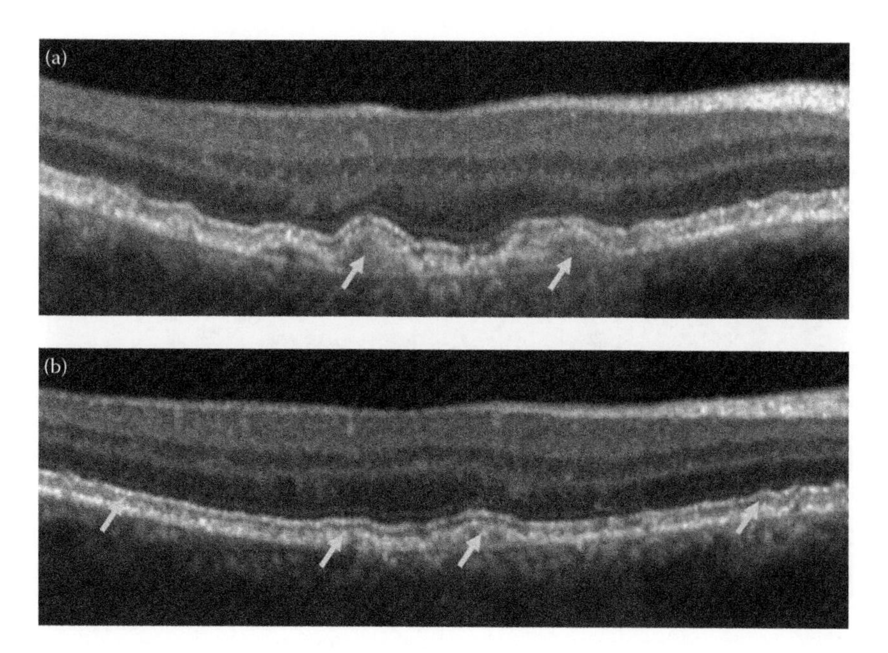

FIGURE 14.13
B-scans (SD-OCT) for retina of two patients with age-related macular degeneration (AMD) (dry type). Focal areas of sub-retinal pigment epithelium (RPE) deposits (arrows in (a)) can be seen pushing the inner segment–outer segment (IS/OS) junction and distorting the REP layer. The focal sub-RPE deposits are termed drusen. Scan (b) demonstrates diffuse sub-RPE deposits. The deposits in such case are called basal laminar drusen. The exact significance of drusen on the long-term prognosis of dry AMD is not very well characterized but thought of as a good biomarker for the development of the disease. The development of SD-OCT may help understand such role in the near future.

disruption of the IS/OS junction can be followed after the surgery to ensure recovery with restoration of IS/OS integrity and resolution if there is intraretinal fluid.

Many case reports are being published every day highlighting potential uses of SD-OCT in evaluation of various retinal diseases and conveying a wealth of new findings that are revolutionizing our understanding of the phagological processes underlying various retinal diseases and strongly impacting the way clinicians diagnose, monitor, and treat various conditions. For example, SD-OCT was used to visualize PR abnormalities in a rare case of cone/rod dystrophy-6 where minute disruptions of IS/OS junction were the hallmark of the disease [31], a rare case of nodular sclerochoroidopathy mimicking choroidal malignancy was reported [20], manifestations of intraocular lymphoma were characterized [39], and a rare case of sclerochoroidal calcifications from patients with hypercalcemia was identified and reported [67].

14.7.3 Quantitative Assessment of Retina

14.7.3.1 OCT-Generated Thickness Maps

Before the introduction of SD-OCT, the only commercially available system was Stratus TD-OCT (Carl Zeiss Meditec, Dublin, CA). To measure retinal thickness, the Stratus OCT systems use a scan protocol called the fast macular scan, which consists of six radial lines centered on the fovea (Figure 14.15) with a total of 768 A-scans to produce a thickness map

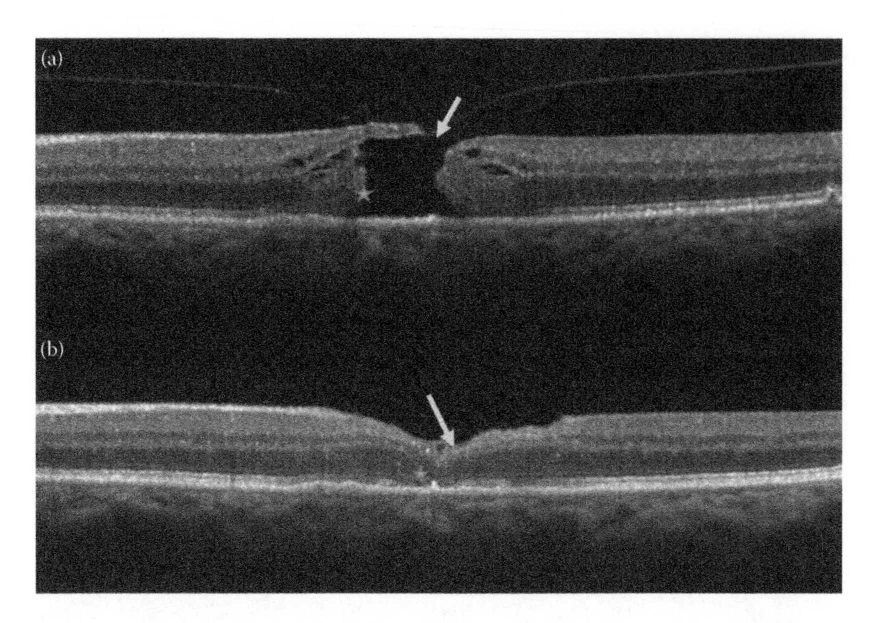

FIGURE 14.14
B-scans (SD-OCT) for retina from a patient with macular hole. Prior to surgery (a), you can see the retinal break (arrow) that was caused by the vitreomacular traction (VMT) with disruption of the integrity of inner segment–outer segment (IS/OS) junction (star). After the surgery (b), the continuity of the retina is restored (arrow) and the IS/OS junction appears to be healing.

with a diameter of 6 mm (27 A-scans/mm^2). The thickness map generated by OCT follows a pattern that was designed by the Early Treatment Diabetic Retinopathy Study (ETDRS) protocols (Figure 14.15). In such scanning protocol, the central macular thickness (CMT) is defined as the mean thickness within the innermost circle of the ETDRS pattern, which has a diameter of 1000 μm. Since the density of measuring points is dependent on the distance from the center, only measurements inside the central 1000 μm diameter area are based on a sufficient number of A-scans (128 A-scans).

The new SD-OCT devices use a rectangular scan pattern that covers adjustable area of the retina. The area of interest is scanned by a series of horizontal or vertical raster scans with variable density (Figure 14.15). Scanning using raster scans rather than radial lines results in a uniform density of A-scans within the scan area. However, the number of A-scans/mm^2 differs considerably between instruments and may be as high as 2000 A-scans/mm^2. In addition to the obvious differences between TD- and SD-OCT devices, different SD-OCT devices have slightly different acquisition protocols and interpolation and segmentation algorithms. Hence, average thickness measurement is expected to be different for different SD-OCT devices. After the introduction SD-OCT, various studies have been published to compare retinal thickness measurements between instruments in healthy eye as well as in disease [19,27,37,61]. Such studies have demonstrated an excellent correlation between the measurements of retinal thickness among various OCT instruments. Despite those high correlations, the retinal thickness was, however, significantly different from one machine to another, with poorer agreement between the TD- and SD-OCT devices. Leung et al. [37] reported the 95% limits of agreement between Stratus and 3D-OCT to be 3.9–37.8 μm. Such poor agreements are considered too large to allow the devices be used interchangeably [14,27,37]. The disagreement of retinal thickness measurements among TD-OCT and SD-OCT technologies are even worse when eyes with retinal

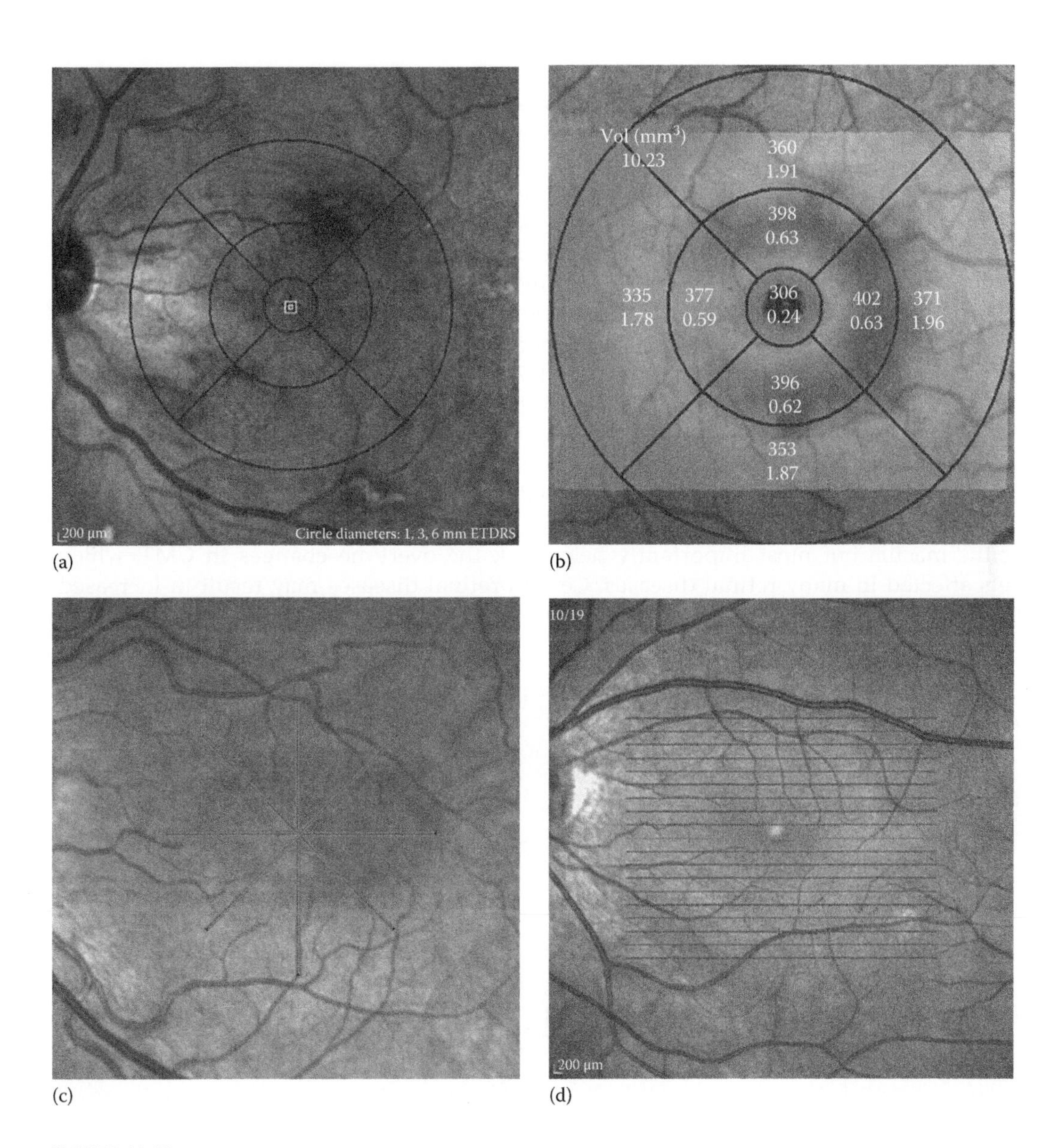

FIGURE 14.15
(See color insert.) Quantitative scan patterns to measure macular thickness. The circles of the early treatment diabetic retinopathy study (ETDRS) grid (a) are 1, 3, and 6 mm in diameter. Thickness map within the central 6 mm of the retina is calculated from the absolute values measured and is presented in a false color scale (b). To calculate the thickness map, TD-OCT uses a scan pattern made of six radial scan lines intersecting at the center of the fovea (c). The average thickness of the areas in between is interpolated from the measurements of the six lines. SD-OCT devices adopted different approach with a scan pattern made of series of horizontal or vertical raster line scans (d).

diseases are compared. In patients with diabetic macular edema (DME), Ibrahim et al. found a mean difference in the CMT values of the 62.5 µm (SE ± 1.2) [27]. Among SD-OCT devices, the disagreements of the CMT values were less pronounced, nevertheless significant. Lammer et al. reported the average difference in thickness measurements between Cirrus and Spectralis SD-OCT to be 19 µm and between Spectralis and 3D OCT to be 55 μm [36]. Several reasons have been identified to cause such discrepancy among measurements; the most notable of which is the different locations of the segmentation lines that are used to calculate retinal thickness. Whereas all instruments agree on the placement of the inner line at the level of the ILM, each instrument had different location for the outer line. For example, Stratus OCT places the posterior (outer) segmentation line along the junction between the inner and outer segments of the retinal PR (IS/OS junction), whereas Spectralis OCT (Spectralis HRA+OCT, Heidelberg Engineering, Vista, CA) places it along the posterior border of the RPE layer. As a result, the Spectralis OCT includes more tissue to the measured thickness as it adds the RPE layer and the outer segments of the PRL. Ibrahim et al. have determined that Spectralis OCT measurements of the CMT can be given by the linear equation $y = (1.029x) + 72.49$, where x is the CMT as measured by the Stratus OCT. The authors has postulated that the intercept in the equation (72.49 μm) can be largely explained by the differences in the measured tissue between both devices, whereas the slope in the equation largely represents the differences in interpolation algorithms and scanning protocols between both devices [27].

OCT thickness maps of the central retina help quickly assess the structural integrity of the macula but most importantly help track the overtime changes in CMT, which gets affected in many retinal diseases. Certain retinal diseases may result in increased thickness such as macular edema (Figure 14.16) and choroidal neovascular membranes

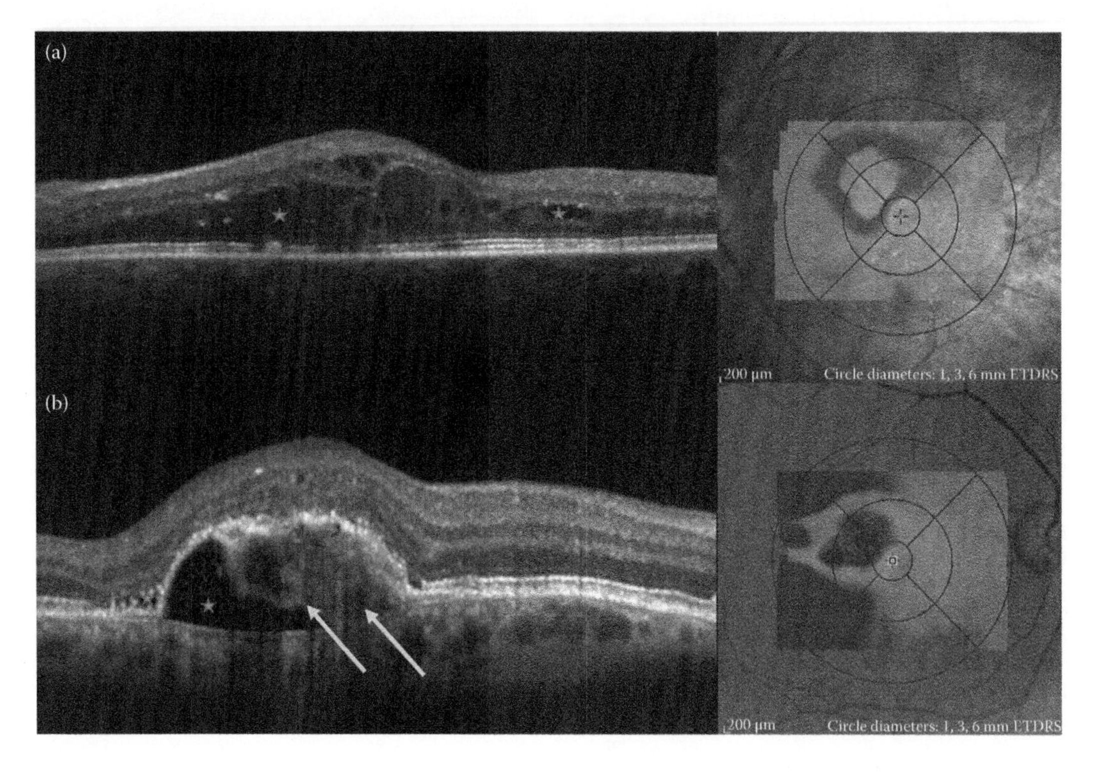

FIGURE 14.16
B-scans and thickness maps of SD-OCT from patients with diabetic macular edema (DME) (a) and neovascular age-related macular degeneration (b). Please note the presence of intraretinal fluid (edema) (stars) that results in increasing the full thickness of the retina as can be noted in the thickness maps to the right of each B scan. Please note, that the images on the right are actually color coded maps. Subretinal neovascular tissue (CNV) can also be observed in (b) (arrows).

(CNVs) (Figure 14.16). Macular edema is a common cause of visual loss. Abnormal fluid accumulation within the retina and a concomitant increase in retinal thickness usually result from the breakdown of the blood–retinal barrier. This process can be found in those with diabetic retinopathy, retinal vein occlusion, uveitis, and active CNV, among others. Traditional methods for evaluating macular edema, such as slit-lamp biomicroscopy, stereoscopic photography, and fluorescein angiography, are relatively insensitive to small changes in retinal thickness and are qualitative at best [37,51].

Exudative macular degeneration (neovascular AMD) is another disease that can cause increased central macular thickness through leaking of fluids into the intraretinal and subretinal spaces and/or through the formation of a neovascular membrane (CNV) that grows underneath the retina adding to the retinal thickness (Figure 14.17). Treatment decisions in exudative AMD usually rely on the presence of fluid accumulation in B-scans, the higher the number of B-scans in 3D scans obtained with SD-OCT,

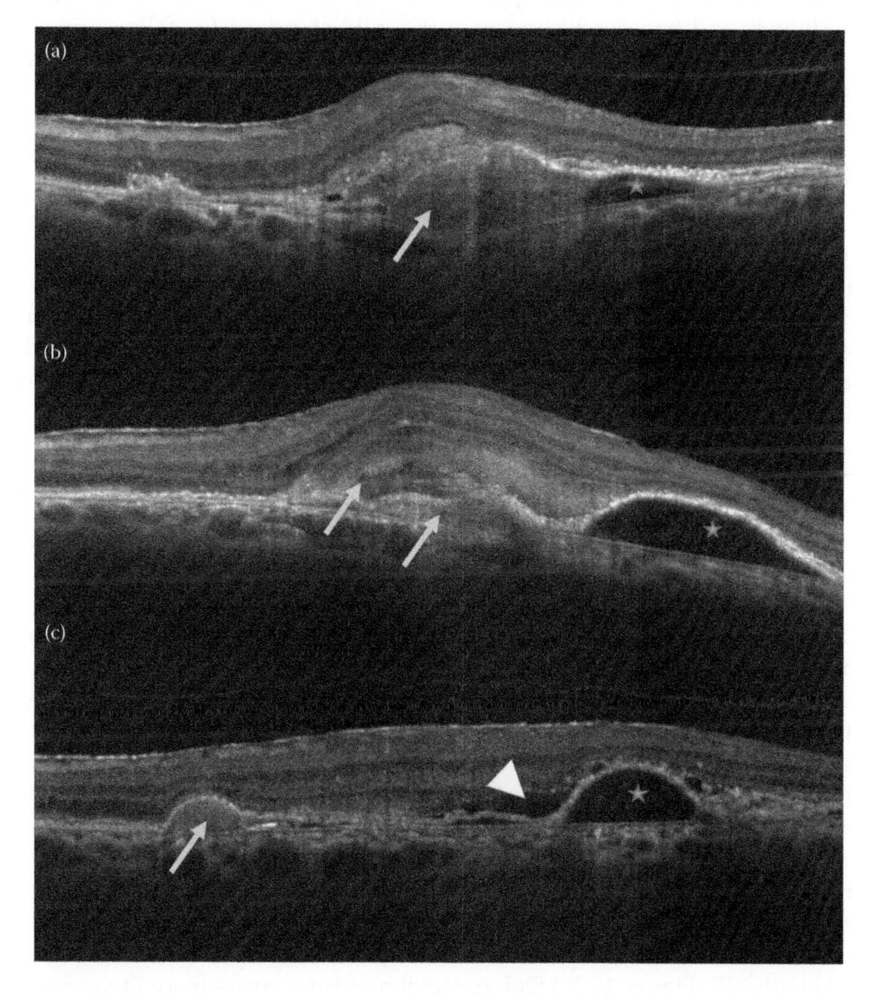

FIGURE 14.17
Series of B-scans of SD-OCT from patient neovascular AMD. Please note the presence of subretinal (stars) and intraretinal (arrowhead) fluid collections that results in increasing the full thickness of the retina. Subretinal neovascular tissue (CNV) can also be observed in all three cuts with variable size (long arrows), which depends on the level of the section.

the higher the chances to detect the presence of intra- and/or subretinal fluid accumulation leading to a higher sensitivity to the disease activity [62]. Nevertheless, quantitative assessment of the disease using CMT and thickness maps is one of the outcome variable in major clinical trials. Correct identification of the posterior segmentation line in such disease category is very difficult and it is more than likely that the automated algorithms of almost all SD-OCT devices misplace such line due to great distortion of the outer retinal layers by the abnormal CNV tissue. Misplacement of the segmentation lines results in erroneous calculation of CMT and in such category of diseases where distortion of either inner or out retinal interface is expected, manual review and correction of segmentation lines are mandatory. Manual correction of segmentation lines can be a daunting and time-consuming task especially in OCT devices that yield as many as 512 raster lines.

The introduction of OCT has enabled clinicians to reliably detect and measure small changes in macular thickness and to quantitatively evaluate the efficacy of different therapeutic modalities and has quickly become the gold standard for follow-up of patients with macular edema. CMT as measured by OCT has become a major outcome variable in almost all clinical trials that are currently undergoing.

14.7.3.2 Quantitative Assessment of Retinal Layers

One of the problems of using CMT as a universal parameter for quantitative assessment of retinal integrity is the fact that retinal thickness varies among normal individuals with a mean 266 μm (SD ± 21 μm) as measured by SD-OCT [27]. With such large range of normal retinal thickness, certain retina can lose up to 80 μm of total thickness before it falls below normal range and, likewise, other retina can gain up to 80 μm of additional thickness before it exceeds the upper boundary of normal CMT. Such fact represents a problem in diseases where the retinal pathology is subtle, symmetric, and/or limited to few layers as is the case in diseases like retinal dystrophies (e.g., retinitis pigmentosa [RP]) and multiple sclerosis (MS). RP is a genetic degenerative disorder that primarily affects the PRs (PRL) and RPE layers. Structural changes in the outer retinal layers in RP patients have not been well investigated *in vivo* because conventional examination such as slit-lamp biomicroscopy and binocular indirect ophthalmoscopy cannot identify those specific changes in details. MS is an immune-mediated disorder of the central nervous system and is the most common nontraumatic cause of neurological disability in early to middle adulthood. The etiology of retinal changes in MS is thought to be secondary to optic nerve demyelination. In such category of diseases, it is important to be able to quantify the thickness of individual retinal layers.

Despite the dire need for a software that automatically allow the segmentation of individual retinal layer, none of the studies that provide such feature currently exist on a commercial level. Researchers, however, have been using semiautomated algorithms to allow such segmentation in laboratory settings.

Ibrahim et al. have used a semiautomated algorithm provided by Heidelberg Engineering Inc., as an add-on feature to the Spectralis OCT software (v5.2) to quantify the thickness of individual retinal layers in normal retina (Figure 14.18), eyes with RP (Figure 14.19), and patients with MS (Figure 14.20) [26]. Individual retinal layers were identified and segmentation lines were drawn along the anterior and posterior borders of the RPE, inner border of OPL, inner border of IPL, and ILM. Placement of the segmentation lines at the aforementioned locations allowed the calculation of average thicknesses of RPE, PRL, BPL, and the combined ganglion cell and NFLs GCL/NFL in 5 mm centered on the fovea

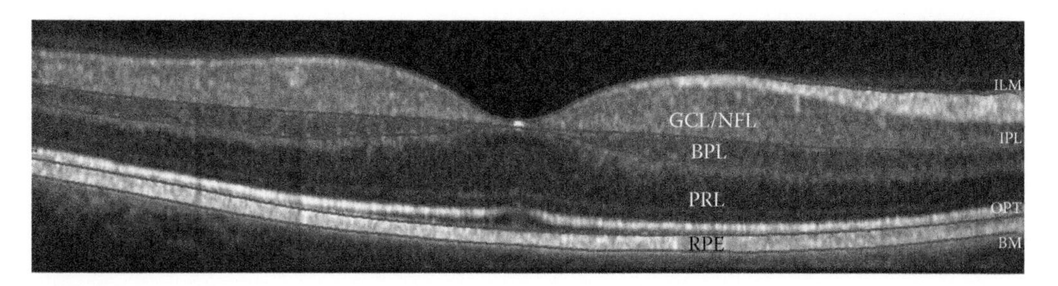

FIGURE 14.18
A horizontal SD-OCT line scan passing through the fovea in a normal eye. Segmentation lines were placed to measure the thickness of retinal pigment epithelium (RPE), photoreceptor layer (PRL), bipolar cell layer (BPL), and ganglion cells/nerve fiber complex (GCL/NFL).

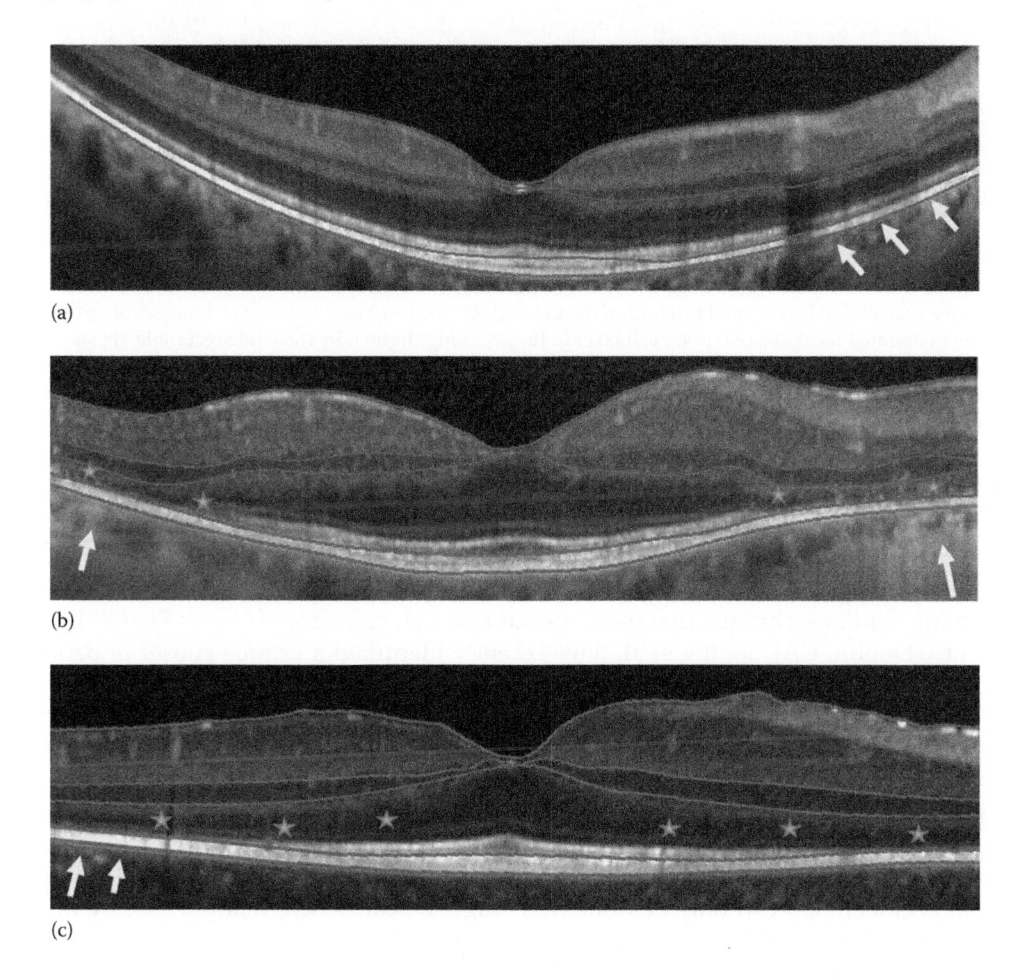

FIGURE 14.19
A horizontal line scan passing through the fovea in patients with retinitis pigmentosa (RP). (a) shows normal full retinal thickness (FRT) in all subfields. Analysis of individual layers, however, demonstrated focal loss of retinal pigment epithelium (RPE) nasal field (arrows). (b) shows significant focal thinning of FRT at peripheral subfields. Segmentations demonstrates severe thinning of the photoreceptor layer (PRL) and RPE layer in other fields where FRT is normal. (c) shows significant focal thinning of FRT in the peripheral temporal subfield (arrows). PRL however showed widespread severe thinning in areas where FRT was normal.

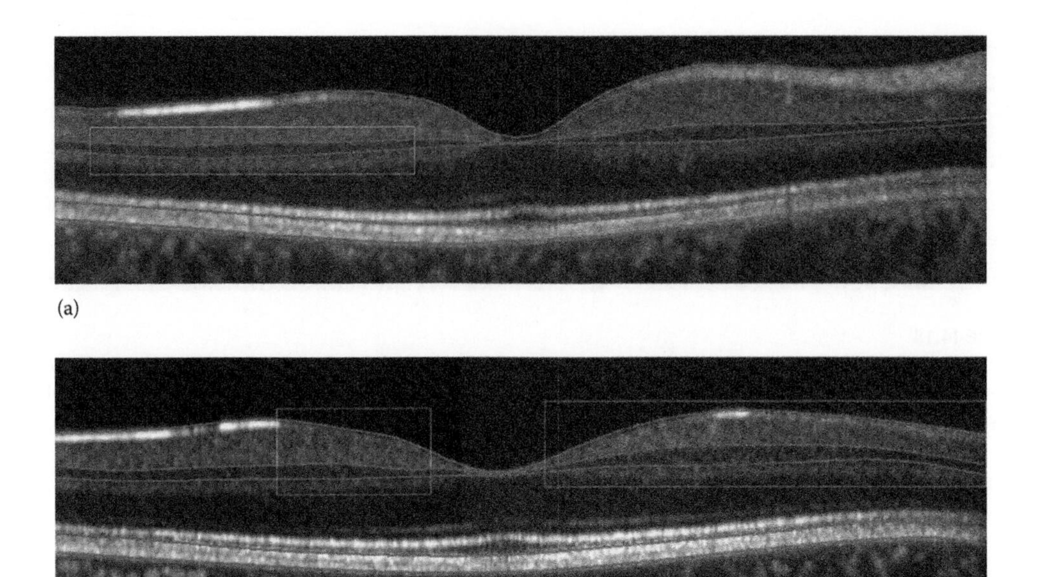

FIGURE 14.20
A horizontal line scan passing through the fovea in patients with multiple sclerosis (MS). (a) shows an OCT scan from a patient that had normal full retinal thickness (FRT) in all subfields. However, analysis of individual layers demonstrated focal loss of bipolar cell layer in the areas highlighted by the white rectangle. (b) shows an OCT scan from a patient with MS that has significant thinning of the overall retinal thickness (2.4–3.6 SD below normal). The loss of retinal tissue was exclusive to the ganglion cell and nerve fiber layers complex (GCL/NFL) with all other retinal layer within the range of normal thickness in all subfields.

[26]. In patients with RP, Ibrahim et al. have demonstrated significant thinning of PR and RPE layer in various subfields in all patients despite the fact that 52% of patients had normal full retinal thickness (FRT) in the central 5 mm of the retina. Patients with MS have demonstrated significant thinning in GCL/RNFL layer and in 53% of the study sample. Employing similar technique that used special research software of Cirrus SD-OCT (Carl Zeiss Ltd. Dublin, CA), Saidha et al. have recently identified a unique subset of patients with MS in whom there appears to be disproportionate thinning of the inner and ONLs [47]. In a case report using similar technique to that of Saidha et al., Oh et al. have reported *in vivo* demonstration of homonymous hemimacular loss of retinal ganglion cells after a thalamic lesion [43].

Segmentation of retinal layers can be of tremendous value for both researchers and retina clinicians. However, manual segmentation has many drawbacks that render its regular use for diagnosis and monitoring of retinal diseases an impractical notion. For example, manual segmentation can only be done in a single B-scan where manual placing of the segmentation lines would not consume valuable time. However, doing the same on a scan that has 512 raster lines, such as the case in some of SD-OCT scanning protocols, or even in a scan that has 25 raster lines, like the default scanning protocol in the Heidelberg Spectralis, would not be time efficient for clinic patients or clinical trials that have thousands of OCT scans. Automatic segmentation, on the other hand, is facing significant difficulties in developing algorithms that would accurately identify the interfaces between various retinal layers in normal as well as pathological retina.

14.8 Developments and Future Directions

Several developments have been considered and suggested for OCT technique and instrumentation in order to improve the results. Among these are attempts to increase depth and axial resolution, find better choices of emission wavelengths for choroid imaging, and develop several processing algorithms that would allow more accurate placement of segmentation lines and autosegmentation of individual retinal layers.

Faster scanning techniques, especially SS-OCT, have been an exciting topic of research recently owing to the high speed of acquisition that can be achieved using this technique [46]. The ability to scan deeper ocular structures is also another field of research interest. Most of the research in this arena is trying to achieve deeper penetration of ocular tissue through using different light sources with longer wavelengths that are closer to the near infrared spectrum while avoiding absorption by the ocular structures such as aqueous and vitreous humor. A wavelength of 1040 nm has been suggested to be a good fit toward that goal [58]. Other methods included the utilization of one-micron adaptive optics OCT for simultaneous high-resolution retinal imaging and high-penetration choroidal imaging [35]. Other trials rely on enhanced depth imaging techniques using current OCT setups to achieve adequate penetration to scan deeper ocular structures [3,28,55,63,67]. EDI is a technique that is developed by Spaide et al. and achieves deeper penetration of the ocular tissue through moving the OCT scanning head to a position where the light beam incident on the deeper ocular structures lies in a plane where $OPD = 0$ [52].

Finally, the ability to scan wider areas of the retina within reasonable time is also one of the future directions for OCT technology. Needless to say, such ability relies largely on the scanning speeds. Toward that direction, Klein et al. and Neubauer et al. have been able in 2011 to obtain OCT scans covering 70° field of view (regular OCT obtain as large as 20°) in as little as 3 s duration using SS-OCT [32,42].

OCT technology has certainly revolutionized diagnostic and monitoring approaches for retinal diseases. As advancements and developments continue to occur, it is most likely that the spectrum of OCT use will remain protean, allowing the clinicians to obtain additional information about ocular structures in a more efficient condition and providing the patients with the best possible management.

References

1. Brockhurst, R. J. and M. A. Sandberg (2007). Optical coherence tomography findings in occult macular dystrophy. *Am J Ophthalmol* **143**(3): 516–518.
2. Channa, R., M. Ibrahim, Y. Sepah, P. Turkcuoglu, J. H. Lee, A. Khwaja, E. Hatef, M. Bittencourt, J. Heo, D. V. Do, and Q. D. Nguyen (2012). Characterization of macular lesions in punctate inner choroidopathy with spectral domain optical coherence tomography. *J Ophthalmic Inflamm Infect* **2**(3): 113–120.
3. Chhablani, J., G. Barteselli, H. Wang, S. El-Emam, I. Kozak, A. L. Doede, D. U. Bartsch, L. Cheng, and W. R. Freeman (2012). Repeatability and reproducibility of manual choroidal volume measurements using enhanced depth imaging optical coherence tomography. *Invest Ophthalmol Vis Sci* **53**(4): 2274–2280.

4. Chinn, S. R., E. A. Swanson, and J. G. Fujimoto (1997). Optical coherence tomography using a frequency-tunable optical source. *Opt Lett* **22**(5): 340–342.
5. Choma, M., M. Sarunic, C. Yang, and J. Izatt (2003). Sensitivity advantage of swept source and Fourier domain optical coherence tomography. *Opt Express* **11**(18): 2183–2189.
6. Do, D. V., M. Cho, Q. D. Nguyen, S. M. Shah, J. T. Handa, P. A. Campochiaro, I. Zimmer-Galler, J. U. Sung, and J. A. Haller (2007). Impact of optical coherence tomography on surgical decision making for epiretinal membranes and vitreomacular traction. *Retina* **27**(5): 552–556.
7. Drexler, W., U. Morgner, R. K. Ghanta, F. X. Kartner, J. S. Schuman, and J. G. Fujimoto (2001). Ultrahigh-resolution ophthalmic optical coherence tomography. *Nat Med* **7**(4): 502–507.
8. Drexler, W., U. Morgner, F. X. Kartner, C. Pitris, S. A. Boppart, X. D. Li, E. P. Ippen, and J. G. Fujimoto (1999). In vivo ultrahigh-resolution optical coherence tomography. *Opt Lett* **24**(17): 1221–1223.
9. Dubois, A., G. Moneron, K. Grieve, and A. C. Boccara (2004). Three-dimensional cellular-level imaging using full-field optical coherence tomography. *Phys Med Biol* **49**(7): 1227.
10. Fercher, A. F., C. K. Hitzenberger, G. Kamp, and S. Y. El-Zaiat (1995). Measurement of intraocular distances by backscattering spectral interferometry. *Opt Commun* **117**(1–2): 43–48.
11. Fercher, A. F., K. Mengedoht, and W. Werner (1988). Eye-length measurement by interferometry with partially coherent light. *Opt Lett* **13**(3): 186–188.
12. Finger, R. P., P. Charbel Issa, U. Kellner, S. Schmitz-Valckenberg, M. Fleckenstein, H. P. Scholl, and F. G. Holz (2010). Spectral domain optical coherence tomography in adult-onset vitelliform macular dystrophy with cuticular drusen. *Retina* **30**(9): 1455–1464.
13. Flournoy, P. A., R. W. McClure, and G. Wyntjes (1972). White-light interferometric thickness gauge. *Appl Opt* **11**(9): 1907–1915.
14. Forooghian, F., C. Cukras, C. B. Meyerle, E. Y. Chew, and W. T. Wong (2008). Evaluation of time domain and spectral domain optical coherence tomography in the measurement of diabetic macular edema. *Invest Ophthalmol Vis Sci* **49**(10): 4290–4296.
15. Fujimoto, J. G. (2003). Optical coherence tomography for ultrahigh resolution in vivo imaging. *Nat Biotechnol* **21**(11): 1361–1367.
16. Fujimoto, J. G. (2003). Optical coherence tomography: Principles and applications. *Rev Laser Eng* **31**(10): 635–642.
17. Golubovic, B., B. E. Bouma, G. J. Tearney, and J. G. Fujimoto (1997). Optical frequency-domain reflectometry using rapid wavelength tuning of a Cr4+:forsterite laser. *Opt Lett* **22**(22): 1704–1706.
18. Gregori, N. Z., B. L. Lam, G. Gregori, S. Ranganathan, E. M. Stone, A. Morante, F. Abukhalil, and P. R. Aroucha (2013). Wide-field spectral-domain optical coherence tomography in patients and carriers of X-linked retinoschisis. *Ophthalmology* **120**(1): 169–174.
19. Hatef, E., A. Khwaja, Z. Rentiya, M. Ibrahim, M. Shulman, P. Turkcuoglu, Y. Sepah et al. (2012). Comparison of time domain and spectral domain optical coherence tomography in measurement of macular thickness in macular edema secondary to diabetic retinopathy and retinal vein occlusion. *J Ophthalmol* **2012**: 354783.
20. Hatef, E., J. Wang, M. Ibrahim, P. Turkcuoglu, A. Khwaja, R. Channa, E. P. Suan, C. Dibernado, Y. J. Sepah, D. V. Do, and Q. D. Nguyen (2010). Nodular sclerochoroidopathy simulating choroidal malignancy. *Ophthalmic Surg Lasers Imaging* **41**(Online): e1–e5.
21. Hee, M. R., J. A. Izatt, E. A. Swanson, D. Huang, J. S. Schuman, C. P. Lin, C. A. Puliafito, and J. G. Fujimoto (1995). Optical coherence tomography of the human retina. *Arch Ophthalmol* **113**(3): 325–332.
22. Hitzenberger, C., P. Trost, P. W. Lo, and Q. Zhou (2003). Three-dimensional imaging of the human retina by high-speed optical coherence tomography. *Opt Express* **11**(21): 2753–2761.
23. Howland, H. C. and B. Howland (1977). A subjective method for the measurement of monochromatic aberrations of the eye. *J Opt Soc Am* **67**(11): 1508–1518.
24. Hu, Z., Y. Pan, and A. M. Rollins (2007). Analytical model of spectrometer-based two-beam spectral interferometry. *Appl Opt* **46**(35): 8499–8505.
25. Huang, D., E. A. Swanson, C. P. Lin, J. S. Schuman, W. G. Stinson, W. Chang, M. R. Hee et al. (1991). Optical coherence tomography. *Science* **254**(5035): 1178–1181.

26. Ibrahim, M. A., A. K. Bittner, M. G. Bittencourt, Y. J. Sepah, D. V. Do, and Q. D. Nguyen (2012). Segmentation of retinal layers in normal eyes, eyes with retinitis pigmentosa, and eyes of patients with multiple sclerosis. *ARVO Meet Abstr* **53**(6): 4095.
27. Ibrahim, M. A., Y. J. Sepah, R. C. Symons, R. Channa, E. Hatef, A. Khwaja, M. Bittencourt, J. Heo, D. V. Do, and Q. D. Nguyen (2012). Spectral- and time-domain optical coherence tomography measurements of macular thickness in normal eyes and in eyes with diabetic macular edema. *Eye (Lond)* **26**(3): 454–462.
28. Ikuno, Y., I. Maruko, Y. Yasuno, M. Miura, T. Sekiryu, K. Nishida, and T. Iida (2011). Reproducibility of retinal and choroidal thickness measurements in enhanced depth imaging and high-penetration optical coherence tomography. *Invest Ophthalmol Vis Sci* **52**(8): 5536–5540.
29. Ishihara, K., M. Hangai, M. Kita, and N. Yoshimura (2009). Acute Vogt-Koyanagi-Harada disease in enhanced spectral-domain optical coherence tomography. *Ophthalmology* **116**(9): 1799–1807.
30. Kellner, U., S. Kellner, and S. Weinitz (2008). Chloroquine retinopathy: Lipofuscin- and melanin-related fundus autofluorescence, optical coherence tomography and multifocal electroretinography. *Doc Ophthalmol* **116**(2): 119–127.
31. Kim, B. J., M. A. Ibrahim, and M. F. Goldberg (2011). Use of spectral domain OCT to visualize photoreceptor abnormalities in cone/rod dystrophy-6. *Retin Cases Brief Rep* **5**(1): 56–61.
32. Klein, T., L. Reznicek, W. Wieser, C. M. Eigenwillig, B. Biedermann, A. Kampik, R. Huber, and A. S. Neubauer (2011). Extraction of arbitrary OCT scan paths from 3D ultra high-speed ultra wide-field swept source OCT. *ARVO Meet Abstr* **52**(6): 1328.
33. Klein, T., W. Wieser, C. M. Eigenwillig, B. R. Biedermann, and R. Huber (2011). Megahertz OCT for ultrawide-field retinal imaging with a 1050 nm Fourier domain mode-locked laser. *Opt Express* **19**(4): 3044–3062.
34. Krivosic, V., R. Tadayoni, P. Massin, A. Erginay, and A. Gaudric (2009). Spectral domain optical coherence tomography in type 2 idiopathic perifoveal telangiectasia. *Ophthalmic Surg Lasers Imaging* **40**(4): 379–384.
35. Kurokawa, K., K. Sasaki, S. Makita, M. Yamanari, B. Cense, and Y. Yasuno (2010). Simultaneous high-resolution retinal imaging and high-penetration choroidal imaging by one-micrometer adaptive optics optical coherence tomography. *Opt Express* **18**(8): 8515–8527.
36. Lammer, J., C. Scholda, C. Prunte, T. Benesch, U. Schmidt-Erfurth, and M. Bolz (2011). Retinal thickness and volume measurements in diabetic macular edema: A comparison of four optical coherence tomography systems. *Retina* **31**(1): 48–55.
37. Leung, C. K., C. Y. Cheung, R. N. Weinreb, G. Lee, D. Lin, C. P. Pang, and D. S. Lam (2008). Comparison of macular thickness measurements between time domain and spectral domain optical coherence tomography. *Invest Ophthalmol Vis Sci* **49**(11): 4893–4897.
38. Lexer, F., C. K. Hitzenberger, A. F. Fercher, and M. Kulhavy (1997). Wavelength-tuning interferometry of intraocular distances. *Appl Opt* **36**(25): 6548 6553.
39. Liu, T., M. Ibrahim, M. Bittencourt, Y. Sepah, D. Do, and Q. Nguyen (2012). Retinal optical coherence tomography manifestations of intraocular lymphoma. *J Ophthalmic Inflamm Infect* **2**(4): 215–218.
40. Mohammad, S., I. Gottlob, A. Kumar, M. Thomas, C. Degg, V. Sheth, and F. A. Proudlock (2011). The functional significance of foveal abnormalities in albinism measured using spectral-domain optical coherence tomography. *Ophthalmology* **118**(8): 1645–1652.
41. Mundt, G. H., Jr. and W. F. Hughes, Jr. (1956). Ultrasonics in ocular diagnosis. *Am J Ophthalmol* **41**(3): 488–498.
42. Neubauer, A. S., L. Reznicek, T. Klein, W. Wieser, C. M. Eigenwillig, B. Biedermann, A. Kampik, and R. Huber (2011). Ultra high-speed ultrawide field swept source OCT reconstructed fundus image quality. *ARVO Meet Abstr* **52**(6): 1327.
43. Oh, J., E. S. Sotirchos, S. Saidha, M. Ibrahim, Y. Sepah, Q. D. Nguyen, and P. A. Calabresi (2013). In vivo demonstration of homonymous hemimacular loss of retinal ganglion cells due to a thalamic lesion using optical coherence tomography. *JAMA Neurol* **70**(3): 410–411.

44. Podoleanu, A., J. Rogers, D. Jackson, and S. Dunne (2000). Three dimensional OCT images from retina and skin. *Opt Express* **7**(9): 292–298.
45. Podoleanu, A. G. (2012). Optical coherence tomography. *J Microsc* **247**(3): 209–219.
46. Potsaid, B., B. Baumann, D. Huang, S. Barry, A. E. Cable, J. S. Schuman, J. S. Duker, and J. G. Fujimoto (2010). Ultrahigh speed 1050 nm swept source/Fourier domain OCT retinal and anterior segment imaging at 100,000 to 400,000 axial scans per second. *Opt Express* **18**(19): 20029–20048.
47. Saidha, S., E. S. Sotirchos, M. A. Ibrahim, C. M. Crainiceanu, J. M. Gelfand, Y. J. Sepah, J. N. Ratchford et al. (2012). Microcystic macular oedema, thickness of the inner nuclear layer of the retina, and disease characteristics in multiple sclerosis: A retrospective study. *Lancet Neurol* **11**(11): 963–972.
48. Schmidt-Erfurth, U., R. A. Leitgeb, S. Michels, B. Povazay, S. Sacu, B. Hermann, C. Ahlers, H. Sattmann, C. Scholda, A. F. Fercher, and W. Drexler (2005). Three-dimensional ultrahigh-resolution optical coherence tomography of macular diseases. *Invest Ophthalmol Vis Sci* **46**(9): 3393–3402.
49. Seo, J. H., Y. S. Yu, J. H. Kim, H. K. Choung, J. W. Heo, and S. J. Kim (2007). Correlation of visual acuity with foveal hypoplasia grading by optical coherence tomography in albinism. *Ophthalmology* **114**(8): 1547–1551.
50. Serranho, P., A. M. Morgado, and R. Bernardes (2012). Optical coherence tomography: A concept review. In *Optical Coherence Tomography*, R. Bernardes and J. Cunha-Vaz, eds., Springer, Berlin, Germany, pp. 139–156.
51. Shahidi, M., Y. Ogura, N. P. Blair, M. M. Rusin, and R. Zeimer (1991). Retinal thickness analysis for quantitative assessment of diabetic macular edema. *Arch Ophthalmol* **109**(8): 1115–1119.
52. Spaide, R. F., H. Koizumi, and M. C. Pozonni (2008). Enhanced depth imaging spectral-domain optical coherence tomography. *Am J Ophthalmol* **146**(4): 496–500.
53. Swanson, E. A., J. A. Izatt, M. R. Hee, D. Huang, C. P. Lin, J. S. Schuman, C. A. Puliafito, and J. G. Fujimoto (1993). In vivo retinal imaging by optical coherence tomography. *Opt Lett* **18**(21): 1864–1866.
54. Thrane, L., H. T. Yura, and P. E. Andersen (2000). Analysis of optical coherence tomography systems based on the extended Huygens? Fresnel principle. *J Opt Soc Am A* **17**(3): 484–490.
55. Tian, J., P. Marziliano, M. Baskaran, T. A. Tun, and T. Aung (2013). Automatic segmentation of the choroid in enhanced depth imaging optical coherence tomography images. *Biomed Opt Express* **4**(3): 397–411.
56. Tomlins, P. H. and R. K. Wang (2005). Theory, developments and applications of optical coherence tomography. *J Phys D Appl Phys* **38**(15): 2519.
57. Tsunoda, K., K. Fujinami, and Y. Miyake (2011). Selective abnormality of cone outer segment tip line in acute zonal occult outer retinopathy as observed by spectral-domain optical coherence tomography. *Arch Ophthalmol* **129**(8): 1099–1101.
58. Unterhuber, A., B. Povazay, B. Hermann, H. Sattmann, A. Chavez-Pirson, and W. Drexler (2005). In vivo retinal optical coherence tomography at 1040 nm—Enhanced penetration into the choroid. *Opt Express* **13**(9): 3252.
59. Wieser, W., B. R. Biedermann, T. Klein, C. M. Eigenwillig, and R. Huber (2010). Multi-megahertz OCT: High quality 3D imaging at 20 million A-scans and 4.5 GVoxels per second. *Opt Express* **18**(14): 14685–14704.
60. Wojtkowski, M., R. Leitgeb, A. Kowalczyk, T. Bajraszewski, and A. F. Fercher (2002). In vivo human retinal imaging by Fourier domain optical coherence tomography. *J Biomed Opt* **7**(3): 457–463.
61. Wolf-Schnurrbusch, U. E., L. Ceklic, C. K. Brinkmann, M. E. Iliev, M. Frey, S. P. Rothenbuehler, V. Enzmann, and S. Wolf (2009). Macular thickness measurements in healthy eyes using six different optical coherence tomography instruments. *Invest Ophthalmol Vis Sci* **50**(7): 3432–3437.
62. Wolf, S. and U. Wolf-Schnurrbusch (2010). Spectral-domain optical coherence tomography use in macular diseases: A review. *Ophthalmologica* **224**(6): 333–340.

63. Wong, I. Y., H. Koizumi and W. W. Lai (2011). Enhanced depth imaging optical coherence tomography. *Ophthalmic Surg Lasers Imaging* **42**(Suppl.): S75–S84.
64. Xu, H., L. Ying, P. Lin, and J. Wu (2013). Optical coherence tomography for multifocal vitelliform macular dystrophy. *Optom Vis Sci* **90**(1): 94–99.
65. Yi, K., M. Mujat, B. H. Park, W. Sun, J. W. Miller, J. M. Seddon, L. H. Young, J. F. de Boer, and T. C. Chen (2009). Spectral domain optical coherence tomography for quantitative evaluation of drusen and associated structural changes in non-neovascular age-related macular degeneration. *Br J Ophthalmol* **93**(2): 176–181.
66. Yohannan, J., M. Bittencourt, Y. J. Sepah, E. Hatef, R. Sophie, A. Moradi, H. Liu, M. Ibrahim, D. V. Do, E. Coulantuoni, and Q. D. Nguyen (2013). Association of retinal sensitivity to integrity of photoreceptor inner/outer segment junction in patients with diabetic macular edema. *Ophthalmology* **120**(6): 1254–1261.
67. Yohannan, J., R. Channa, C. W. Dibernardo, I. E. Zimmer-Galler, M. Ibrahim, Y. J. Sepah, M. Bittencourt, D. V. Do, and Q. D. Nguyen (2012). Sclerochoroidal calcifications imaged using enhanced depth imaging optical coherence tomography. *Ocul Immunol Inflamm* **20**(3): 190–192.
68. Yu, J., Y. Ni, P. A. Keane, C. Jiang, W. Wang, and G. Xu (2010). Foveomacular schisis in juvenile X-linked retinoschisis: An optical coherence tomography study. *Am J Ophthalmol* **149**(6): 973–978 e972.

15

Role of Optical Coherence Tomography in Anterior Segment Imaging

Tin Aung Tun, Sze-Yee Lee, Rachel Nge, and Louis Tong

CONTENTS

15.1 Introduction

Optical coherence tomography (OCT) is a noncontact and noninvasive investigation for in vivo imaging of the ocular tissues at a microscopic level. Measurements at micrometer scale and visualization of structures in the anterior eye are required in the study of the pathophysiology of anterior eye diseases and therapies. OCT is widely used nowadays and has evolved from time domain to Fourier domain recently. Soon after the introduction of the use of OCT in retinal imaging in 1991, Izatt et al. reported that OCT is capable of the imaging of the cornea and anterior segment (anterior segment OCT [AS-OCT]). OCT has become a powerful tool to assist in the diagnosis of various ocular diseases [26,29].

In order to produce 2D images of biological tissues in a way that is analogous to ultrasound biomicroscopy, OCT uses low-coherence interferometry that compares the echo time delay and intensity of the reflected and backscattering light from a sample and a reference mirror to determine the longitudinal depth of the sample. OCT uses two infrared wavelengths—840 and 1310 nm, mainly—but studies at 1050 nm were demonstrated recently [60]. For anterior segment imaging, a wavelength of 840 nm provides higher resolution, while 1310 nm gives better penetration due to lesser backscattering effect of light at longer wavelength. Therefore, 840 nm produces better results for corneal imaging with higher resolution, while 1310 nm is used for anterior chamber biometry and angle assessment with higher depth imaging.

In the time domain system, an optical signal is produced from a superluminescent diode to a sample in one interferometer arm and a reference mirror that is varying in the other arm. Due to the mechanical movement of the reference mirror, time domain systems have a limited speed (maximum 2000 A-scans per second). Visante AS-OCT (Carl Zeiss Meditec, Dublin, CA), slit lamp-mounted AS-OCT and, slit lamp OCT (SL-OCT) (Heidelberg Engineering, GmbH, Dossenheim, Germany) are commercially available time domain OCTs.

The basic principle of Fourier domain systems is similar to time domain. Fourier domain system uses a fixed reference plane, whereas time domain system does not. The spectrometer detects the signals from the sample and reference mirror. The axial depth of tissue is measured by Fourier transformation of the interference spectrum data and Fourier domains have a faster scan speed (≥20,000 A-scans per second) compared to time domains. A few Fourier/spectral domain OCTs in the market are available to image the anterior segment with the aid of an external adaptor. RTVue OCT (Optovue, Fremont, CA) and Cirrus HD-OCT (Carl Zeiss Meditec, Dublin, CA) are widely used for anterior segment imaging.

Another form of Fourier domain OCT is the swept source OCT that uses a monochromatic tunable fast-scanning laser source and a photodetector for the receiving of wavelength-resolved interference signals. The CASIA (Tomey, Nagoya, Japan) is a commercially available swept source OCT used for anterior segment imaging [40]. By increasing the signal/noise ratio combined with high-speed scanning, Fourier domains are able to reduce motion artifacts and produce high-quality images. The specifications of commercially available AS-OCTs are mentioned in Table 15.1.

In this section, we will introduce the clinical and research applications of OCT to understand anatomical structures and function of an anterior segment of the eye. We will cover the usage of AS-OCT in corneal and glaucoma imaging by explaining the pathophysiology of the diseases or conditions and the usefulness of AS-OCT in these conditions.

15.2 Corneal Imaging

The cornea is the transparent tissue at the anterior eye that provides two-thirds of the refractive power required for clear vision. Its transparency is crucial in maintaining vision; therefore, the cornea possesses several features to ensure it retains its function [33].

TABLE 15.1

Comparison of Commercially Available AS-OCTs

	Time Domain OCTs		**Fourier Domain OCTs**		
	Visante OCT	**SL-OCT**	**Cirrus HD-OCT**	**RTVue FD-OCT**	**CASIA SS-OCT**
Manufacturer	Carl Zeiss Meditec	Heidelberg Engineering	Carl Zeiss Meditec	Optovue	Tomey
Wavelength of light source	1,310 nm	1,310 nm	840 nm	840 nm	1,310 nm
Axial resolution	18 μm	<25 μm	5 μm	5 μm	<10 μm
Scan length	16 mm (LD) 8 mm (HD)	15 mm	3 mm	6 mm (CAM-L) 3 mm (CAM-S)	16 mm (LD) 8 mm (HD)
Image acquisition speed	2,000 A-scans per second	200 A-scans per second	27,000 A-scans per second	26,000 A-scans per second	30,000 A-scans per second

Note: LD, low density; HD, high density; CAM-S, cornea anterior module—short; CAM-L, cornea anterior module—long.

However, in diseases where the cornea is implicated, its transparency may decrease. Regularity of the tears and corneal surface may also be significantly affected, while changes in corneal curvature will alter the refractive power.

The cornea is made up of five layers: (from the most superficial) the epithelium, Bowman's membrane, stroma, Descemet's membrane, and the endothelium.

The epithelium works closely with the precorneal tear film. Together, they primarily serve two functions: (1) acting as a protective barrier against external insults' penetration to deeper layers and (2) forming a smooth optical surface for the refraction of light entering the eye [11]. The epithelium itself has several layers of cells, with the deepest layer (the basal cells) constantly multiplying and migrating outward to become the wing cells and then the outermost superficial cells. Therefore, fresh cells can be produced to replace the outer layers of the epithelium when it is damaged.

The Bowman's membrane separates the epithelium from the stroma, which forms 90% of the entire corneal thickness. The stroma is made up of approximately 200 layers of collagen fibrils. The same type of collagen fibers can be found in the sclera; however, the regular arrangement of these collagen fibers in the corneal stroma gives it its transparency. In diseases of the stroma, such as keratoconus and stromal dystrophies, the arrangement of collagen fibrils has been disrupted. Corneal thinning or swelling can occur as a result of the disorganized fibers and affects both its transparency and optical refractive power.

The Descemet's membrane separates the stroma and endothelium. It is secreted by the single layer of endothelial cells to allow the latter's adherence to the cornea. The endothelium actively maintains the relative dehydration of the stroma. In cases where the Descemet's membrane and endothelium are detached or diseased, usually due to mechanical forces during ocular surgery, excess fluid enters into the stroma and causes corneal edema (swelling of the cornea; Section 15.2.1) [54].

The conventional method of corneal examination is with slit lamp biomicroscopy, a readily available instrument that all eye care practitioners have in their practice. However, the relatively low magnification of slit lamp biomicroscopy (most only up to 40×) may make it challenging to detect minute changes in corneal thickness and curvature. The high magnification and resolution of AS-OCT allow not just a closer look at the cornea but also a larger field of view than that of slit lamp biomicroscopy with the same magnification.

The cross-sectional images produced by AS-OCT also enable clinicians to detect corneal morphology changes easily. In addition, visible light emitted by the slit lamp may be irritating to the patient at the brightness level necessary to examine the corneal layers. OCT utilizes wavelengths not visible to the human eye and therefore eliminates this problem.

Mapping of the corneal curvature and thickness through the entire cornea without contact makes it a convenient modality for use in the clinic and in research. The quality of AS-OCT images is hardly affected by corneal opacities such as scars or excessive inflammatory cells. Such opacities would have hindered the observer's view through a slit lamp biomicroscope [31]. Diagnosis and monitoring of corneal diseases can be simplified with AS-OCT imaging. The newer models possess resolutions high enough to even differentiate the various corneal layers. AS-OCT imaging in corneal diseases will be further discussed in Section 15.2.2.

15.2.1 Corneal Thickness Measurement

Corneal edema is the swelling of the cornea. Like the swelling in other parts of the body, it is a clinical manifestation of an underlying condition such as inflammation in response to infection, ocular surgeries, and an endothelial or Descemet's membrane defect. Endothelial diseases such as Fuchs' endothelial dystrophy and increased acidosis of the cornea due to contact lens wear also cause corneal edema [14,25,69].

Small magnitudes of corneal edema usually do not cause any symptoms or give rise to any clinical signs. However, when the swelling is sufficiently heightened, corneal edema can be detected as a slight decrease in corneal transparency or folds and striae in the stroma. Unfortunately, these signs are extremely subtle and easily missed. The increase in corneal thickness during edema is also tricky to detect as the change is usually not apparent on slit lamp biomicroscopy.

Corneal ultrasound pachymetry is currently the most used method and arguably the gold standard for measuring corneal thickness [59]. However, this method requires the instillation of local anesthesia and the contact between a probe and the cornea, which may cause some discomfort for the patient. In addition, the region of the cornea measured is dependent on the operator's positioning of the probe, which is done manually, giving a higher chance of error.

Mapping the corneal thickness using AS-OCT has been extensively studied. Most studies agreed that this method is highly repeatable and reproducible, with negligible inter-examiner variability. The sole measurement of the epithelium thickness is also possible [28,41,49,78]. In addition, no contact between the scanning device and the cornea is necessary unlike ultrasound pachymetry.

A good correlation between AS-OCT corneal thickness measurements and the ultrasound methods has been reported, further supporting its use over ultrasound due to the relative convenience of the former. However, although correlated, an agreement between the raw values of measurements is not fully established. Different methods of measurements therefore should not be used interchangeably [41,59,99].

Wolf et al. reported that normal corneas can range in thickness from 427 to 620 μm (mean of 537 μm). The assessment of corneal thickness is not only vital to determine the presence of corneal edema. Corneal thickness directly affects the measurement of the intraocular pressure (IOP), which is one of the parameters measured for the evaluation of glaucoma (Section 15.3). The normal IOP is in the range of 10–21 mmHg. However, IOP measurements will be underestimated in thinner corneas and overestimated in thicker ones. Studies have estimated that for every 10 μm of corneal thickness, the IOP will be recorded as 0.3–1.0 mmHg higher than the actual pressure, depending on the method of IOP measurement used [13,34,91].

During the measurement of corneal thickness, clinicians have to bear in mind that the corneal thickness may vary throughout the day. Overnight corneal swelling has been documented to be a 5.5% increase in corneal thickness [15,23]. Feng et al. evaluated the diurnal variation in corneal thickness using AS-OCT and found that the corneal epithelial thickness and entire corneal thickness increase by 8.1% and 5.5%, respectively, after 10 h of eye closure by patching the eye. On the other hand, the control eye from the same patient was not patched, and thicknesses only increased insignificantly by 2.4% and 0.4%. The measurements in the patched eye returned to their preclosure values after 4 h of normal eye opening [15].

Corneal thickness measurements with AS-OCT have become extremely common and may be beneficial in cases where contact methods of measurements are not feasible, such as poor patient cooperation, young children, and patients with drug allergy to anesthetic. This method of corneal thickness measurement also requires less training of the operator and is much quicker to learn than other methods such as ultrasound and in vivo confocal microscopy.

15.2.2 Corneal Diseases

As the first refractive surface at which incident light comes into contact, the corneal integrity directly impacts the vision. Gross signs of corneal diseases such as opacities and increase in inflammatory cells can usually be visualized with the slit lamp biomicroscopy. However, subtle changes such as corneal thinning and changes in the cellular level may not be as apparent. High-resolution and high-magnification imaging, such as in vivo confocal microscopy, would be beneficial in this case. However, the need for the contact between a probe and the cornea might pose a problem. The cornea is the most sensitive part of the human body, and the sensitivity may be heightened in corneal diseases. The use of a contact method may add on to patient discomfort even with the application of topical anesthesia.

The noncontact method of AS-OCT imaging offers two advantages: no patient discomfort and no risk of further corneal damage by a contact probe. The latter is particularly advantageous in postoperative cases where there may be mechanical weakness of the globe due to the presence of a recent surgical wound. Real-time and highly magnified images of the cross sections of the cornea may therefore be valuable in assessing these fine changes and used to monitor and diagnose diseases.

15.2.2.1 Corneal Ectasia

Corneal ectasia is a degenerative noninflammatory thinning of the cornea. There are several forms of such thinning, keratoconus being the most common. An eye with keratoconus starts to thin at stoma, usually slightly inferotemporal to the central cornea, reforming into a conical shape. The posterior surface first increases in curvature before the anterior surface curvature steepens. Frequent fluctuations in refractive status can therefore occur due to the change in curvatures.

Since corneal thickness and curvature mapping is not a routine clinical examination, keratoconus can be easily missed and be mistaken for other causes of refractive error change. While glasses and contact lens can still correct the vision temporarily, it is usually not until further changes in refractive power that keratoconus is suspected. In addition,

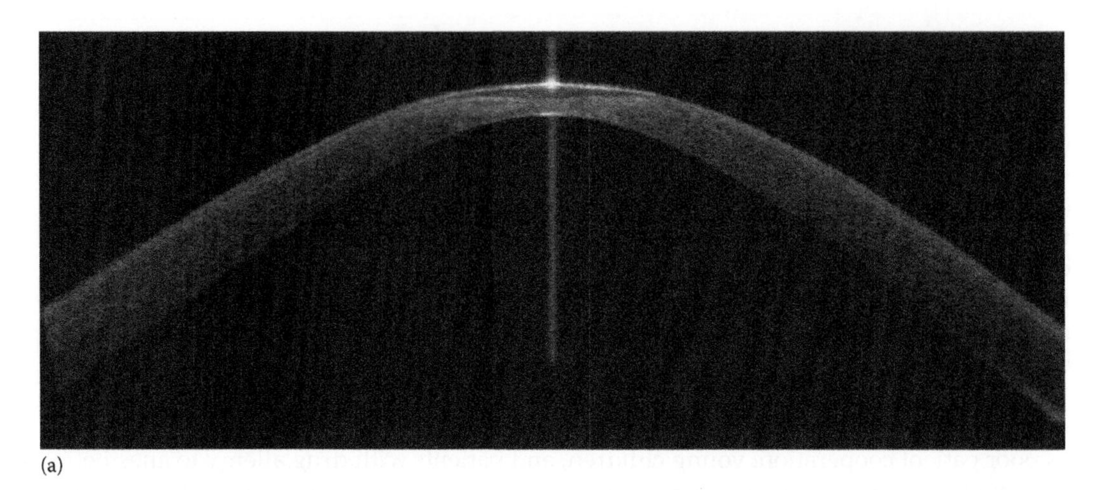

(a)

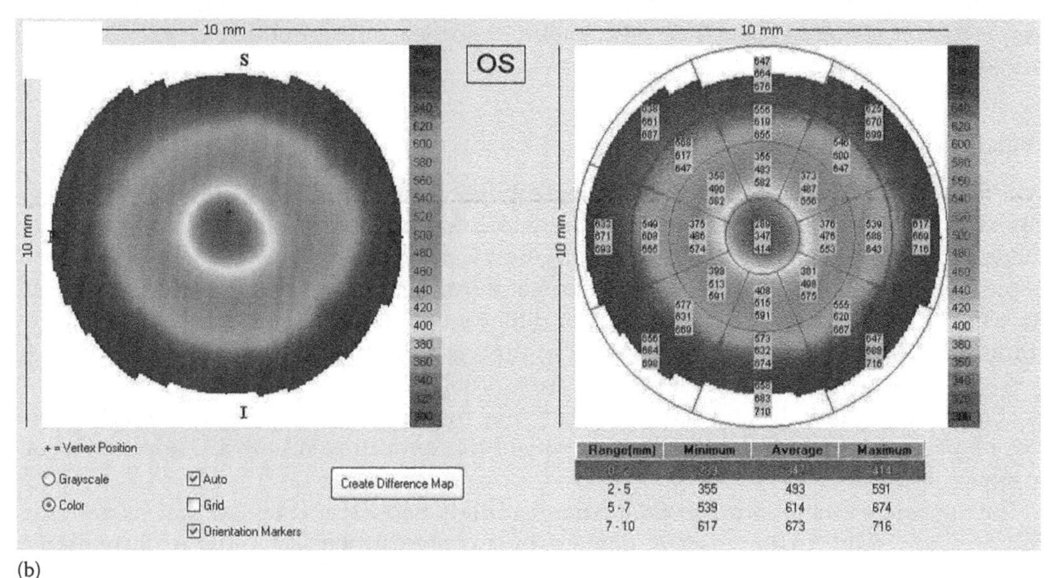

(b)

FIGURE 15.1
Keratoconus. A raw AS-OCT scan of a keratoconic cornea (a) and color-coded thickness map (b).

clinical signs such as Fleisher ring, Munson's sign, and corneal thinning and steepening are subtle, becoming apparent on slit lamp biomicroscopy only in the moderate to advanced stages.

AS-OCT imaging provides a quick method of screening for the disease by utilizing the corneal thickness mapping feature. On the raw AS-OCT image of a keratoconic eye, the central cornea is seen to be steeper and thinner than the periphery (Figure 15.1). The newer models of AS-OCT provide operators with four parameters specific to keratoconus evaluation: (1) difference in average thickness between the inferior and superior halves of the cornea, (2) difference in average thickness between the inferotemporal and superonasal halves of the cornea, (3) minimum corneal thickness, and (4) difference between the minimum and maximum thickness. These parameters allow clinicians to identify local and global thinning, as well as asymmetry. The cutoff values of these four parameters to diagnose keratoconus have been published [42]. An abnormal value for any one of the four parameters indicates a suspected keratoconus and two or more abnormal parameters indicate a definite diagnosis of corneal ectasia [65].

Management of keratoconus largely depends on the severity of the disease and the rate of progression, which can be monitored using AS-OCT imaging. As mentioned earlier, glasses and soft contact lens can be used in the early stage to correct the vision. Rigid contact lenses may be used to control progression in the early to moderate stages. Toward the advanced stages, corneal grafting may be warranted as a final resort (Section 15.2.3.2). It is much preferable to slow down disease progression and delay the need for corneal grafting due to the long-term complications of keratoplasty that may follow. Intrastromal corneal ring (ISCR) implantation is a method used to control the progression of keratoconus.

15.2.2.1.1 *Intrastromal Corneal Rings*

ISCRs are small devices that are implanted into the cornea to flatten the central cornea while providing a biomechanical support for the tissue. Typically, two of these devices, ranging 0.25–0.45 mm in thickness, are implanted, forming a ring shape (Figure 15.2a and b). Reported visual outcome and control of disease progression of ISCR is good, with the risk of serious complications generally not more than 2% [2,70]. Although complication rates are low, continued monitoring of the ISCR is important.

OCT imaging can provide vital and more accurate information with a single scan. The depth of the ISCRs and corneal thickness map can be obtained from AS-OCT imaging. Lai et al. reported that qualitative slit lamp observations of the ISCR depth were not correlated to AS-OCT measurements. They postulated that the slit lamp observation of depth is dependent on the observer's technique [37]. Recently, Gorgun et al. reported using AS-OCT that depths of the ISCR are much shallower than what was targeted [20]. Quantitative measurement of the ICSR depth is important as shallow ISCR may cause tension and a breakdown of the epithelium and the anterior stroma, causing another pathological process similar to keratoconus.

15.2.2.1.2 *Acute Hydrops*

The use of AS-OCT to evaluate and monitor the treatment outcome in hydrops has been documented. Hydrops is a complication of advanced keratoconus. The most serious consequence of corneal ectasia is acute hydrops. This is when a focal area of the cornea thins to the extent that the posterior surface (the endothelium and Descemet's membrane) ruptures and the aqueous in the anterior chamber enters into the stroma. Acute hydrops is extremely painful and significantly affects the vision. It is easily recognizable on slit lamp biomicroscopy coupled with patient's history of corneal ectasia and symptoms, the corneal opacity being most apparent at the area of focal thinning. However, the opacity hinders the clinician's view of the ruptured posterior surface.

In a case report, the acute hydrops was due to pellucid marginal degeneration—a crescent-shaped thinning of the peripheral cornea usually starting at the inferior. The use of AS-OCT allowed the clinicians to observe the resolution of the hydrops after treatment from a cross-sectional view. The quantitative documentation of the extent of hydrops was possible with AS-OCT [88].

15.2.2.2 Descemet's Membrane Detachment

Descemet's membrane detachment (DMD) is the separation of the Descemet's membrane after, or during, an intraocular surgery. Although rare, it is a serious complication that

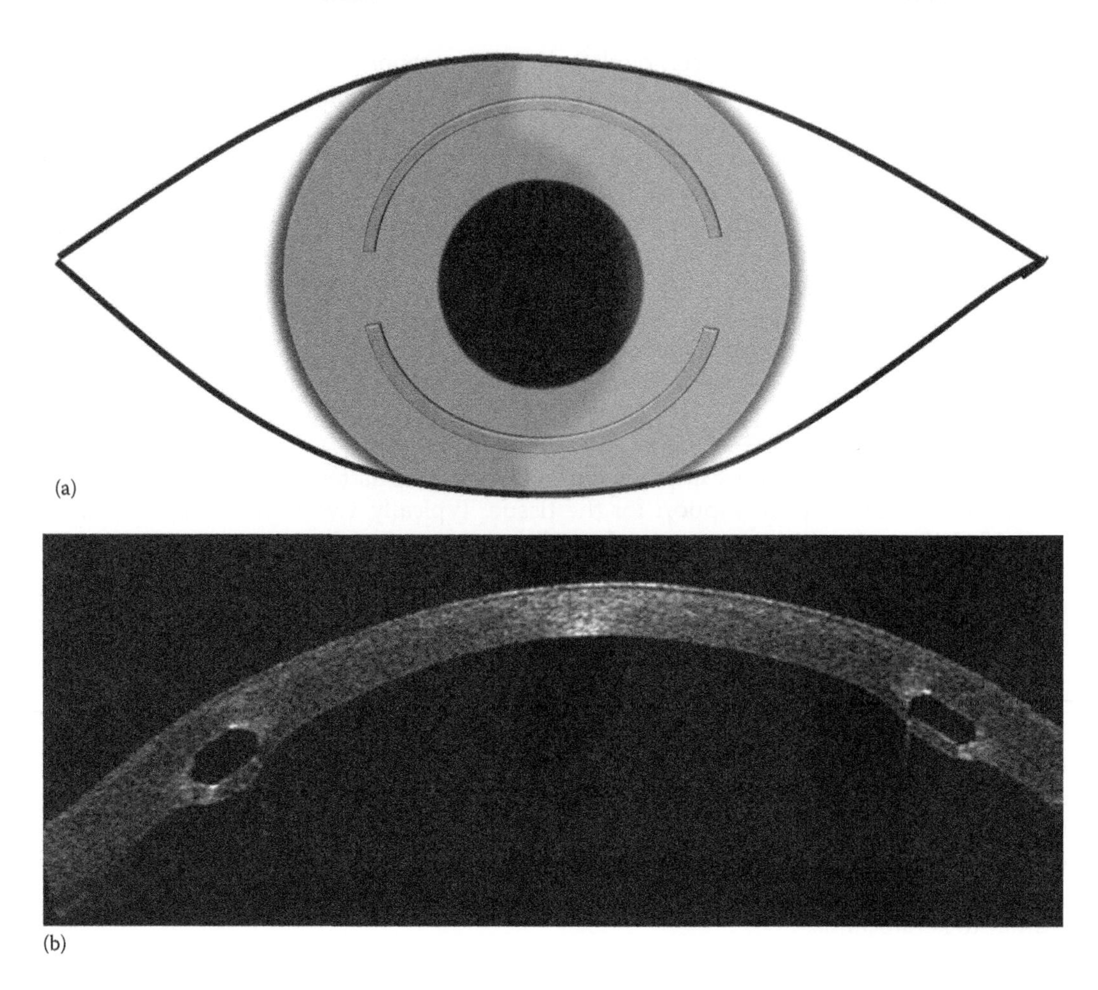

(a)

(b)

FIGURE 15.2
ISCRs. A schematic diagram of ISCR from the front view of the eye. Two semicircle ISCRs are implanted to form a circle shape (a). An AS-OCT cross-sectional scan of ISCRs in a cornea (b).

leads to an acute corneal edema and loss of vision. DMD has been reported to occur after various types of intraocular surgeries, not exhaustively including cataract extraction surgery, corneal grafting, glaucoma surgery (e.g., iridectomy, trabeculectomy), and anterior vitrectomy [45]. DMD is possibly caused by the mechanical forces of the blade during incision of the cornea, with suggested risk factors of shallow anterior chamber and the type or method of incision.

In patients with DMD, the cornea is usually very edematous, and thus, it is hard to visualize the Descemet's membrane and endothelium with the slit lamp biomicroscope. In addition, DMD usually follows uneventful intraocular surgeries; thus, there are few clinical indications that point toward the diagnosis of DMD [1]. Other methods of detecting DMD reported include ultrasound biomicroscopy, gonioscopy, and in vivo confocal microscopy [1]. However, these methods require direct contact between the imaging probe and the cornea.

Clinicians have utilized AS-OCT to image the Descemet's membrane and detect DMD through extremely edematous corneas [12,43]. DMD can be seen as a thin line at the

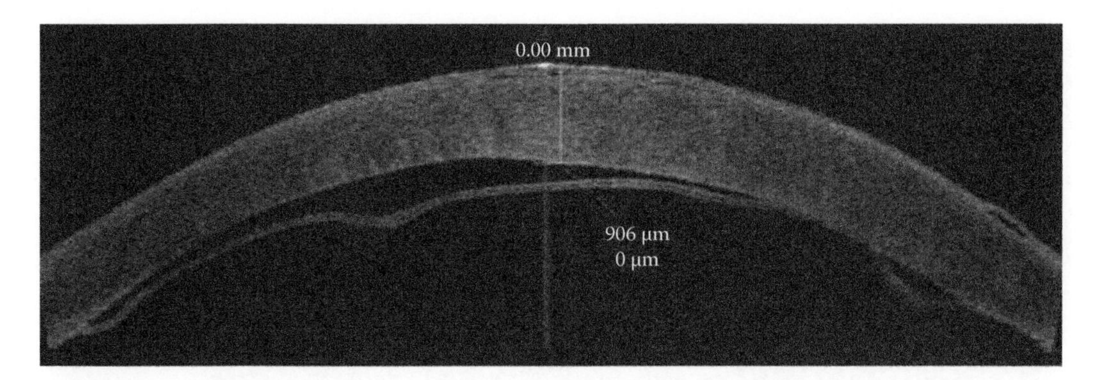

FIGURE 15.3
DMD. A raw AS-OCT scan shows the swelling of cornea with DMD, with a CCT of 906 μm.

posterior surface separated from the rest of the cornea. The extent and location of the detachment can be imaged, thus allowing the appropriate management to be implemented. Monitoring of patients after DMD treatment is also feasible with AS-OCT (Figure 15.3).

15.2.3 Ocular Surgeries

With the advances in technology, ocular surgeries have better outcomes. However, every surgery carries a certain amount of risk regardless of the success rates. Better understanding of individual patient's ocular status may help surgeons in the prediction of success rates and decision of the best management either surgical or nonsurgical treatments.

15.2.3.1 Corneal Refractive Surgeries

Corneal refractive surgery is an alternative to wearing glasses or contact lens to correct for one's refractive error. It involves the removal of a part of the corneal tissue to modify the shape of the cornea and change its refractive power. The success rates of refractive surgery are high, which can be partially attributed to the exclusion of patients who have the risk factors of serious complications, such as corneal ectasia, to undergo the procedure.

Keratoconus or other types of corneal ectasia are a few of the main contraindications for conventional refractive surgery (laser-assisted in situ keratomileusis [LASIK]) as they can hasten the progression of the disease. Reports of patients developing keratoconus after corneal refractive surgery have been documented. These patients exhibited subtle signs of keratoconus on topography (inferior corneal steepening) and no remarkable slit lamp biomicroscopy findings [7,76]. In the report by Schmitt-Bernard et al., the patient eventually had to undergo corneal grafting due to severe scarring 4 years after refractive surgery.

Preoperative factors that put patients at higher risk of corneal ectasia after surgery include abnormal corneal topography (possibly already suggesting an early form of corneal ectasia such as those in the case reports), high refractive error to be corrected, and thin corneas [66,67]. With the ability to detect early corneal thinning and changes in corneal curvature, AS-OCT may be useful in screening for corneal ectasia prior to corneal refractive surgery. Thin stromal beds after surgery are also a risk factor for postsurgical ectasia [66]. Since AS-OCT is noncontact in nature and high in resolution, high-magnification flap

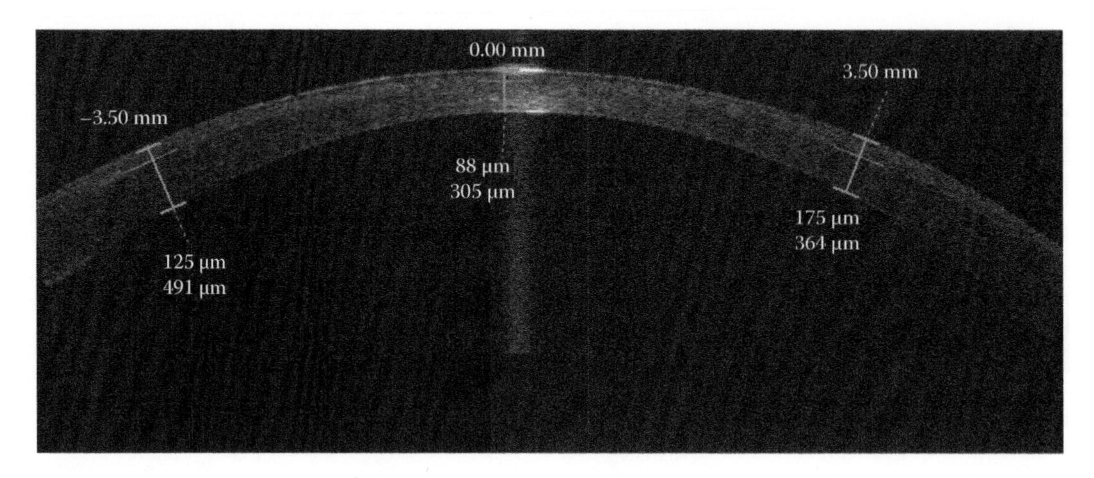

FIGURE 15.4
Post-LASIK cornea. Measurements made by AS-OCT show thickness of flap and residual stroma bed. In each measured point on the cornea, numbers above the cornea represent eccentricity from the central cornea; numbers below the cornea are the thickness measurements of the flap and stromal bed.

and stroma bed evaluation can be done immediately after surgery to aid the clinicians to roughly assess the risk of ectasia (Figure 15.4).

In a case report by Izquierdo et al., a patient with residual refractive error was considered for enhancement LASIK surgery. However, AS-OCT imaging revealed an abnormally thick flap with a thin stromal bed after surgery. LASIK was contraindicated in this case as the stromal bed was too thin to undergo further ablation. Photorefractive keratectomy, the refractive procedure where the superficial cornea is modified rather than the stroma, was performed instead [30].

Moreover, AS-OCT contributes a role in refractive surgery by providing accurate measurements of biometric of anterior chamber dimensions (Section 15.3.2). Due to the increased usage of refractive phakic and pseudophakic intraocular lens (IOL) in the correction of myopia, anterior chamber biometry and horizontal visible iris diameter measurement have become a critical assessment for that purpose. With AS-OCT, the quantitative assessment of the safety margin for phakic IOL can be performed before and after operation, and the position and alignment of phakic IOL can also be visualized postoperatively (Figure 15.5).

15.2.3.2 Corneal Grafting

Corneal grafting is the replacement of diseased corneal tissue with a healthy donor tissue to restore, at least partially, the vision. It is indicated in corneal diseases where the vision has been significantly affected and the cornea is unable to heal. Advanced keratoconus, corneal dystrophies, and severe corneal scarring due to infections or inflammation are common indications for corneal grafting.

Corneal grafting may refer to the transplant of the entire corneal thickness (penetrating keratoplasty [PK]) or just the diseased layers of the cornea (lamellar keratoplasty). Lamellar keratoplasty is currently being favored over PK due to the closed globe nature of the surgical procedure. However, in cases where most or all of the corneal layers have been implicated by the disease, PK would still be warranted.

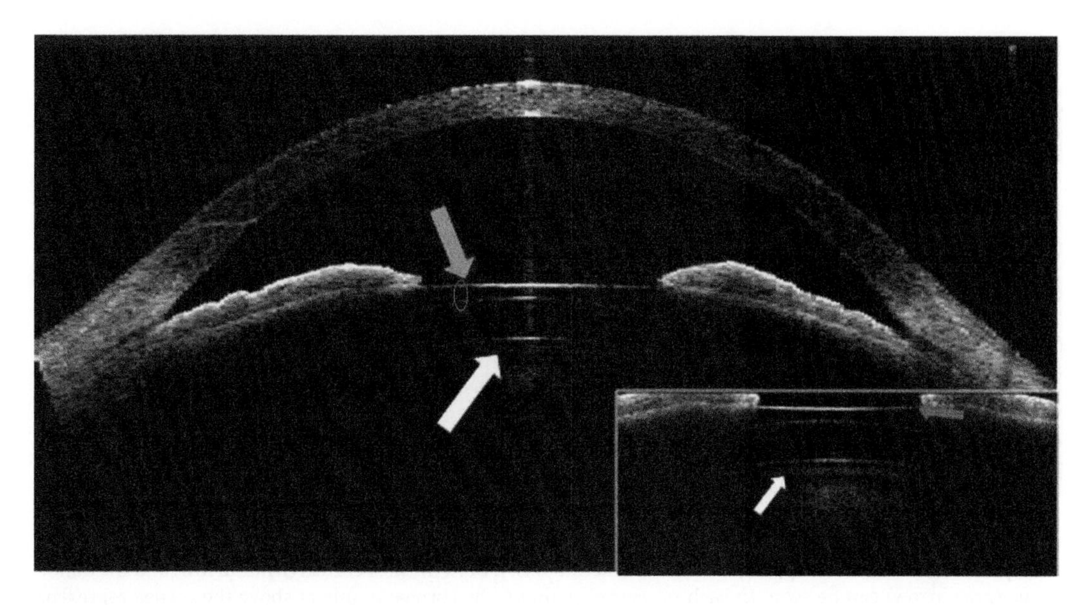

FIGURE 15.5
Phakic IOL. The IOL (encircled, denoted by gray arrow) is implanted on top of the original crystalline lens (white arrow: anterior surface of crystalline lens).

OCT is a useful tool for the preoperative assessment for keratoplasties. The in-depth assessments of the depths of the pathological lesion(s) allow clinicians to know whether all layers are involved, thus allowing a decision to be made between PK and lamellar keratoplasty. Lim et al. used AS-OCT to confirm the integrity of the endothelial layer in a patient with neurotrophic keratitis. This led them to perform a deep anterior lamellar keratoplasty (DALK) to specifically replace the stroma. In a patient with bullous keratopathy, AS-OCT revealed a homogenous appearance of the stroma, and endothelial irregularities corresponding to large areas of endothelial cell loss were observed. A Descemet's stripping endothelial keratoplasty (DSEK) was therefore performed to specifically replace the diseased endothelium [43].

Postoperatively, graft alignment, corneal thickness, corneal layer evaluation, and other complications such as graft detachment can be imaged with AS-OCT (Figure 15.6). Postoperative complications that have been reported using AS-OCT imaging include secondary glaucoma, microperforation (leading to an apparent second anterior chamber), DMD, and iris apposition [43,65].

This technique is especially useful when corneal edema or opacities limit the view of the deeper layers and anterior chamber. A partial DMD and fluid accumulation were detected with AS-OCT through a hazy cornea after DSEK in a report by Kymionis et al. It was later determined that the graft failure was due to inadequate Descemet's membrane stripping [36]. Lim et al. noticed the accumulation of fluid in the deep stromal layer after DSEK with AS-OCT. However, alignment of the graft was good and the poor endothelium function was therefore concluded to be due to the fluid accumulation. A second surgery was performed and the patient's vision significantly improved after the surgery [43].

AS-OCT is a complementary tool for pre- and postoperative assessment especially in patients whose corneas are hazy after surgery. Visualization of the functional anatomy of the deeper layers such as the Descemet's membrane and endothelium is also made easier with AS-OCT.

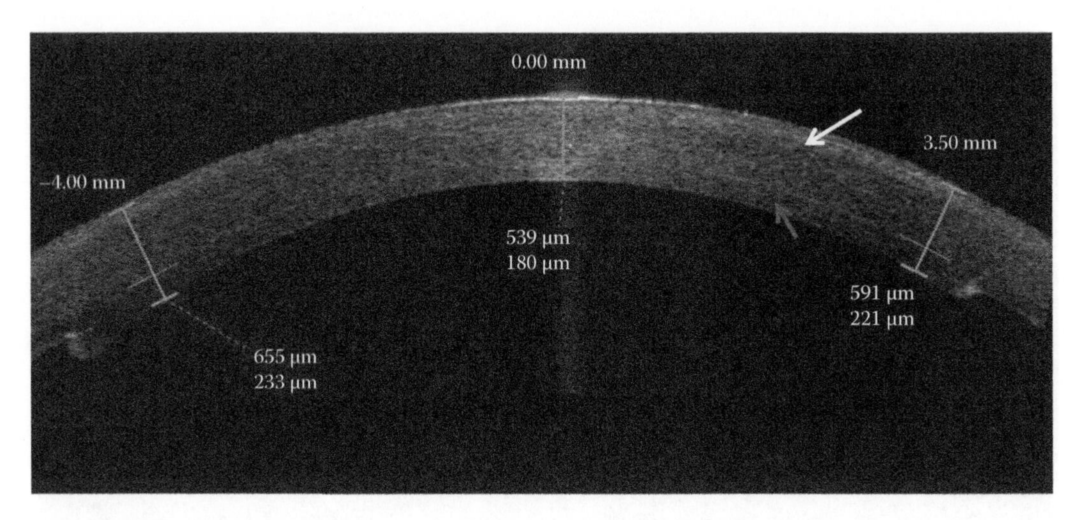

FIGURE 15.6
Postoperative Descemet's stripping endothelium keratoplasty. Both the host cornea (white arrow) and the donor tissue (gray arrow) can be seen. In each measured point on the cornea, numbers above the cornea represent eccentricity from the central cornea; numbers below the cornea are the thickness measurements of the host and donor tissues.

15.2.3.3 Cataract Extraction Surgery

A cataract refers to the opacified crystalline lens in the eye, causing blurring of vision that is uncorrectable by glasses especially in the moderate stages. It remains the leading cause of blindness worldwide; responsible for 50% of the visual impairment globally, this number being higher in the developing countries [18,32,68,85].

Techniques in cataract extraction surgery are constantly evolving. The currently most performed method is phacoemulsification. This procedure involves making an incision at the peripheral cornea and inserting an ultrasonic probe through the incision to break the cataract into small fragments. The chipped cataract fragments are removed from the eye by the probe or by aspiration and an IOL is implanted in its place.

Surgeons generally prefer to make smaller incisions (approximately 1–4 mm) during phacoemulsification due to the better predictability of surgically induced astigmatism, quicker duration of wound healing, reduced risk of wound leak, and lack of bleeding [24]. Small incisions are also usually self-healing. As reported by Schallhorn et al., there was no significant difference in wound architecture between corneal incisions that received suturing and those that did not [75]. The independence from wound sutures reduces the risk of infection [31]. Smaller incisions were also reported and that healing was faster. However, the size of incision may be limited by the surgeon's technique and experience [81].

Architecture of incision can be evaluated by AS-OCT after cataract extraction surgery. Incision wound size and angle position can be accurately measured. Angle position of the wound after surgery gives the surgeon an idea of the angle of blade insertion during surgery. In patients with higher IOPs, wound closure was better when incisions were made at 46° to the corneal surface of the incision site or less, whereas angles from 48° to 84° worked best in patients with lower IOPs [81]. Incision angle and size measurements may therefore be valuable for future research on wound healing, and AS-OCT imaging may be the best method for this evaluation (Figure 15.7).

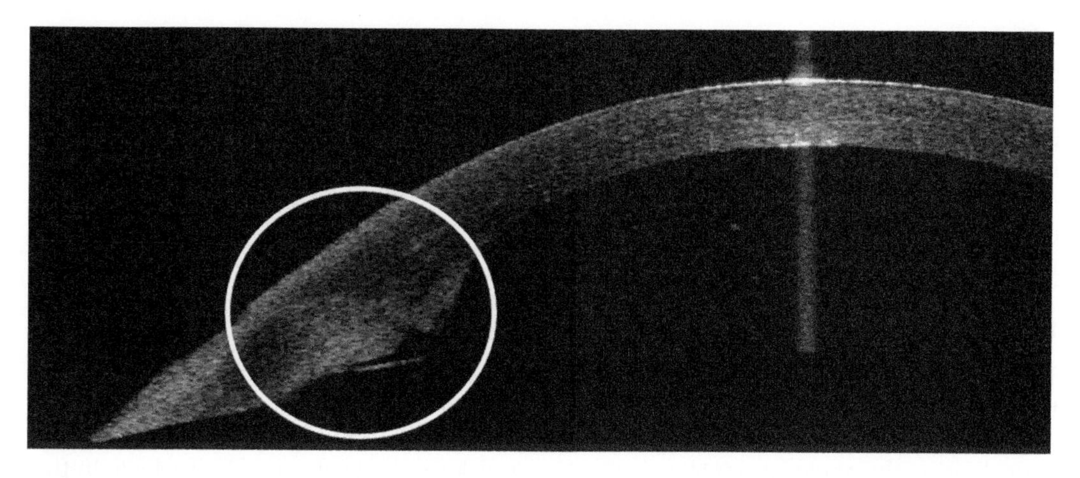

FIGURE 15.7
Clear corneal incision wound from cataract extraction surgery. The wound area (circled in white) is edematous and seen to be thicker than the rest of the cornea.

Other focal corneal complications at the site of incision have also been reported with AS-OCT evaluation. Xia et al. documented bubble formation in the epithelium, edema, endothelial apposition, and DMD at the site of incision 1 day after surgery. They noted that patients who had endothelial apposition had a larger extent of focal corneal edema (mean increase ± SD, 0.43 ± 0.14 mm) than the patients without (0.35 ± 0.13 mm) [96].

The aforementioned complications would have been difficult to detect with slit lamp biomicroscopy. Similarly, wound size and angle would not have been measured accurately with the routine methods of postoperative eye examination. AS-OCT imaging can provide scans through the entire cornea to screen for subtle abnormalities such as epithelial bubbles and localized edema, so as to call for early intervention if warranted.

15.3 Glaucoma Imaging

Glaucoma can be regarded as a group of eye diseases that damage the optic nerve due to elevated or inappropriate IOP. The damage is irreversible and will eventually cause blindness if untreated. Glaucoma is the second leading cause of blindness globally, after cataract [68]. Cedrone et al. reported that the highest prevalence of primary open-angle glaucoma (POAG) is in African origin population and primary angle-closure glaucoma (PACG) is commonest in Asians [5]. It is important to identify whether the angle is open or closed because of the possibility of an acute episode, a medical emergency, in closed angles. Moreover, the managements of POAG and PACG are different. Preventive interventions such as laser peripheral iridotomy have been introduced to control progress to glaucoma in narrow angles such as in primary angle-closure suspect and primary angle closure, but this form of treatment is irrelevant in open-angle glaucoma.

The current reference method for evaluation of anterior chamber angle is gonioscopy. However, it is still very much a difficult and subjective method due to various factors, such as the lens used, the illumination of examination room, the techniques and the skill of the observer, inadvertent pressure on the cornea, and moderate intra- and interobserver reproducibility. Therefore, objective evaluation of anterior chamber angle with ultrasound biomicroscopy, AS-OCT, or Eyecam is developed. AS-OCTs are widely used in both clinic and research settings because the examination is rapid, is noncontact in nature, and does not require a skilled operator as compared to ultrasound biomicroscopy or Eyecam.

15.3.1 Anterior Chamber Angle

The cross-sectional image of anterior chamber angle could be acquired with AS-OCT, and this can be used to grade the anterior chamber angle. The low intra- and interobserver variability in anterior chamber angle measurements with AS-OCTs proves its reliability in evaluating the angle and detecting a patient's risk for angle closure [39,48,64,82]. In the detection of angle closure, AS-OCT showed as high sensitivity as gonioscopy, which is the current gold standard. In fact, AS-OCT might be a suitable screening tool to detect angle-closure glaucoma suspects [51].

Sakata et al. reported that AS-OCT predicted more closed angles than gonioscopy, especially in the superior and inferior quadrants [71]. This may be attributed to the fact that AS-OCT provides only cross-sectional views in the analysis of an angle, whereas gonioscopy gives the visibility of the angle in its entirety. Swept source domain OCT, which is a form of Fourier domain OCT, can image anterior chamber angle in 128 cross sections across the whole anterior segment in 2.4 s [44]. This provides cross-sectional images of the anterior segment of just 2°–3° apart, thus may be used as a digital gonioscopy.

If posterior trabecular meshwork is not visible in gonioscopy, the angle is graded as closed. However, the scleral spur, where the inner surface of cornea and sclera meet, is the only visible landmark to grade open or closed angle in AS-OCT images (Figure 15.8a and b). This is another factor that contributes to the discrepancy of findings between gonioscopy and AS-OCT due to the usage of different anatomy landmarks to define a closed angle. Sakata et al. reported that scleral spur could be identified in 72% of the images, and the percentage of visibility of scleral spur was lesser in superior and inferior quadrants compared to nasal and temporal ones. The scleral spur was more difficult to identify in a closed angle than open. The trabecular meshwork is visible in high-resolution scan with Fourier/spectrum domain OCTs. However, deciding where the posterior part ends is complicated [71].

To quantify the anterior chamber angle, angle opening distance (AOD), trabecular iris space area (TISA), and angle recess area (ARA) at 250, 500, and 750 μm were introduced [57,58]. AOD is defined as the perpendicular distance from trabecular meshwork to iris, anterior to scleral spur. TISA is a trapezoidal area with the following boundaries: AOD anteriorly, a perpendicular line drawn from scleral spur posteriorly, inner surface of cornea or trabecular meshwork superiorly, and peripheral iris inferiorly. ARA is a triangular area bounded by trabecular meshwork, anterior iris surface, and AOD (Figure 15.9a).

Although these quantitative measurements of angle are used mostly in the research field, these findings may assist in the prediction and diagnosis of angle-closure glaucoma. Radhakrishnan et al. reported that 190 μm is the cutoff value for AOD500 and 0.11 mm^2 is the cutoff value for TISA500 in detecting an occludable angle [63]. A study by Narayanaswamy et al. found that the diagnostic performances of AOD500, AOD750, and

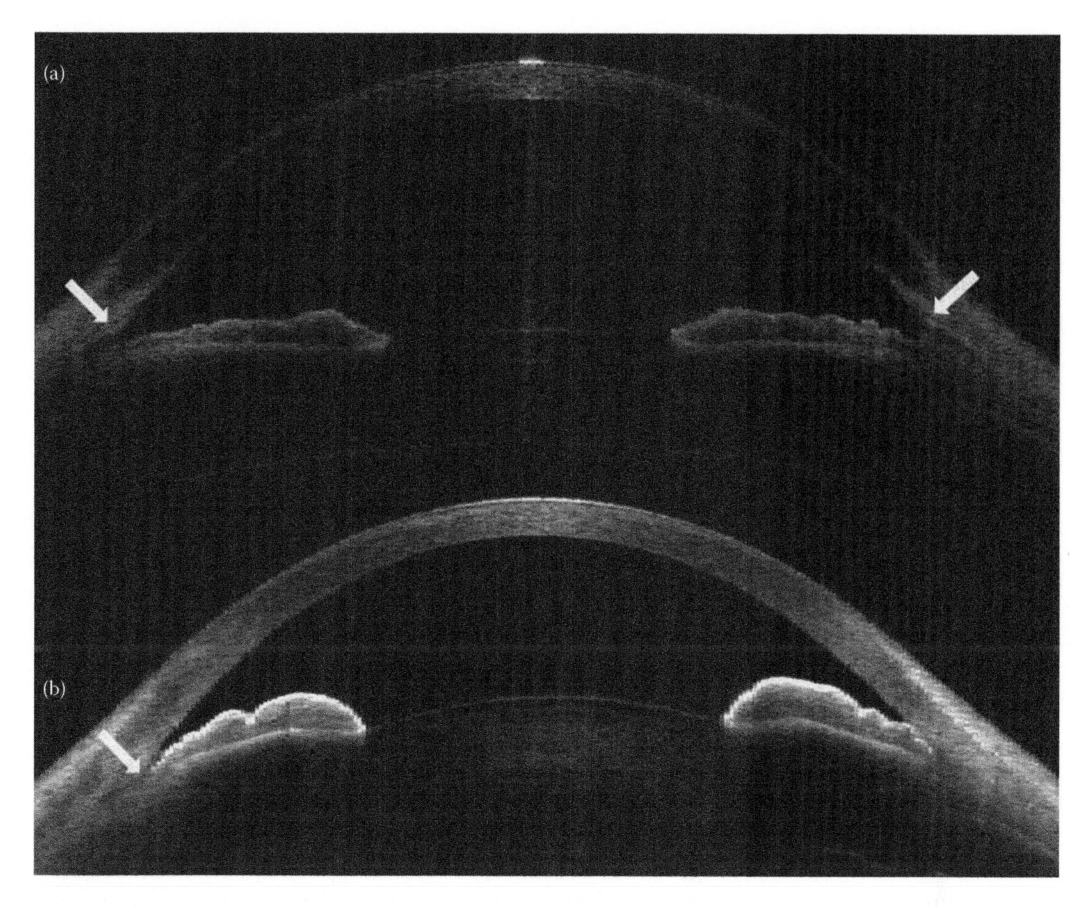

FIGURE 15.8
An opened anterior chamber angle (a) and a closed angle (b). The white arrows in both images indicate the location of the scleral spurs. The location of the scleral spur is not detected in the right-hand side angle in (b) and can be graded as closed. Other features of angle closer in this image are the semidilated pupil, shallow anterior chamber, and thickened iris.

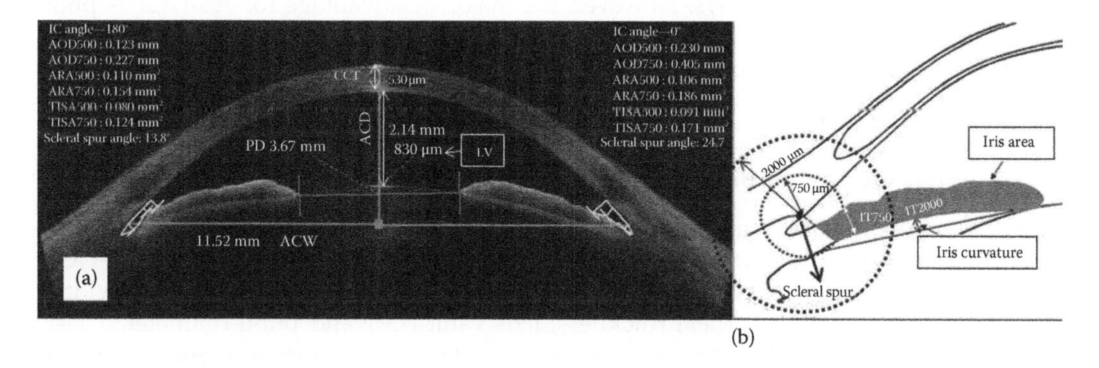

FIGURE 15.9
Quantitative measurements of anterior chamber angle. Measuring of anterior chamber biometry and angle parameters (a) and iris parameters (b) is displayed. CCT, central corneal thickness; ACD, anterior chamber depth; PD, pupil diameter; LV, lens vault; AOD, angle opening distance; TISA, trabecular iris space area; ARA, angle recess area; ACW, anterior chamber width; IT, iris thickness.

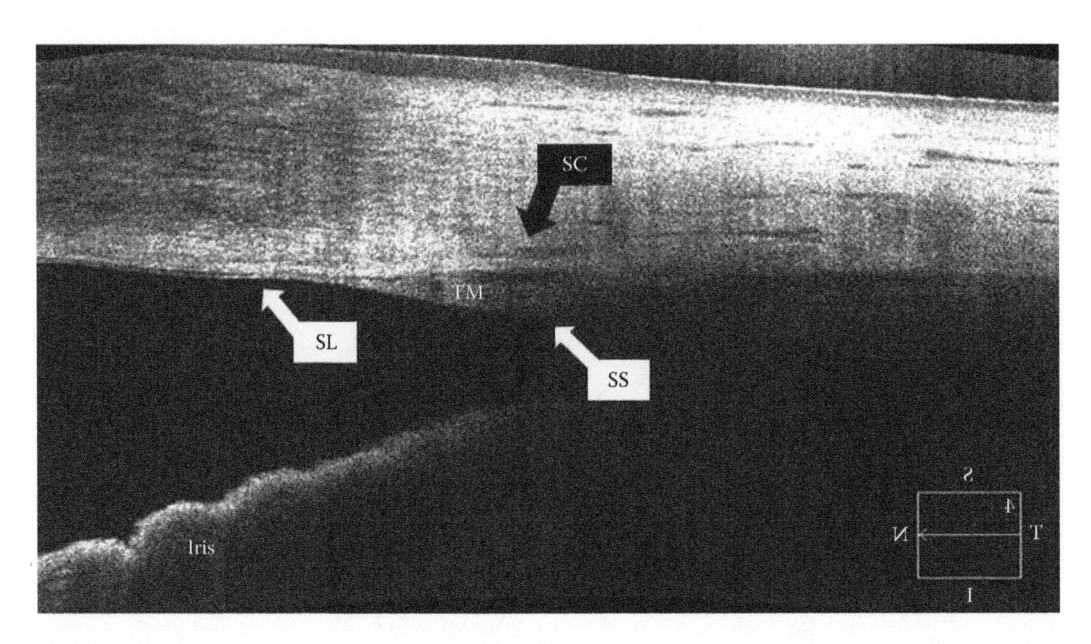

FIGURE 15.10
Anatomical details of anterior chamber angle. SL, Schwalbe's line; SC, Schlemm's canal; SS, sclera spur; TM, trabecular meshwork.

TISA750 were better than other parameters [50]. However, the contour of the iris might influence AOD750 and might give a false interpretation of angle status.

Recently, Fourier domain OCTs provide the visualization of the anatomic details of anterior chamber angle with high axial resolution of 5 µm in spectrum domain and less than 10 µm in swept source domain. Several studies reported high identification rate of Schwalbe's line (SL), Schlemm's canal (SC), trabecular meshwork, and scleral spur in Fourier domain OCTs (Figure 15.10) [61,87,93]. Without any discomfort, AS-OCTs enable identification of dynamic changes of the SC and trabecular meshwork in vivo. With non-contact, rapid scanning in a sitting position, AS-OCT is widely used as compared to ultrasound biomicroscopy nowadays. However, the major disadvantage for AS-OCT is poor visualization of the structures behind the heavily pigmented epithelial layer of the iris so that several secondary causes of angle closure such as plateau iris, ciliary body cyst or tumor, and lens subluxation are not detected.

15.3.2 Anterior Chamber Biometry

AS-OCT images the entire anterior segment and is able to provide an accurate anterior chamber biometry without any distortion as seen in ultrasound biomicroscopy. AS-OCT can yield the measurements such as anterior chamber depth; anterior chamber width, area, and volume; central corneal thickness; lens vault (LV); and pupil diameter. These parameters have shown the association with angle closure as reported by multiple studies (Figure 15.9a) [17,53,94]. Two studies showed that LV, which is the anterior portion of crystalline lens, was independently associated with angle closure [52,55]. The eyes found to have angle closure were noted to have thicker lenses with larger LV as compared to normal eyes in Chinese and Japanese populations. Moreover, obtaining an accurate anterior chamber biometry is important for refractive surgeries (Section 15.2.3.1).

15.3.3 Iris

Characteristics of the iris play a key role in the pathogenesis of glaucoma. The iris is a dynamic tissue that changes the configurations responding to the illumination or accommodation. There are three iris configurations: (1) flat, (2) anterior bowing (convex), and (3) posterior bowing (concave). Since the cross-sectional iris image has been captured with AS-OCT, the dynamic changes of iris configuration were observed. A study reported that three dynamic iris patterns (convex to convex, concave to convex, and concave to concave) were found in response to light [6]. The convex to convex configuration was found in older subjects and subjects with shorter axial length and with narrow angles. Moreover, the speed of pupil constriction was found to be slower in closed angle when compared to open-angle eyes [100].

AS-OCT is able to assess not only the iris curvature and configurations but also the measurements of iris thickness (IT) and cross-sectional areas. As the illumination used in AS-OCT is minimal, assessment of the thickness, cross-sectional area, and volume of the iris is possible under physiological dilated pupil condition in a dark room. The iris volume was found to be reduced when the pupil was dilated due to eliminating of extracellular fluid [62]. The increased IT and iris curvature toward the trabecular meshwork in the dim light condition are associated with acute attacks of angle closure. Quantitative iris measurements such as IT at 750 and 2000 μm from the scleral spur, maximum IT, and cross-sectional area were independently associated with narrow angles, especially in women and older subjects (Figure 15.9b) [89,90].

15.3.4 Ciliary Body

There are three components to the ciliary body: (1) the ciliary muscle, (2) the ciliary processes (pars plicata), and (3) the pars plana. The ciliary muscle comprises a ring of striated smooth muscle, which plays an important role in the accommodative function of the eye for viewing objects at varying distances [16]. The contraction and relaxation of the muscle lead to an alteration of the lens shape and thus the focus of the eye. It also extends anteriorly to provide attachment for the iris, which forms the pupillary diaphragm. The muscle is supplied by the anterior ciliary arteries and has both parasympathetic and sympathetic innervations. The ciliary processes can be found arranged in a circular ring behind the iris. These processes function in the production of aqueous humor. The pars plana structure is a continuation of the choroid, lined by a layer of epithelium that continues with the retina at the ora serrata.

Plateau iris is the occurrence of a closure of the anterior chamber angle secondary to a large or an anteriorly situated ciliary body. This phenomenon alters the position of the peripheral iris against the trabecular meshwork, thus giving rise to angle-closure glaucoma.

However, detection of the anterior rotation of the ciliary body in plateau iris using AS-OCT proved to be difficult as reported by Salim [72]. In fact, the use of AS-OCT in the visualization of ciliary body, let alone the diagnosis of other ciliary body pathologies such as ciliary body tumors, ciliary effusions, and cyclodialysis clefts, is still very much limited due to the blockage of the infrared light by the pigments located in the iris epithelial layer. In this case, ultrasound biomicroscopy is still the preferred imaging method for ciliary body pathologies. The measurement of ciliary body thickness in children at 1, 2, and 3 mm posterior to the scleral spur has been reported but deciding where the lower border of ciliary body under the iris was complicated [3,46].

15.3.5 Glaucoma Surgeries

The use of AS-OCT is not only limited to the study of pathophysiology of glaucoma. It also assists in the postoperative management of glaucoma. In order to reduce the IOP and prevent further damage to the optic nerve in glaucoma, there are procedures to facilitate the outflow of aqueous humor. As a noncontact investigation, AS-OCTs are widely used in postsurgical assessment compared to ultrasound biomicroscopy.

15.3.5.1 Laser Peripheral Iridotomy and Iridoplasty

By utilizing a focused beam of light, laser iridotomy makes a hole at the iris periphery or iris base, while iridoplasty causes contraction burns in the iris base around the eye. The aim of this surgical procedure is to physically retract an apposition of the iris away from the trabecular meshwork. Laser peripheral iridotomy is known to be the standard treatment for acute angle-closure glaucoma. A study showed that subjects with primary angle closure or PACG had significant reduction in IOP after iridotomy alone or iridotomy with iridoplasty [80]. By equalizing the hydrostatic pressure between the anterior and posterior chambers of the eye, iridotomy reverses the anterior bowing of iris configuration and opens the angle. AS-OCT aids in diagnosis and monitoring of effectiveness of the treatment. The patency of peripheral iridotomy can also be imaged using AS-OCTs (Figure 15.11).

15.3.5.2 Trabeculectomy

Trabeculectomy is a filtering surgery that removes part of the trabecular meshwork, creating a drainage channel from the anterior chamber to the space under the conjunctiva together with iridectomy [4]. This procedure allows the flow of aqueous humor into a cavity located on the surface of the eye, known as a bleb. The fluid is then slowly absorbed by the conjunctiva. Using AS-OCT, the outcomes of this surgical procedure can be monitored by assessing the bleb morphology.

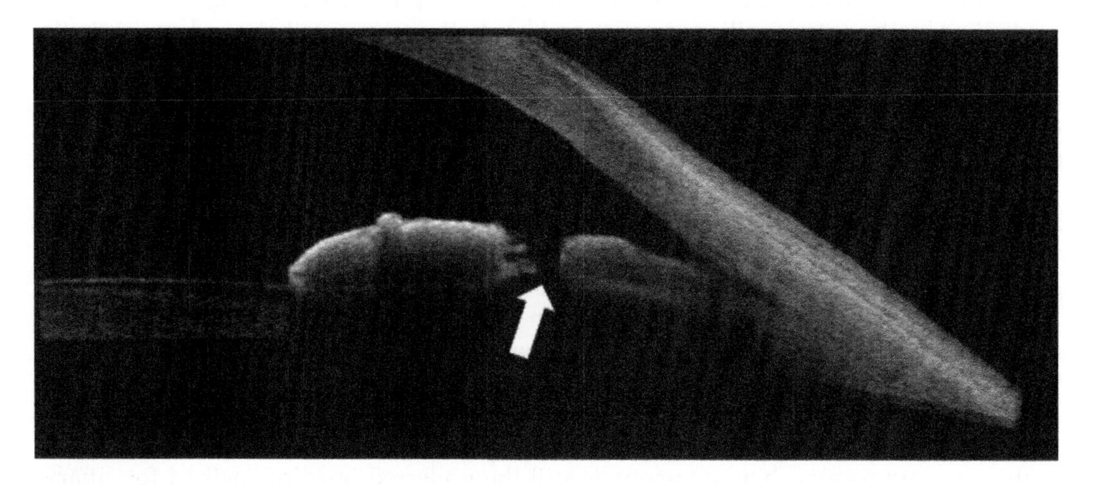

FIGURE 15.11
Peripheral iridotomy. The AS-OCT scan shows a patent iridotomy (white arrow).

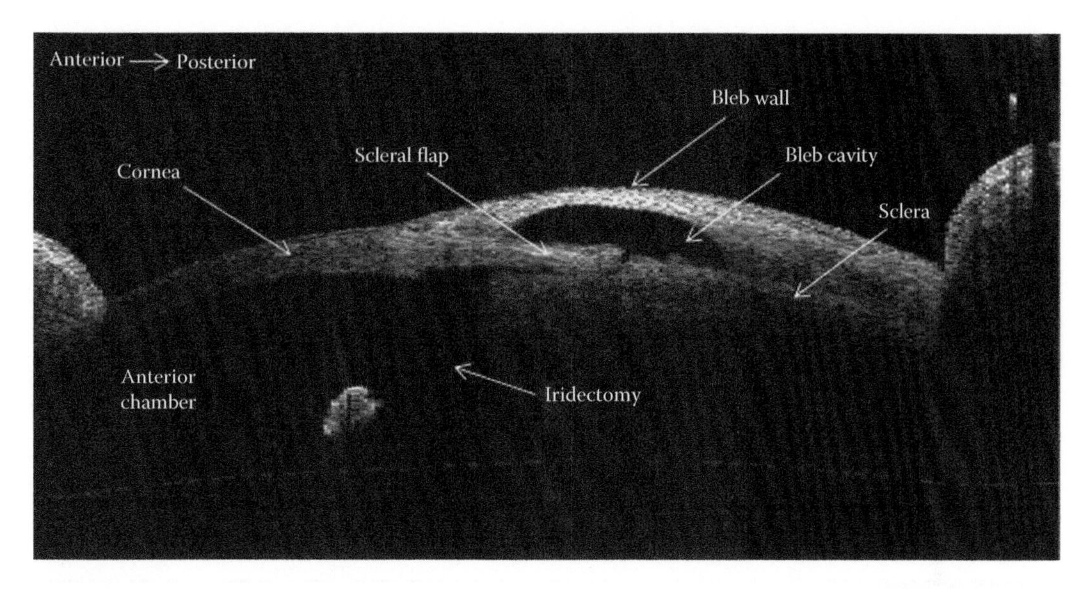

FIGURE 15.12
Trabeculectomy bleb. A large cystic space can be seen within this particular bleb in this AS-OCT scan; the bleb is therefore likely to be functioning well.

As no direct contact with AS-OCT scanning device prevents direct trauma and potential infection to the bleb, it has a significant benefit over ultrasound microscopy in the evaluation of blebs and scanning could be done as early as days after surgery. The qualitative assessments such as the detection of the presence or absence of cavity and microcyst, cystic space in the bleb wall, scleral flap apposition, patency of the internal ostium, and scarring can be obtained with the use of AS-OCT. It also allows quantitative measurements to be made such as the height of the bleb, cross-sectional area of the bleb, and height of the wall, which can be obtained with AS-OCT (Figure 15.12) [79].

The internal bleb morphology is the important indicator of bleb function and bleb-related complications such as bleb leak, inflammation, and scarring. AS-OCT aids the visualization of internal bleb anatomy that is inferred from clinical examination. Moreover, for failing filtering bleb, SL-OCT-guided bleb needling with antifibrotic agent provides good accuracy because the target area is imaged real time, and well-focused visualization during intervention causes minimal damage to the surrounding tissues [9].

15.3.5.3 Tube Shunt Surgery

Tube shunt surgery is an alternative option for the treatment of glaucoma in cases when there is failure of the trabeculectomy due to extensive scarring. Gedde et al. reported that tube shunt surgery had a higher success rate than trabeculectomy with mitomycin C in a 3-year follow-up study [19]. The positioning of the filtering devices in relation to the surrounding structures could be assessed with AS-OCT (Figure 15.13) [73]. Chua et al. used AS-OCT to detect the obstruction of the glaucoma drainage device caused by the iris tissue and enable the surgeon to perform another iridectomy precisely, avoiding the tube and reducing the IOP [8].

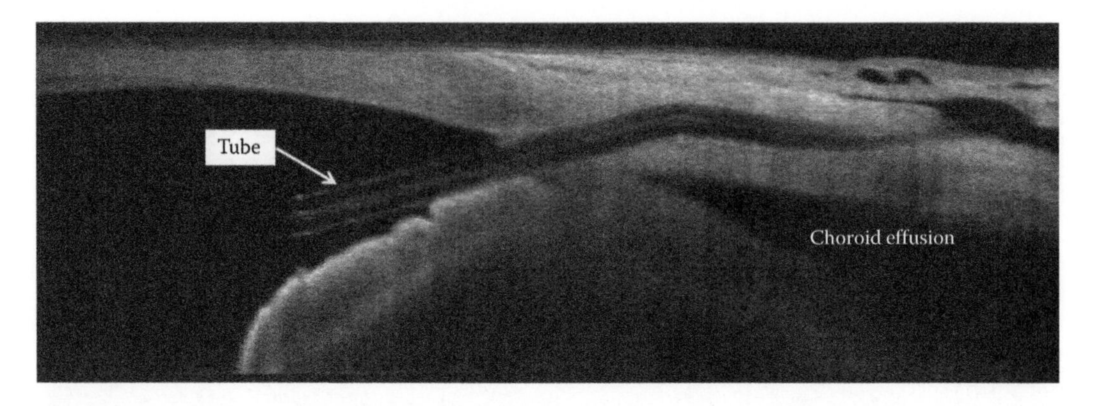

FIGURE 15.13
Filtering tube after a tube shunt surgery. The AS-OCT scan shows the position of tube and choroidal effusion after the surgery. The diverted fluid under the conjunctiva indicates that the shunt is functioning well.

15.4 Miscellaneous

AS-OCTs are mainly used to aid the diagnosis of corneal diseases and glaucoma and to monitor the outcomes and complications of corneal and glaucoma surgeries (Sections 15.2 and 15.3). However, it has been found that AS-OCT may be useful in the visualization of other structures of the eye as discussed further in the following.

15.4.1 Crystalline Lens

The crystalline lens is a transparent structure that lies suspended behind the iris, supported by zonular fibers arising from the ciliary body [77]. It consists of a hard nucleus surrounded by fiber mass, known as the cortex, and enveloped by an outermost layer of elastic membrane called the capsule. The lens is known for its role in the accommodation and refraction of the eye. It loses its accommodative function with age. In the event of cataract formation, the lens can be removed and replaced.

The Lens Opacification Classification System III (LOCS III) is a widely used lens grading system. A study showed that quantitative measurements of nucleus density of the lens on AS-OCT were reliable and there was a correlation with LOCS III nuclear opalescence and nuclear color score [92]. AS-OCTs proved to be useful in the detection of delamination of anterior lens capsule and provide insight into the etiology of capsular bag distension syndrome [83,84]. Moreover, lens thickness measurement using AS-OCT was comparable with A-scan ultrasonography [97]. AS-OCT appears to be an alternative method to assess the lens in vivo when a noncontact technique is needed.

15.4.2 Tear Film

The tear film coats the cornea and conjunctiva and serves to continuously lubricate these tissues. Other roles of the tear film include the delivery of oxygen and other nutrients, as well as providing immunological protection [86]. In patients with dry eye, the amount of tears can be reduced by either a decrease in its production or increase in tear evaporation. Dry eye may cause significant discomfort to the patients. Artificial tear lubricants are the first line of treatment for dry eye and are usually sufficient to control the symptoms. In severe cases, significant inflammation may occur that may lead to a decrease in visual quality [38].

The tear film is a very dynamic structure. The slightest ocular discomfort, yawning, or prolonged eye opening without blinking can stimulate the glands to elicit a reflex production of tears almost instantly as a protective mechanism. It is therefore rather difficult to obtain accurate measurements of the physiological tear film parameters.

Current commonly used methods of tear film evaluation include Schirmer's test, tear break up time, and tear meniscus height measurement with slit lamp biomicroscopy. The outcomes of these tests are dependent on the experience of the clinician and unfortunately would only be able to provide the single parameter that they are designed to test. Tear film decay time, which is taken as the time from eye opening to the next blink, is also not measureable with these tests. AS-OCT imaging can provide all these information of the tear film while allowing the patient to blink normally during measurements [56].

Tear meniscus height, area, and curvature can be measured from the AS-OCT scans of tear film (Figure 15.14). Multiple quick scans performed in a short time or a video enables the clinician to observe the decay of the tear film over a period of time. For example, tear parameters (height, area, radius, and volume) are largest after a blink and start to shrink almost immediately [56]. The decrease in volume is significantly steeper in patients with dry eye, even though most dry eye patients may have started off with smaller values of tear film parameters [27,35,74].

The noncontact nature of AS-OCT makes it useful in evaluating the dynamic tear film, especially in research studies where the most accurate measurements are preferred. AS-OCT allows the effect of dry eye treatment on the tear meniscus to be evaluated

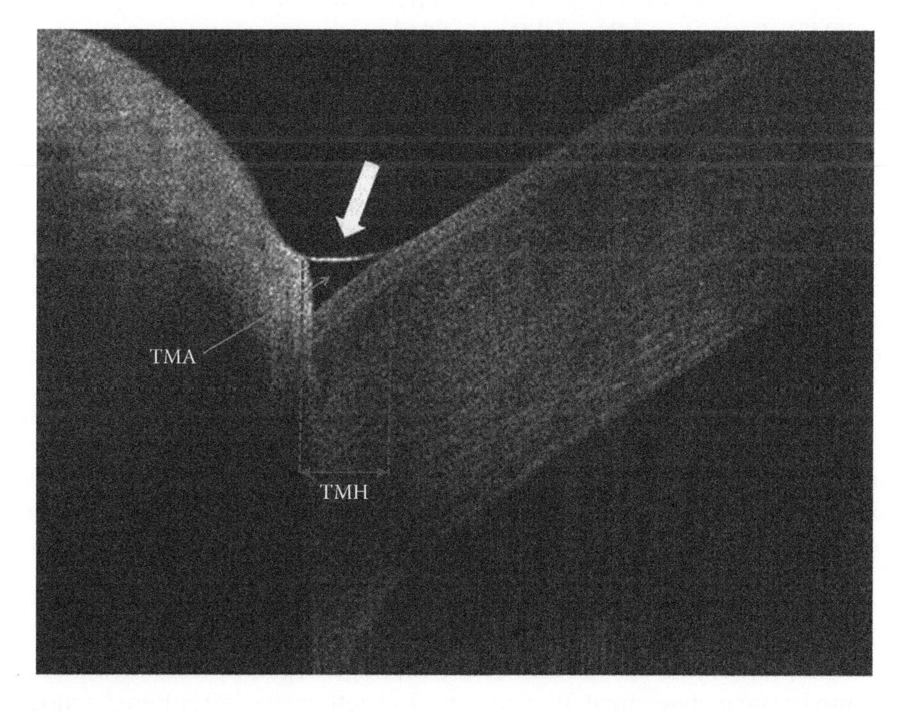

FIGURE 15.14
Tear meniscus. Tear meniscus parameters can be measured using this AS-OCT scan. TMH, tear meniscus height; TMA, tear meniscus area. Tear meniscus curvature can be measured as the radius of the hyperreflective line (white arrow). Surrounding are the lower lid (to the left) and the cornea (to the right).

effectively. During tear film image acquisition, the operator has to remind the patient to blink as per normal so as to not stimulate reflex tearing and result in an overestimation of the tear volume.

15.4.3 Conjunctivochalasis

The conjunctiva is the thin transparent mucous membrane that lines the exposed surface of the globe all the way to the inner surface of the eyelids. It is an important source of immunological defense against external insults. In some cases, the conjunctiva may become loose and forms redundant folds. These folds interfere with the normal spreading of the tear film, causing symptoms similar to those of dry eye, including excessive tearing [10]. There is currently no clear etiology and pathophysiology of conjunctivochalasis.

Conjunctivochalasis can be identified with the slit lamp, especially with the instillation of fluorescein. The fluorescein shows the irregularity of the tear film that coats the redundant folds. In moderate to advanced conjunctivochalasis, the tear meniscus is nonuniform, usually being higher at the center, obscuring the inferior 1–2 mm of the cornea [10].

The grading of conjunctivochalasis is problematic. This is partially due to its tendency to apparently change in severity at different gazes and with digital pressure. Grading systems have been developed but a universal consensus is still lacking [98]. A standard and objective method of grading is therefore warranted.

The role of AS-OCT in tear meniscus evaluation has been discussed in Section 15.4.2. Its application in the tear meniscus can be further extended to evaluating conjunctivochalasis. Cross-sectional AS-OCT scans showed the prolapse of the conjunctiva into the tear meniscus, causing the meniscal cross-sectional area to be filled by conjunctival tissue (Figure 15.15) [21]. Gumus and Pflugfelder reported an increase in severity of conjunctivochalasis with age, even in healthy eyes, supporting the use of AS-OCT in the objective and quantitative assessment of conjunctivochalasis [22].

15.4.4 Ocular Injuries

Injuries to the eye are usually sustained while carrying out manual labor or engaging in a high-impact sport; majority of these patients are therefore young males. Such injuries can range from intraocular foreign body to a full penetration of the eye [46,47]. Vision can be significantly affected and severe symptoms such as photophobia and pain may be experienced in the more serious cases. Rapid diagnosis is therefore crucial for the implementation of the best management.

OCT's value in the evaluation of ocular injuries has been reported by Wylegala et al. Patients presenting with various types of ocular injury went through AS-OCT imaging at first presentation and in subsequent follow-ups. In a patient who suffered from blurred vision following a car accident, AS-OCT imaging (together with gonioscopy) revealed a piece of glass in the anterior chamber. The corneal thickness was able to be measured with AS-OCT for the planning of the surgery to remove the glass piece [95].

Blood in the anterior eye may hinder slit lamp view of the lens and iris. In a patient whose eye was hit by a ball, AS-OCT revealed an acute angle closure with pupillary block with blood infiltration into the cornea. These findings, together with the elevated IOP, indicated immediate management for glaucoma. In another eye that suffered a mechanical trauma, a dislocated crystalline lens was able to be visualized with AS-OCT despite the blood in the anterior chamber [95].

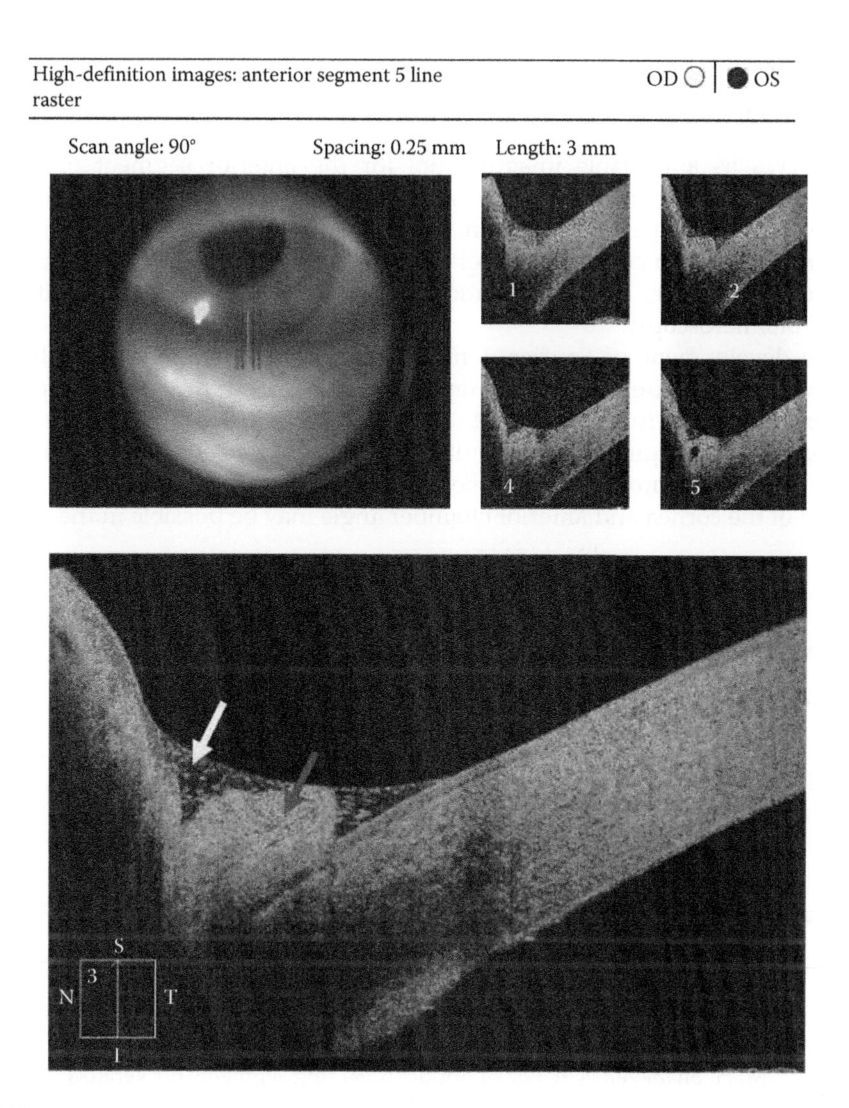

FIGURE 15.15
(See color insert.) Conjunctivochalasis taken by a Cirrus OCT. A high-definition colored scan taken by a Cirrus OCT shows the cross-sectional view of the conjunctivochalasis (red arrow) surrounded by the tear meniscus (white arrow). The tear meniscus height and volume appear to be greater than they are with the conjunctivochalasis. Surrounding are the lower lid (to the left) and the cornea (to the right).

Ocular surface burns can cause the growth of the conjunctiva tissue and vessels over the cornea. This is another example of AS-OCT's value in visualizing beyond such opacities. Information on the anterior chamber was important in deciding whether it is safe to perform corneal grafting to restore vision. In penetrating injuries, localization of the wound and monitoring of its healing after treatment can be done with AS-OCT [95].

In ocular injuries, contact methods of imaging may not be advisable due to the intense pain that a patient may feel and the possibility of causing further damage to the already weakened eye. The ability of AS-OCT to image through opacities such as blood, together with its noncontact nature, makes it a valuable tool to assess ocular injuries.

15.5 Future Directions and Summary

AS-OCT serves as a valuable imaging tool for the anterior segment of the eye. Its noncontact nature allows the operator to safely examine the eye multiple times during or immediately after a surgery. In addition, its high resolution, rapid scanning speed, and ability to image through certain extent of opacities make it a valuable tool for documenting disease progressions and therapeutic outcomes, as well as being an alternative to ultrasound biomicroscopy.

Since the development of Fourier domain OCTs, a large volume of high-resolution images have been captured. Due to its rapid scanning speed, there are less motion artifacts and better-quality images are able to be produced. The resolution of an image has been improved by averaging those of multiple cross sections. Moreover, 3D models of the cornea and anterior chamber could also be reconstructed from those obtained data. A 360° observation of the cornea and anterior chamber angle may be possible in the near future.

Acknowledgment

The authors would like to acknowledge Mr. Lakshmanasamudram S. Mohanram (Figures 15.2b and 15.5) for illustrations in this chapter.

References

1. Al-Mezaine, H. S. (2010). Descemet's membrane detachment after cataract extraction surgery. *Int Ophthalmol* 30(4): 391–396.
2. Alio, J. L., M. H. Shabayek et al. (2006). Intracorneal ring segments for keratoconus correction: Long-term follow-up. *J Cataract Refract Surg* 32(6): 978–985.
3. Bailey, M. D., L. T. Sinnott et al. (2008). Ciliary body thickness and refractive error in children. *Invest Ophthalmol Vis Sci* 49(10): 4353–4360.
4. Cairns, J. E. (1968). Trabeculectomy. Preliminary report of a new method. *Am J Ophthalmol* 66(4): 673–679.
5. Cedrone, C., R. Mancino et al. (2008). Epidemiology of primary glaucoma: Prevalence, incidence, and blinding effects. *Prog Brain Res* 173: 3–14.
6. Cheung, C. Y., S. Liu et al. (2010). Dynamic analysis of iris configuration with anterior segment optical coherence tomography. *Invest Ophthalmol Vis Sci* 51(8): 4040–4046.
7. Chiang, R. K., A. J. Park et al. (2003). Bilateral keratoconus after LASIK in a keratoconus patient. *Eye Contact Lens* 29(2): 90–92.
8. Chua, J., J. S. Mehta et al. (2009). Use of anterior segment optical coherence tomography to assess secondary glaucoma after penetrating keratoplasty. *Cornea* 28(2): 243–245.
9. Dada, T., S. Vengayil et al. (2008). Slitlamp-optical coherence tomography-guided needling of failing filtering blebs. *Arch Ophthalmol* 126(2): 284–286.
10. Di Pascuale, M. A., E. M. Espana et al. (2004). Clinical characteristics of conjunctivochalasis with or without aqueous tear deficiency. *Br J Ophthalmol* 88(3): 388–392.

11. Dohlman, C. H. (1971). The function of the corneal epithelium in health and disease. The Jonas S. Friedenwald Memorial Lecture. *Invest Ophthalmol* 10(6): 383–407.
12. Doors, M., T. T. Berendschot et al. (2010). Value of optical coherence tomography for anterior segment surgery. *J Cataract Refract Surg* 36(7): 1213–1229.
13. Doughty, M. J. and M. L. Zaman (2000). Human corneal thickness and its impact on intraocular pressure measures: A review and meta-analysis approach. *Surv Ophthalmol* 44(5): 367–408.
14. Edelhauser, H. F. (2006). The balance between corneal transparency and edema: The Proctor Lecture. *Invest Ophthalmol Vis Sci* 47(5): 1754–1767.
15. Feng, Y., J. Varikooty et al. (2001). Diurnal variation of corneal and corneal epithelial thickness measured using optical coherence tomography. *Cornea* 20(5): 480–483.
16. Fisher, R. F. (1986). The ciliary body in accommodation. *Trans Ophthalmol Soc UK* 105(Pt 2): 208–219.
17. Foo, L. L., M. E. Nongpiur et al. (2012). Determinants of angle width in Chinese Singaporeans. *Ophthalmology* 119(2): 278–282.
18. Foster, A. and G. J. Johnson (1990). Magnitude and causes of blindness in the developing world. *Int Ophthalmol* 14(3): 135–140.
19. Gedde, S. J., J. C. Schiffman et al. (2009). Three-year follow-up of the tube versus trabeculectomy study. *Am J Ophthalmol* 148(5): 670–684.
20. Gorgun, E., R. B. Kucumen et al. (2012). Assessment of intrastromal corneal ring segment position with anterior segment optical coherence tomography. *Ophthalmic Surg Lasers Imaging* 43(3): 214–221.
21. Gumus, K., C. H. Crockett et al. (2010). Anterior segment optical coherence tomography: A diagnostic instrument for conjunctivochalasis. *Am J Ophthalmol* 150(6): 798–806.
22. Gumus, K. and S. C. Pflugfelder (2013). Increasing prevalence and severity of conjunctivochalasis with aging detected by anterior segment optical coherence tomography. *Am J Ophthalmol* 155(2): 238.e232–242.e232.
23. Harper, C. L., M. E. Boulton et al. (1996). Diurnal variations in human corneal thickness. *Br J Ophthalmol* 80(12): 1068–1072.
24. Hoffman, R. S., I. H. Fine et al. (2003). *Incision Construction. Phacoemulsification: Principles and Techniques,* L. Buratto, L. Werner, D. J. Apple, and M. Zanini (eds.). Thorofare, NJ: SLACK Incorporated, pp. 265–277.
25. Holden, B. A., G. W. Mertz et al. (1983). Corneal swelling response to contact lenses worn under extended wear conditions. *Invest Ophthalmol Vis Sci* 24(2): 218–226.
26. Huang, D., E. A. Swanson et al. (1991). Optical coherence tomography. *Science* 254(5035): 1178–1181.
27. Ibrahim, O. M., M. Dogru et al. (2010). Application of visante optical coherence tomography tear meniscus height measurement in the diagnosis of dry eye disease. *Ophthalmology* 117(10): 1923–1929.
28. Ishibazawa, A., S. Igarashi et al. (2011). Central corneal thickness measurements with Fourier-domain optical coherence tomography versus ultrasonic pachymetry and rotating Scheimpflug camera. *Cornea* 30(6): 615–619.
29. Izatt, J. A., M. R. Hee et al. (1994). Micrometer-scale resolution imaging of the anterior eye in vivo with optical coherence tomography. *Arch Ophthalmol* 112(12): 1584–1589.
30. Izquierdo, L., Jr., M. A. Henriquez et al. (2008). Detection of an abnormally thick LASIK flap with anterior segment OCT imaging prior to planned LASIK retreatment surgery. *J Refract Surg* 24(2): 197–199.
31. Jancevski, M. and C. S. Foster (2010). Anterior segment optical coherence tomography. *Semin Ophthalmol* 25(5–6): 317–323.
32. Javitt, J. C. and F. Wang (1996). Blindness due to cataract: Epidemiology and prevention. *Annu Rev Public Health* 17: 159–177.
33. Klintworth, G. K. (1977). The cornea—Structure and macromolecules in health and disease. A review. *Am J Pathol* 89(3): 718–808.

34. Ko, Y. C., C. J. Liu et al. (2005). Varying effects of corneal thickness on intraocular pressure measurements with different tonometers. *Eye (Lond)* 19(3): 327–332.
35. Koh, S., C. Tung et al. (2010). Simultaneous measurement of tear film dynamics using wavefront sensor and optical coherence tomography. *Invest Ophthalmol Vis Sci* 51(7): 3441–3448.
36. Kymionis, G. D., L. H. Suh et al. (2007). Diagnosis of residual Descemet's membrane after Descemet's stripping endothelial keratoplasty with anterior segment optical coherence tomography. *J Cataract Refract Surg* 33(7): 1322–1324.
37. Lai, M. M., M. Tang et al. (2006). Optical coherence tomography to assess intrastromal corneal ring segment depth in keratoconic eyes. *J Cataract Refract Surg* 32(11): 1860–1865.
38. Lemp, M. A., C. Baudouin et al. (2007). The definition and classification of dry eye disease: Report of the Definition and Classification Subcommittee of the International Dry Eye WorkShop (2007). *Ocul Surf* 5(2): 75–92.
39. Leung, C. K., H. Li et al. (2008). Anterior chamber angle measurement with anterior segment optical coherence tomography: A comparison between slit lamp OCT and Visante OCT. *Invest Ophthalmol Vis Sci* 49(8): 3469–3474.
40. Leung, C. K. and R. N. Weinreb (2011). Anterior chamber angle imaging with optical coherence tomography. *Eye (Lond)* 25(3): 261–267.
41. Leung, D. Y., D. K. Lam et al. (2006). Comparison between central corneal thickness measurements by ultrasound pachymetry and optical coherence tomography. *Clin Exp Ophthalmol* 34(8): 751–754.
42. Li, Y., D. M. Meisler et al. (2008). Keratoconus diagnosis with optical coherence tomography pachymetry mapping. *Ophthalmology* 115(12): 2159–2166.
43. Lim, L. S., H. T. Aung et al. (2008). Corneal imaging with anterior segment optical coherence tomography for lamellar keratoplasty procedures. *Am J Ophthalmol* 145(1): 81–90.
44. Liu, S., M. Yu et al. (2011). Anterior chamber angle imaging with swept-source optical coherence tomography: An investigation on variability of angle measurement. *Invest Ophthalmol Vis Sci* 52(12): 8598–8603.
45. Marcon, A. S., C. J. Rapuano et al. (2002). Descemet's membrane detachment after cataract surgery: Management and outcome. *Ophthalmology* 109(12): 2325–2330.
46. McGwin, G., Jr. and C. Owsley (2005). Incidence of emergency department-treated eye injury in the United States. *Arch Ophthalmol* 123(5): 662–666.
47. McGwin, G., Jr., A. Xie et al. (2005). Rate of eye injury in the United States. *Arch Ophthalmol* 123(7): 970–976.
48. Muller, M., G. Dahmen et al. (2006). Anterior chamber angle measurement with optical coherence tomography: Intraobserver and interobserver variability. *J Cataract Refract Surg* 32(11): 1803–1808.
49. Muscat, S., N. McKay et al. (2002). Repeatability and reproducibility of corneal thickness measurements by optical coherence tomography. *Invest Ophthalmol Vis Sci* 43(6): 1791–1795.
50. Narayanaswamy, A., L. M. Sakata et al. (2010). Diagnostic performance of anterior chamber angle measurements for detecting eyes with narrow angles: An anterior segment OCT study. *Arch Ophthalmol* 128(10): 1321–1327.
51. Nolan, W. P., J. L. See et al. (2007). Detection of primary angle closure using anterior segment optical coherence tomography in Asian eyes. *Ophthalmology* 114(1): 33–39.
52. Nongpiur, M. E., M. He et al. (2011). Lens vault, thickness, and position in Chinese subjects with angle closure. *Ophthalmology* 118(3): 474–479.
53. Nongpiur, M. E., L. M. Sakata et al. (2010). Novel association of smaller anterior chamber width with angle closure in Singaporeans. *Ophthalmology* 117(10): 1967–1973.
54. Nouri, M., R. Pineda, Jr. et al. (2002). Descemet membrane tear after cataract surgery. *Semin Ophthalmol* 17(3–4): 115–119.
55. Ozaki, M., M. E. Nongpiur et al. (2012). Increased lens vault as a risk factor for angle closure: Confirmation in a Japanese population. *Graefes Arch Clin Exp Ophthalmol* 250(12): 1863–1868.
56. Palakuru, J. R., J. Wang et al. (2007). Effect of blinking on tear dynamics. *Invest Ophthalmol Vis Sci* 48(7): 3032–3037.

57. Pavlin, C. J. and F. S. Foster (1992). Ultrasound biomicroscopy in glaucoma. *Acta Ophthalmol Suppl* 70(204): 7–9.
58. Pavlin, C. J., K. Harasiewicz et al. (1991). Clinical use of ultrasound biomicroscopy. *Ophthalmology* 98(3): 287–295.
59. Piotrowiak, I., B. Soldanska et al. (2012). Measuring corneal thickness with SOCT, the Scheimpflug system, and ultrasound pachymetry. *ISRN Ophthalmol* 2012.
60. Potsaid, B., B. Baumann et al. (2010). Ultrahigh speed 1050 nm swept source/Fourier domain OCT retinal and anterior segment imaging at 100,000 to 400,000 axial scans per second. *Opt Express* 18(19): 20029–20048.
61. Quek, D. T., A. K. Narayanaswamy et al. (2012). Comparison of two spectral domain optical coherence tomography devices for angle-closure assessment. *Invest Ophthalmol Vis Sci* 53(9): 5131–5136.
62. Quigley, H. A., D. M. Silver et al. (2009). Iris cross-sectional area decreases with pupil dilation and its dynamic behavior is a risk factor in angle closure. *J Glaucoma* 18(3): 173–179.
63. Radhakrishnan, S., J. Goldsmith et al. (2005). Comparison of optical coherence tomography and ultrasound biomicroscopy for detection of narrow anterior chamber angles. *Arch Ophthalmol* 123(8): 1053–1059.
64. Radhakrishnan, S., J. See et al. (2007). Reproducibility of anterior chamber angle measurements obtained with anterior segment optical coherence tomography. *Invest Ophthalmol Vis Sci* 48(8): 3683–3688.
65. Ramos, J. L., Y. Li et al. (2009). Clinical and research applications of anterior segment optical coherence tomography—A review. *Clin Exp Ophthalmol* 37(1): 81–89.
66. Randleman, J. B., B. Russell et al. (2003). Risk factors and prognosis for corneal ectasia after LASIK. *Ophthalmology* 110(2): 267–275.
67. Randleman, J. B., M. Woodward et al. (2008). Risk assessment for ectasia after corneal refractive surgery. *Ophthalmology* 115(1): 37–50.
68. Resnikoff, S., D. Pascolini et al. (2004). Global data on visual impairment in the year 2002. *Bull World Health Organ* 82(11): 844–851.
69. Rodrigues, M. M., J. H. Krachmer et al. (1986). Fuchs' corneal dystrophy. A clinicopathologic study of the variation in corneal edema. *Ophthalmology* 93(6): 789–796.
70. Ruckhofer, J., J. Stoiber et al. (2001). One year results of European Multicenter Study of intrastromal corneal ring segments. Part 2: Complications, visual symptoms, and patient satisfaction. *J Cataract Refract Surg* 27(2): 287–296.
71. Sakata, L. M., R. Lavanya et al. (2008). Comparison of gonioscopy and anterior segment ocular coherence tomography in detecting angle closure in different quadrants of the anterior chamber angle. *Ophthalmology* 115(5): 769–774.
72. Salim, S. (2012). The role of anterior segment optical coherence tomography in glaucoma. *J Ophthalmol* 2012: 476801.
73. Sarodia, U., E. Sharkawi et al. (2007). Visualization of aqueous shunt position and patency using anterior segment optical coherence tomography. *Am J Ophthalmol* 143(6): 1054–1056.
74. Savini, G., P. Barboni et al. (2006). Tear meniscus evaluation by optical coherence tomography. *Ophthalmic Surg Lasers Imaging* 37(2): 112–118.
75. Schallhorn, J. M., M. Tang et al. (2008). Optical coherence tomography of clear corneal incisions for cataract surgery. *J Cataract Refract Surg* 34(9): 1561–1565.
76. Schmitt-Bernard, C. F., C. Lesage et al. (2000). Keratectasia induced by laser in situ keratomileusis in keratoconus. *J Refract Surg* 16(3): 368–370.
77. Sebruyns, M. (1951). The ultrastructure of the cornea and the lens studied by means of the electronic microscope. *Am J Ophthalmol* 34(10): 1437–1442.
78. Sin, S. and T. L. Simpson (2006). The repeatability of corneal and corneal epithelial thickness measurements using optical coherence tomography. *Optom Vis Sci* 83(6): 360–365.
79. Singh, M., P. T. Chew et al. (2007). Imaging of trabeculectomy blebs using anterior segment optical coherence tomography. *Ophthalmology* 114(1): 47–53.

80. Sun, X., Y. B. Liang et al. (2010). Laser peripheral iridotomy with and without iridoplasty for primary angle-closure glaucoma: 1-year results of a randomized pilot study. *Am J Ophthalmol* 150(1): 68–73.
81. Taban, M., B. Rao et al. (2004). Dynamic morphology of sutureless cataract wounds—Effect of incision angle and location. *Surv Ophthalmol* 49 (Suppl. 2): S62–S72.
82. Tan, A. N., L. D. Sauren et al. (2011). Reproducibility of anterior chamber angle measurements with anterior segment optical coherence tomography. *Invest Ophthalmol Vis Sci* 52(5): 2095–2099.
83. Tan, D. K., T. Aung et al. (2012). Novel method of assessing delamination of the anterior lens capsule using spectral-domain optical coherence tomography. *Clin Ophthalmol* 6: 945–948.
84. Tan, Y. L., L. S. Mohanram et al. (2012). Imaging late capsular bag distension syndrome: An anterior segment optical coherence tomography study. *Clin Ophthalmol* 6: 1455–1458.
85. Thylefors, B., A. D. Negrel et al. (1995). Global data on blindness. *Bull World Health Organ* 73(1): 115–121.
86. Tiffany, J. M. and A. J. Bron (1978). Role of tears in maintaining corneal integrity. *Trans Ophthalmol Soc UK* 98(3): 335–338.
87. Usui, T., A. Tomidokoro et al. (2011). Identification of Schlemm's canal and its surrounding tissues by anterior segment Fourier domain optical coherence tomography. *Invest Ophthalmol Vis Sci* 52(9): 6934–6939.
88. Vanathi, M., G. Behera et al. (2008). Intracameral SF6 injection and anterior segment OCT-based documentation for acute hydrops management in pellucid marginal corneal degeneration. *Cont Lens Anterior Eye* 31(3): 164–166.
89. Wang, B., L. M. Sakata et al. (2010). Quantitative iris parameters and association with narrow angles. *Ophthalmology* 117(1): 11–17.
90. Wang, B. S., A. Narayanaswamy et al. (2011). Increased iris thickness and association with primary angle closure glaucoma. *Br J Ophthalmol* 95(1): 46–50.
91. Wolfs, R. C., C. C. Klaver et al. (1997). Distribution of central corneal thickness and its association with intraocular pressure: The Rotterdam Study. *Am J Ophthalmol* 123(6): 767–772.
92. Wong, A. L., C. K. Leung et al. (2009). Quantitative assessment of lens opacities with anterior segment optical coherence tomography. *Br J Ophthalmol* 93(1): 61–65.
93. Wong, H. T., M. C. Lim et al. (2009). High-definition optical coherence tomography imaging of the iridocorneal angle of the eye. *Arch Ophthalmol* 127(3): 256–260.
94. Wu, R. Y., M. E. Nongpiur et al. (2011). Association of narrow angles with anterior chamber area and volume measured with anterior-segment optical coherence tomography. *Arch Ophthalmol* 129(5): 569–574.
95. Wylegala, E., D. Dobrowolski et al. (2009). Anterior segment optical coherence tomography in eye injuries. *Graefes Arch Clin Exp Ophthalmol* 247(4): 451–455.
96. Xia, Y., X. Liu et al. (2009). Early changes in clear cornea incision after phacoemulsification: An anterior segment optical coherence tomography study. *Acta Ophthalmol* 87(7): 764–768.
97. Zeng, Y., Y. Liu et al. (2009). Comparison of lens thickness measurements using the anterior segment optical coherence tomography and A-scan ultrasonography. *Invest Ophthalmol Vis Sci* 50(1): 290–294.
98. Zhang, X., Q. Li et al. (2011). Assessing the severity of conjunctivochalasis in a senile population: A community-based epidemiology study in Shanghai, China. *BMC Public Health* 11: 198.
99. Zhao, P. S., T. Y. Wong et al. (2007). Comparison of central corneal thickness measurements by visante anterior segment optical coherence tomography with ultrasound pachymetry. *Am J Ophthalmol* 143(6): 1047–1049.
100. Zheng, C., C. Y. Cheung et al. (2012). Pupil dynamics in Chinese subjects with angle closure. *Graefes Arch Clin Exp Ophthalmol* 250(9): 1353–1359.

16

Anterior Segment Imaging with Anterior Segment Optical Coherence Tomography

Zheng Ce and Paul Tec Kuan Chew

CONTENTS

16.1 Introduction

Anterior segment optical coherence tomography (ASOCT) is a new type of optical imaging modality that performs high-resolution, faster scanning speed, and cross-sectional imaging of the anterior chamber of the eye. Optical coherence tomography (OCT) was first described by Huang et al. in 1991 [1]. The first in vivo ASOCT imaging of the human eye was demonstrated in 1994 [2]; soon the commercially available ASOCT system was reported in 2003. Its important clinical and research applications, such as anterior chamber angle evaluation, filtering bleb imaging, and corneal pachymetry, have made the largest clinical and research impact in ophthalmology.

The principle of OCT is analogue to ultrasound imaging. However, unlike ultrasound that measures the delay time of the reflected sound wave, OCT imaging is to measure the delay of light (typically infrared) reflected from tissue structures. As the reflection intensity cannot be measured electronically due to extremely fast speed (300,000 km/s) of light, OCT employs low-coherence interferometry to compare the delay of tissue reflections against a reference reflection. A beam splitter of the interferometer is used

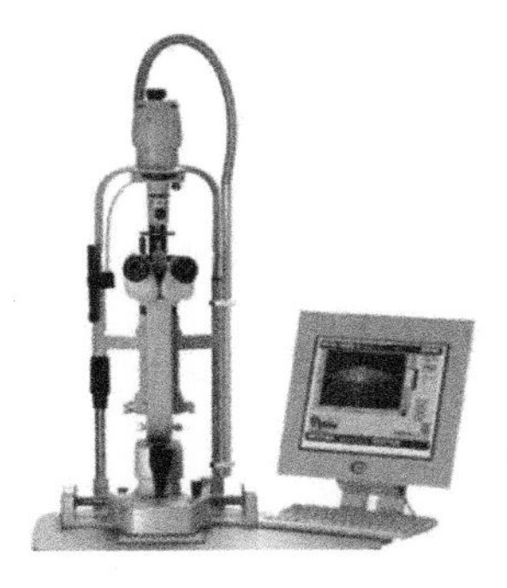

Slit-Lamp OCT (SLOCT) (Heidelberg Engineering, GmbH, Dossenheim, Germany)

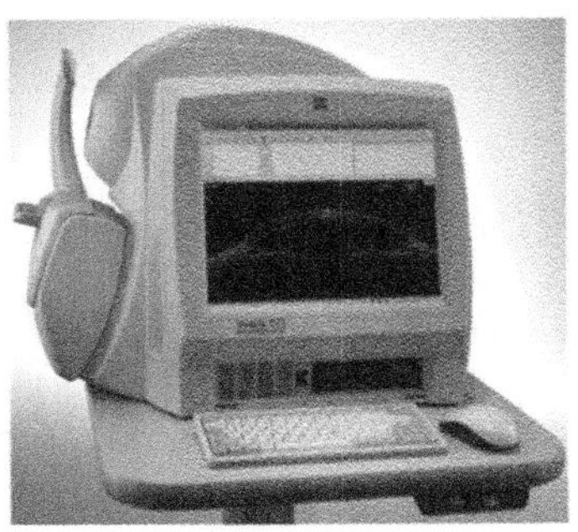

ZEISS Visante^{TM} OCT (Carl Zeiss Meditec, Dublin, CA)

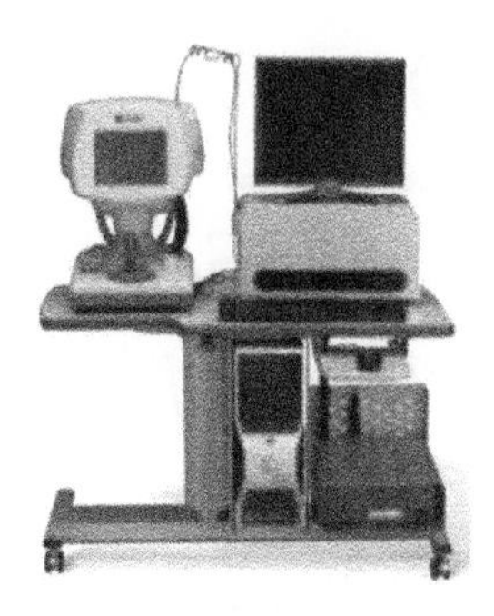

Casia SS-1000 OCT (Tomey, Nagoya, Japan)

FIGURE 16.1
Commercially available ASOCT models.

to split low-coherence infrared light into two components—one is directed to a movable mirror in the reference arm (time-domain [TD] OCT) and the other to the object of interest in the sample arm. The reflected signals from these two components are then superimposed at the interferometer. An OCT image is composed by combining a series of axial scans (A scans) that contains information on the strength of reflected signal as a function of depth. For TDOCT, the scanning speed is limited by the mechanical movement of mirror in the reference arm. Recently, the development of OCT hardware, such as spectral-domain OCT (SDOCT) and swept-source OCT (SSOCT), allows a faster scanning speed (30,000 A scans per second) and higher-resolution imaging of anterior segment than conventional TD-ASOCT (2,000 A scans per second), which results in the ability to visualize not only cross-sectional but also 3D structure of anterior segment. SDOCT improved the scanning speed considerably by using a stationary reference mirror, which is supposed to have no mechanical limitations. Currently, SDOCT uses a broad bandwidth light source and detects the interference spectra with a spectrometer. In contrast to SDOCT, SSOCT obtains time-encoded spectral information by using a monochromatic laser source. Interference signal is detected with a photodetector. One advantage of SSOCT is that most systems are now operating at longer wavelengths (1300 nm) that penetrates more deeply through the iris and sclera and may be useful for imaging of anterior segment.

At present, three ASOCT models are commercially available the ZEISS Visante™ OCT (Carl Zeiss Meditec, Dublin, CA), the Slit-Lamp OCT (SLOCT) (Heidelberg Engineering, GmbH, Dossenheim, Germany), and Casia SS-1000 OCT (Tomey, Nagoya, Japan). The former two OCTs are TDOCT, and the last one is SSOCT (Figure 16.1).

16.2 Clinical and Research Applications of ASOCT

16.2.1 ASOCT Application of Angle-Closure Glaucoma

As a major form of glaucoma that can cause irreversible blindness, primary angle-closure glaucoma (PACG) is more common in Asia [3], compared with primary open-angle glaucoma (POAG), which is the predominant form among Caucasians and Africans [4,5]. In China, nearly 3.5 million people are found to have PACG, and 28 million have a narrow or occludable drainage angle, which is the anatomical trait predisposing to PACG [6]. Although the number of PACG is only 30% higher than the POAG in China, PACG causes 10 times blindness than POAG [5]. Similar destructive condition was also found in other Asian countries; it has been reported that nearly half of PACG patients in South India were found to be blind in one or both eyes [7].

It is important to detect anatomically narrow angles early, as the subsequent prevention of visual loss from PACG depends on an accurate assessment of the anterior segment. Traditionally, the anterior segment and iridocorneal angle are evaluated with the help of a slit lamp and gonioscope. So far, gonioscopy is still the gold standard for assessing angle structures and configuration. However, it is a contact method by placing a gonioscope lens on a patient's eye and requires a subjective assessment. Classifications of angle grading depend on varying grading schemes, like Shaffer or Spaeth gonioscopic grading system. Although the Shaffer angle width appears to be commonly reported in research, no single scheme is used clinically. Furthermore, being a subjective method, gonioscopy is prone to potential measurement errors due to unavoidable light falling on the pupil. There are only rare small sample studies in reproducibility of gonioscopy with moderate agreement reported. Modern imaging devices such as ultrasound biomicroscopy (UBM), scanning peripheral anterior chamber depth (ACD) analyzer, and ASOCT facilitate objective and quantitative assessment of anterior chamber angle.

However, UBM is limited by being a close-contact immersion technique, which can cause artifacts and overestimate the angle measurement. As a noncontact, noninvasive, and fast method, ASOCT allows objective high-resolution visualization and reproducible measurement of the anterior segment structures (Figure 16.2). Using ASOCT, novel biometric risk factors associated with closed angle, including smaller anterior chamber width (ACW), area (ACA), and volume (ACV), and increased lens vault (LV) have recently been described. More recently, some authors also suggested that some dynamic physiological behavior of anterior segment may also be independent risk factors for closed angle by analyzing ASOCT videography.

Surgical treatment for glaucoma includes laser peripheral iridotomy (LPI) or trabeculectomy. Trabeculectomy, with its many modifications, has become the standard glaucoma filtration procedure. A fistula is created to allow aqueous outflow from the anterior chamber to the sub-Tenon space and form a bleb. Therefore, investigating bleb morphology is an important clinical parameter after trabeculectomy, and a functional bleb was used to be evaluated directly under slit lamp, which lacks capability to image intrableb structures and functions. ASOCT is a promising modality to image and assess trabeculectomy blebs (Figure 16.3). Singh et al. found that failure of filtration usually has a low bleb with some unique characteristics, like apposition of the scleral flap to its bed or apposition of conjunctiva–episclera to sclera, ostial occlusion [8]. Recently, the SSOCT offers considerably faster scanning speed than TDOCT and enables a 3D analysis intrableb structure. LPI has replaced incisional surgical iridectomy and is the recommended first-line treatment in the management of PACG [9]. After LPI, static and dynamic changes in ACA in angle-closure eyes have been described in a number of studies using ASOCT [10,11]. Our study group recently reported that the pupil constricts faster in response to illumination in patients with angle closure after LPI using ASOCT videography. Moreover, dynamic changes in the iris, particularly in thickness, were faster after LPI, and more rapid widening of the angle was likewise noted after the procedure. These findings are likely to be due to relief of pupil block after LPI.

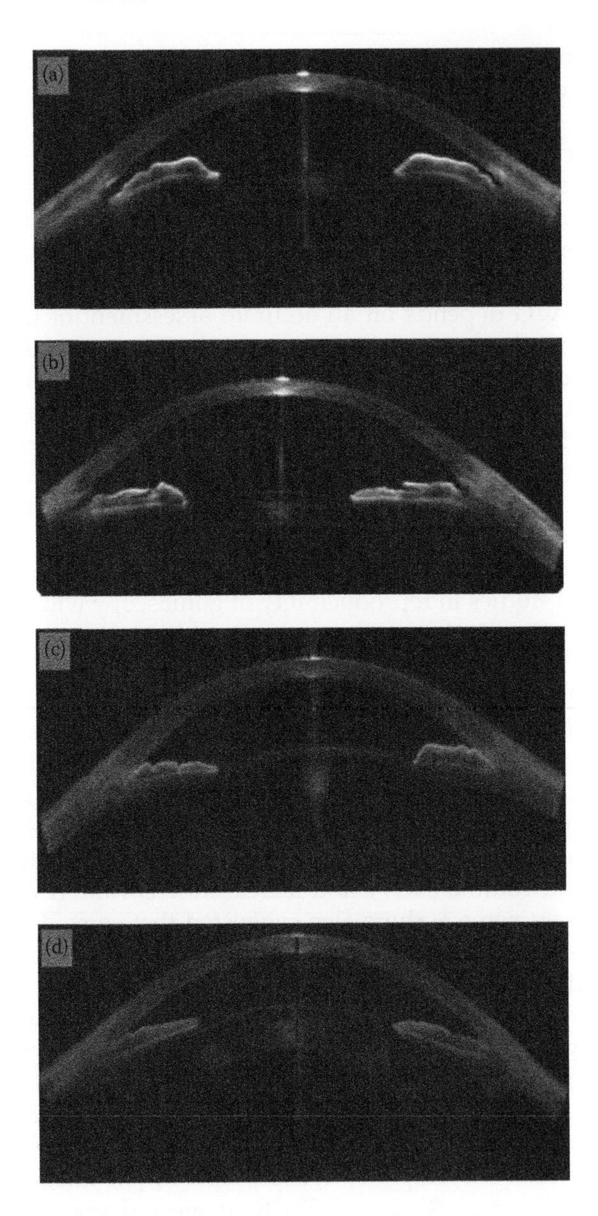

FIGURE 16.2
Nasal–temporal ASCOT images showing four mechanisms of PAC: (a) pupil block, (b) plateau iris configuration, (c) thick peripheral iris roll, and (d) exaggerated LV.

16.2.2 ASOCT Application of Corneal Abnormalities

ASOCT accurately maps corneal thickness in clear and opacified corneas. As a noncontact, noninvasive, and fast method, it allows the examiner to precisely map the corneal lesions, such as corneal degenerations, corneal scars, corneal dystrophies, the thickness of the cornea, the degree of epithelial hyperplasia, as well as scleral melts. The value of ASOCT in congenital corneal opacities is its ability to give structural information through opaque corneas in higher resolution than ultrasound and its applicability to do so without general

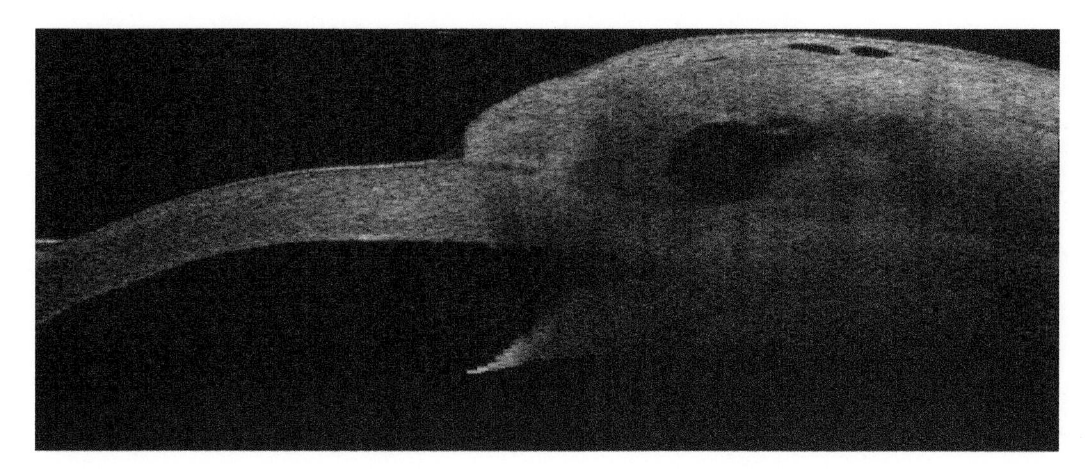

FIGURE 16.3
ASOCT imaging of trabeculectomy blebs.

anesthesia. This allows early assessment and follow-up of the eye-specific risk factors of the surgical interventions.

Majander et al. reported 14 eyes with congenital corneal opacities could be imaged using ASOCT [12]. The ease of use of ASOCT allows frequent imaging, even at every checkup, and thereby insight into the poorly understood natural history of congenital corneal opacities.

Keratoconus is another example for clinical and research application of ASOCT. As a bilateral progressive ectatic corneal disease, keratoconus is characterized by thinning and apical protrusion of the corneal [13]. In general, the focal thinning of cornea occurs in the inferotemporal position, and ASOCT pachymetry can detect this characteristic corneal thinning pattern to diagnose keratoconus.

LASIK, commonly referred to as laser in situ keratomileusis, is one of the most popular laser refractive surgeries in the world. In the early postoperative period, ASOCT has shown to be able to visualize LASIK flaps to evaluate the performance of microkeratome or femtosecond laser being used. Using Visante ASOCT, Ventura et al. compared ASOCT pachymetry between preoperative and postoperative measurements, and they found results correlate well with laser ablation settings [14].

16.2.3 ASOCT Application of Anterior Segment Tumors

Imaging technologies for anterior segment tumor evaluation provide useful information with regard to tumor size, shape, internal features, and extension, all of which help the clinician to make an accurate diagnosis and plan for treatment. Pavlin et al. reported the comparison of UBM and ASOCT in 18 eyes with anterior segment tumors, including 5 iris pigment epithelial cysts, 8 iris tumors, and 5 ciliary body tumors [15]. It seems that UBM has a better ability to penetrate through the lesion into the eye, providing better images of the posterior margin as well as the entire tumor configuration compared with ASOCT. However, ASOCT proved to be better for imaging the anterior surface of tumors, as well as imaging conjunctival lesions [16]. This is related to the fact that ASOCT has higher image resolution, with the capacity to achieve 18 μm in the high-quality mode, and that conjunctival lesions are superficial and in many cases, nonpigmented.

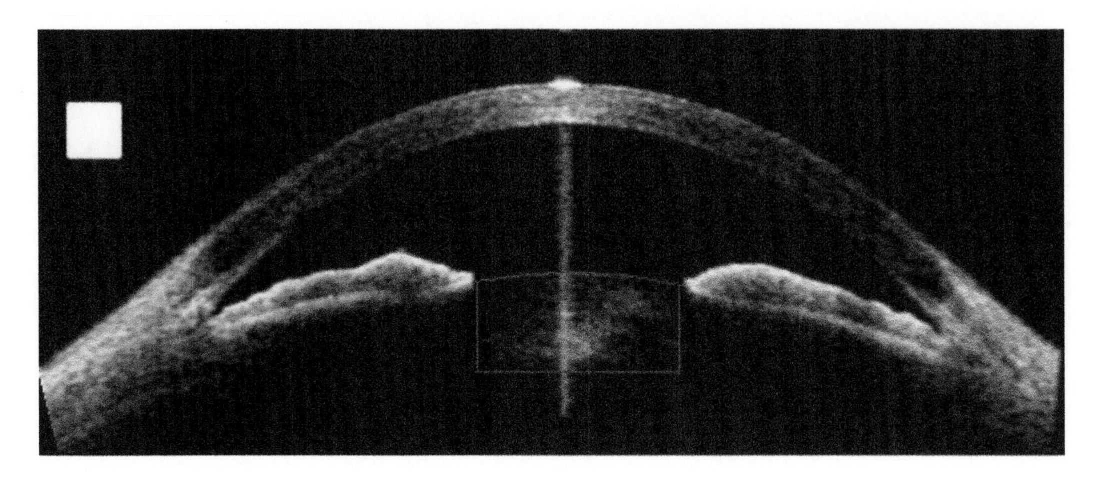

FIGURE16.4
ASOCT imaging of lens opacification (encircle with gray line).

16.2.4 ASOCT Application of Cataract

A cataract is the opacity of lens of the eyes. It is a major blinding disease in all over the world. It has been estimated that more than half of Americans with age above 80 have a cataract. So far, the Lens Opacities Classification System III (LOCS III), a well-recognized cataract classification system, is a subjective method based on the standard color photographics. Several authors have reported cataract density measurement using ASOCT (Figure 16.4). Leung et al. reported a significant correlation between the ASOCT nuclear cataract density measurement and the LOCS III system.

Cataract removal (phacoemulsification or small-incision cataract surgery) is the most common operation to improve visual acuity. More than 90% of cases have better vision after cataract surgery. The clear corneal incision (CCI; sutureless temporal CCIs) is a preferred technique of phacoemulsification used today. One concern when performing CCIs in phacoemulsification is that pathogens may enter into the anterior chamber after surgery as CCIs may possibly permit fluid from the extraocular to intraocular through a wound as corneal incision may work as a valve. ASOCT has been shown to be useful in evaluating phacoemulsification incision structure, like main incisions or CCI. Calladine reported that, under ASOCT image, CCI structural integrity may decrease due to endothelial gaping and loss of coaptation in the immediate postoperative period [17]. Chee et al. further compared wound characteristics and integrity in different sizes of CCIs (2.2 or 2.65 mm) using ASOCT. They found that both 2.2 and 2.65 mm CCIs clinically were competent [18].

16.3 Clinical Imaging Analysis of ASOCT

16.3.1 ASOCT Image Analysis Program

Computer medical imaging has become an essential component in both clinic and research area. The advance of medical imaging modalities, like ASOCT, provides better imaging of anterior segment of the eye. This allows clinician or research scientist to precisely measure biometric parameters that can only be hypothesized previously by traditional angle assessing methods. Not surprisingly, computer imaging processing can do medical image analysis faster without compromising measurement reproducibility. Moreover, newly developed computer algorithm accompanied with advanced imaging modalities can go even beyond just recording what clinicians and research scientist have observed. For example, the imaging of dynamic anterior segment feature in our group study was recorded via videography.

Unfortunately, the built-in software of the commercial ASOCT device, like Zeiss Visante ASOCT or SSOCT, is time-consuming and offers a limited function for quantitative measurement of biometric parameters. Sunita et al. had reported a software based on MATLAB® [19]. The operator had to manually mark both anterior and posterior corneal surface and the anterior iris surface firstly with mouse. Program only calculated the quantitative parameters after the operator marked the scleral spur (SS), which may unavoidably compromise the final result. Console et al. developed another semiautomated ASOCT program (Zhongshan Angle Assessment Program [ZAAP], Guangzhou, China) that measures biometric parameters once the SS is marked [20]. Manual identification of SS may compromise the reproducibility of anterior chamber angle measurements since SS shows low reflectivity in most of ASOCT images. Further studies need to be done to develop totally automated analysis, which may bring great advantage in both clinic and research area.

In this chapter, we described a customized software (Anterior Segment Analysis Program or ASAP) for ASOCT image processing. ASAP was coded as a plug-in software under the ImageJ (version 1.44x) framework by using its built-in editor and Java compiler.

ImageJ is a public domain Java image processing program inspired by NIH Image for Windows, Mac OS, Mac OS X, and Linux. ImageJ can be freely downloaded from the web link http://rsb.info.nih.gov/ij/ [21]. As a powerful scientific image processing platform, ImageJ provides a comprehensive set of digital image processing functions that allow developers to customize image acquisition, analysis, and processing for their own purpose. The applications of ImageJ on ASOCT image include biometric parameter measurement, in vivo 3D anterior chamber imaging, and dynamic ASOCT videography analysis [22,23].

The basic function of ASAP covers displaying, filtering, mathematical morphology, segmentation, and measurement of ASOCT images. The detail of ASAP will be described later in this chapter. Figure 16.5 shows ASAP's user interface.

16.3.2 Speckle Noise Model and Contract Adjustment of ASOCT Images

Visante ASOCT has a built-in function to optimize the image quality by adjusted saturation and noise. Unfortunately, such a function cannot be applied to raw images, which were directly captured from the ASOCT screen. This makes boundary detection and measurement problematic and unreliable.

Due to the coherence nature of the OCT technique, speckle noise gives the OCT image a granular pattern. The mean (average) filter, which is good at removing salt and pepper noise [24], was used in this software for image low-pass filtering. This technique replaces each pixel with the mean value in its 3 × 3 neighborhood. For each pixel in the selection, the nine pixels in the 3 × 3 neighborhood must be sorted, and the mean value will replace the center pixel. Therefore, histogram equalization can be applied to enhance and standardize image contrast. Histogram modeling techniques (e.g., histogram equalization)

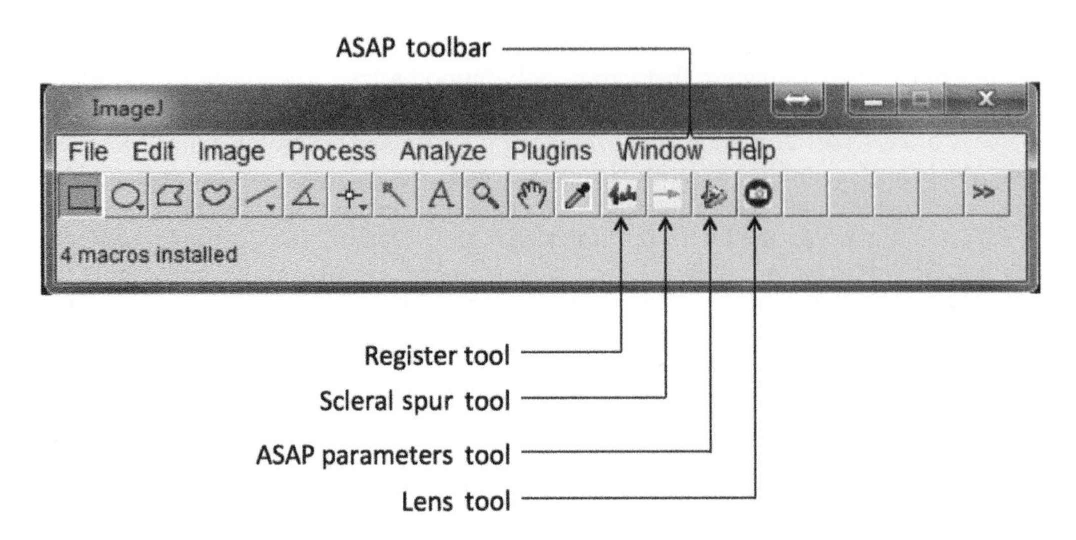

FIGURE 16.5
User interface of a customized software based on Image J (ASAP).

modify the dynamic range and contrast of intensity histogram into a desired shape that allows comparison and correction of nonlinear effects introduced by ASOCT display system [25].

16.3.3 "Dewarp" to Correct OCT Image Distortion

The unprocessed ASOCT image is distorted by the scan geometry and refraction at corneal interfaces. For accurate measurement of ASOCT images, a correction (dewarping) algorithm is needed to correct the beam refraction and to transform optical delay into physical lengths. The image misalignment in OCT was mainly due to two factors: the scan geometry and refraction on corneal interfaces. The detailed algorithms for dewarping ASOCT images have been described by Westphal et al. [26]. Briefly, it involves two steps.

First, the Visante ASOCT used in our study had a rectangular scan geometry probe. As OCT measures the optical delay rather than the physical distance, the refractive indices of human eyes are important to convert optical group delays to actual physical dimensions. The velocity of light varies according to the density of the medium through which it travels. It is the velocity of the medium that determines the delay of wave packets and the interferometry signal peaks in OCT. The denser the medium, the slower the light passing through it. A comparison of the velocity of light in vacuum and in another medium gives a measure of the optical density of that medium. This measurement is called the absolute refractive index, n, of the medium.

$$\text{Absolute refractive index} = \frac{\text{Velocity of light in vacuum}}{\text{Velocity of light in medium}}. \tag{16.1}$$

OCT records the optical path length that the light travels, so the optical delays must be converted to reflect the actual physical dimension.

$$\text{Physical distance} = \frac{\text{Optical path length}}{\text{Refractive index of the medium}}. \tag{16.2}$$

Moreover, as ASOCT uses light to probe the eye, the light changes its propagation direction at the interface between air and cornea due to refraction. Refraction happens when light passes from one transparent medium into another of different optical density (also referred to as refractive index). Image distortions due to refraction may also occur at other tissue index transition surfaces such as the cornea–aqueous interface. It causes significant image distortion. A forward transformation using Snell's law was used to correct the refraction and transition of the group index at the interface [27].

According to Snell's law,

$$n_1 \sin \theta_1 = n_2 \sin \theta_2 \tag{16.3}$$

where

n_1 is the refractive index of the first medium, which equals 1 for air
n_2 is the refractive index of the second medium, which is 1.389 for human air–cornea interface at 1.3 μm wavelength [28]

As refraction occurs in both the air–cornea and endothelium–aqueous interface, a further dewarping process has to be done for correcting image misalignment with 1.32 for human endothelium [19] (Figure 16.6).

16.3.4 Segmentation of ASOCT Images

Image segmentation is the division of an image into regions or categories corresponding to different objects or parts of objects.

Segmentation is often the critical step in ASOCT image analysis because anterior segment is composed of several different anatomical structures, like corneal, iris, and lens. Therefore, it is important to separate different anatomical structures before quantitative measurement. A good segmentation will make other stages in image analysis simpler.

16.3.4.1 Corneal Boundary

So far, ASOCT systems have capability of differentiating three corneal structures clearly. The highest reflectivity is found at the epithelium–Bowman's layer and at the Descemet's endothelial layer, whereas lower reflectivity is observed in the corneal stroma. The development of SDOCT even allows one to visualize more detailed structures including epithelium–Bowman's layer interface, the termination of the Descemet's membrane (Schwalbe line [SL]), and trabecular meshwork. An ASOCT image of a section of normal human cornea is shown in Figure 16.7. The following algorithms were developed to automatically identify the corneal boundary (Figure 16.8):

1. Detect and delete the vertical flare based on the corneal vertex. When the laser light passes through the corneal vertex, the light reflected from the corneal vertex was strong enough to saturate the dynamic range of the OCT system. Such a vertical flare in the ASOCT image provides useful information to locate the corneal vertex but also produces an artifact signal noise for identifying the corneal boundary.

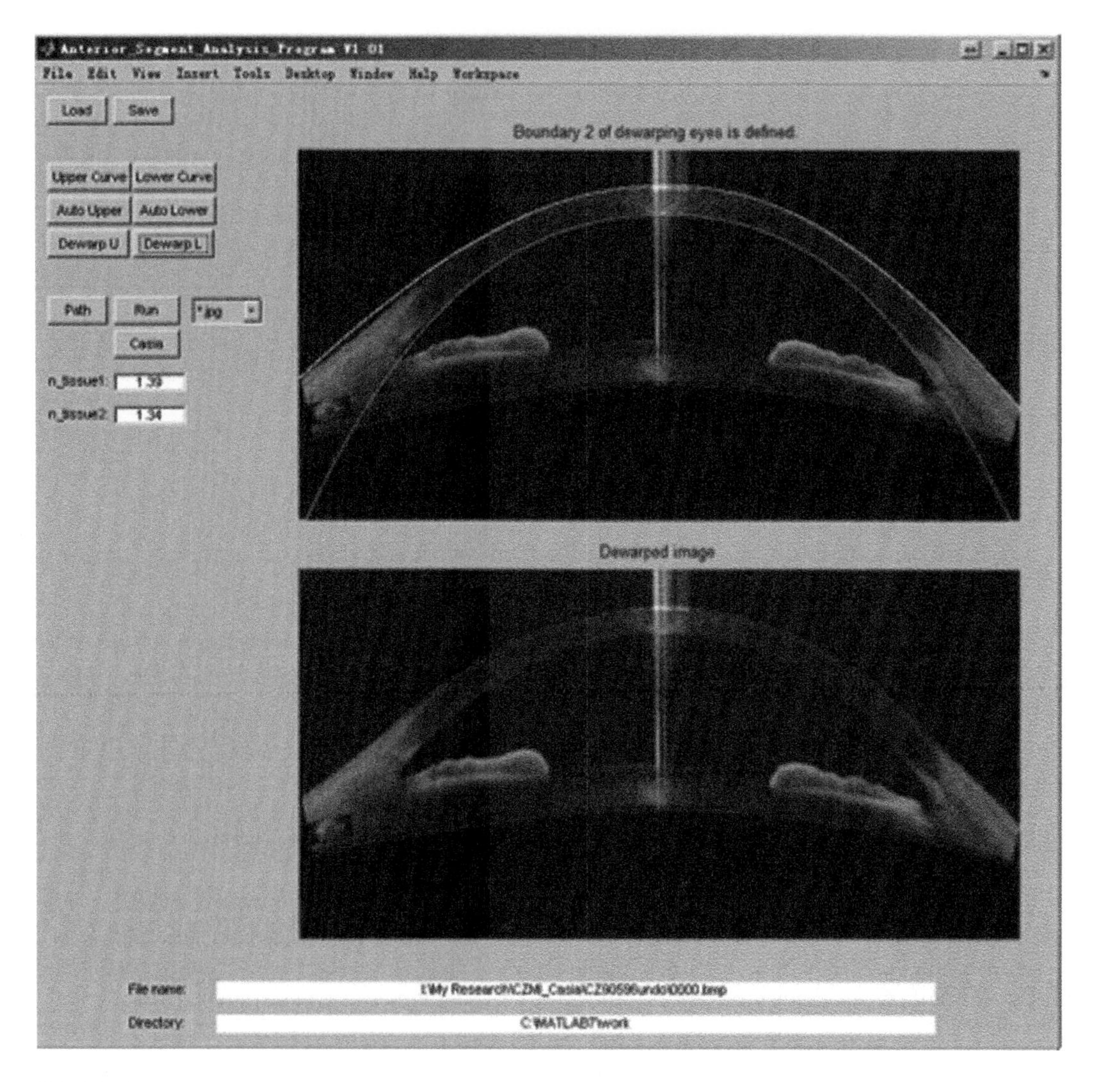

FIGURE 16.6
"Dewarp" to correct the image distortion due to refraction both at the air–cornea interface (refractive index = 1.389) and at the endothelium–aqueous boundary (refractive index = 1.32).

2. A binary ("0" or "1" pixels) thresholded image is obtained with a threshold of ((255 – t)*0.3), where t is the mean of the background noise. The algorithm will divide each pixel as either 1's (tissue that is normally brighter than background noise) or 0's (open space) based on the calculated threshold value.
3. The raw curve of corneal boundary is identified and refined using spline fitting.

16.3.4.2 Iris Boundary

Iris boundary detection was more challenging than the corneal boundary especially the posterior iris boundary. One reason is that the light back reflection occurred at the posterior iris–aqueous interface is much weaker than that of the air–tear/cornea interface. Moreover, the highly reflecting iris pigment epithelium attenuates the incident light and

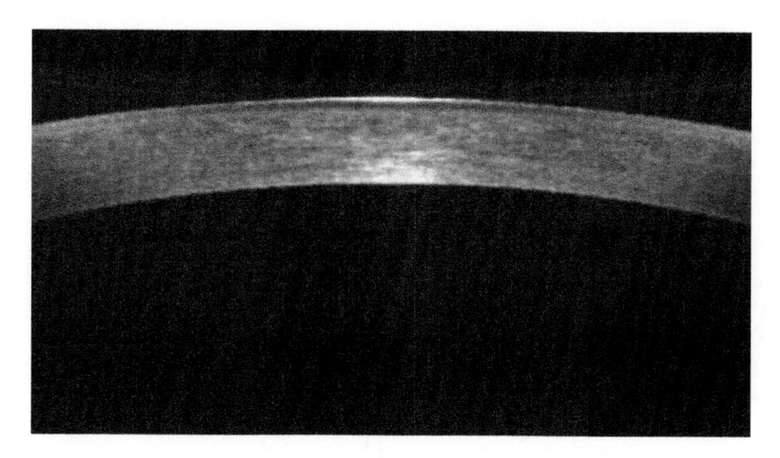

FIGURE 16.7
ASOCT image of normal human cornea.

prevents visualization of the ciliary body and posterior chamber structure, which were shadowed in ASOCT images.

A pseudocolor image processing was used to identify the iris boundary. A pseudocolor algorithm changes each grayscale pixel value to a color pixel value according to a table or function produced by computer algorithm. Depending on pseudocolor algorithm used, pseudocoloring may increase the information contents of the original image. The following algorithms were developed to automatically identify the iris boundary:

1. The raw image is extracted from the 8-bit grayscale (intensities from 0 to 255) image.
2. Lookup tables of 16 colors are used to transform grayscale image into pseudocolor image.
3. The pseudocolor image is further split into three 8-bit grayscale images that contain the red, green, and blue components of the original image. The red component is extracted as iris showing higher signal density in this component.
4. A binary ("0" or "1" pixels) thresholded image is calculated based on the red component images with a threshold of t, the mean of the background noise.
5. The curve of the iris boundary is identified (Figure 16.9).

16.3.5 Measurement

Quantitative analysis of ASOCT images has largely remained undeveloped. The application of quantitative ASOCT image analysis techniques should yield significant information about mechanisms of PAC or PACG. In this chapter, we described ASOCT biometric measurement by an ImageJ program. As described earlier, ASAP was designed to automatically calculate the parameters of ASOCT images after marking of the SSs by the observer. Anatomically, SS represents the origin of the longitudinal ciliary muscle fibers and is the landmark of the trabecular meshwork base. In ASOCT images, SS often appears as an inward wedge shaped although it is actually a ring of circularly oriented collagen bundles in the inner aspect of the sclera. As scleral bed has different curvature compared to posterior surface of corneal, the SS was more often defined as a point to represent such

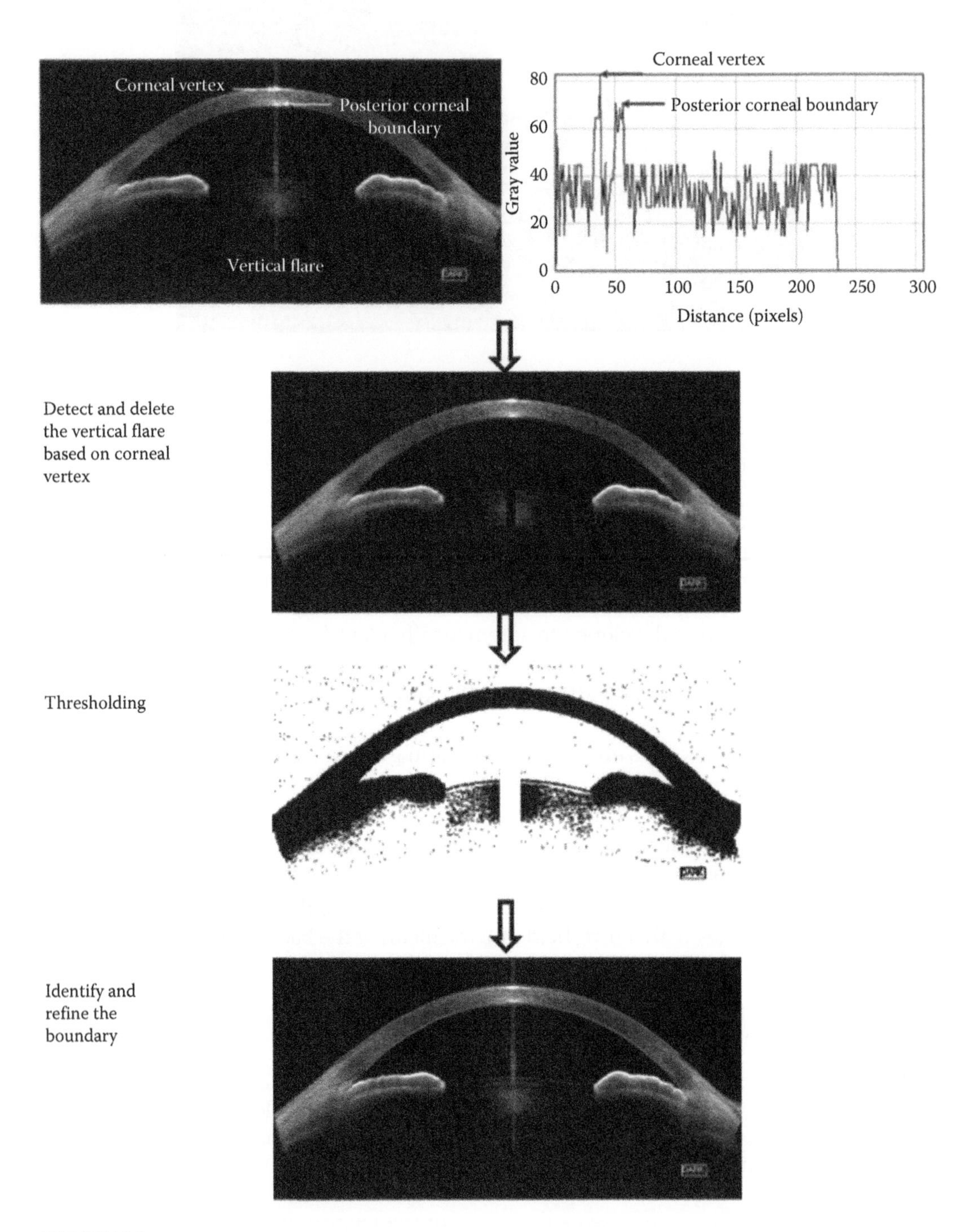

FIGURE 16.8
Flowchart of the segmentation algorithm for identifying the corneal boundary.

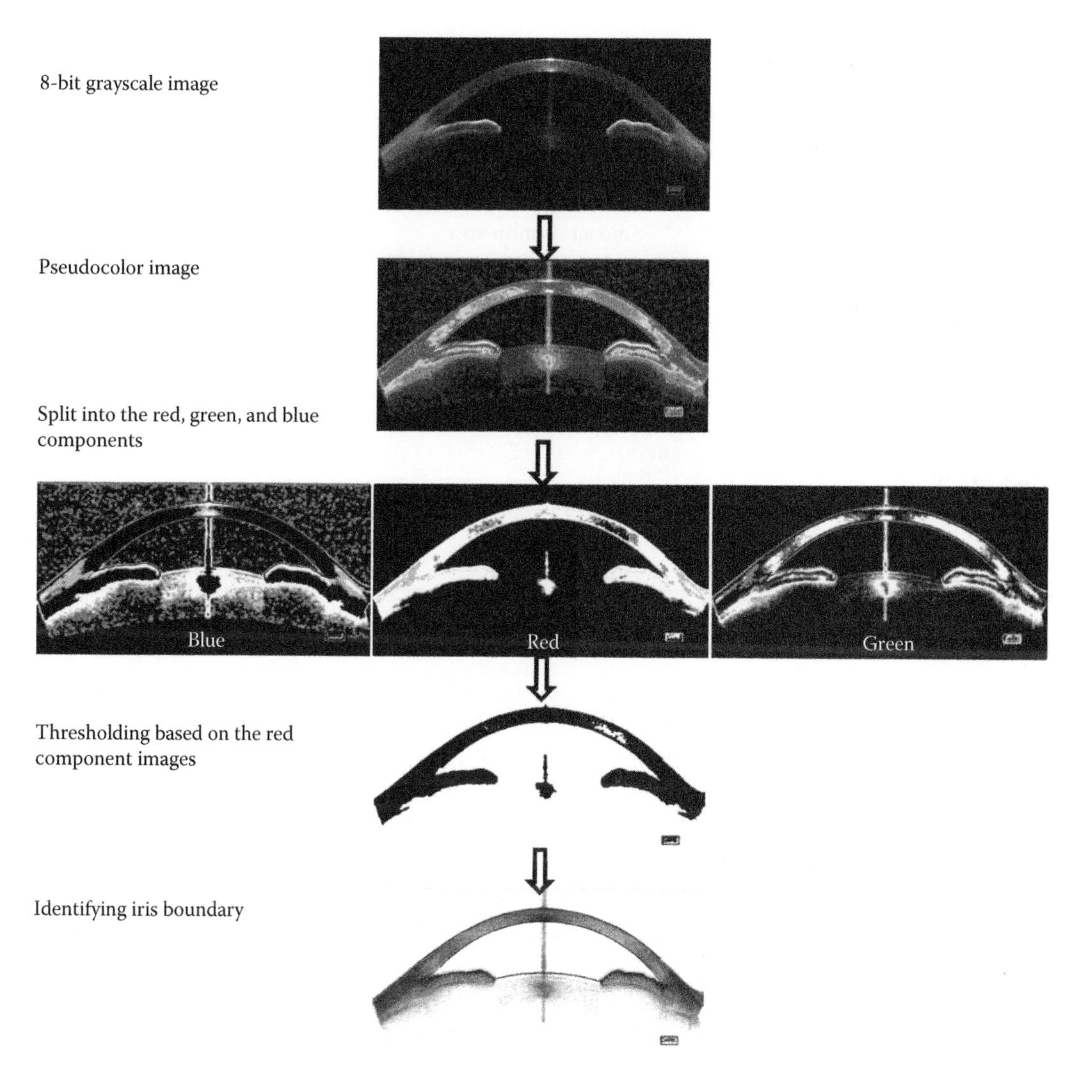

FIGURE 16.9
(See color insert.) Flowchart of the segmentation algorithm for identifying the iris boundary.

curvature change in ASOCT images [29]. The following are the definitions for some important ASOCT parameters (Figure 16.10):

1. Angle opening distance (AOD_{500} or AOD_{750}) was calculated as the perpendicular distance between the trabecular meshwork and the anterior iris surface at 500 or 750 μm anterior to the SS.
2. Iris thickness at 750 (IT_{750}) was measured 750 μm anterior to the SS.
3. Iris area (IA) was defined as the cumulative cross-sectional area of the full length of the iris.
4. ACA was defined as the cumulative cross-sectional area bounded superiorly by corneal endothelium and inferiorly by the lens–iris diaphragm.
5. ACW was calculated as the distance between 2 SSs.

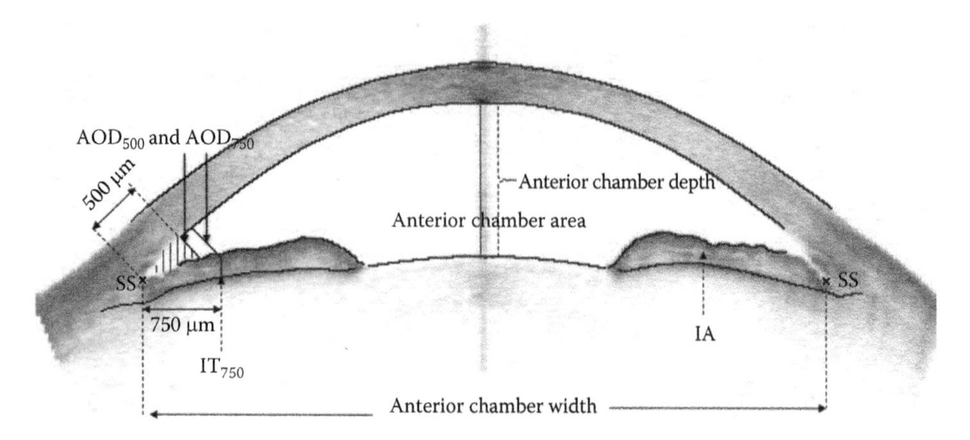

FIGURE 16.10
ASOCT image showing the measurements of some clinical important parameters.

16.4 Future Direction and Summary

With the improvement of ASOCT technology from TD to SD technology, novel anterior segment structure assessment (like 3D measurement) can be performed with reliable measurement, and this improvement should bring not only increased image-acquisition speeds but also promise of improved diagnostics, disease follow-up, surgical planning, and outcome monitoring and enhance the response to therapy. Furthermore, the incorporation of newly developed computer imaging processing into ASOCT instruments has boosted both basic medical research and clinic work.

In summary, ASOCT is applicable to assess a wide variety of anterior segment conditions. As a noncontact method, ASOCT would become an essential tool for screening some eye diseases, like PAC, corneal lesions, and lens opacity. Information obtained could be used in the assessment of the guidelines for medical or surgical treatment.

References

1. Huang D, Swanson EA, Lin CP, Schuman JS, Stinson WG, Chang W, Hee MR et al.: Optical coherence tomography. *Science* 1991, 254(5035):1178–1181.
2. Izatt JA, Hee MR, Swanson EA, Lin CP, Huang D, Schuman JS, Puliafito CA, Fujimoto JG: Micrometer-scale resolution imaging of the anterior eye in vivo with optical coherence tomography. *Arch Ophthalmol* 1994, 112(12):1584–1589.
3. Foster PJ, Johnson GJ: Glaucoma in China: How big is the problem? *Br J Ophthalmol* 2001, 85(11):1277–1282.
4. Quigley HA, Congdon NG, Friedman DS: Glaucoma in China (and worldwide): Changes in established thinking will decrease preventable blindness. *Br J Ophthalmol* 2001, 85(11): 1271–1272.
5. Quigley HA, Broman AT: The number of people with glaucoma worldwide in 2010 and 2020. *Br J Ophthalmol* 2006, 90(3):262–267.
6. Quigley HA: Number of people with glaucoma worldwide. *Br J Ophthalmol* 1996, 80(5):389–393.

7. Klein BE, Klein R, Sponsel WE, Franke T, Cantor LB, Martone J, Menage MJ: Prevalence of glaucoma. The Beaver Dam Eye Study. *Ophthalmology* 1992, 99(10):1499–1504.
8. Singh M, Chew PT, Friedman DS, Nolan WP, See JL, Smith SD, Zheng C, Foster PJ, Aung T: Imaging of trabeculectomy blebs using anterior segment optical coherence tomography. *Ophthalmology* 2007, 114(1):47–53.
9. Nolan WP, Foster PJ, Devereux JG, Uranchimeg D, Johnson GJ, Baasanhu J: YAG laser iridotomy treatment for primary angle closure in east Asian eyes. *Br J Ophthalmol* 2000, 84(11): 1255–1259.
10. How AC, Baskaran M, Kumar RS, He M, Foster PJ, Lavanya R, Wong HT, Chew PT, Friedman DS, Aung T: Changes in anterior segment morphology after laser peripheral iridotomy: An anterior segment optical coherence tomography study. *Ophthalmology* 2012, 119(7):1383–1387.
11. See JL, Chew PT, Smith SD, Nolan WP, Chan YH, Huang D, Zheng C, Foster PJ, Aung T, Friedman DS: Changes in anterior segment morphology in response to illumination and after laser iridotomy in Asian eyes: An anterior segment OCT study. *Br J Ophthalmol* 2007, 91(11):1485–1489.
12. Majander AS, Lindahl PM, Vasara LK, Krootila K: Anterior segment optical coherence tomography in congenital corneal opacities. *Ophthalmology* 2012, 119(12):2450–2457.
13. Krachmer JH, Feder RS, Belin MW: Keratoconus and related noninflammatory corneal thinning disorders. *Surv Ophthalmol* 1984, 28(4):293–322.
14. Ventura BV, Moraes HV, Jr., Kara-Junior N, Santhiago MR: Role of optical coherence tomography on corneal surface laser ablation. *J Ophthalmol* 2012, 2012:676740.
15. Pavlin CJ, Vasquez LM, Lee R, Simpson ER, Ahmed, II: Anterior segment optical coherence tomography and ultrasound biomicroscopy in the imaging of anterior segment tumors. *Am J Ophthalmol* 2009, 147(2):214.e2–219.e2.
16. Shields CL, Belinsky I, Romanelli-Gobbi M, Guzman JM, Mazzuca D, Jr., Green WR, Bianciotto C, Shields JA: Anterior segment optical coherence tomography of conjunctival nevus. *Ophthalmology* 2011, 118(5):915–919.
17. Calladine D, Packard R: Clear corneal incision architecture in the immediate postoperative period evaluated using optical coherence tomography. *J Cataract Refract Surg* 2007, 33(8):1429–1435.
18. Chee SP, Ti SE, Lim L, Chan AS, Jap A: Anterior segment optical coherence tomography evaluation of the integrity of clear corneal incisions: A comparison between 2.2-mm and 2.65-mm main incisions. *Am J Ophthalmol* 2010, 149(5):768.e1–776.e1.
19. Radhakrishnan S, See J, Smith SD, Nolan WP, Ce Z, Friedman DS, Huang D, Li Y, Aung T, Chew PT: Reproducibility of anterior chamber angle measurements obtained with anterior segment optical coherence tomography. *Invest Ophthalmol Vis Sci* 2007, 48(8):3683–3688.
20. Console JW, Sakata LM, Aung T, Friedman DS, He M: Quantitative analysis of anterior segment optical coherence tomography images: The Zhongshan Angle Assessment Program. *Br J Ophthalmol* 2008, 92(12):1612–1616.
21. Eliceiri KW, Rueden C: Tools for visualizing multidimensional images from living specimens. *Photochem Photobiol* 2005, 81(5):1116–1122.
22. Burger W, Burge MJ: *Digital Image Processing: An Algorithmic Approach Using Java*. Springer, Berlin, Germany, 2007.
23. Dougherty G: *Digital Image Processing for Medical Applications*. Cambridge University Press, Cambridge, U.K., 2009.
24. Davies ER: *Machine Vision: Theory, Algorithms, Practicalities*. Elsevier, Amsterdam, the Netherlands, 2005.
25. Jain AK: *Fundamentals of Digital Image Processing*. Prentice Hall, Upper Saddle River, NJ, 1989.
26. Westphal V, Rollins A, Radhakrishnan S, Izatt J: Correction of geometric and refractive image distortions in optical coherence tomography applying Fermat's principle. *Opt Express* 2002, 10(9):397–404.
27. Sarunic MV, Asrani S, Izatt JA: Imaging the ocular anterior segment with real-time, full-range Fourier-domain optical coherence tomography. *Arch Ophthalmol* 2008, 126(4):537–542.

28. Lin RC, Shure MA, Rollins AM, Izatt JA, Huang D: Group index of the human cornea at 1.3-microm wavelength obtained in vitro by optical coherence domain reflectometry. *Opt Lett* 2004, 29(1):83–85.
29. Sakata LM, Lavanya R, Friedman DS, Aung HT, Seah SK, Foster PJ, Aung T: Assessment of the scleral spur in anterior segment optical coherence tomography images. *Arch Ophthalmol* 2008, 126(2):181–185.

17

Cyst Detection in OCT Images for Pathology Characterization

Ana González, Beatriz Remeseiro, Marcos Ortega, Manuel G. Penedo, and Pablo Charlón

CONTENTS

17.1 Introduction

From the early 1990s computational performance has been improving and numerous diagnostic techniques have been incorporated into clinical practice, improving the study and monitoring of many diseases in all areas of health. In the study of the eye, and more specifically the study of pathologies affecting the retina, using many of these techniques has become essential for diagnosis, treatment, and monitoring. Correct interpretation and understanding of these techniques is very important for the clinical practice of health professionals dedicated to visual care.

Currently, in the study of retinal pathology, optical coherence tomography (OCT), which provides a large amount of information, has become an essential test. Because of OCT, it is possible to detect, investigate, and understand the pathological changes, and monitor diseases or the effectiveness of treatments. One of the retinal alterations, which is present in a wide variety of pathologies, is the cystoid macular edema (CME), whose presence significantly affects visual function. It is easily detectable using OCT and can guide the therapeutic approach to be followed in those pathologies with intraretinal cysts. This makes detection and monitoring of CME interesting to specialists.

17.1.1 Optical Coherence Tomography Images

OCT retinal images are used by experts to diagnose pathologies, as the images are captured in a noninvasive, contactless method that gives a cross sectional image of the retina and its structures in real-time fashion [18]. The principle of OCT is based on interferometry and the images are generated by measuring the reflectance of light from translucent materials such as the retina. Light is reflected and backscattered from refractive index interfaces within the retina according to the optical properties of each interface. In this way, it allows the visualization of each layer and the structures present on them, as Figure 17.1 shows. Therefore OCT is particularly effective in identifying retinal morphology that explains disease pathogenesis and heralds disease progression. OCT has progressed in recent years, especially since the detection of the spectral domain (SD), and presents a higher potential to be used in ophthalmic clinical examinations because it shows extremely high sensitivity and image-acquisition speed. Both these characteristics are essential for ophthalmic applications [28].

At present, several diseases can be diagnosed with an OCT retinal analysis: OCT layer-thickness information is particularly useful in diagnosing and treating eye diseases like glaucoma [4], macular degeneration [13], and diabetic retinopathy [20]. Experts also found that a high-speed retinal thinning is correlated with multiple sclerosis [1]. The presence of cystic structures may denote inflammation and diabetes [21].

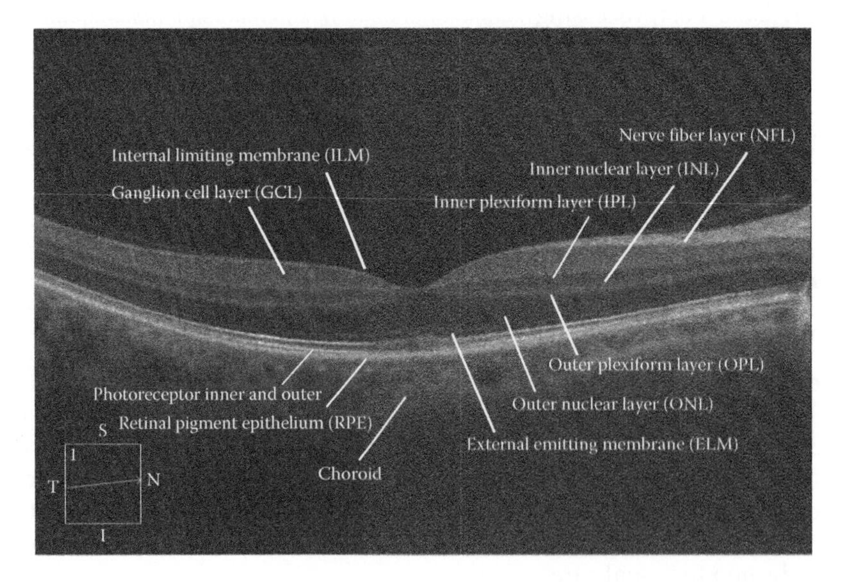

FIGURE 17.1
Identification of the retinal layers on a OCT image.

17.1.2 Cystoid Macular Edema

CME consists of the accumulation of fluid between the outer plexiform and inner nuclear layers in the retina. It is a nonspecific response, a consequence of the rupture of the blood–retinal barrier. It often produces vision loss in a wide variety of eye conditions.

17.1.2.1 Blood–Retinal Barrier Functions

The blood–retinal barrier is located at two levels: between tight junctions of endothelial cells on the retinal vessel walls (inner blood–retinal barrier) and between tight junctions of the retinal pigment epithelium (RPE) (outer blood–retinal barrier). Active transport of electrolytes and molecules from the retina to the choroid happens through the RPE. This helps to maintain the extracellular space volume, which is severely disrupted by the failure of any or both blood–retinal barriers, resulting in the accumulation of plasma, specially proteins and serum. This plasma accumulation is often located at the level of the macular area between the outer plexiform and inner nuclear layers, and it is called cystoid macular edema if it affects the extra-foveal capillaries or diffuse edema if the accumulation of plasma is more widespread.

17.1.2.2 Pathophysiology and Histopathology of Cystoid Macular Edema

The pathophysiology of CME is not entirely clear. For Gass [8], the main thing is the increase in the extracellular fluid of the retina. This accumulation of fluid between the outer plexiform and inner nuclear layers takes the form of cysts (Figure 17.2) of varying size depending on the age and severity of the process that creates them. For other researchers the primary focus would be the deterioration of the integrity of the Müller cells [26,27],

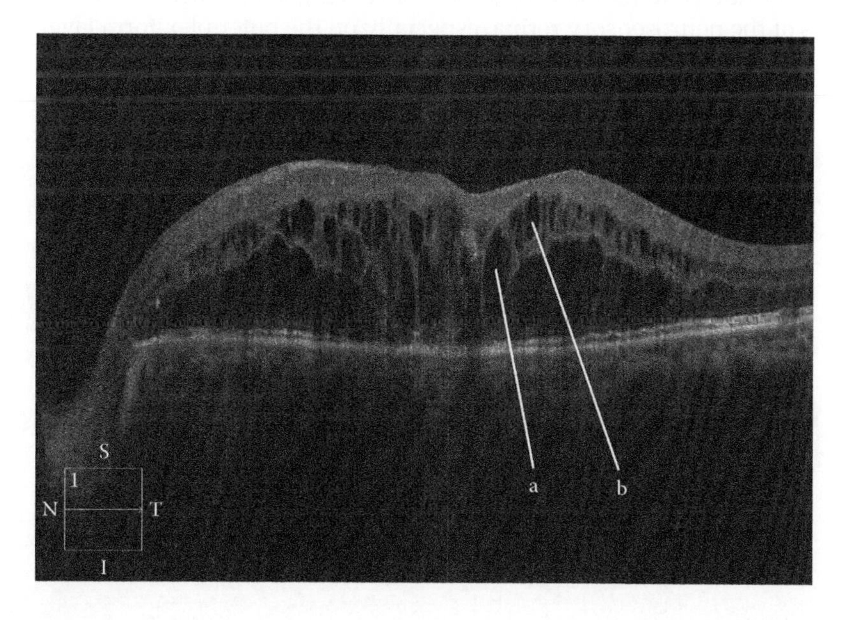

FIGURE 17.2
Cystoid macular edema (CME) on a OCT image. (a) Cysts distributed in the outer nuclear layer. (b) Cysts distributed in the inner nuclear layer.

whose function may be affected by inflammatory, ischemic, or genetic processes [16]. The degeneration of these cells produces a swelling, which results in the formation of cystic spaces. Histopathologically, CME is associated with a localized loss of photoreceptors [22–24] and degenerative changes in the pigment epithelium.

17.1.2.3 Breakdown Mechanisms of the Blood–Retinal Barrier

Goldberg [9] described a variety of processes that could modify the behavior of the blood–retinal barrier, which affect different structures in the eye: the *vitreous* (epiretinal membranes, vitritis, cyclitis, etc.), the *retina* (diabetes, venous thrombosis, hypertension, macroaneurysms, telangiectasias, tumors, retinitis pigmentosa, inflammatory processes such as phlebitis, arteritis, post-surgical recovery [Figure 17.3]), or the *choroid* (tumors, subretinal neovascularization, choroiditis, etc.). These processes must be distinguished from the following processes that do not have liquid leaks at extracellular level, but result in changes in the macula, which adopts a cystic appearance—epiretinal membranes without secondary exudation, degenerative cystic formations, retinitis pigmentosa, retinoschisis, Goldman-Favre disease or toxicity of the retinal pigment epithelium.

17.1.2.4 OCT Diagnosis of Cystoid Macular Edema

OCT technology has revolutionized opthalmic diagnostic imaging, given that it is a fast, quantifiable, reproducible, and innocuous technique. However, the data obtained by OCT are common irrespective of the cause of CME. This lack of specificity makes fluorescein angiography (Figure 17.4) the first choice when a diagnostic test is done. The findings in the images obtained by OCT which correspond to any CME, show macular thickness with formation of rounded and nonreflective areas of varying size, which are placed on the different layers of the neurosensory retina, especially on the outer plexiform layer.

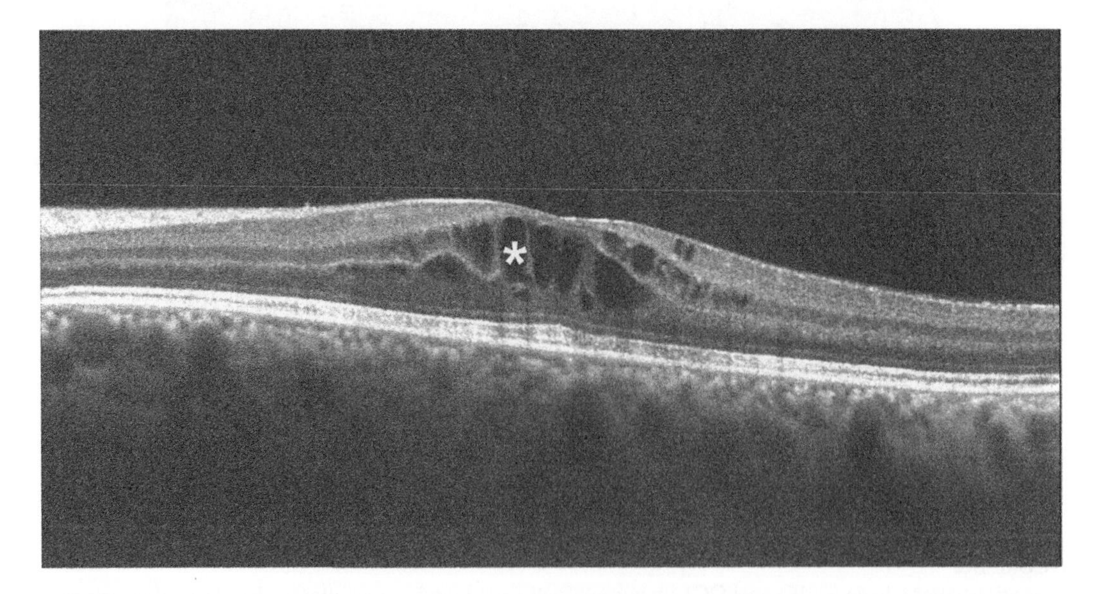

FIGURE 17.3
Intraretinal cystic lesions in OCT image caused by pseudophakic macular edema after cataract surgery with intraocular lens implantation.

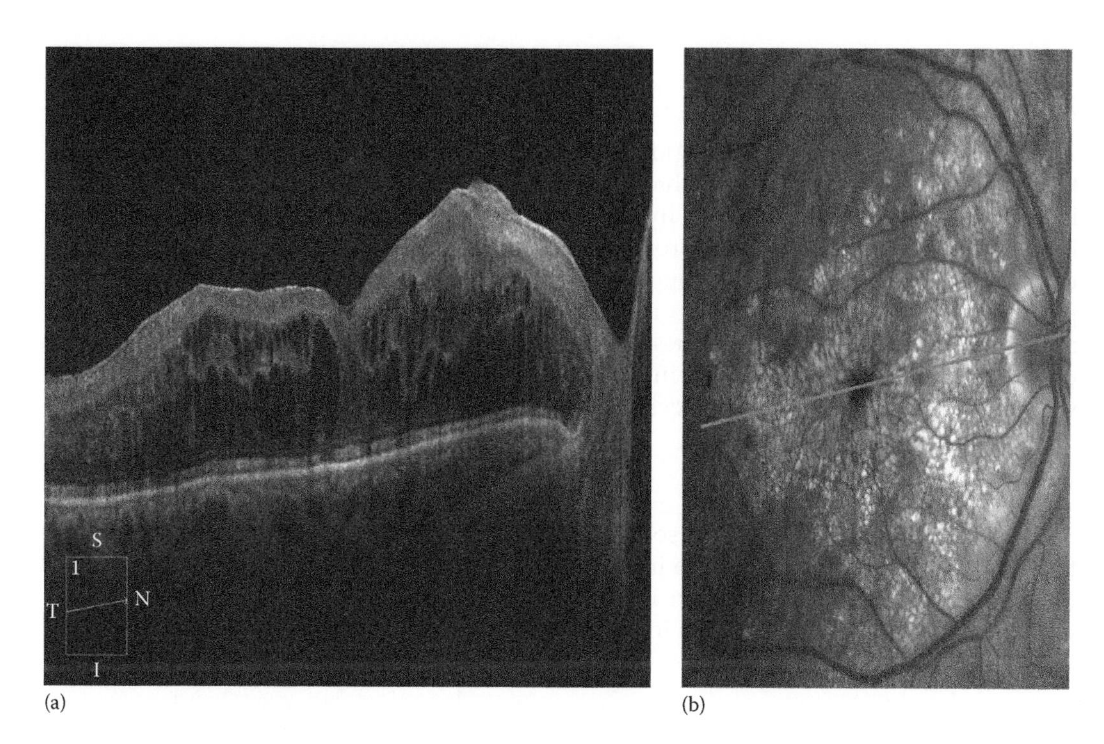

FIGURE 17.4
(See color insert.) (a) Cystoid macular edema (CME) on a OCT image. (b) Fluorescein angiography, where petaloid placement of the cysts is appreciable, as well as other vascular disorders that provide information for more accurate diagnosis.

The great advantage of OCT over other diagnostic techniques in CME is that it can provide quantitative data, which allows optimal monitoring of treatment response.

17.1.3 Automatic Cyst Detection in OCT Images

Although some image-processing techniques to detect anomalies in the macula [15] automatically have been developed in the opthalmologic environment, there is no previous work establishing a global quantitative method for automatic cyst detection, independent of the kind of cyst. This, therefore, is the aim of this work. Given the different problems that OCT retinal images present, cyst detection is not of immediate importance. First, it is possible to find different pathologies in the same patient, resulting in several alterations in the retinal image that should be taken into account. Some parts of the image may be of poor quality due to the capture process. A high variability in shape, size, and orientation in the cyst is possible, and they can be situated on different layers of the retina, presenting different intensity properties. There are also other structures, such as vessel shades, on the image with similar properties. There are even situations where the expert cannot determine with sufficient confidence if a suspicious region is a cyst.

Section 17.2 explains a methodology for an automatic detection of candidate regions to be identified as cysts, in OCT retinal images. In this case, HD-OCT images have been considered, which are obtained by combining the information extracted from a sequence of more than 20 images.

17.2 Methodology

The detection of cyst candidate regions has some complexity involved. Our proposal for this task is composed of different phases, as Figure 17.5 shows: first, a preprocessing of the image is needed. In this phase, the image is enhanced and the region of interest is delimited to perform the cyst location process. In the second phase, a watershed algorithm is used with the purpose of detecting candidate regions. The last phase is a classification process, which is applied over texture descriptors extracted from the regions to identify real cysts. The steps involved in these phases are detailed in the following sections. The necessity of these steps is reflected in Figure 17.6, where an original OCT image is shown, with the region of interest and the cysts present on it.

17.2.1 Preprocessing

The capture process gives rise to some deficiencies, so an enhanced process is applied to remove noise and normalize the images. After that, it is possible to delimit the region of interest. In this case, this region is determined by the bounding layers of the retina, which are considerably appreciable in OCT images. Boundary layers, the internal limiting

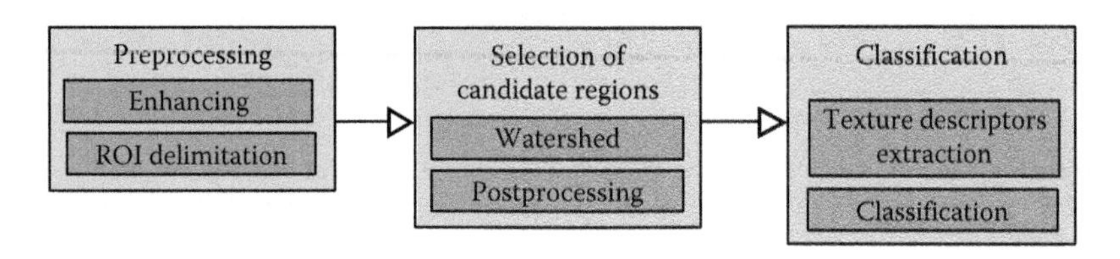

FIGURE 17.5
Phases in the methodology followed.

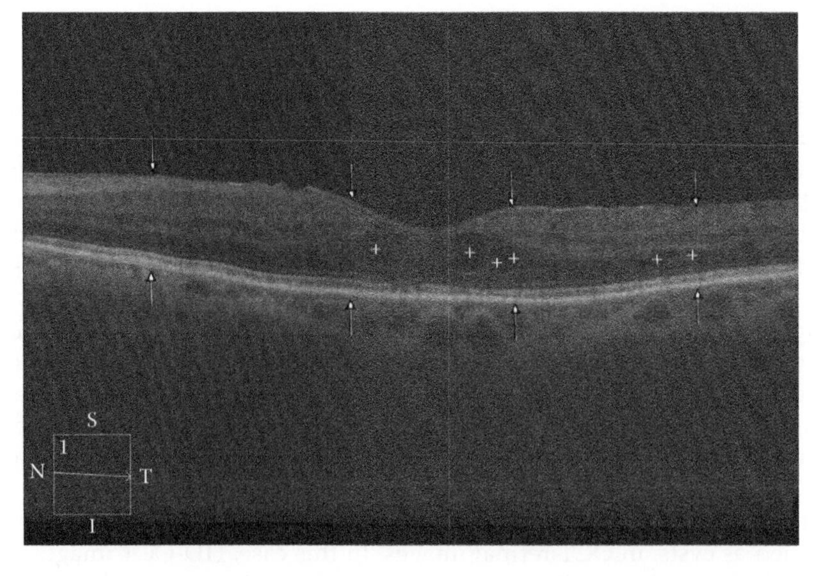

FIGURE 17.6
Example of OCT retinal image: region of interest is delimited by arrows. Cysts are marked in white crosses.

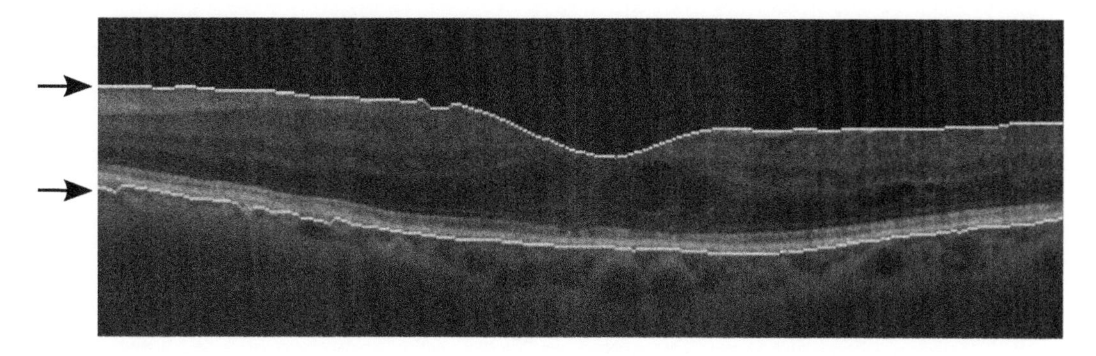

FIGURE 17.7
Region of interest is delimited on the image presented in Figure 17.6. Boundary layers of the retina are highlighted and identified by arrows.

membrane (ILM) and the RPE, must be segmented in order to delimit the area of interest where the search will be conducted. For this task, the methodology proposed in [11] is taken into account. It involves transforming the segmentation task into that of finding a minimum-cost closed set in a geometric graph [14], which is built on information from the edge and the region, taking into account some surface smoothness and interaction constraints.

In this task, the main problem is the designing of the cost functions to be used to segment a particular layer. This work [10] presents suitable cost functions to segment the top boundary of the ILM layer, as well as the bottom boundary of the RPE layer. Figure 17.7 shows the segmentation of the boundary layers, used to reduce the region of interest.

17.2.2 Selection of Candidate Regions

As the methodology exposed in Figure 17.5 presents, the selection of candidate regions is done in two steps: first, dark areas on the image are identified using a flooding algorithm and then, some of these areas are excluded automatically based on their properties. The process is presented in the next sections.

17.2.2.1 Flooding

Once the area of interest is bounded, cyst searching begins. These structures can be presented in different layers in the retina, especially in the outer nuclear layer (ONL). Cysts are darker regions in a lighter environment, but their shape is variable (they are usually elliptic but might conform to other shapes too). In addition, their orientation and size are not constant. The presence of other structures with similar characteristics, such as retinal folds or vessels shades, complicates the detection of cyst. The approach for this task is to locate dark areas in the image using the watershed algorithm [3,25].

The watershed algorithm is based on the idea that a gray-level image can be represented as a topographic relief, where the gray level of a pixel is interpreted as its altitude in the relief. The process starts with placing a water source in each regional minimum in the image, then the relief is flooded from sources. Barriers are built where different sources meet (Figure 17.8). When the process ends, a large set of basins have been found. Looking at an excessive number of basins is usually avoided by using information from the gradient image to know which barriers are significant.

However, using the gradient image does not work in this problem, because there is not enough information about the edges in the images, especially on the ONL, which is too

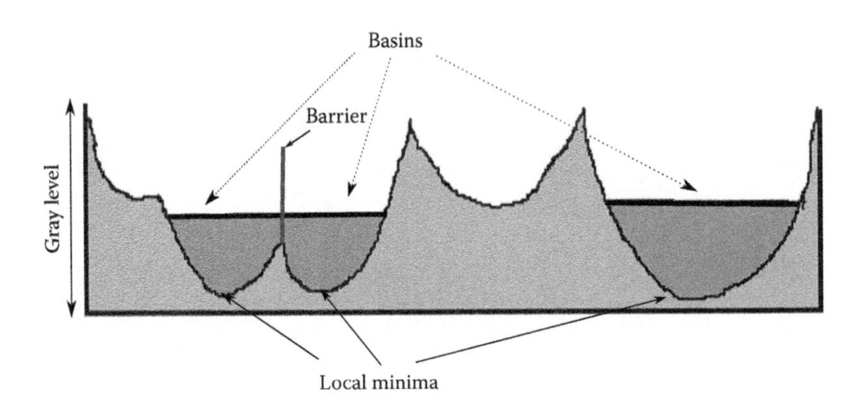

FIGURE 17.8
Schema of watershed process: basins are flooded and barriers are built where two of them meet.

dark to present abrupt transitions when a cyst is found. Therefore, a modification is introduced in the algorithm, to consider the merging of basins during the first l levels of flooding. If two regions get connected in a few flooding steps and they share a considerable connected area, it suggests those areas should conform to only one region and the separation between these basins in the watershed algorithm must be ignored. In the implementation of the algorithm, this situation is controlled by p_{con}, which represents the minimum percent of connected pixels that the regions must have, with respect to their own size.

To avoid degeneration of the regions with excessive flooding, the process is interrupted when a percent of the darkest pixels in the image has been covered. This way, we avoid flooding useless regions in the image and decrease the number of candidate regions, given that cysts always correspond to dark areas in the image. The number of regions to flood is also reduced if only regions with pixels whose intensities are below a threshold are included in the flooding. Thus, the flooding starts at the gray level which covers the p_{ini} percent of darkest pixels in the image, and it ends when p_{end} percent have been flooded.

At the end of this phase, a set of candidate areas has been extracted by the watershed algorithm, as Figure 17.9 shows in different colors. This set includes cyst regions and other regions in the image whose intensities make them similar to cysts. Therefore, a postprocessing of the regions to reduce the number of initial candidates is discussed next.

17.2.2.2 Postprocessing

A large set of candidate regions is obtained during the watershed process, containing a high number of false positives. As they often share intensity properties, a merging process is applied over them at this stage, with the purpose of unification. Additionally, some rules are applied later to discard regions that, from domain knowledge, can be disregarded as cyst candidates.

- *Region merging*: In this step, connected regions with similar intensities are merged. For merging, two similarity measures between regions are considered: intensity average and dispersion. This way, two regions are merged if their intensity averages i_{a1}, i_{a2} and dispersions i_{d1}, i_{d2} are close enough (considering thresholds i_a and i_d, respectively):

$$|i_{a1} - i_{a2}| < i_a \quad \&\& \quad |i_{d1} - i_{d2}| < i_d$$

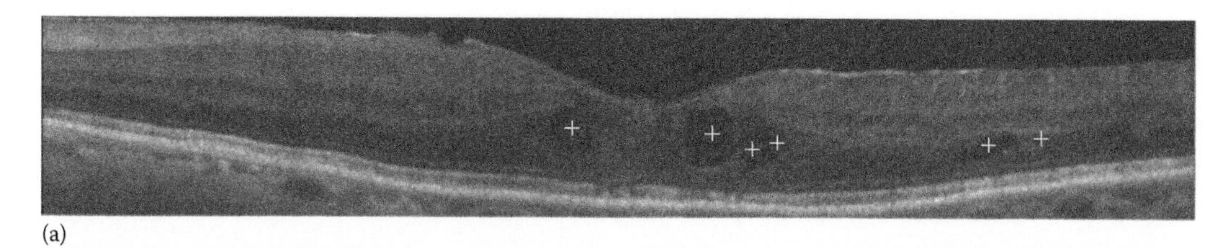

(a)

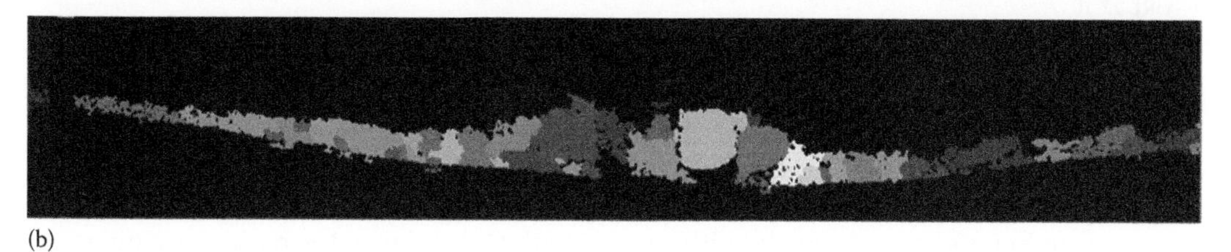

(b)

FIGURE 17.9
Candidate regions selected for an example image: (a) original image marked by an expert (white crosses) and (b) flooded regions.

- *Discarding candidate regions:* After the watershed process and the unification, a set of candidate regions with the appropriate size to be studied is obtained. In this set, there are regions associated with cysts, but there are still a large number of regions which do not correspond to cystic structures. To reduce the number of candidate regions and to enhance the performance in the classification stage, different kind of features that cysts should satisfy have been studied. These features have given rise to rules for discarding regions:
  - *Very small regions*: This feature has been included in a very relaxed way, given that not all cysts have the same size. A region will be discarded if

$$n_r < n_{min} \quad \&\& \quad (h_r < h_{min} \| w_r < w_{min})$$

    where
    n_r is the number of pixels in the region
    h_r and w_r its height and width, respectively
    n_{min}, h_{min}, w_{min} are the thresholds which control these parameters
  - *Regions which are too elongated in the horizontal dimension*: As in the case of the previous rule, this condition is not satisfied strictly, although cysts do not usually have this shape. Thus, considering the dimensions w_r and h_r of the regions, the rectangle r which bounds the region and the percent p_r of occupation of the region over r, that will be excluded if

$$w_r > t_1 * h_r \| (w_r > t_2 * h_r \quad \&\& \quad p_r > p_{occ})$$

    where t_1, t_2, and p_{occ} work as thresholds for the dimensions and the percent of occupation.

    Some examples of this kind of regions, as well as those discarded using the previous rule, are shown in Figure 17.10.
  - *Regions that in a few flooding levels are not dense enough*: During the watershed process, flooding in the cyst regions is regular. They usually start flooding

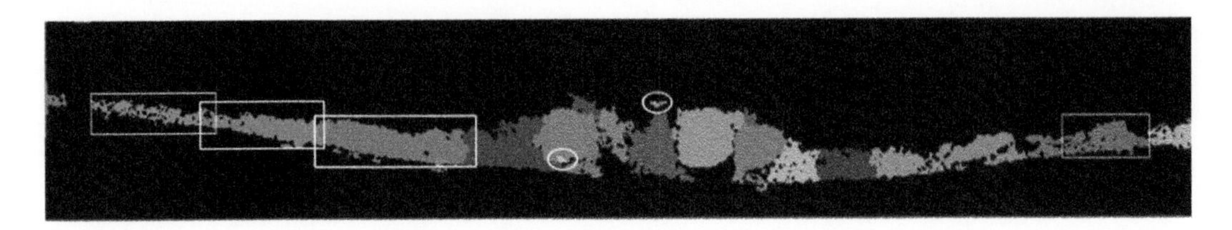

FIGURE 17.10
Example of regions to be discarded: too small areas (white circles) and too elongated areas (white rectangles).

with a considerable size and then grow in a regular way. To evaluate this behavior, the configuration of the candidate region at level l_{ref} in the flooding process is studied. If it is composed of many small disconnected clusters, the number and size of which (with respect to the total size of the region) are given by rc_n and rc_s, satisfying

$$rc_n > c_n \quad \&\& \quad rc_s > c_s$$

where c_n and c_s are certain thresholds, then it is probably not a cyst, given that cysts usually grow, after some flooding levels, from the inner part of the region toward the outside, as Figure 17.11 presents.

- *Regions located right next to the sides of the image*: Cysts are not usually located right next to the image boundaries, therefore, the proximity and size of these regions are controlled by thresholds d_{side} and s_{side}.
- *Regions located right next to boundary top layer*: Regions detected at this part of the image usually correspond to imperfections in the segmentation of the top boundary layer. Threshold d_{top} controls the proximity of these regions.
- *Regions on the bottom part of the ONL, even in contact with RPE layer*: There are often cysts on the ONL, but they are not connected, in general with the RPE. In order to apply this rule, a suitable approach for the top boundary of RPE has been done, drawn on the methodology that was used in Section 17.2.1, but by designing the appropriate cost function for this layer. Once this layer

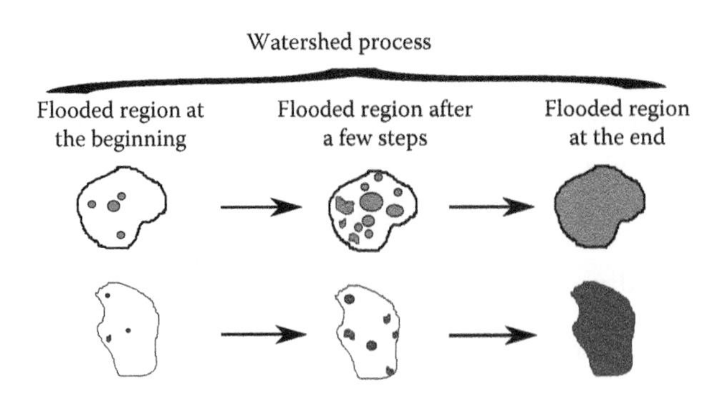

FIGURE 17.11
Details of the state for two regions in a few levels of flooding: no cystic regions usually present the behavior of the darker region (below).

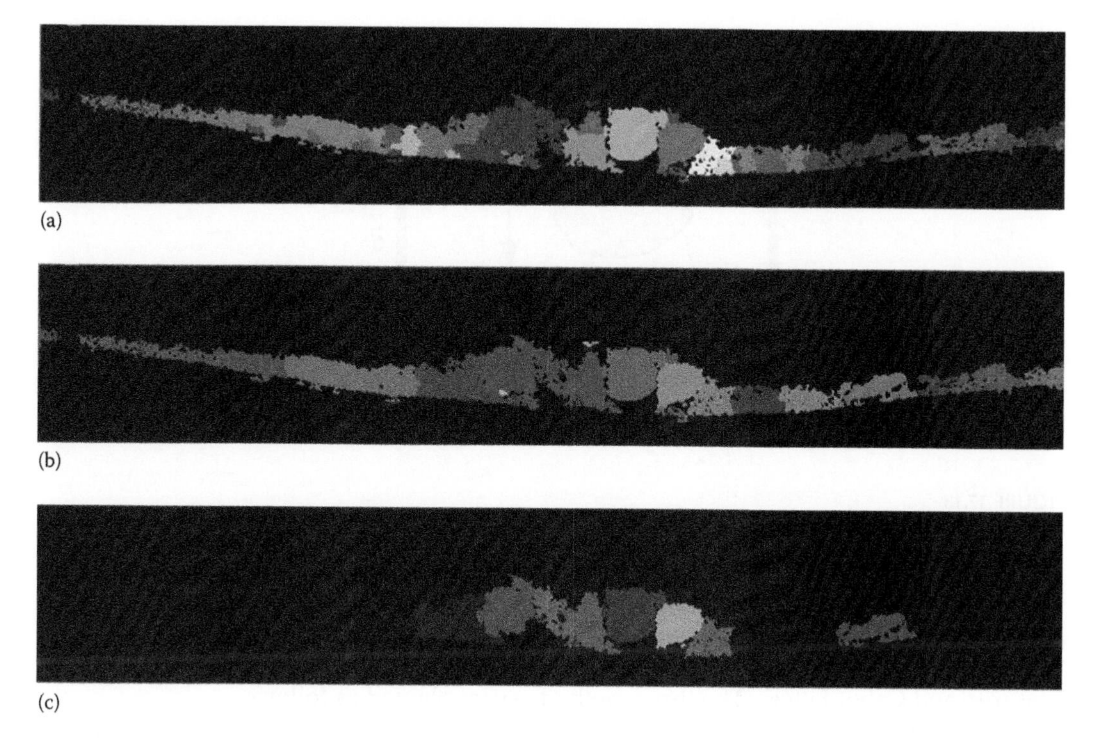

FIGURE 17.12
(a) Regions obtained by watershed process, (b) merged regions, and (c) remaining regions after applying discarding rules.

is detected, it is possible to discard regions with height h_r and a percent p_r of pixels close enough to the layer, in the following way:

$$h_r > h_{max} \quad \&\& \quad p_r > p_{near}$$

where p_{near} and h_{max} represent the thresholds which control these parameters.

The number of candidate regions at the end of the postprocessing has decreased considerably. Figure 17.12 presents the process detailed in this section, applied over the image used in the previous step, where all the regions detected are painted using different intensities.

17.2.3 Classification of Candidate Regions

At the previous stage, a number of regions that did not correspond to cysts were removed. However, other regions with properties similar to cysts still remained. Given that, in general, cysts are mainly dark regions in a lighter environment, an analysis based on texture descriptors should be done using that information. To extract the descriptors, a window over the image, centered in each region, is used. The dimensions h_{win}, w_{win} for this window are obtained scaling the region ones h_{reg}, w_{reg} in f_h and f_w factors, as Figure 17.13 shows. Thus, a portion of the environment is included. The problem arises when two regions are overlapped in the same window because they are located together. In this case, the window is automatically cut to exclude the information of the other region.

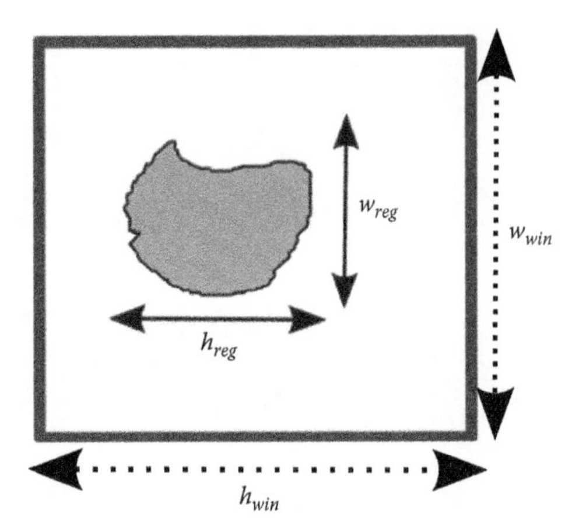

FIGURE 17.13
Diagram showing the window (square) built over a candidate region, with $(h_{win}, w_{win}) = (f_h, f_w) * (h_{reg}, w_{reg})$.

17.2.3.1 Texture Analysis

The texture descriptors considered in this work are Markov Random Fields, Co-occurrences Features, and Gabor Filters. The three methods are explained as follows:

Markov Random Field (MRF) [2] is a two-dimensional lattice of points where each point has a value that depends on its neighboring values. Therefore, a MRF generates a texture model by expressing the gray value of each pixel in an image as a function of the gray values in its neighborhood. The values that define this function are called parameters of the model.

In this case, the neighborhood of a pixel is defined as the set of pixels within a distance d, using the *Chebyshev distance*. Thus, for each input image, the parameters of the model must be calculated. The directional variances proposed in [5] are obtained using those parameters, resulting in the feature vector. If a distance d is considered, $4d$ defines the descriptor. By means of their concatenation, the vector of each distance can be combined with the vector of any other distances.

Co-occurrence Features, proposed by Haralick et al. [12], are extended and effective texture descriptors. The computation is based on the conditional joint probabilities of all pairwise combinations of gray levels, given an interpixel distance d and an orientation θ. This method generates a set of Gray Level Co-occurrence Matrices (GLCM) and extracts several statistics from their elements $P_{\theta,d}(i, j)$.

When a distance $d = 1$ is used, a total of four orientations (0°, 45°, 90°, and 135°) are considered, as Figure 17.14 shows, and four matrices are generated. For a distance $d > 1$, the number of orientations increases as also the number of matrices. In general, the number of orientations for a distance d is $4d$. From each co-occurrence matrix a set of 14 statistics proposed by Haralick et al. [12], are computed, representing features such as homogeneity or contrast. The mean and range across matrices are obtained, resulting in a set of 28 features, which will be the descriptor of the input image.

Gabor Filters are complex exponential signals modulated by Gaussians [7] and they are widely popular in texture analysis. A two-dimensional Gabor Filter [6], using Cartesian coordinates in the spatial domain and polar coordinates in the frequency domain, is defined as:

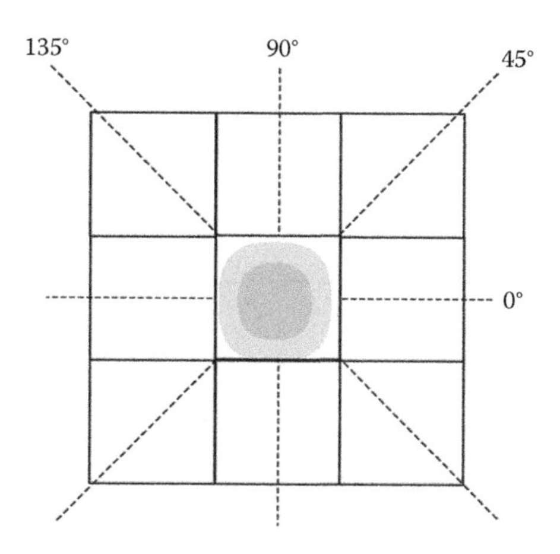

FIGURE 17.14
Orientations considered for distance $d = 1$ in co-occurrence features.

$$g_{x_0,y_0,f_0,\theta_0} = exp\{i[2\pi f_0(x\cos\theta_0 + y\sin\theta_0)\varphi]\}gauss(x,y)$$

where

$$gauss(x,y) = a\,exp\{-\pi[a^2(x\cos\theta_0 + y\sin\theta_0)^2 + b^2(x\sin\theta_0\cos + y\theta_0)^2]\}$$

with a and b modeling the shape of the filter and x_0, y_0, f_0, and θ_0 representing the location in the spatial and frequency domains, respectively.

A bank of 16 Gabor Filters centered at 4 frequencies and 4 orientations have been used in this work. Each input image is mapped to 16 result images, one per frequency-orientation pair. Thus, the descriptor of each output image is its uniform histogram with nonequidistant bins.

17.2.3.2 Classifiers

After extracting descriptors, they are passed to a classifier, which will determine if a region must be considered as a cyst or should be ignored. Several machine learning algorithms [17] can be applied to the problem of classifying texture descriptors in categories. Three popular algorithms have been selected and are briefly described as follows:

- *Support Vector Machine (SVM)*: SVM is a supervised learning method that is based on statistical learning theory. It constructs an n-dimensional hyperplane that optimally separates the data into classes. Thus, data are represented as points in space and examples from different classes are mapped so that they are separated by a distance that is as high as possible.
- *Naive-Bayes*: Naive-Bayes is a simple probabilistic classifier based on the Bayesian theorem and the maximum posteriori hypothesis that can predict class membership probabilities. This classifier assumes that, given the class variable, a particular feature of the class being present (or not) is not related to the presence (or absence) of any other feature.

- *Random-Forest*: Random-Forest is an ensemble classifier including the individual decision trees where each one depends on the values of a random vector. This vector is sampled independently and with the same distribution for all trees in the forest.

17.3 Results

The methodology presented in the previous section has been tested on 30 HD-OCT retinal gray-scale images from patients with diabetic retinopathy, where 5 of them do not present any cystic structure. The number of cysts present on them, excluding those regions that the expert himself cannot mark as cyst with certainty, is 109. The number of candidate regions generated at the each step of this method is given in Table 17.1. Parameters for each phase have been extracted empirically after some initial tests and they are given in Table 17.2. In the classification stage, a 10-fold cross validation [19], extended to validate a model, has been performed for testing to generalize results for larger datasets.

TABLE 17.1

Number of Candidate Regions Remaining after Each Stage of the Method

Stage	Cyst	No Cyst
Watershed	109	2194
Merge	109	933
Discarding	83	122

TABLE 17.2

Values for Parameters in Each Stage of the Method

Flooding		Postprocessing		Classification	
Parameter	Value	Parameter	Value	Parameter	Value
l	5	i_a	3	f_h	1
p_{con}	20	i_d	6	f_w	2
p_{ini}	5	n_{min}	10		
p_{end}	25	w_{min}	10		
		t_1	2.5		
		t_2	2		
		p_{occ}	0.6		
		l_{ref}	5		
		c_n	20		
		c_s	0.25		
		s_{side}	0.5		
		d_{side}	30		
		d_{top}	3		
		p_{near}	10		
		h_{max}	30		

TABLE 17.3

Accuracy (%) for the Three Descriptors Using SVM Classifier

	1	2	3	4	5
Markov Random Fields					
1	65.85	**66.34**	61.46	60.68	60.00
2		64.39	60.98	60.00	60.00
3			60.98	60.00	59.51
4				59.51	59.51
5					59.51
Co-Occurrence Features					
1	80.00	80.00	80.49	80.49	79.02
2		80.98	81.95	81.46	80.00
3			80.49	80.98	80.00
4				**82.93**	79.51
5					80.00
Gabor Filters					
Number of bins					
3	80.98				
5	80.49				
7	81.46				
9	**82.44**				
11	81.46				
13	79.51				
15	80.00				

Notes: Markov random fields and co-occurrences features: cell(i, j) depicts results obtained combining the distances ranging from i to j. Gabor filters: Results for different number of bins. Best rate achieved using each method has been given in bold.

The results are presented as follows: as a first experiment, the three texture descriptors are evaluated using the SVM classifier. In the case of Markov Random Fields and Co-Occurrences Features, each distance has been analyzed separately, and in combination. The combination of adjacent distances has been achieved through the concatenation of their descriptors. With regard to Gabor Filters, the experiment consists in creating the uniform histogram that defines the descriptor, using a different number of bins. The results using SVM are exposed in Table 17.3. The best rate in classification for each method is highlighted, although the behavior is quite stable for each one, without dependence on the distances considered (Markov Random Fields and Co-Occurrences Features) or the number of bins (Gabor Filters). It is possible to observe that rates obtained using Markov Random Fields are lower than with the other two methods, which present similar results, with over 80% accuracy.

With the purpose of analyzing more deeply the two methods which present better rates, Co-Occurrences Features and Gabor Filter, they are evaluated using other classifiers: Naive-Bayes and Random-Forest. The results obtained are given in Tables 17.4 and 17.5.

TABLE 17.4

Accuracy (%) Using Naive-Bayes and Random-Forest Classifiers for Co-Occurrences Features

	1	2	3	4	5
Naive-Bayes					
1	70.73	70.24	71.71	72.20	71.22
2		72.68	72.20	72.68	71.71
3			72.68	71.71	71.71
4				**73.17**	72.68
5					71.71
Random-Forest					
1	73.66	73.66	73.17	76.10	75.61
2		77.07	77.07	**78.05**	73.66
3			75.61	72.68	76.59
4				74.15	74.64
5					75.61

Note: Cell(i, j) depicts results obtained combining the distances ranging from i to j. Best rate achieved using each method has been given in bold.

TABLE 17.5

Accuracy (%) Using Naive-Bayes and Random-Forest Classifiers for Gabor Filters, Considering Different Number of Bins

Number of Bins	Naive-Bayes	Random-Forest
3	73.17	74.63
5	76.56	75.12
7	76.58	**80.49**
9	76.10	78.56
11	**79.02**	77.56
13	76.10	79.02
15	77.07	74.63

Note: Best rate achieved using each method has been given in bold.

The best rate has been highlighted for each one, but in general, using these classifiers provides lower accuracy than using SVM.

Although accuracy is given for each classifier and the performed tests, the effectiveness of this method should be measured taking into account two measures: First, the number of cysts with respect to all those classified as cysts, and second, the number of cysts detected with respect to the number of real cysts present in the set. These measures correspond to the precision and recall of the system, which can be computed based on the confusion matrix for the best case achieved, SVM with Co-Occurrences Features with distance 4, which is shown in Table 17.6.

TABLE 17.6
Confusion Matrix Obtained with Co-Occurrences Features and Distance 4 Using SVM Classifier

	Cyst	No Cyst
Cyst	64	19
No cyst	16	106
Precision	80.00	
Recall	77.11	

It is important to note that, without the discarding step, more variety would be included in the classifier, probably providing worse results. Nevertheless, the accuracy would remain stable in the best case, but it would be computed over a higher number of regions, so the real precision would be lower. Therefore, the process of discarding regions as a step in classification is essential. All these analyses show that this methodology is a good approach to this problem, given that results in classifications are around 80% precise.

Despite the results being very promising, the behavior of the proposed methodology should be improved if we take into account the following aspects: distinguishing categories of cysts based on their location on the image is important, given that, after experiments, it has been observed that their properties are different if they are located on the top layers, where detection is more immediate, than on the ONL layer. Shades and other conflictive structures also need to be detected to reduce the number of candidates.

References

1. P. Albrecht, M. Ringelstein, A.K. Mueller, N. Keser, T. Dietlein, A. Lappas, A. Foerster, H.P. Hartung, O. Aktas, and A. Methner. Degeneration of retinal layers in multiple sclerosis subtypes quantified by optical coherence tomography. *Multiple Sclerosis Journal*, 18(10):1422–1429, 2012.
2. J. Besag. Spatial interaction and the statistical analysis of lattice systems. *Journal of the Royal Statistical Society, Series B*, 36:192–236, 1974.
3. S. Beucher and C. Lantuejoul. Use of watersheds in contour detection. *International Workshop on Image Processing*, 1979.
4. C. Bowd, R.N. Weinreb, J.M. Williams, and L.M. Zangwill. The retinal nerve fiber layer thickness in ocular hypertensive, normal, and glaucomatous eyes with optical coherence tomography. *Archives of Ophthalmology*, 118(1):22–26, 2000.
5. E. Cesmeli and D. Wang. Texture segmentation using Gaussian–Markov, random fields and neural oscillator networks. *IEEE Transactions on Neural Networks*, 12(2):394–404, 2001.
6. J.G. Daugman. Uncertainty relation for resolution in space, spatial frequency, and orientation optimized by two-dimensional visual cortical filters. *Journal of the Optical Society of America A: Optics, Image Science, and Vision*, 2(7):1160–1169, 1985.
7. D. Gabor. Theory of communication. *Journal of the Institute of Electrical Engineering*, 93:429–457, 1946.
8. J.D.M. Gass. *Stereoscopic Atlas of Macular Diseases*. St. Louis, MO: Mosby, 1987.
9. M.F. Goldberg. Diseases affecting the inner blood–retinal barrier. In J.G. Cunha Vaz (ed.). *The Blood Retinal Barriers*. New York: Plenum Publishing Corporation, pp. 309–363, 1979.

10. A. Gonzalez, M. Ortega, and M.G. Penedo. Cost function selection for a graph-based segmentation in OCT retinal images. *14th International Conference on Computer Aided Systems, Eurocast 2013*, 2013.
11. M. Haeker, M. Sonka, R. Kardonc, V.A. Shah, X. Wu, and M.D. Abràmof. Automated segmentation of intraretinal layers from macular optical coherence tomography images. *Proceedings of the SPIE: Medical Imaging*, 6512:651214, 2007.
12. R.M. Haralick, K. Shanmugam, and I. Dinstein. Textural features for image classification. *IEEE Transactions on Systems, Man, and Cybernetics*, 3:610–621, 1973.
13. P.A. Keane, P.J. Patel, S. Liakopoulos, F.M. Heussen, S.R. Sadda, and A. Tufail. Evaluation of age-related macular degeneration with optical coherence tomography. *Survey of Ophthalmology*, 57(5):389–414, 2012.
14. K. Li, X. Wu, D.Z. Chen, and M. Sonka. Optimal surface segmentation in volumetric images—A graph-theoretic approach. *Proceedings of the IEEE Transactions on Pattern Analysis and Machine Intelligence*, 28(1):119–134, 2006.
15. Y.-Y. Liu, M. Chen, H. Ishikawa, G. Wollstein, J. Schuman, and J.M. Rehg. Automated macular pathology diagnosis in retinal OCT images using multi-scale spatial pyramid and local binary patterns in texture and shape encoding. *Medical Image Analysis*, 15(5):748–759, 2011.
16. K.U. Loeffler, Z.L. Li, G.A. Fishman, and M.O. Tso. Dominantly inherited cystoid macular edema, a histopathologic study. *Ophthalmology*, 99(9):1385–1392, 1992.
17. T. Mitchell. *Machine Learning*. New York: McGraw Hill, 1997.
18. O. Puzyeyeva, W.C. Lam, J.G. Flanagan et al. High-resolution optical coherence tomography retinal imaging: A case series illustrating potential and limitations. *Journal of Ophthalmology*, 2011:764183, 2011.
19. J. Rodriguez, A. Perez, and J. Lozano. Sensitivity analysis of *k*-fold cross-validation in prediction error estimation. *IEEE Transactions on Pattern Analysis and Machine Intelligence*, 32:569–575, 2010.
20. H. Sanchez-Tocino, A. Alvarez-Vidal, M.J. Maldonado, J. Moreno-Montañes, and A. Garcia-Layana. Retinal thickness study with optical coherence tomography in patients with diabetes. *Investigative Ophthalmology and Visual Science*, 43(5):1588–1594, 2002.
21. G. Tremolada, L. Pierro, U. De Benedetto, S. Margari, M. Gagliardi, G. Maestranzi, G. Calori, M. Lorenzi, and R. Lattanzio. Macular micropseudocysts in early stages of diabetic retinopathy. *Retina*, 31(7):1352–1358, 2011.
22. M.O. Tso. Pathological study of cystoid macular edema. *Transactions of the Ophthalmological Society of the United Kingdom*, 100:408–413, 1980.
23. M.O. Tso. Pathology and pathogenesis of cystoid macular edema. *Ophthalmologica*, 183:46–54, 1981.
24. M.O. Tso. Pathology of cystoid macular edema. *Ophthalmology*, 89(8):902–915, 1982.
25. L. Vincent and P. Soille. Watershed in digital spaces: An efficient algorithm based on inmersion simulations. *Proceedings of the IEEE Transactions on Pattern Analysis and Machine Intelligence*, 13(6):583–598, 1991.
26. J.R. Wolter. The histopathology of cystoid macular edema. *Albrecht von Graefes Archiv für klinische und experimentelle Ophthalmologie*, 216(2):85–101, 1981.
27. M. Yanof, B.S. Fine, A.J. Brucker, and R.C. Eagle Jr. Pathology of human cystoid macular edema. *Survey of Ophthalmology*, 28(Suppl.):505–511, 1984.
28. Z. Yaqoob, J. Wu, and C. Yang. Spectral domain optical coherence tomography: A better OCT imaging strategy. *Biotechniques*, 39(6 Suppl.):S6–S13, 2005.

18

Scanning Laser Ophthalmoscope Fundus Perimetry: The Microperimetry

Millena G. Bittencourt, Daniel Araújo Ferraz, Hongting Liu, Mostafa Hanout, Yasir J. Sepah, Diana V. Do, and Quan Dong Nguyen

CONTENTS

18.1 Introduction

Visual perception is the ultimate outcome of a variety of discriminative functions of the visual system in which the macular function plays a great role. For many years, physicians relied on best-corrected visual acuity (VA) measurements and retinoscopy to assess macular dysfunction. It is well known, however, that VA cannot fully distinguish deterioration of macular function. Throughout the ophthalmic history, several clinical examinations were designed to aid in the assessment of the various aspects of the visual function. Some of them are still in use such as contrast sensitivity, reading speed, macular recovery function, low-luminance VA, and color acuity, among others. However, no other functional test has shown the same ability of localizing retinal function depression as perimetry does.

By definition, perimetry is a systematic and quantitative evaluation of the retinal sensitivity to different intensities of light at different locations inside the retina field. The technology can also quantify the extension and patterns of the visual field [1–5].

The selection of the area of interest, usually ranging from 10° to 30° of eccentricity in old perimeters and 10° to 90° of eccentricity in modern devices, is the first step to conduct the exam [6,7]. To test the selected area, a computer projects a light stimulus onto a background with fixed luminance via a mirror unit. Patients are then instructed to press a button every time a stimulus is noticed. The patient's response is then recorded and matched with the time of the stimulus presentation. The macular threshold to light, the percentage of correct responses, as well as false-positive and false-negative ones are provided in the test report [1,2].

For many years, standard perimeters used a cupola of 600 mm of diameter as background, setting it 30 cm distant from the patient's eye [6]. Recently, modern perimeters introduced a liquid crystal display (LCD), set in the patient's infinite point of vision, to project the stimuli onto the patient retina.

To assess the retina sensitivity, a light stimulus is presented repeatedly in the patient's visual field while the patient is steadily focusing at a projected target. The stimuli can be offered in different grid patterns and luminance levels. Every point in the grid pattern is tested multiple times with decrement or increment staircase stimuli intensity until a threshold can be found for each point. Consequently, the retinal light sensitivity is determined as the lowest intensity of light at which a stimulus can be detected 50% of the time [1,2,8]. The first well-defunded perimeter was the manual Goldmann perimeter. The information provided by the Goldmann perimeter changed the approach of diseases in neuroophthalmology, glaucoma, and retina, among other ophthalmology subfields.

Many diseases located in the retina, in the optic nerve, or even in the brain visual cortex can lead to a decrease in the sensitivity to light. In addition, they can constrict the visual field in different fashions. More modern perimeters offer a wide range of settings to permit the evaluation of diseases characteristics. It allows customization of the stimulus size, stimulus color, test strategy, area and density of pattern, kinetics of the stimulus (static or in motion), and background chromaticity [1,2,8]. These test settings are more often customized to sell clinical parameters, such as the patient's age, differential diagnosis, and stage of disease, which can affect the results if ignored. An ingenious combination of settings can also enhance the probability of detecting subtle and initial disease changes.

The better understanding of the physiopathology of retinal diseases generated a continuous demand for more advanced perimetric evaluation. From this chain reaction, various perimeters have reached the market. Among them, the manual Goldmann perimetry and the standardized automated full threshold static cupola perimetry became the gold standard test [8]. The settings adopted in the most common perimeters are described in Table 18.1.

The perimetry has conveyed nondoubtful contributions to the diagnosis and follow-up of patients. Although well established in the clinical setting, the precise evaluation of macular disorders with conventional perimetry was yet a challenge until the 1980 [9]. At that time, the accuracy of the conventional visual field was based on the assumption that the gaze fixation during the examination was stable and located centrally at the fovea. The devices did not detect the eye movements and in those cases with compromised gaze fixation or lack of attention by the patient would have the stimulus presented in a more extensive area than planned for the test. The evaluation of the ability to hold steady fixation, which is a fundamental aspect of good visual function, could not be conducted by means of standard perimetry [10]. In addition, standard perimetry showed several other limitations such as the inability to detect the preferred retinal locus (PRL) (nonfoveal, well-defined region of retina used to fixate a target), the lack of accurate retest examination over

TABLE 18.1

Standard Perimeters Characteristics

	HFA II Series	Octopus 300 PRO/900	Easy Field, Center Field	Humphrey Matrix	M730
Maximum temporal range (°)	30 and 90	30 and 90	30	30	15 and 30
Threshold test library	24-2, 30-2, 10-2, 60-4, Macula, nasal step	Physiological glaucoma test, physiological macular test 5°/12°/30°, 32, ST, LVS, LVC, 07, D1, N1, BT, BG, FG, Esterman, country-dependent static expert opinion test, country-dependent automated kinetic test	Glaucoma staging program, progression report threshold noiseless trend (TNT), glaucoma staging system 2 (GSS2)	Glaucoma Hemifield test (GHT), serial field overview	Test fields, central 22A 22°, central 30°, flicker test 15°–22°, macula test 22°, flashscan 22°–30°
Threshold test strategy	SITA Standard, SITA Fast, full threshold, FastPac SITA-SWAP	Tendency-oriented perimetry (TOP), 2–3 min, dynamic (adaptive step size, 5–8 min), normal (4-2-1 bracketing, 8–12 min), low-vision Goldmann V (LVS), 2-LT, 1-LT	Classical (4–2) threshold, fast threshold, adapted to surroundings, age- or suprathreshold-oriented screening (2/3 zone, quantify defects)	MOBS, ZEST	Fast threshold, threshold, screening (deprecated), three zones, fixed level, age related
Background illumination	31.5 asb	0, 4, 31, and 314 asb	10 cd/m² (32 asb)	100 cd/m² (320 asb)	3.2 cd/m² (10 asb)
Stimulus generation	Threshold related, single intensity	Direct projection system, mirror projection system	Direct projection system	Frequency doubling sinusoidal gratings	Rear projection light-emitting diode
Stimulus intensity	10,000 asb	0.08–4,000 asb (47 dB)	0.1–3,180 cd/m² (10,000 asb)	10,000 asb	0.03–1,000 asb
Stimulus size	Goldman I–V	Goldmann I–V	Goldmann III	Goldmann III, V	Goldmann size III (0.43°)

(continued)

TABLE 18.1 (continued)

Standard Perimeters Characteristics

	HFA II Series	Octopus 300 PRO/900	Easy Field, Center Field	Humphrey Matrix	M730
Stimulus duration	200 ms	100, 200, 500, 1,000 ms	100, 200, 500	300 ms	0.1–9.9 s
Stimulus color	White-on-white, red-, or blue-on-white, blue-on-yellow	White-on-white, red-on-white, blue-on-yellow (SWAP) testing	White	Frequency doubling	Pale green—wavelength 565 nm, half bandwidth 28 nm
Fixation control	Heijl–Krakau blind-spot monitor, video eye monitor, gaze tracking, head tracking, vertex monitoring remote video eye monitor capability	Automatic eye tracking with fixation control using the pupil as landmark	Charged coupled device camera, via central threshold, Heijl–Krakau	Heijl–Krakau blind-spot monitor, video eye monitor	*Heijl–Krakau* blind-spot method, automatic tracking during test with visual and audible warning of fixation errors. Fixation camera included for clinician reference
Kinetic testing	Yes	Yes	No	Yes	Yes
Custom testing	Yes	Yes	No	Yes	Yes
Other	—	Flicker perimetry, Goldmann kinetic both manual and semiautomated, low-vision testing, TOP strategy for threshold testing	—	—	

SITA standard: A threshold testing method, which collects the same amount of information in half the time as the original Humphrey® full threshold standard algorithm, without compromising test reproducibility.

SITA fast: A threshold testing method that collects the same amount of information in half the time as FastPac, without compromising test reproducibility.

the same area, the unreliability in patients with low VA, and the inability to detect retinal threshold over discrete retinal lesions smaller than 5° [8].

The fundus perimetry technology emerged to offer accurate identification of functional impaired areas within the macula. The development of the confocal scanning laser ophthalmoscopy (cSLO), the eye-tracking systems, and the fixation assessment were essential to develop this new perimetry modality [8,11–13].

The cSLO technology utilizes infrared (IR) low-energy laser source and horizontal and vertical scanning mirrors to perusal a specific region of the retina and create raster images viewable on a screen [14]. The retina is imaged in real time with a high degree of spatial sensitivity as the confocal nature of the optics ensures that the light reflectance correspond to the same focal plane. The defocused light is almost completely suppressed, thus overcoming the interference of reflected light from the optical media anterior to the retina, such as the lens or the cornea. Although the cSLO provided good quality of spatial imaging, the device was not able to handle the eye movement confounders [14].

Posteriorly, an eye-tracking system was incorporated into the SLO and automated macular perimeter to compensate the eye movements [15,16]. The system consisted in using predefined landmarks in the retina as a reference point to identify bidimensional dislocations during the exam. Each landmark dislocation measured in the Cartesian axis or degrees was compared with its original locations, allowing the correction of stimulus presentation in real time and same frequency of the eye movements. In addition, the Cartesian coordinates could also be used to calculate the bivariate contour ellipse area (BCEA), which measures the area of the PRL [10,17,18]. The eye-tracking system, however, worked under a maximum limit of eye movement (frequency and length), and its speed was crucial to achieve perfect eye tracking.

Since the first SLO fundus perimetry device, the technology of these machines has considerably changed to improve the exam duration, image resolution, follow-up retest, speed of the tracking system, and analytic software. There were three generations of SLO fundus perimetry since 1982 and, for didactic purpose, will be described in their chronological sequence of appearance.

18.2 Evolution of Fundus Perimetry Technology

18.2.1 First Generation of SLO Fundus Perimetry

18.2.1.1 Rodenstock SLO (Model 101; Rodenstock, Ottobrunn, Germany)

The first fundus perimetry with the scanning laser ophthalmoscope reached the market in 1982 as a promising technique that allows the correlation between morphologic appearance of the fundus and its function [9,11,13]. The real-time video image of the retina showing the location that each test stimulus felt in the macular was the greatest advance over the conventional 10° perimetry (Goldman, Humphrey, and Octopus) [9,11–13].

The SLO fundus perimetry was obtained using two laser sources simultaneously projected onto the retina [11,12,19–21]. The first laser source was a modulated helium–neon IR laser beam (633 nm) used to project the stimulus, while the second source, an IR diode laser (780 nm), was used to scan the retina and detect real-time fundus images [19]. The background luminance was set in 10 cd/m^2, and the stimulus intensity varied in 0.1 logarithmic steps from the brightest luminance, 0 dB (71 cd/m^2), to the lowest luminance, 35 dB

[22]. Computer-controlled modulation of the scanning laser beam generated the variance in the stimulus luminance [11]. The stimulus size followed the same Goldmann III size available in the Octopus perimetry (0.410) with a presentation time of 120 ms. It used a cross as a target, which was directly projected onto the retina using a monitor display [21].

From 1982 to 2003, the Rodenstock SLO-101 was the only fundus perimeter available and quickly became a well-established instrument to assess fundus sensitivity. The system required manual input of stimulus presentation, intensity, and location by a skilled technician. Using a frozen image, the stimulus placement was manually adjusted for changes in retinal landmark location at the time of each stimulus presentation, by placing a cursor on a retinal landmark on the frozen image and allowing correction of the eye movement. At the conclusion of testing, the perimetry result was displayed on the retinal image frame.

Some researchers developed computer programs to automate some aspects of this process [22]. Although the instrument was not specifically designed to measure fixation, different methods have been described to allow its quantification [19,23].

Because there was no fundus tracking, the device did not allow automated follow-up examination, which made the correspondence between function and retinal location only approximate. Similarly, the evaluation of patients with unstable fixation and low vision was limited and led to some unexplainable results reported by some authors [16]. The instrument was particularly noisy and difficult to use and was limited to red stimuli.

Although the instrument is no longer commercially available since 2003, many machines are still in use in research facilities and low-vision clinics.

18.2.2 Second Generation of SLO Fundus Perimetry

18.2.2.1 Nidek MP1 Microperimeter (Nidek Technologies, Padova, Italy)

NIDEK MP-1 (MP-1, NIDEK Technologies Srl, Rome, Italy; holding company, NIDEK Co., Ltd., Japan)

In 2002, the MP-1 microperimeter produced by NIDEK Technologies reached the market, being described in the literature by Nishida et al. in the same year [24]. It was the first time that a commercial microperimeter was garnished with true eye-tracking system, replacing the manual correction for eye movements (Figure 18.1) [16,25].

The device is composed of an IR fundus camera, which acquires real-time fundus images in up to 450 of view (768 × 576 pixels resolution). An LCD with set luminance of 1.27 cd/m^2 (4 asb) presents the fixation target and the stimuli, which is generated and controlled by a computer [15]. Stimulus intensity varies in 1 dB (0.1 log) steps from 0 to 20 dB, where 0 dB represents the brightest luminance (127 cd/m^2) [18].

For each eye, the assessment began with the fundus camera capturing a reference image with 1 pixel (0.1°) resolution, which allows the examiner to select the closest high-contrast retinal landmark to the area of interest. Once the test starts, the software calculates the shift between the reference image and the real-time fundus image at 40 ms (25 Hz) rate, acquiring over 750 x and y coordinates for gaze fixation [10,18]. The stimuli presentation is then corrected to fit the patient's eye movement and ensure that it will fall in the programmed area of interest. A conventional fundus camera is used to take a full color image at the end of the assessment, and the visual field map is superimposed onto the retinal image, providing the spatial correlation between the anatomic landmarks and visual sensitivity maps [15,16,25–27]. The device software also allows customization of the test parameters; the overlay of the fixation test results onto the fundus

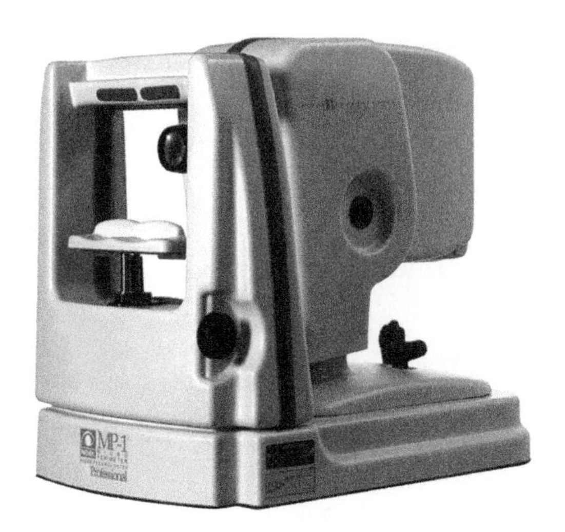

FIGURE 18.1
MP-1, NIDEK Technologies Srl, Rome, Italy.

image, retest of the same area scanned in a previous visit, and automated comparison between exams.

Another advantage provided by the eye-tracking system is the automated fixation analysis with built-in software (Navis software version 3.6; Nidek Technologies Srl). The fixation semiquantitative analysis described by Fujii et al. and a quantitative analysis are available [22,28].

Following the semiquantitative fixation classification proposed by Fujii et al., the fixation pattern is graded based on two variables: fixation location (defined as the position of fixation with respect to the center of the foveal avascular zone) and fixation stability (defined as the ability of the eye to maintain fixation in the PRL). The recorded fixation can be classified into three categories:

- Stable: if more than 75% of the fixation points are inside the 2° diameter circle
- Relatively unstable: if less than 75% are inside the 2° diameter circle but more than 75% inside the 4° diameter circle
- Unstable: if less than 75% of the fixation points are inside the 4° diameter circle [15,22]

The quantitative assessment of retinal fixation first described by Steinman in 1965 is automatically provided [17]. The author's work quantifies fixation stability as the BCEA (Figure 18.2) that provides the best fit to the boundary of one standard deviation (1-SD, 63%), two standard deviations (2-SD, 95.4%), and three standard deviations (3-SD, 99.6%) of the fixation points acquired during the test [23,28,29].

Physicians interested in the study of psychophysics parameters incorporated the technology employed in the MP-1 microperimetry rapidly. Moreover, macular sensitivity and gaze fixation were then reliable parameters reachable in the daily clinics context. Some fields have shown great benefits from the information provided by the biofeedback module for fixation location. Low-vision rehabilitation can be enhanced with training sessions for fixation relocation [30]. This can be achieved through an auditory biofeedback system

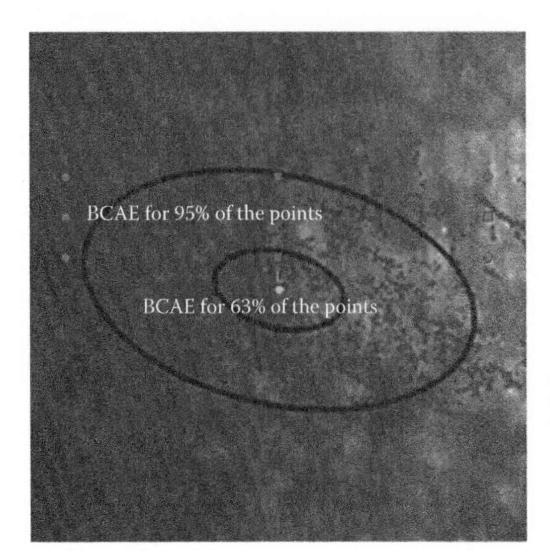

Bivariate contour eillpse area:
63% BCEA: 2.0° x 1.1°, area = 6.9°², angle = −12.0°
95% BCEA: 5.9° x 3.3°, area = 62.2°², angle = −12.0°

FIGURE 18.2
Fixation stability plot acquired with MAIA™ microperimeter. The BCEA is automatically calculated. (Courtesy of Marco Morales, CenterVue Inc., Padova, Italy, 2013.)

that trains patients with central vision loss to relocate the PRL to a more suitable location and improve fixation concomitantly [30].

18.2.3 Third Generation of SLO Fundus Perimetry

18.2.3.1 Optos OCT SLO (Optos, Dunfermline, Scotland, UK)

OPTOS OCT/SLO Microperimeter (OCT/SLO; OTI/OPTOS, Miami, FL)

In 2006, the Spectral OCT/SLO (OPKO/OTI, Miami, FL) became available [31]. It was the first time that the SLO fundus perimetry and optical coherence tomography (OCT) were provided by a single machine. In 2011, the technology was purchased by OPTOS, Inc., having the name of the device changed to OPTOS OCT/SLO (Figure 18.3). The OPTOS OCT SLO received the Food and Drug Administration (FDA) 510 k for the SLO and OCT systems in November of 2008 (information provided by OPTOS, Inc.). The microperimetry module received the FDA 510 k in March of 2013.

As the Nidek MP-1, the OCT SLO microperimeter apparatus employs automated examination with an eye-tracking system. Regression or progression of visual function of a specific region can be accurately performed using the system's vascular pattern alignment algorithm [32]. The same algorithm is used to provide accurate point-to-point registration and orientation of sensitivity map, SLO fundus image, and an OCT thickness map (Figures 18.4 and 18.5) [31,33]. Likewise, cross-sectional OCT images are simultaneously displayed in the vertical and horizontal axis, allowing the reader to analyze the retinal layers in the OCT at a specific sensitivity point [13,31,33]. Because the SLO confocal fundus image and OCT image share the same pixel-to-pixel correspondent optics, registration and orientation are very precise.

The OCT SLO microperimeter imaging system is capable of obtaining images at twice the original time-domain OCT technology, with axial resolution of 5 μm versus 10 μm and at speeds that are up to 32 times faster (64 Hz vs. 2 Hz). The SD-OCT module produces

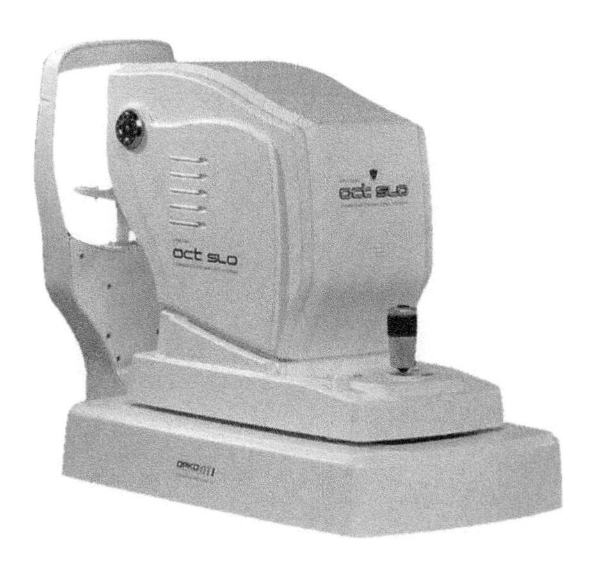

FIGURE 18.3
OPTOS OCT/SLO® microperimeter.

27,000 A-scans per second creating a retinal thickness map with 200 scan lines, 200 A-scans per line, for a total of 40,000 A-scans in the area scanned [32]. A sequence of B-scans produces the macular topography, which can be appreciated in 5-by-5 or 8-by-8 cubed grids over 6-by-6 mm [32,34]. Retinal thickness is defined as the distance between the internal limiting membrane (internal reference) and the outer segment of the photoreceptors layer. Such higher-speed and higher-resolution imaging system minimizes movement artifacts and allows fast and accurate acquisition of different imaging modalities to be performed quickly and with greater accuracy [31].

The threshold strategy for measuring retinal sensitivity is similar to standard automated perimetry [31,32,35]. The display type for this instrument is a color organic light-emitting diode screen with 10 cd/m^2 (31 asb) background illumination [31]. The stimulus range above background extends from 1.25 cd/m^2 (20 dB) to 125 cd/m^2 (0 dB). The luminance of each point tested starts at 10 dB, with subsequent change in the staircase strategy of 1 dB (0.1 log) stimulus attenuation or increase depending on the subjects' response. The final retinal sensitivity score is depicted in dB scale, which ranges from 0 to 20 dB [31–34,36,37]. A sensitivity map is created with the pattern displayed over the corresponding IR scanning laser image of the retina. The built-in software automatically provides the fixation scatter plot by analyzing the gaze distribution in x and y (2D) plan. The fixation data can be collected during a regular perimetry scan or during a fixation specific test.

18.2.3.2 Macular Integrity Assessment: MAIA Microperimeter (CenterVue S.p.A, Padova, Italy)

The macular integrity assessment (MAIA) device was first introduced in 2009 and received the FDA clearance in 2012 (Figure 18.6). The machine employs a scanning laser ophthalmoscope with an IR super luminescent diode source with 850 nm [38].

The fundus images generated have a 25 μm optical resolution producing high-quality images. As in previous technologies, anatomical landmarks are used to track and quantify

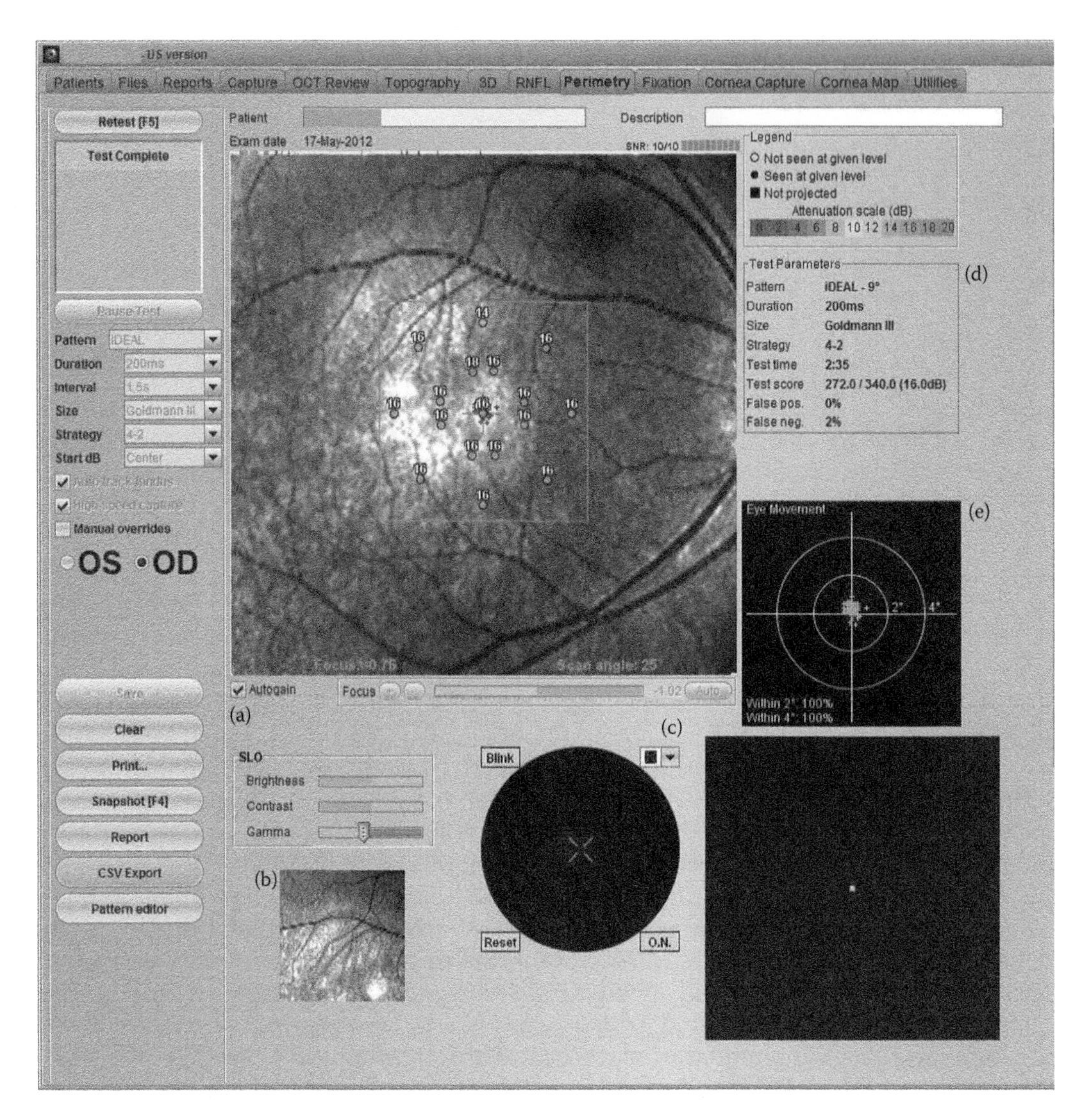

FIGURE 18.4
The OPTOS OCT/SLO software interface showing (a) fundus SLO image and sensitivity pattern; (b) retinal landmarks (vessels) tracked during the exam; (c) target shape, color, and location presented during the exam; (d) exam setting; and (e) fixation map.

the corresponding eye movements at a 25 Hz frequency. MAIA has a background luminance of 1.27 cd/m^2 (4 asb) and maximum stimuli luminance set at 319 cd/m^2 (1000 asb) [39,40]. A broad stimuli scale, ranging from 0 to 36 dB, with dynamic stimulus range of 3.6 log units, offers good contrast staircase as compared to other devices with the same background luminance. Perimetric stimuli are automatically projected in random order, corrected by the eye-tracking system, to measure threshold sensitivity. Only two fixation targets and five grid patterns are available, but custom grids can be drawn to assess areas of interest [41,42].

The device was released with normative database allowing a good number of comparisons with patients' findings. The results are averaged and compared with normative data,

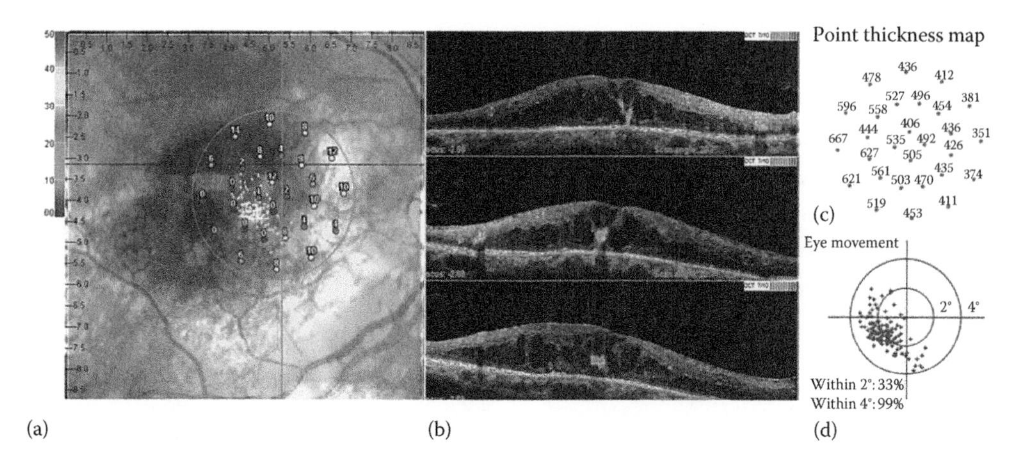

FIGURE 18.5
(a) Topography with the superimposed sensitivity map, (b) OCT, (c) thickness map, and (d) fixation map acquired in patients with diabetic macular edema with the OPTOS OCT/SLO microperimeter.

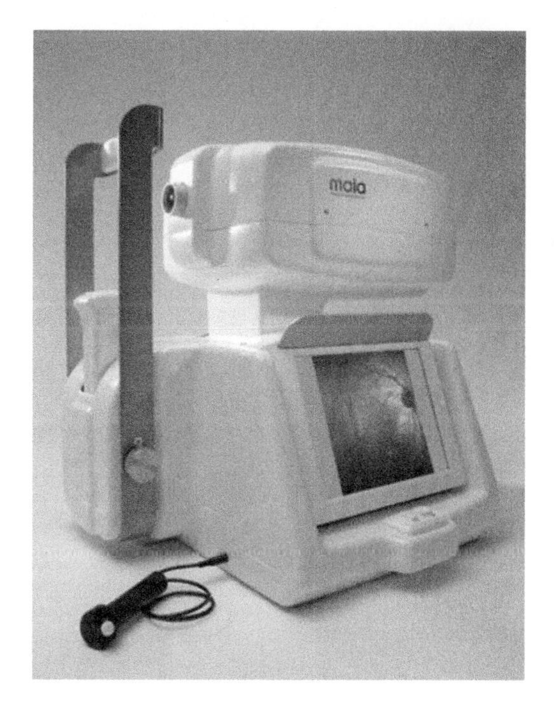

FIGURE 18.6
MAIA™ microperimeter. (Courtesy of CenterVue Inc., Padova, Italy.)

which allows the calculation of threshold and fixation indexes, showing the likelihood of abnormal results. In addition to the indexes, user-friendly built-in software produces plots of fixation target, PRL, and fixation distribution facilitating the understanding of fixation loss and allowing fixation training by using a biofeedback module [38]. Automatic quantification of BCEA is also available for 63% and 95% of the points (Figures 18.2 and 18.7)

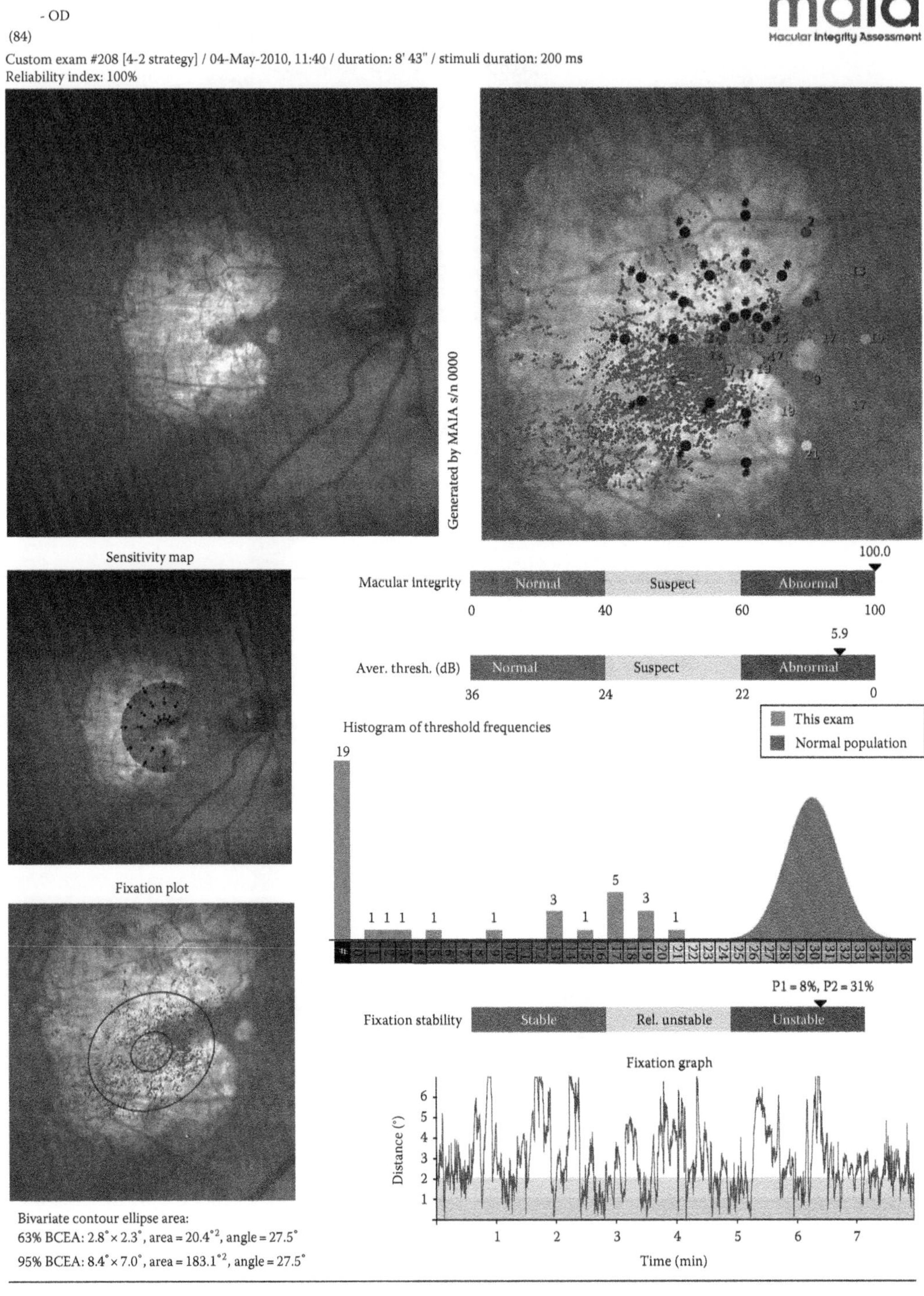

FIGURE 18.7
(See color insert.) MAIA perimetry report. (Courtesy of Marco Morales, CenterVue Inc., Padova, Italy, 2013.)

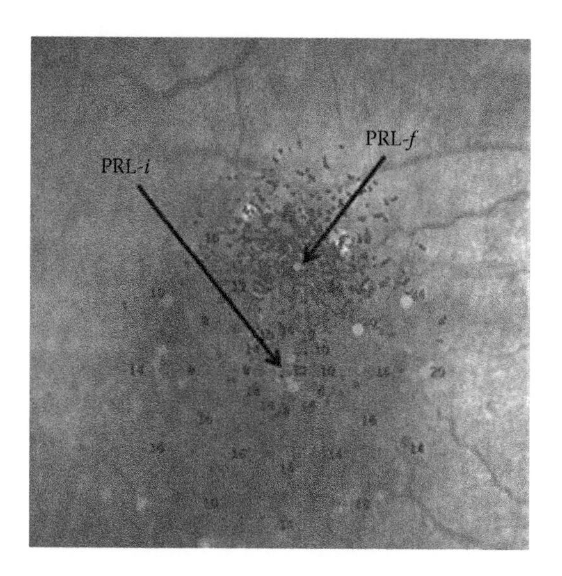

FIGURE 18.8
Image of MAIA exam with projection strategy nominated SF. The SF strategy projects only 0 dB stimuli; it covers 10° (diameter) with an examination time of 1.5 min. This strategy allows fast identification (less than 2 min) of deep scotomata in the retina. (Courtesy of Marco Morales, CenterVue Inc., Padova, Italy, 2013.)

[40,43]. Furthermore, MAIA has a projection strategy nominated scotoma finder (SF) that allows fast identification of deep scotomata in the retina. The SF strategy projects only 0 dB stimuli and covers an area of 10° (diameter) with an examination time of 1.5 min (Figure 18.8) [38]. As in previous technologies, good test–retest accuracy provides longitudinal monitoring of diseases.

18.3 Comparison of Different Microperimeters

Microperimetry provides important information of visual function that cannot be assessed by other means. The precise structural and functional correlation, which makes this technology a unique tool to diagnose, monitor, and tailor treatment, may not show the same results across the available devices. Moreover, the design choices made by manufacturers play an important role in the ability of each device to evaluate specific features of visual function. Although direct comparison among the three commercial options is yet to be addressed, comparisons between pairs of devices are abundant in the literature, especially for the first and second generation of microperimeters [3,15,16,26,44,45]. Table 18.2 summarizes the characteristics of MP-1, OPTOS OCT/SLO, and MAIA microperimeters.

18.3.1 Macular Threshold

The understanding of the psychophysics behind any perimetric test is crucial to the interpretation of the results. The contrast between background and the stimulus luminance,

TABLE 18.2

Scanning Laser Ophthalmoscope Fundus Perimeters (Microperimeters) Characteristics

	MP-1	OPKO®	MAIA™
Working distance	47.1 mm		33 mm
Field of view	36° × 44°	37°	36° × 36°
Visual field	Up to 22.5°	Up to 20°	20° × 20°
Background luminance	1.27 cd/m² (4 asb)	10 cd/m² (31 asb) observation: equal to Humphrey	1.27 cd/m² (4 asb)
Stimulus size	Goldman: I, II, III, IV, and V	Goldman: I, II, III, IV, and V	Goldman III
Stimulus duration	100–2000 ms	200–300 ms	
Stimulus pattern (grid)	MacTel and custom	Polar 3, 4, 5; Humphrey modified 10-2; square 5 × 5 and 7 × 7; peripapillary; custom	20°; 10°; 6°; 10-2 custom
Stimulus presentation	Static and kinetic	Static	Static
Stimulus maximum intensity (cd/m²)	127 (400 asb)	125 (396.7 asb)	318
Stimulus dynamic range (log units)	2	2	3.6
Stimulus attenuation scale (dB)	0–20	0–20	0–36
Threshold strategy	4-2-1, 4-2; fast, raw, manual	4-2-1, 4-2; fast, 0/10/16	Suprathreshold (fast test) or a 4-2 (expert test)
Target size	The dimension and the color of all targets can be customized	The dimension and the color of all targets can be customized	Two targets
Target shape	Single cross, four crosses, circle	Cross, circle, dot, and custom targets	
Fixation stability	Fixation plot Semiquantitative classification: Fuji classification Automated quantitative assessment BCEA Low-vision rehabilitation module	Fixation plot Semiquantitative classification: Fuji classification	Fixation plot Semiquantitative classification: Fuji classification Automated quantitative assessment: BCEA Fixation graphic interpolating distance (degrees) × minute Low-vision rehabilitation module
Follow-up test	Yes	Yes	Yes
Refractive error correction	Patient refractive error should be entered	Automatic correction	Automatic correction
Minimum pupil diameter required (mm)	4	2.5	2.5
Distance detection	Purkinje bright spot created by IR rays reflected on the cornea	Move the scanning head to align the patient's eye until the three dots of light on the patient's cornea are in sharp focus	Automatic focus

TABLE 18.2 (continued)

Scanning Laser Ophthalmoscope Fundus Perimeters (Microperimeters) Characteristics

	MP-1	OPKO®	MAIA™
Eye true track (Hz)	25	25	25
Imaging speed (Hz)	25	64	25
Images coregistration	Can merge images from any source (OCT, fundus autofluorescence, and fluorescein angiography) with the sensitivity map	SLO fundus image, OCT, and fundus perimetry are obtained and coregistered simultaneously by a single machine. Because the SLO confocal fundus image and OCT image share the same pixel-to-pixel correspondent optics, registration and orientation are precise	—

Note: The luminance values refer to the white background and white stimuli. No nominal data are provided for the red background and stimuli.

in addition to the dynamic range of stimulus variation, interferes in the visual perception, and therefore, the normal distribution of the macula threshold is not expected to show the same interval among the machines. Using the standard Humphrey field analyzer (HFA) as a reference, the MP-1 microperimeter offers a dim maximum stimulus luminance (127×3.183 cd/m^2) with a small dynamic range (2 log units), which means that dimmest light is only approximately 1% of the brightest stimuli. The nominal stimulus intensities of 0 and 20 dB in the MP-1 is roughly equivalent to 14 and 34 dB on the HFA [46]. Interestingly, although the background luminance difference is only 8.73 cd/m^2 between MP-1 and OPTOS device, the stimulus intensity of 0 dB in the OCT SLO microperimeter is equivalent to 13.6 dB in the HFA and 20–33.1 dB [47]. Therefore, the normal threshold distribution in both devices shows a ceiling effect (can easily perceive the dimmest light), and likewise, patients with macular disease show a floor effect (may not be able to see the brightest light) when the devices are compared to HFA [46,47].

The maximum stimulus luminance and dynamic stimulus range in the OCT SLO microperimeter are close to that in the MP-1, approximately 125 cd/m^2 and 2 log units. However, the difference in the background luminance between both devices creates a diverse exam psychophysics. The lower contrast between stimulus and background luminance in spectral device shifts the normal threshold distribution downward when compared to the MP-1 [47,48].

The MAIA microperimeter has the same background luminance as that of MP-1. However, it has higher maximum stimulus intensity (318 cd/m^2; equivalent to 10 dB on the HFA) and better dynamic range of the stimulus, 3.6 log units (Marco Morales, CenterVue Inc., 2011) [42,49].

In previous studies with 31 volunteers, Springer et al. found the average light sensitivity to be 19.1 ± 0.5 dB with the MP-1 [39,44]. Shah et al. found a mean overall threshold of the 18.33 dB (range: 13.0–19 dB) in 66 healthy eyes [25]. Sabates and collaborators studied 169 healthy eyes measuring the macular threshold and found an overall mean of 17.9 ± 1.2 dB. Similarly, a study with 200 normal patients conducted by Vujosevic and coauthors found an overall mean sensitivity of 29.78 + 1.71 with the MAIA device [39].

As a direct comparison of results acquired with these three devices is not possible, some reports using conversion formulas have shown good correlations between machines and conventional perimetry [4,47]. The conversion to HFA equivalent values can be accomplished by using the formula

TABLE 18.3

Stimuli Intensity Dynamic Range

	HFA (dB)	Octopus (dB)	MAIA (dB)	MP1 (dB)	Spectral OCT/SLO (dB)
Apostilb	—	—	—	—	—
0.1	50	40	—	—	—
0.4	44	36	36	—	—
1	40	30	30	—	—
4	34	24	24	20	20
10	30	20	20	16	16
100	20	10	10	6	6
400	14	4	4	0	0
1,000	10	0	0	—	—
10,000	0	—	—	—	—

Source: Adapted from material provided by Marco Morales, CenterVue Inc., Padova, Italy.

$$\text{HFA equivalent} = -\left(\log\left(\frac{\mu}{3183}\right) \times 10\right),$$

where
 3183 is the maximum intensity of the HFA perimeter in cd/m^2
 μ is the value of the microperimeter (MP-1 or OCT SLO microperimeter) increment in cd/m^2
 the multiplier 10 converts the value to dB [42]

Table 18.3 shows the equivalence between microperimeters and the HFA (data published by Heijl et al. in 2002, Midena in 2007, Seiple in 2012 and data provided by Marco Morales, CenterVue Inc., personal communication, 2013) [2,47,50].

In previous studies with 50 healthy volunteers and 50 patients with various maculopathies, the mean test–retest variability of MP-1 microperimeter was found to be 0.23 ± 0.55 dB and 0.20 ± 0.9 dB, respectively, with a coefficient of repeatability of 5.56 ± 0.86 dB [18]. Results from a study with 32 normal subjects showed that the mean threshold variability of OCT SLO microperimeter was 0.13 dB between 2 sessions and 0.20 dB among 3 sessions in 16 individuals [13].

18.3.2 Fixation

Fixation stability is an important element of good quality vision. Patients with maculopathies lose the physiological fixation area, which makes them unable to maintain steady fixation. A smaller BCEA correlates to more stable fixation, whereas if the eye uses a broader range of retina points, the BCEA will be larger and fixation unstable [42].

Different methods of assessment may yield different BCEA values; for example, previous comparisons between SLO-101 and MP-1 in healthy eyes have revealed that BCEA areas measured with the SLO-101 can be 0.25–2.25 times smaller than with the eye-tracking system devices [16,51,28].

Both MP-1 and MAIA provide automatic quantitative analysis of fixation by means of BCEA. BCEA quantification of fixation stability using the OCT SLO microperimeter is possible by manual exportation of the bidimensional (x and y location) of every fixation point collected during the fixation exam. Henceforth, the global BCEA value is calculated using the formula

$$\text{BCEA} = 2k\pi\sigma_H\sigma_V(1-\text{p}2)1/2,$$

where

σ_H is the standard deviation of point location over the horizontal meridian (x)
σ_V is the standard deviation of point location over the vertical meridian (y)
ρ is the product-moment correlation of these two position components [17,28]

The value k is dependent upon the probability (p) area chosen (e.g., 63%, 68%, or 95%):

$$p = 1 - e - k,$$

where e is the base of the natural logarithm. Different authors have used different values of p, such as 63% [52], 68% [53,54], or 95% [55].

Several research groups have shown that this older method of calculating fixation instability is more closely related to other characteristics of visual function, such as reading speed, and have criticized the use of the semiquantitative classification defined by Fujii [19,22,29,56]. Both MP-1 and MAIA are garnished of a biofeedback module that facilitates the training of patients with unstable fixation as it identifies with accuracy the patient's PRL.

18.3.3 Coregistration

Topographic maps acquired with microperimetry permits precise mapping of the central visual field with precise correlation to the anatomy observed on clinical examination. It can be achieved with the three commercial microperimeters [15,16,25–27,32,42,49]. However, only the MP-1 and OPTOS OCT/SLO software allows coregistration with images other than fundus SLO. In the MP-1, an IR camera with much lower resolution and high noise ratio than scanning laser-based systems is used to capture the fundus images used for coregistration [32,57]. To improve the quality of the image, pupil dilation is required. The software comports imported images for coregistration, although some degree of inconsistency can be found among images from different optical systems [32,57]. In the OPTOS OCT/SLO, the images of the fundus and organic light emitting diode are coherent, thus, eliminating concerns of misalignment [41]. In addition, the use of the same optical apparatus to obtain SLO, microperimetry, and OCT images in the OPTOS device is a great advantage for coregistration as the amount of distortions is reduced across images facilitating an accurate record [32].

Woods et al. tested the coregistration of stimulus presentation and retinal imaging with MP-1 in a small sample size study and found repeatable spatial alignment errors of 0.5°. Measurement errors associated with different operators, subjects, and different images were less than 0.2°. He postulated that even small tilts of the head might produce apparent changes in foveal location [41].

The coregistration of images is also used in the retesting function of MP-1, spectral OCT/SLO, and MAIA. It is probably one of the major add-ons of this technology, allowing precise monitoring of function at a specific location in the retina.

18.3.4 Other Characteristics

The perimetric strategy of the current software version of the MP-1 starts at the threshold level that is chosen before the examination for each stimulus. Although the examiner can define the initial stimuli attenuation value, there are no adaptive test strategies, for example, the Swedish interactive threshold algorithm (SITA), that shortens the lengthy staircase threshold procedure. In addition, the instrument tests the same luminance levels at all test locations before moving on to the next luminance level [15,16,26,44]. Likewise, the OPTOS OCT/SLO microperimeter offers different starting threshold levels. However, the lack of adaptive strategies can increase the testing time in up to 10 min, which elevates the changes of *fatigue effect* and consequently produces artificially reduced sensitivity measurements [58]. The fast threshold examination available in MAIA was designed to decrease the time required to run the test. The examination takes approximately 3 min to be completed, but the sensitivity of the test to detect subtle changes has not been analyzed yet.

Another advantage of MAIA is the normative database incorporated in the software, which automatically compares the patient's data to the normal range. The likelihood of abnormal results is provided making the results' interpretation easier.

18.4 Applicability in Specific Diseases

The ability of measuring focal deterioration of macular function, in addition to precise follow-up testing, made microperimetry an assessment extensively investigated in the recent years. Taking into consideration only the last 5 years, over 293 articles related to microperimetry were indexed in Pubmed. The reliability of the test was evaluated in a number of diseases.

In a longitudinal study, 38 patients with ABCA4-associated retinal degeneration (RD) or with retinitis pigmentosa (RP) were studied with microperimetry. The repeatability of macular threshold measurement in the foveal–papillary axis did not vary significantly, even as a function of the sensitivity slope, eccentricity from the fovea, age, fixation location, or instability [59]. These findings demonstrate that microperimetry offers accurate results in patients with residual macular function. Furthermore, Liu et al. found that patients with various maculopathies and stable VA may show intervisit variations of macular threshold significantly greater than the intrinsic intersession variance across examinations (2.43 dB), inferring that patients could not be stable as predicted by VA and retinoscopy [48].

Studies dedicated to the study of macular threshold and macular fixation in the context of residual visual functions and functional vision after macular vision loss have shown that three major components can be used as reliable parameters of functional vision: scotoma characteristics, PRLs, and oculomotor control [28,60]. For example, recently published data showed that BCEA is strongly correlated with reading performance [28]. Rohrschneider et al. demonstrated that in late stages of Stargardt disease, a deep central scotoma typically shifts the PRL to the upper border of the visual field defect or even located further superior at the retina, which means movement of the scotoma upward in the visual field [61]. Recently published data have also demonstrated early relative scotoma correlated with increased fundus autofluorescence in early age-related macular degeneration (AMD) [27]. Likewise, Ota and colleagues identified direct correlation between retina sensitivity decrease and structural changes after resolution of the macular edema associated with retinal vein occlusion (RVO).

On the affected side, the mean retinal sensitivity within the area of deteriorated inner segment and outer segment junction (IS/OS junction) of the photoreceptor layer was significantly less (3.8 ± 4.8 dB) than that within areas with complete IS/OS (10.1 ± 6.4 dB, $p < 0.001$). Similarly, mean retinal sensitivity within nonperfused areas was extremely low (0.3 ± 1.3 dB), compared with that in perfused retina (10.9 ± 5.9 dB, $p < 0.001$) [62]. Similar results were found by Yohannan et al. in patients with diabetic macular edema [36].

The list of studies using microperimetry to monitor surgical and pharmacological therapies is extensive. Acosta et al. were one of the first to use microperimetry to describe dense scotoma over all macular holes and movement of the PRL to the upper border of the macular hole [56]. Comparable results were obtained by other authors and further revealed that retinal sensitivity provides accurate determination of visual recovery after anatomical correction of macular hole [63–66]. The follow-up of treatment modalities of AMD such as surgical strip-off of neovascular membranes, autologous retinal pigment epithelium (RPE)–choroidal sheet transplantation, and photodynamic therapy (PDT) have also been reported [56,67,68]. In patients with central serous chorioretinopathy, even after months of anatomical resolution of the macular fluid and recovery of VA, fundus perimetry may still show diminished differential light threshold, granting mandatory monitoring of functional impairment in these patients [69].

18.5 Conclusion

In summary, all currently available microperimeters have strengths and weaknesses. Certain aspects of the examination still require further improvements, including test strategies, test dynamic range, precise coregistration with other structural tests, and availability of extensive normative database. Despite the limitations commonly inherited in test modalities, microperimetry has contributed new parameters to aid in the diagnosis, monitoring, and rehabilitation of various ocular diseases.

References

1. Anderson DR: *Perimetry with and without Automation.*, 2nd edn. St Louis, MO: Mosby, 1987.
2. Heijl A, Patella V: *Essential Perimetry: The Field Analyzer Primer.* Dublin, CA: Carl Zeiss Meditec Inc., 2002.
3. Midena E, Radin PP, Convento E, Cavarzeran F: Macular automatic fundus perimetry threshold versus standard perimetry threshold. *Eur J Ophthalmol* 2007, 17(1):63–68.
4. Ratra V, Ratra D, Gupta M, Vaitheeswaran K: Comparison between Humphrey Field Analyzer and Micro Perimeter 1 in normal and glaucoma subjects. *Oman J Ophthalmol* 2012, 5(2):97–102.
5. Johnson CA, Wall M, Thompson HS: A history of perimetry and visual field testing. *Optom Vis Sci* 2011, 88(1):E8–E15.
6. Meditec CZ: Perimetry brochure. 2002. Available at http://www.meditec.zeiss.com/88256DE3007B916B/0/2A853BEEDCDF977CC1257BEA004A7414/$file/effective_perimetry_the_field_analyzer_primer.pdf.
7. Octopus® 900 brochure. HAAG-STREIT Diagnostics, Switzerland. http://www.haag-streit.com/products/perimetry/octopusr-900.html, accessed March, 2013.

8. Crossland MD, Engel SA, Legge GE: The preferred retinal locus in macular disease: Toward a consensus definition. *Retina* 2011, 31(10):2109–2114.
9. Mainster MA, Timberla ke GT, Webb RH, Hughes GW: Scanning laser ophthalmoscopy. Clinical applications. *Ophthalmology* 1982, 89(7):852–857.
10. Subramanian V, Jost RM, Birch EE: A quantitative study of fixation stability in amblyopia. *Invest Ophthalmol Vis Sci* 2013, 54(3):1998–2003.
11. Andersen MV: Scanning laser ophthalmoscope microperimetry compared with Octopus perimetry in normal subjects. *Acta Ophthalmol Scand* 1996, 74(2):135–139.
12. Menke MN, Sato E, Van De Velde FJ, Feke GT: Combined use of SLO microperimetry and OCT for retinal functional and structural testing. *Graefes Arch Clin Exp Ophthalmol* 2006, 244(5):634–638.
13. Anastasakis A, McAnany JJ, Fishman GA, Seiple WH: Clinical value, normative retinal sensitivity values, and intrasession repeatability using a combined spectral domain optical coherence tomography/scanning laser ophthalmoscope microperimeter. *Eye (Lond)* 2011, 25(2): 245–251.
14. Webb RH, Hughes GW: Scanning laser ophthalmoscope. *IEEE Trans Biomed Eng* 1981, 28(7):488–492.
15. Midena E, Radin PP, Pilotto E, Ghirlando A, Convento E, Varano M: Fixation pattern and macular sensitivity in eyes with subfoveal choroidal neovascularization secondary to age-related macular degeneration. A microperimetry study. *Semin Ophthalmol* 2004, 19(1–2):55–61.
16. Rohrschneider K, Springer C, Bultmann S, Volcker HE: Microperimetry—Comparison between the micro perimeter 1 and scanning laser ophthalmoscope—Fundus perimetry. *Am J Ophthalmol* 2005, 139(1):125–134.
17. Steinman RM, Cushman WB, Martins AJ: The precision of gaze. A review. *Hum Neurobiol* 1982, 1(2):97–109.
18. Chen FK, Patel PJ, Xing W, Bunce C, Egan C, Tufail AT, Coffey PJ, Rubin GS, Da Cruz L: Test-retest variability of microperimetry using the Nidek MP1 in patients with macular disease. *Invest Ophthalmol Vis Sci* 2009, 50(7):3464–3472.
19. Rohrschneider K, Fendrich T, Becker M, Krastel H, Kruse FE, Volcker HE: Static fundus perimetry using the scanning laser ophthalmoscope with an automated threshold strategy. *Graefes Arch Clin Exp Ophthalmol* 1995, 233(12):743–749.
20. Rohrschneider K, Bethke-Jaenicke C, Becker M, Kruse FE, Blankenagel A, Volcker HE: Fundus-controlled examination of reading in eyes with macular pathology. *Ger J Ophthalmol* 1996, 5(5):300–307.
21. Varano M, Scassa C: Scanning laser ophthalmoscope microperimetry. *Semin Ophthalmol* 1998, 13(4):203–209.
22. Fujii GY, De Juan E, Jr., Humayun MS, Sunness JS, Chang TS, Rossi JV: Characteristics of visual loss by scanning laser ophthalmoscope microperimetry in eyes with subfoveal choroidal neovascularization secondary to age-related macular degeneration. *Am J Ophthalmol* 2003, 136(6):1067–1078.
23. Crossland MD, Culham LE, Rubin GS: Fixation stability and reading speed in patients with newly developed macular disease. *Ophthalmic Physiol Opt* 2004, 24(4):327–333.
24. Nishida Y, Murata T, Yoshida K, Sawada T, Kani K: An automated measuring system for fundus perimetry. *Jpn J Ophthalmol* 2002, 46(6):627–633.
25. Shah VA, Chalam KV: Values for macular perimetry using the MP-1 microperimeter in normal subjects. *Ophthalmic Res* 2009, 41(1):9–13.
26. Sawa M, Gomi F, Toyoda A, Ikuno Y, Fujikado T, Tano Y: A microperimeter that provides fixation pattern and retinal sensitivity measurement. *Jpn J Ophthalmol* 2006, 50(2):111–115.
27. Midena E, Vujosevic S, Convento E, Manfre A, Cavarzeran F, Pilotto E: Microperimetry and fundus autofluorescence in patients with early age-related macular degeneration. *Br J Ophthalmol* 2007, 91(11):1499–1503.
28. Crossland MD, Dunbar HM, Rubin GS: Fixation stability measurement using the MP1 microperimeter. *Retina* 2009, 29(5):651–656.

29. Amore FM, Fasciani R, Silvestri V, Crossland MD, de Waure C, Cruciani F, Reibaldi A: Relationship between fixation stability measured with MP-1 and reading performance. *Ophthalmic Physiol Opt* 2013, 33(5):611–617.
30. Tarita-Nistor L, Gonzalez EG, Markowitz SN, Steinbach MJ: Plasticity of fixation in patients with central vision loss. *Vis Neurosci* 2009, 26(5–6):487–494.
31. Landa G, Rosen RB, Garcia PM, Seiple WH: Combined three-dimensional spectral OCT/SLO topography and microperimetry: Steps toward achieving functional spectral OCT/SLO. *Ophthalmic Res* 2010, 43(2):92–98.
32. Sabates FN, Vincent RD, Koulen P, Sabates NR, Gallimore G: Normative data set identifying properties of the macula across age groups: Integration of visual function and retinal structure with microperimetry and spectral-domain optical coherence tomography. *Retina* 2011, 31(7):1294–1302.
33. Hatef E, Colantuoni E, Wang J, Ibrahim M, Shulman M, Adhi F, Sepah YJ, Channa R, Khwaja A, Nguyen QD et al.: The relationship between macular sensitivity and retinal thickness in eyes with diabetic macular edema. *Am J Ophthalmol* 2011, 152(3):400.e2–405.e2.
34. Kiernan DF, Mieler WF, Hariprasad SM: Spectral-domain optical coherence tomography: A comparison of modern high-resolution retinal imaging systems. *Am J Ophthalmol* 2010, 149(1):18–31.
35. Rohrschneider K, Bultmann S, Springer C: Use of fundus perimetry (microperimetry) to quantify macular sensitivity. *Prog Retin Eye Res* 2008, 27(5):536–548.
36. Yohannan J, Bittencourt M, Sepah YJ, Hatef E, Sophie R, Moradi A, Liu H, Ibrahim M, Do DV, Coulantuoni E et al.: Association of retinal sensitivity to integrity of photoreceptor inner/outer segment junction in patients with diabetic macular edema. *Ophthalmology* 2013, 120(6):1254–1261.
37. Sepah YJ, Hatef E, Colantuoni E, Wang J, Shulman M, Adhi FI, Akhtar A, Ibrahim M, Khwaja A, Channa R et al.: Macular sensitivity and fixation patterns in normal eyes and eyes with uveitis with and without macular edema. *J Ophthalmic Inflamm Infect* 2012, 2(2):65–73.
38. MAIA microperimetry brochure. Centervue S.p.A., Rome, Italy. 2009. http://www.centervue.com/articms/admin/upAllegati/639/1342089423.pdf, accessed March, 2013.
39. Vujosevic S, Smolek MK, Lebow KA, Notaroberto N, Pallikaris A, Casciano M: Detection of macular function changes in early (AREDS 2) and intermediate (AREDS 3) age-related macular degeneration. *Ophthalmologica* 2011, 225(3):155–160.
40. Alexander P, Mushtaq F, Osmond C, Amoaku W: Microperimetric changes in neovascular age-related macular degeneration treated with ranibizumab. *Eye (Lond)* 2012, 26(5):678–683.
41. Woods RL, Vera-Diaz FA, Lichtenstein L, Peli E: Spatial alignment of microperimeters. *Invest Ophthalmol Vis Sci* 2007, 48(5):144.
42. Michael D, Crossland M-LJ, Seiple WH: Microperimetry: A review of fundus related perimetry. In: *Optometry Reports 2012; 2:e2*. Edited by Institute I-E, vol. 2. Valladolid, Spain: University of Valladolid 2012.
43. Vujosevic S, Smolek MK, Lebow KA, Notaroberto N, Pallikaris A, Casciano M: Detection of macular function changes in early (AREDS 2) and intermediate (AREDS 3) age-related macular degeneration. *Ophthalmologica* 2011, 225(3):155–160.
44. Springer C, Bultmann S, Volcker HE, Rohrschneider K: Fundus perimetry with the Micro Perimeter 1 in normal individuals: Comparison with conventional threshold perimetry. *Ophthalmology* 2005, 112(5):848–854.
45. Schmitz-Valckenberg S, Ong EE, Rubin GS, Peto T, Tufail A, Egan CA, Bird AC, Fitzke FW: Structural and functional changes over time in MacTel patients. *Retina* 2009, 29(9):1314–1320.
46. Acton JH, Bartlett NS, Greenstein VC: Comparing the Nidek MP-1 and Humphrey field analyzer in normal subjects. *Optom Vis Sci* 2011, 88(11):1288–1297.
47. Seiple W, Rosen RB, Castro-Lima V, Garcia PM: The physics and psychophysics of microperimetry. *Optom Vis Sci* 2012, 89(8):1182–1191.
48. Liu HBM, Agbedia O, Moradi A, Sepah YJ, Ferraz DF, Ibrahim MA, Sophie R, Ansari M, Nguyen QD: Longitudinal changes in retinal sensitivity among patients with maculopathy. *ARVO Meeting* 2013, Seattle, WA, Program number: 5026.

49. Salvatore S, Librando A, Esposito M, Vingolo EM: The Mozart effect in biofeedback visual rehabilitation: A case report. *Clin Ophthalmol* 2011, 5:1269–1272.
50. Midena E: *Microperimetry and the Fundus: An Introduction to Microperimetry*. Thorofare, NJ: SLACK Inc., 2007.
51. Crossland MD, Rubin GS: The use of an infrared eyetracker to measure fixation stability. *Optom Vis Sci* 2002, 79(11):735–739.
52. Kosnik W, Fikre J, Sekuler R: Visual fixation stability in older adults. *Invest Ophthalmol Vis Sci* 1986, 27(12):1720–1725.
53. Culham L, Fitzke FW, Timberlake GT, Marshall J: Assessment of fixation stability in normal subjects and patients using a scanning laser ophthalmoscope. *Clin Vision Sci* 1993, 8:551–561.
54. Nachmias J: Two-dimensional motion of the retinal image during monocular fixation. *Journal of the Optical Society of America* 1959, 49:901–908.
55. Schuchard RA, Raasch TW: Retinal locus for fixation: Pericentral fixation targets. *Clin Vision Sci* 1992, 7:511–520.
56. Acosta F, Lashkari K, Reynaud X, Jalkh AE, Van de Velde F, Chedid N: Characterization of functional changes in macular holes and cysts. *Ophthalmology* 1991, 98(12):1820–1823.
57. MP-1 microperimeter brochure. NIDEK TECHNOLOGIES Srl, Rome, Italy. Rev.041115. http://www.nidektechnologies.it/ProductsMP1All.htm, accessed March, 2013.
58. Gonzalez de la Rosa M, Pareja A: Influence of the "fatigue effect" on the mean deviation measurement in perimetry. *Eur J Ophthalmol* 1997, 7:29–34.
59. Cideciyan AV, Swider M, Aleman TS, Feuer WJ, Schwartz SB, Russell RC, Steinberg JD, Stone EM, Jacobson SG: Macular function in macular degenerations: Repeatability of microperimetry as a potential outcome measure for ABCA4-associated retinopathy trials. *Invest Ophthalmol Vis Sci* 2012, 53(2):841–852.
60. Schmidt-Erfurth UM, Elsner H, Terai N, Benecke A, Dahmen G, Michels SM: Effects of verteporfin therapy on central visual field function. *Ophthalmology* 2004, 111(5):931–939.
61. Rohrschneider K, Gluck R, Blankenagel A, Volcker HE: Fixation behavior in Stargardt disease. *Ophthalmologe* 1997, 94(9):624–628.
62. Ota M, Tsujikawa A, Ojima Y, Miyamoto K, Murakami T, Ogino K, Akagi-Kurashige Y, Muraoka Y, Yoshimura N: Retinal sensitivity after resolution of the macular edema associated with retinal vein occlusion. *Graefes Arch Clin Exp Ophthalmol* 2012, 250(5):635–644.
63. Sjaarda RN, Frank DA, Glaser BM, Thompson JT, Murphy RP: Resolution of an absolute scotoma and improvement of relative scotomata after successful macular hole surgery. *Am J Ophthalmol* 1993, 116(2):129–139.
64. Hikichi T, Ishiko S, Takamiya A, Sato E, Mori F, Takahashi M, Yanagiya N, Akiba J, Yoshida A: Scanning laser ophthalmoscope correlations with biomicroscopic findings and foveal function after macular hole closure. *Arch Ophthalmol* 2000, 118(2):193–197.
65. Ergun E, Maar N, Radner W, Barbazetto I, Schmidt-Erfurth U, Stur M: Scotoma size and reading speed in patients with subfoveal occult choroidal neovascularization in age-related macular degeneration. *Ophthalmology* 2003, 110(1):65–69.
66. Richter-Mueksch S, Vecsei-Marlovits PV, Sacu SG, Kiss CG, Weingessel B, Schmidt-Erfurth U: Functional macular mapping in patients with vitreomacular pathologic features before and after surgery. *Am J Ophthalmol* 2007, 144(1):23–31.
67. Muller S, Ehrt O, Gundisch O, Eckl-Titz G, Scheider A: Functional results after surgical extraction or photocoagulation of choroid neovascularization (CNV) in age-related macular degeneration. *Ophthalmologe* 2000, 97(2):142–146.
68. Joussen AM, Heussen FM, Joeres S, Llacer H, Prinz B, Rohrschneider K, Maaijwee KJ, van Meurs J, Kirchhof B: Autologous translocation of the choroid and retinal pigment epithelium in age-related macular degeneration. *Am J Ophthalmol* 2006, 142(1):17–30.
69. Ozdemir H, Karacorlu SA, Senturk F, Karacorlu M, Uysal O: Assessment of macular function by microperimetry in unilateral resolved central serous chorioretinopathy. *Eye (Lond)* 2008, 22(2):204–208.

19

In Vivo Confocal Microscopy: Imaging of the Ocular Surface

Sze-Yee Lee, Shakil Rehman, and Louis Tong

CONTENTS

19.1 Introduction

Imaging biological tissue at higher resolution and greater depths is required in many applications. Optical microscopy is used to visualize structure and function of biological tissue, organelles, and cells. Confocal microscopy is a high-resolution optical microscopic modality that is used to obtain 3D images of thick samples. A unique property of confocal microscopy is optical sectioning that allows one to obtain images of thin sections of a tissue without excision, thereby helping to visualize the tissue without a biopsy. Confocal microscopy can provide images in real time and in vivo that can be used in the diagnosis of disease and other pathological conditions. In vivo confocal microscopy has become a mature technology and has found its way into clinical settings, where it is used in visualization and diagnostics on a routine basis.

Confocal microscopy is based on scanning a tightly focused laser spot (or a line) onto the specimen, and the reflected or scattered light is used to make an image in a raster scan. 2D images of very thin sections of a tissue are collected at various depths, owing to the property of rejecting the out-of-focus light in a confocal microscope. These optically sectioned images are later recombined digitally to obtain 3D images.

The first confocal microscope was developed in 1961 [95] followed by a spinning disk confocal microscope [120]. Theoretical analysis and modelling for the image formation in a confocal microscope was done in 1978 [136,137]. Confocal imaging was soon applied to imaging biological specimens [3] and application of confocal microscope in imaging the human and rabbit corneas was reported in 1985 [77]. A slit scanning confocal microscope was developed in 1969 by employing an oscillating two-sided mirror for simultaneous scanning and descanning of the sample. This microscope helped imaging living neural tissue [85,146].

Confocal laser scanning microscope was later implemented in ophthalmology [31,169]. The first commercial confocal microscope was developed in 1987, which has now become a vital imaging tool in research laboratories, biomedical imaging facilities, and industrial applications. Confocal microscopy is now used in ophthalmology in clinical settings as a scanning laser ophthalmoscope. Slit scanning in vivo confocal microscope (IVCM) and laser scanning IVCM are now commercially available from a number of providers and are routinely used in clinical settings.

A confocal microscope can be used in reflection or transmission mode depending on the application. The transmission type of confocal imaging is used for thin samples that otherwise cannot be imaged in vivo. The reflection mode of confocal imaging is used for live tissue and in vivo imaging and can provide 3D images of samples at high resolution than is possible with widefield microscopes. The imaging contrast in a confocal microscope is obtained from variations in the index of refraction or fluorophores that are used as contrast agents for obtaining information at cellular level.

A major advantage of confocal images is to provide histological information without prior staining and excising the tissue, giving clinicians an extra control over diagnosis. IVCM in ophthalmology is used for obtaining useful information about the structure and function of cornea and other ocular surface structures, along with quantitative diagnosis of cell morphology, cell count, and infections. This chapter will discuss more of the applications of IVCM in both clinical and research practices.

19.2 Imaging of Various Structures in the Ocular Surface

IVCM allows detailed observation of specific ocular surface structures in health and disease. This section discusses in detail the capabilities of IVCM in observing various aspects of the ocular surface (Figure 19.1).

19.2.1 Examination of the Cornea

IVCM is a very valuable tool in providing information on the anatomical structure of the cornea. This avascular and transparent tissue is constructed from regularly arranged collagen fibrils. Its unique structure, together with the precorneal tear film, is responsible for two-thirds of the optical power, refracting the light that enters into the eye. Briefly, the cornea comprises of five layers: the outermost epithelial layer, the Bowman's membrane, the stromal layer, the Descemet's membrane, and the innermost endothelial layer. The stromal layer is separated from the epithelium and endothelium by the Bowman's membrane and Descemet's membrane, respectively (Figure 19.2). IVCM allows clinicians to measure the

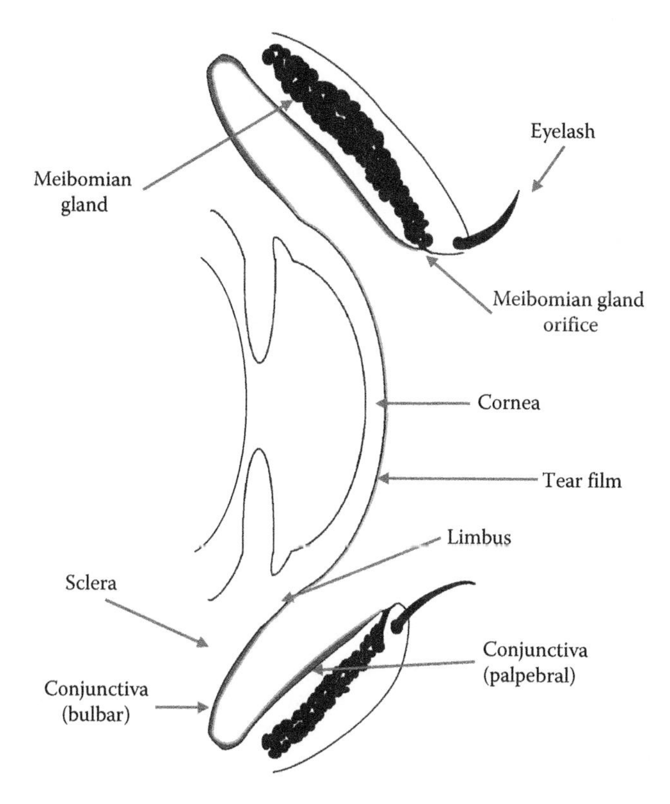

FIGURE 19.1
Structures of the ocular surface.

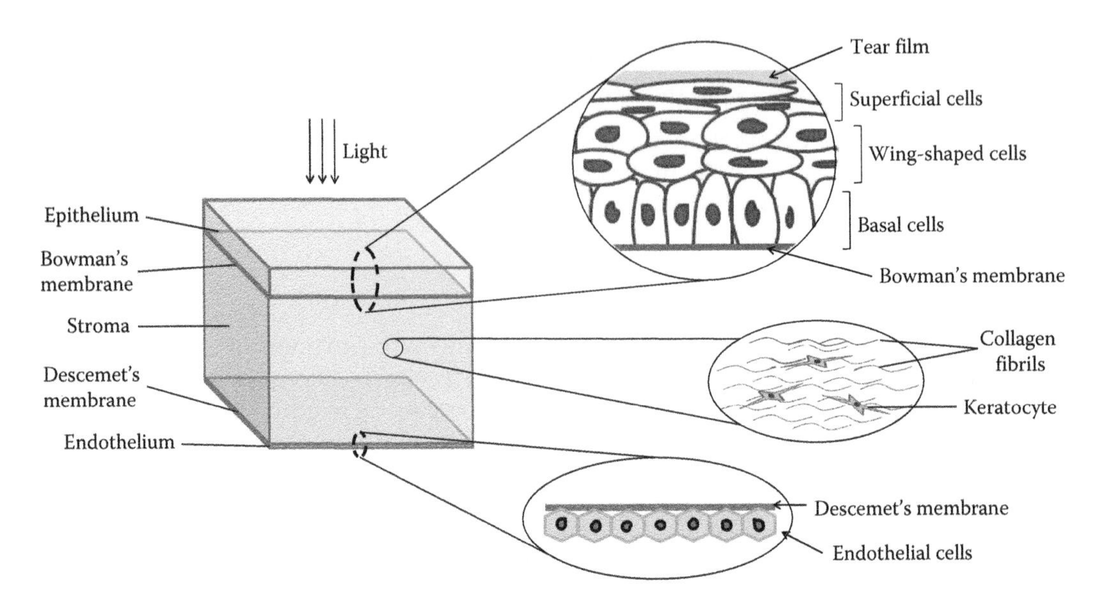

FIGURE 19.2
The five layers of the cornea.

thickness of each individual layer and monitor for changes that may occur with corneal diseases, aging, or contact lens wear [180].

19.2.1.1 Epithelium

The epithelial layer consists of five to six cell layers: one layer of cylindrical-shaped basal cells adjacent to the Bowman's membrane, two to three layers of wing-shaped cells, and two layers of superficial cells in contact with the precorneal tear film (Figure 19.2). The cylindrical basal cells secrete collagen that forms the Bowman's membrane. They also undergo mitosis, generating new epithelial cells. The superficial epithelial cells are usually difficult to image with IVCM in the normal cornea; these can be visualized only when there is an abnormal change in morphology such as in contact lens wear. The size, shape, and density of the other cell layers—the wing-shaped cells and basal cells (Figure 19.3)—can be evaluated using IVCM [37].

19.2.1.2 Stroma

The second main layer, the stroma, makes up approximately 90% of the cornea. It consists of about 300 layers of regularly arranged collagen fibers in the central cornea and increases to 500 layers at the edge [16]. The stroma itself contains cellular elements such as keratocytes (Figure 19.4), corneal nerves (Figure 19.5), and other inflammatory cells. These features may alter during corneal diseases and IVCM can aid in the assessment of the fine structures of the stroma.

Keratocytes: Stellate-shaped cells called keratocytes are present throughout the stroma and help to maintain the structure of this layer. In the event of an inflammatory process, the normally passive keratocytes may either transition into repair phenotypes or undergo cell death. The newly formed repair phenotypes can trigger regeneration of the corneal cells

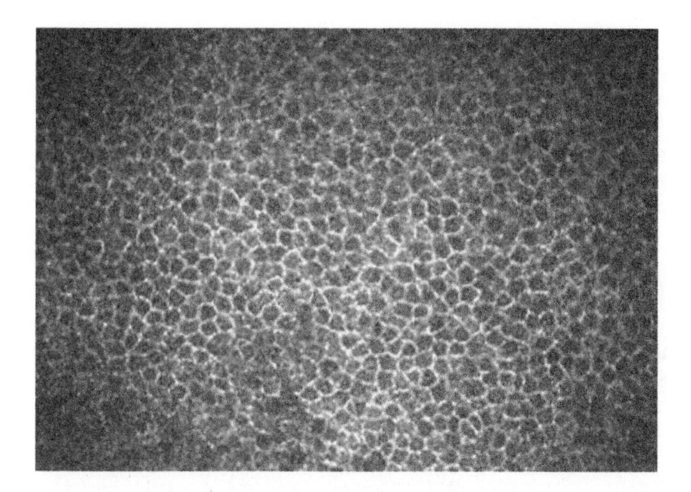

FIGURE 19.3
Basal corneal epithelial cells. A raw IVCM image of the basal epithelial cells in a normal cornea.

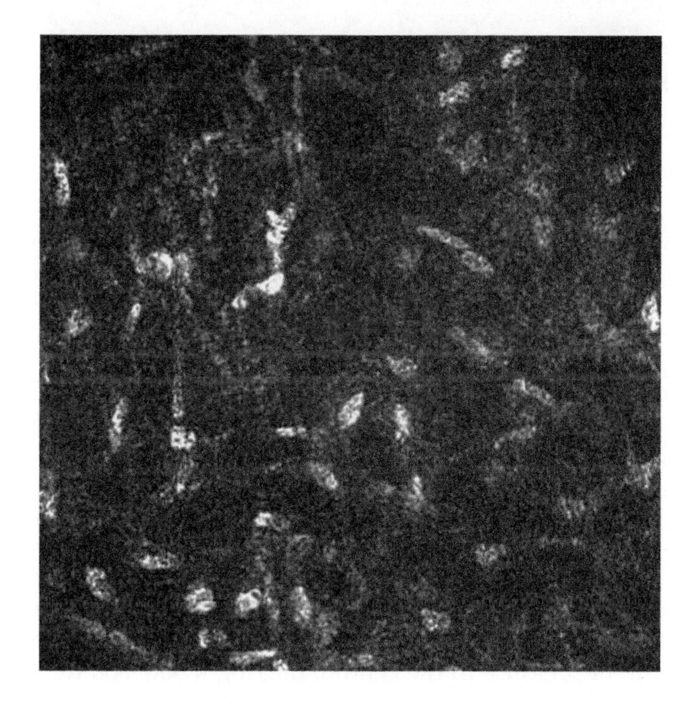

FIGURE 19.4
Corneal stromal keratocytes. A raw IVCM image of the stromal keratocytes (hyperreflective white structures) in a normal cornea.

or the formation of a scar [40]. Death of keratocytes may occur as a response to injury. If the cell death is apoptotic (programmed cell death), it will minimize inflammation and opacification [170].

Keratocyte activity can be evaluated using IVCM. Activated keratocytes, either in the process of transitioning into repair phenotype or cell death, can be noted by an increased reflectivity of their nuclei within the stroma [53]. The number and distribution of

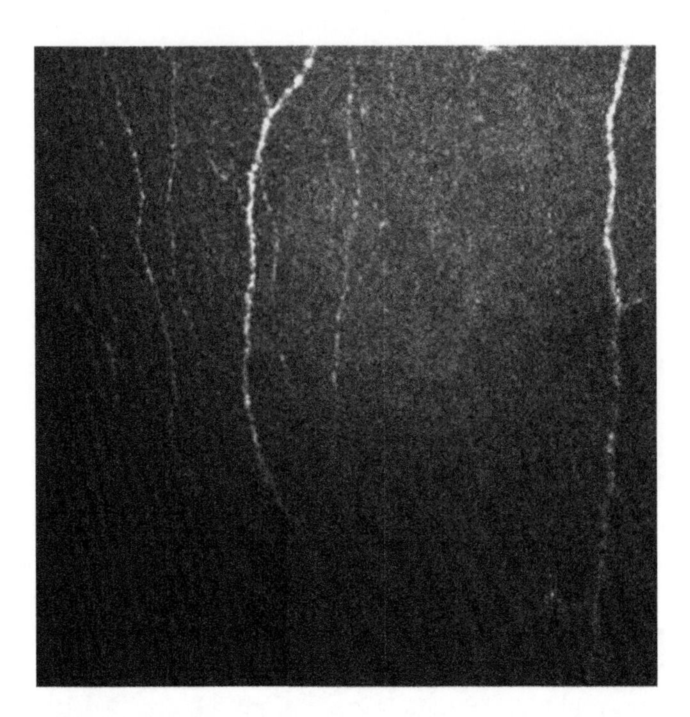

FIGURE 19.5
Corneal stromal nerves. A raw IVCM image of corneal stromal nerves.

keratocytes vary with the health status of the cornea. For instance, a greater density of keratocytes may be found close to a wound site during inflammation compared to the non-inflamed tissue [145,170].

Other inflammatory cells: Among the suprabasal cells, basal cells, and nerve plexus of the cornea, dendritic cells called Langerhans cells are sparsely situated. Langerhans cells are antigen-presenting cells. Like the stromal keratocytes, these resident cells are activated during inflammation and may serve as effective biomarkers for severity of inflammation. These activated cells trigger the infiltration of other immune cells or lymphocytes, resulting in an inflammatory process [164]. In IVCM, the appearance of Langerhans cells varies from small cells with no cellular extensions to larger cells with long processes [53].

Corneal nerves: Approximately 70–80 nerve fibers supply the cornea alone. This makes the cornea the most densely innervated structure in the human body. The normal cornea can detect 10–14 mg/mm^2 of pressure in the central, making it 300–600 times more sensitive than the human skin [94,148]. The remarkable sensitivity of the cornea serves as a protective mechanism in which an immediate reflex to blink or close the eye is triggered with the slightest mechanical stimulation.

Corneal nerve density decreases by approximately 0.9% per year throughout life; thus, corneal sensitivity decreases [93,104,105,131]. Corneal nerves may also be affected by certain types of ocular surgery (e.g., laser-assisted in situ keratomileusis [LASIK]), ocular diseases (e.g., keratoconus), and even systemic diseases (e.g., diabetes) [21,30,32,70,106,116].

Mapping of the corneal nerves throughout the cornea has been done for the normal eye as well as those with ocular conditions. Researchers had to manually combine hundreds of corneal nerve images from adjacent parts of the cornea to form a 2D nerve map. Such a modality has allowed researchers to monitor for long-term changes, such as in keratoconus (Section 19.3.2.4) and orthokeratology contact lens wear (Section 19.3.4.1) [83,115].

Neovascularization: The cornea is normally avascular to preserve its transparency. However, blood vessels may invade the corneal tissue during chronic inflammation or long-term oxygen deficiency (hypoxia). Some of the chronic ocular surface diseases with new blood vessels formation (vascularization) may be viewed using IVCM and will be discussed in the later sections. Blood vessels in the cornea exhibit hyperreflective walls and hyporeflective lumen [103]. Although vascularization produces no symptoms in the early and middle stages, it can be devastating for the vision in advanced cases. An additional imaging tool for documenting progression of corneal vascularization may therefore be valuable.

19.2.1.3 Endothelium

The deepest layer of the cornea, the endothelium, is made up of a single layer of hexagonal-shaped cells (Figure 19.2). The pump function of these cells transports water away from the cornea in order to maintain its transparency and integrity. Diseases affecting the endothelium will therefore eventually cause the cornea to become edematous and lose its transparency. However, unlike the epithelium, these cells do not regenerate even in the event of injury, and the number of cells decreases with age at an average rate of 0.6% per year [14]. In corneal endothelial diseases, such as Fuchs' dystrophy, the manifestations of clinical signs and symptoms are as a result of the inability of endothelial cells to regenerate in the event of excessive cell loss [11].

IVCM can easily detect areas of endothelial cell loss, called guttata, and thus cell density diminishes that occurs in such diseases [100]. In fact, the newer models of IVCM even have an automated cell counting software incorporated into it. The automated method, however, tends to overestimate cell densities as compared to manual counting from a print out of the obtained images. On the other hand, manual counting of cells on the liquid-crystal display, which require the operator to mark each individual cells in the screen, tends to underestimate cell densities [55]. Although the automated cell counting software may not yet be suitable for clinical use, future advances could make it feasible and easier for clinicians to monitor corneal endothelial diseases.

19.2.1.4 Regional Difference

At the edge of the cornea is the limbus (Figures 19.1 and 19.6). This is the transition zone between the cornea and sclera. In recent times, IVCM has aided in the discovery of a novel structure in the ocular surface that has not been previously identified. Deep within the epithelial cells of the normal limbus lays the limbal lacuna. The limbal lacuna was first detected in 2011 with the use of IVCM [177]. Its well-concealed and protected location may suggest its physiological importance in the ocular surface. However, its function is currently unclear and requires further investigation.

IVCM can facilitate the early diagnoses of easily missed pathologies such as limbal stem cell deficiency (LSCD), which will be elaborated on in later sections of the chapter [96,113].

19.2.2 Examination of the Conjunctiva

The conjunctiva is a thin, transparent mucous membrane that forms a continuous lining over the inner surface of the eyelids (palpebral conjunctiva) and the scleral surface

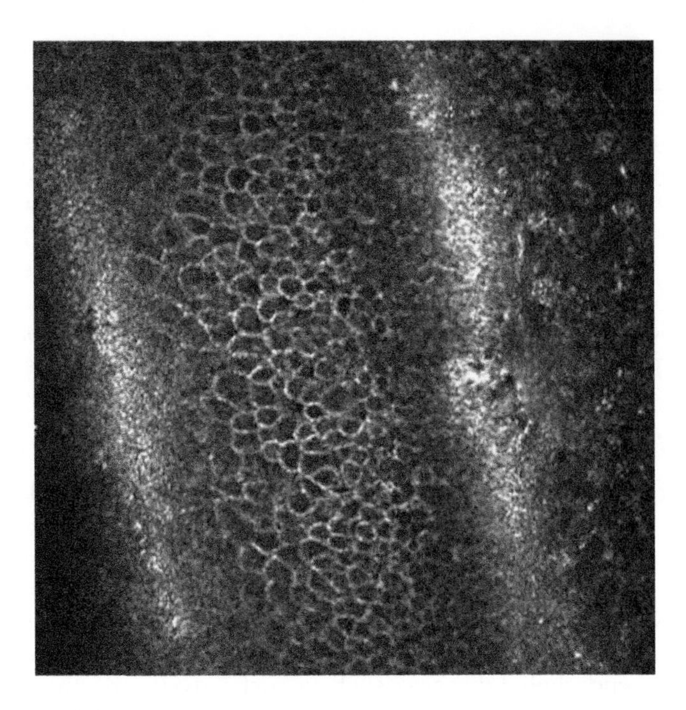

FIGURE 19.6
Limbal epithelial cells. A raw IVCM image of the nasal portion of limbus in a normal patient. The limbus is the transition zone between the conjunctiva (left of the limbus in this image) and cornea (right).

(bulbar conjunctiva) up to the limbus (Figure 19.1). The conjunctiva is an additional immunological defense system against pathogens and aids in the lubrication of the ocular surface.

The conjunctiva has two main layers: the superficial epithelial layer and the stromal layer. The epithelial layer composes of five neatly arranged cell layers and houses the mucus-producing goblet cells that facilitate the spreading of tears over the ocular surface and maintain tear stability. The stromal layer can be subdivided into the adenoid layer, which contains fibrous tissue and immune cells, and the deeper fibrous layer, which contains the blood vessels, nerve fibers, and connective tissue fibers (Figure 19.7).

Impression cytology used to be the most common method for the analysis of conjunctival cells. This technique simply requires the collection of the most superficial cell layer of the conjunctiva with a filter membrane. The acquired cells are then prepared for histological staining to distinguish and observe the epithelial cells, goblet cells, and inflammatory cells of the conjunctiva. Unfortunately, only the most superficial cell layer can be assessed with this method. In addition, with the need to be sent to a lab for processing and analysis, impression cytology may take days to yield results [141].

IVCM, on the other hand, allows the evaluation of deeper cell layers without the need of taking a tissue sample. Furthermore, goblet cells are easily identified as clusters of *giant hyperreflective oval cells* among the significantly smaller epithelial cells in IVCM images [91]. Because of its recognizable structure, goblet cell density can be readily evaluated with IVCM and its findings were shown to be consistent to that made by impression cytology [71]. Images taken by IVCM can also be viewed and analyzed instantly. More clinicians today therefore prefer to employ IVCM over impression cytology for conjunctival evaluation.

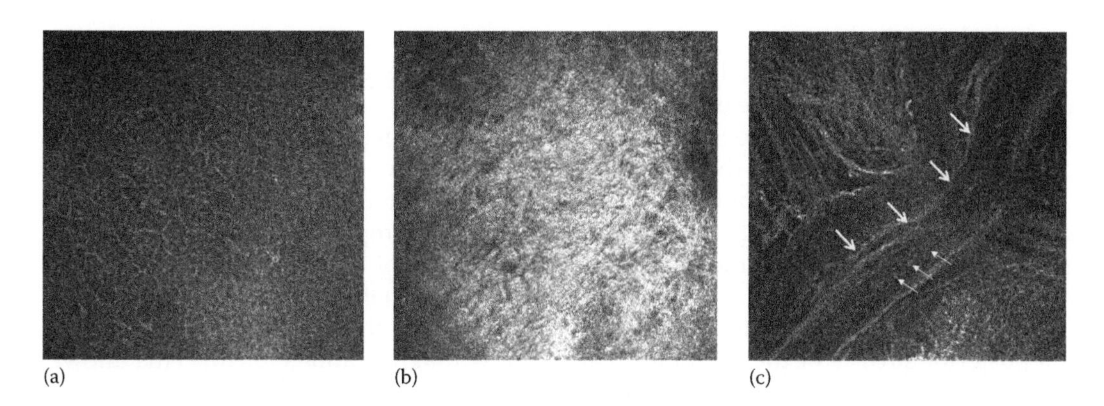

FIGURE 19.7
Various layers of the bulbar conjunctiva. Raw IVCM images of the epithelial layer (a), the stromal adenoid layer (b), and the fibrous layer (c) of a normal bulbar conjunctiva. The fibrous layer has a less homogenous appearance than the adenoid layer. A blood vessel can be seen in this image (open arrows) with blood cells flowing though (block arrows).

IVCM has been a significant instrument in the discovery of conjunctiva-associated lymphoid tissues (CALT). These tissues are lymphatic aggregates embedded in the palpebral conjunctiva and serve as an induction site for the immune defense of the ocular surface. CALT are composed of T and B lymphocytes, macrophages, dendritic cells, and plasma cells [8,60,78].

The use of IVCM for detailed evaluation of the eyelid margins has also been done. The movement of the eyelid (the action of blinking) is crucial for the even distribution of the tear film. IVCM is able to image two unique structures of the palpebral conjunctiva, the lid wiper and the mucocutaneous junction (MCJ) [62]. The lid wiper is the inner border of the eyelid directly in contact with the eyeball. It spreads the tear film evenly over the ocular surface during the upward movement of a blink [63]. The MCJ is the transition zone between the anterior keratinized epithelium (the eyelid skin) and the nonkeratinized mucous membrane epithelium (the conjunctiva). The MCJ plays a role in the mitosis of conjunctival cells that migrate across the palpebral conjunctiva [174].

Abnormalities of the MCJ can be viewed with fluorescein dye staining. For example, patients with dry eye show greater epithelial cell keratinization in this area as compared to normal volunteers. The MCJs in dry eye patients therefore tend to migrate anteriorly from its original position [65]. At the moment, the lid wiper and MCJ may be sufficiently assessed using slit-lamp biomicroscopy. IVCM of the lid wiper and MCJ may not be practical in the clinical setting as yet. The observation of their cellular structures may instead be achieved by IVCM for research purposes.

To summarize, IVCM can be a complementary examination method to current conventional techniques, which can only observe the ocular surface at lower magnifications. Its ability to examine the conjunctiva and analyze the extent of inflammation will be extremely valuable in both research and clinical settings.

19.2.3 Examination of the Meibomian Glands

Meibomian glands are present in the upper and lower eyelids and function to secrete oil, otherwise known as meibum, onto the tear film (Figure 19.1). The meibum forms the outermost lipid layer of the tear film that maintains elasticity of the tear film and the characteristics of tear spreading. Meibum is first produced in the secretory acini, travels through connecting ductules, the central and excretory ducts, and reaches the gland openings or orifices to finally be released into the tear film [17].

The meibomian glands are located within the tarsal plates, further from the superficial eyelid skin and closer to the posterior lid surface (palpebral conjunctiva). Because of this position, visualization of the glands using the commonly available clinical instruments is generally challenging. For example, the slit-lamp biomicroscope can only evaluate gland openings, which gives little information of the integrity of the glands beyond the surface. Infrared meibography is a transillumination technique that brought meibomian gland imaging to the next level. It can image the meibomian glands from the posterior surface of the eyelid at relatively low magnifications [6,123]. This allows qualitative and quantitative assessment of glandular changes, such as loss and twisting of the glands, to be observed [6,124]. Unfortunately, due to its lower magnification and resolution, this technique cannot provide information on the microanatomy of the individual acinus.

Meibomian glands imaging using IVCM was pioneered in 2005 [64]. The high resolution of the IVCM images made the evaluation of individual glandular acinus possible (Figure 19.8). Soon after, novel parameters were developed for the investigation of meibomian glands: the diameter and density of the glandular acinar units [88]. Normal values for these parameters have been described, though not yet established, to be 100–119 units/mm^2 in density and 41–53 µm in diameter [88,162,163]. This method of meibomian gland evaluation expanded further to the introduction of additional parameters: acinar longest diameter, acinar shortest diameter, inflammatory cell density, and acinar unit density [51].

These developments in the IVCM examination of meibomian glands have enabled researchers to identify minute morphological changes in various disease and contact lens wear (Section 19.3.2.1.1).

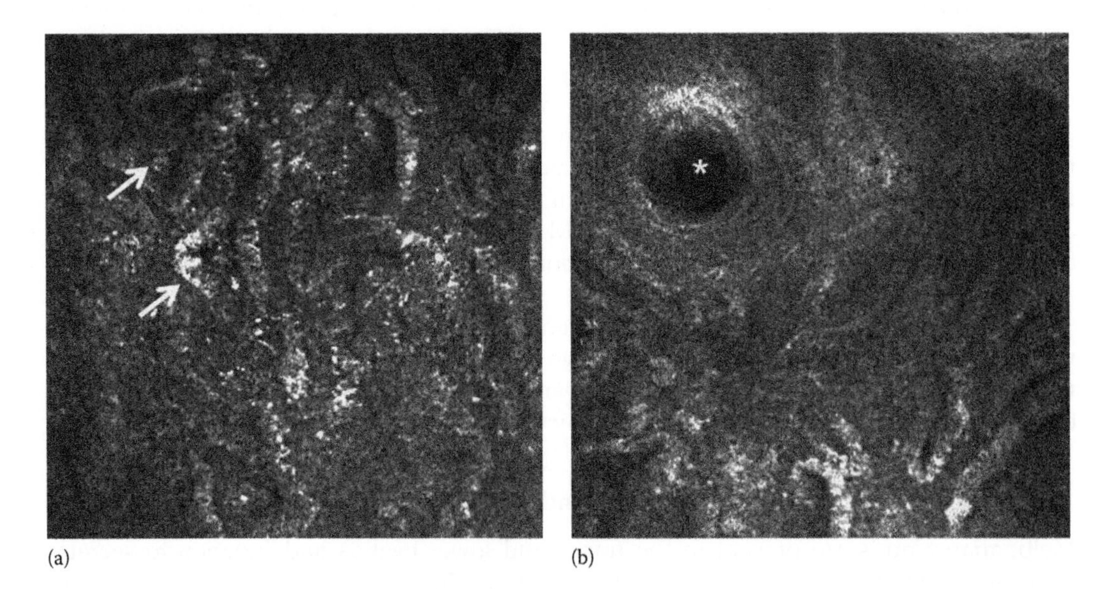

FIGURE 19.8
IVCM images of the meibomian glands. The acini are indicated by the white arrows (a) and a gland orifice (*) (b).

19.3 Clinical Applications

The high resolution and magnification that IVCM can achieve makes it a powerful instrument for the examination of the ocular surface structures. Microscopic details up to the cellular level provided by IVCM that conventional clinical examination tools are unable to offer. As evidenced by research findings, IVCM can be extremely helpful in the diagnosis and monitoring of disease progression. For instance, quantification of cell densities in each layer of the cornea and conjunctiva has enabled researchers to determine the normal parameters for the general population. This information may enable clinicians to identify abnormalities associated with disease or changes with age. The gross morphology of the corneal nerve fiber has also been found to modify with contact lens wear (Section 19.3.4).

Ocular diseases can manifest vague clinical signs. Differential diagnosis of diseases can be made easier with IVCM. For example, corneal edema (the swelling of the cornea) may be due to a defect in the endothelium layer or inflammation. Examination with the slit lamp may be hindered by the relative corneal opacity caused by the edema. In this scenario, IVCM can help to distinguish between an inflammatory cause (identified by the presence of excessive inflammatory cells) and a deficit in the endothelium (identified by an attenuated number of endothelial cells). Pre- and postoperative assessments, such as the morphology of corneal nerves before and after refractive surgery, can also be performed (Section 19.3.3.1).

19.3.1 Infectious Corneal and Conjunctival Diseases

Diseases of the cornea encompass a large array of etiology: from infectious to inflammatory in nature and from genetic to acquired. The major cause of cornea-related blindness arises from infections, especially in developing countries [149]. The natural history of corneal infections is scarring and vascularization, loss of transparency, and finally loss of vision when the cornea opacifies, or alternatively it could perforate, leading to endophthalmitis [171]. Corneal diseases are currently the second most important cause of blindness worldwide [144,171]. Conjunctival diseases usually do not impact the vision until the cornea is involved. Trachoma, discussed in the next section, is a good example of a disease that originates in the conjunctiva and later can impact on the cornea.

19.3.1.1 Trachoma

Trachoma is a major cause of blindness due to infection in the world. The conjunctiva is first infected by the bacteria *Chlamydia trachomatis*; chronic inflammation occurs and results in conjunctival scarring and vascularization. When this inflammatory process implicates the cornea, scarring and vascularization and eventually total opacification of the cornea can be observed [144,149,171].

In studies on patients with active trachoma, abnormal follicular structures and black cystic spaces were seen in the conjunctiva (indicating tissue swelling). Dendritic-like inflammatory cells were easily observed [49]. Additionally, inflammatory cells residing within the superficial trachomatous scars were found within 30 μm from the surface, suggesting a close interaction between these inflammatory cells and the epithelium [50].

A system for the grading of conjunctival inflammation was developed. Characteristic features of trachoma in the palpebral conjunctiva, such as the presence of inflammatory

TABLE 19.1

Grading System for Extent of Conjunctival Scarring in Trachoma

Grade[a]	Description
0	Normal: homogenous, amorphous appearance with occasional fine, wispy strand
1	Heterogeneous appearance with poorly defined clumps or bands present
2	Clearly defined bands of tissue that constitute <50% of the area of the scan
3	Clearly defined bands or sheets of tissue that constitute ≥50% of the area of the scan in which striations are visible

Source: Hu, V.H. et al., *Ophthalmology*, 118(4), 747, 2011.

[a] The higher grade is given if features of different grades are visible.

infiltrates and cells, tissue edema, and papillae, are used as the basis to determine the degree of inflammation. A four-point grading system can be employed to evaluate the extent of conjunctival scarring, ranging from grade 0 to 3 (Table 19.1) [49].

For now, it may not be practical to depend on IVCM for the diagnosis and monitoring of trachoma in developing countries for various reasons. Nevertheless, IVCM will be valuable for research purposes. From investigating the pathophysiology of trachoma to analyzing the extent of inflammation of the disease, IVCM will enable us to broaden our understanding of the disease.

19.3.1.2 Corneal Infections

Mainly four types of microorganisms are responsible for infective keratitis—in order of prevalence—viruses, bacteria, fungi, and amoeba. Risk factors of infective keratitis include, but not limited to, contact lens wear, ocular trauma, and certain systemic diseases [29,79,127,134]. Corneal culture is the current mainstay for the identification of the microorganism responsible for infections. IVCM offers an additional tool to aid in the diagnosis.

Viral keratitis: The most common viral keratitis is caused by the *herpes simplex* virus (HSV). HSV keratitis may be seen in patients with a history of cold sores. Perhaps the most ominous feature of this infection is the virus' ability to survive in its dormant state, residing in the trigeminal nerve (the largest of the cranial nerves; responsible for corneal sensation) and even the corneal tissue itself [58,140]. Because of its stubborn survival ability, complete eradication of the virus is almost impossible and the recurrence of the infection is commonly seen after the initial have apparently resolved.

In active HSV, dendritic cells, easily identified due to its characteristic wire netting, can be detected with IVCM [42]. In the corneal endothelium, the usually neatly arranged cells become irregular as the shapes and sizes of cells change [130]. In the endothelial layer, spaces between cells increase, cell borders become indistinct, large areas of cell loss (guttata), and inflammatory cells can be seen. These changes are not permanent and the endothelium returns to its original appearance when the infection is resolved [43].

The involvement of dendritic cells in HSV keratitis is a sign of inflammation. A decrease in its number is an indication that the infection is resolving [42]. When the disease is in its inactive stage, clinicians would not be expected to detect any abnormalities in the cornea, especially with slit-lamp biomicroscopy. However, corneal changes have been observed in patients with a history of HSV keratitis, even during the inactive stage. IVCM signs that suggest a previous HSV infection include areas with excessive abnormal extracellular matrix, enlarged corneal superficial epithelial cells, and hyperreflective structures among the basal epithelial cells (especially around areas of stromal fibrosis).

In this condition, it may be harder to visualize long nerve fiber bundles, or less nerve fibers could be observed [130]. IVCM can help to determine the chronological process of these changes and, in the future, may be helpful in predicting HSV keratitis recurrence.

Bacterial keratitis: The primary risk factor for bacterial keratitis is contact lens wear, clinical keratitis being relatively rare in non–contact lens wearers. Like most other bacterial infections in other parts of the body, broad-spectrum antibiotics are initially prescribed when bacterial keratitis is suspected. It is not until laboratory reports concerning the class of bacteria involved (gram negative or positive) are available that an antibiotic with a narrower spectrum of microbial action, directed at the causative species, is given.

On slit-lamp biomicroscopy, the corneal ulcer caused by bacterial infection is typically a white lesion near or at the central cornea. The lesion can be seen in IVCM images as a hyperreflective structure with an undefined posterior border, with surrounding edema of the otherwise normal epithelium. Inflammatory activities can be indicated by the presence of leukocytes and Langerhans cells in the posterior epithelium and the stroma surrounding the ulcer [42]. Distinction between gram-positive and gram-negative bacteria, as well as isolation of the responsible bacteria, is currently not possible with IVCM. Corneal scrapping and bacteria culture remain the only way to identify the species involved [158].

Fungal keratitis: Fungal keratitis usually occurs to individuals living or working in tropical areas or plantations, where the most common cause is mechanical trauma to the eye. Such an injury can occur in the scenario of vegetative matter, predisposing the cornea to fungal keratitis in two ways: (1) it induces a corneal defect and (2) introduces fungal microspores onto the eye. The corneal defect would permit the microspores to penetrate into deeper layers [48,129]. Other risk factors include excessive or inappropriate steroid use, and lack of hygiene [151].

In fungal keratitis, inflammation is shown by an increase in dendritic cells and round inflammatory cells detected in the corneal epithelium and stromal infiltrates. The epithelial cells and stroma become disorganized; the latter represents the activation of corneal keratocytes to become fibroblasts [72,166]. The fungus typically presents as long and defined hyperreflective lines in IVCM images (Figure 19.9). The identification of the fungal species is possible with IVCM. Various fungi species exhibit distinct physical properties in IVCM images (Table 19.2), providing a way to immediately isolate the causative fungal species [15]. This may be advantageous as clinical decisions may not be delayed till the availability of microbiology reports.

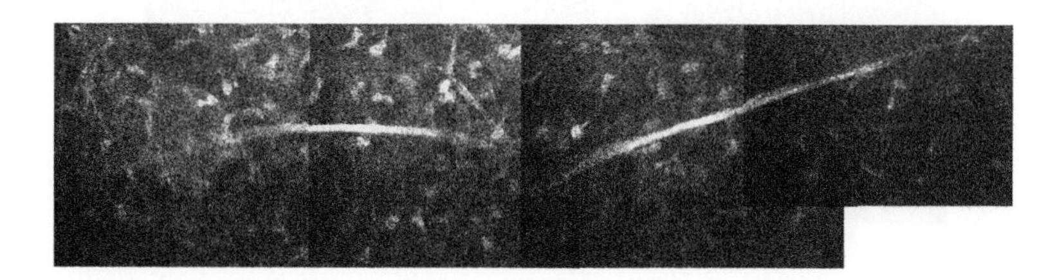

FIGURE 19.9
Fungal keratitis. Four IVCM images are stitched together to form this image of the fungus *Aspergillus fumigatus*, identified as the thick hyperreflective line in the anterior stroma among the keratocytes.

TABLE 19.2

IVCM Findings in Corneas with the Three Types of Infectious Keratitis

Fungi Species	Appearance/Findings
Yeast	
Fusarium solani	High-contrast lines 200–300 μm × 3–5 μm Branches at right angles in the anterior stroma
Candida albicans	High-contrast elongated particles 10–40 μm × 5–10 μm
Filamentous	
Aspergillus fumigatus	High-contrast lines 200–300 μm × 3–5 μm Branches at 45° in the anterior stroma

Amoebic keratitis: Amoebic keratitis, *Acanthamoeba* keratitis in particular, is the rarest but most devastating of corneal infections. The microorganism primarily attacks the corneal nerves first, causing severe pain and eventually a significant loss of vision [35]. Despite the intense pain at the ocular surface caused by *Acanthamoeba* keratitis, patients generally present with only a mild to moderate red eye—an extremely vague clinical sign often overlooked by clinicians. The disproportion between clinical signs and patient symptoms therefore often leave clinicians perplexed, and the disease is easily missed [23].

Using IVCM for rapid and effective diagnosis of *Acanthamoeba* keratitis may be plausible. In its active form (trophozoite), the amoeba presents as a hyperreflective element 24–40 μm in size in the corneal epithelium or stroma, surrounded by edematous tissue. The inactive form of the *Acanthamoeba* (cyst) is a hyperreflective rounded object, 10–28 μm in size in the epithelium or stroma (Figure 19.10). These well-described appearances make it easily recognizable with IVCM [42,67].

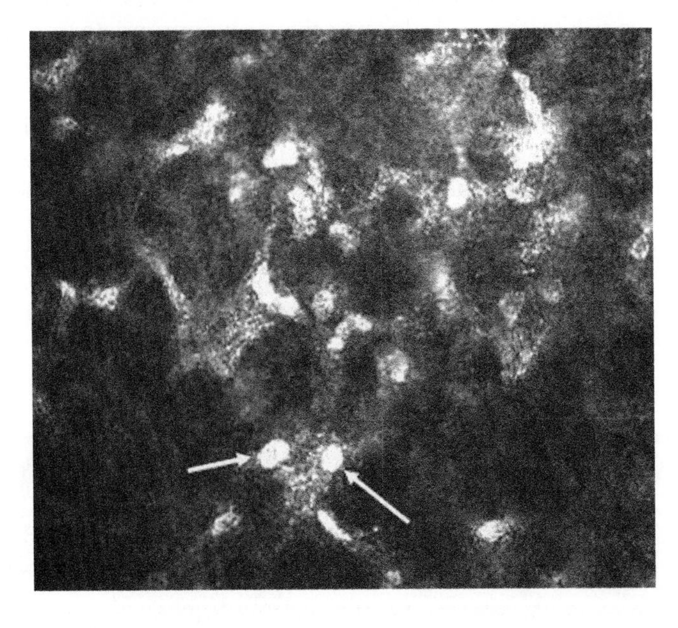

FIGURE 19.10
Acanthamoeba keratitis. The cysts of the *Acanthamoeba* are seen as round hyperreflective structures (arrows) in this raw IVCM image.

Corneal infections: Summary—Corneal scraping and culture is currently the mainstay of identifying the microorganism responsible for the infection. For unusual organisms, this process may take weeks, and time is of the essence in infective keratitis as it can lead to a significant loss of vision in a matter of weeks. Furthermore, cultures may require special culture media and, as reported by studies, only 30%–67% of the collected samples were positive in cultures [56,59,109,176]. Negative cultures obtained may be due to previous antibiotics or attempted treatment.

When IVCM imaging was compared against corneal cultures and corneal smears for the identification of *Acanthamoeba* keratitis, the evidence of the infection from IVCM was perceptible in 48 out of 53 patients (91%). On the other hand, corneal cultures and smears showed positive results in only 30 out of 41 patients (73%) and 23 out of 42 (55%) patients, respectively, compared to clinical criteria [154]. IVCM's accuracy in the identification of microorganism in infective keratitis is fairly high—with sensitivities and specificities of 90%–100% and 84%–100% for *Acanthamoeba* and 90%–94% and 78%–93% for fungi in culture-proven cases [56,154,157].

In a report by Babu and Murthy, IVCM revealed fungal filaments, *Acanthamoeba* cysts, and trophozoites in the cornea of a patient presenting with ocular pain, redness, and blurred vision. Where this was clearly a case of combined fungal and *Acanthamoeba* keratitis when imaged with IVCM, slit-lamp biomicroscopy only revealed a peripheral corneal ulcer and pus in the anterior chamber (hypopyon). This patient was able to receive treatment for both infections in time and the patient's vision was restored [9]. This is a rare example of the limitations of slit-lamp biomicroscopy for rapid and accurate infection diagnosis. By themselves, the presence of hypopyon and corneal ulcer would be unlikely to lead to a suspicion of *Acanthamoeba* involvement.

Ambiguous signs of infective keratitis (such as corneal lesion, red eyes, and tearing) are shared by those caused by different microorganisms. This complicates diagnosis and treatment of the infection. IVCM is therefore a potentially beneficial instrument for the instant identification of the causative microorganism and timely implementation of the appropriate treatment.

19.3.2 Noninfectious Corneal and Conjunctiva Diseases

Noninfectious diseases of the cornea and conjunctiva are usually less acute in nature (with the exception of ocular chemical burns); cellular changes take place over a long period of time. The following sections discuss the role of IVCM in the evaluation in such diseases, including monitoring disease progression, treatment evaluation, and deeper understanding of the pathophysiological processes.

19.3.2.1 Dry Eye

Dry eye is a dysfunction of the tear film and can be caused by either a decrease in tear secretion or, more commonly, an increase in evaporation rates of the tears. The ocular surface is inadequately lubricated due to the compromised tear film and increases inflammatory activity. Subsequently, cell damage of the surface occurs and symptoms of dry eye manifest. Although more common in old age and in women, the prevalence of dry eye is nevertheless extremely high in the general population, ranging from 5% to 35% [80,89]. Individuals with previous ocular surgeries, with systemic diseases, on certain medications, and who wore contact lenses are at higher risks of developing dry eye [1,74].

Slit-lamp biomicroscopy is the usual method of dry eye assessment. Unfortunately, it provides little information on subtle inflammatory process that may occur in the cornea and conjunctiva. Inflammatory cells in the conjunctiva would not have been visible with slit-lamp examination due to the minute size of the inflammatory cells and lack of contrast with the conjunctival tissue. Despite the absence of slit-lamp findings in the conjunctiva, it has been reported that inflammatory cell densities in patients with dry eye (without any other associated inflammatory disorder) are 11 times higher than in normal patients [165].

In the cornea, decreased corneal thickness and epithelial cell density have been found in dry eye patients. Nerve fiber changes were equally notable, with reductions in nerve fiber density, irregular branching patterns of nerve fiber, and increased fiber tortuosity [38,178]. These findings in relation to the nerve fibers are significant; as reported in a study on aqueous tear-deficient dry eye patients, the number of nerve fibers is positively correlated with the amount of corneal cellular damage as evident by slit-lamp biomicroscopy findings [178].

The application of IVCM in dry eye assessment is not limited to the cornea and conjunctiva. As mentioned in Section 19.2.3, the meibomian glands play an important role in tear film function. A dysfunction of the glands may therefore be devastating to the integrity of the tear film.

Meibomian gland dysfunction: In meibomian gland dysfunction (MGD), the glands are obstructed and the biochemistry of the meibum is modified. The inability of the glands to secrete meibum as effectively disturbs the integrity of the tear film lipid layer [61]. MGD is the major cause for evaporative dry eye and is extremely prevalent, affecting 9%–69% of the general population [18,19,54,75,80,89,156].

IVCM has provided clinicians with ways to precisely measure inflammatory cell density, acini density, and acinus diameter. This makes it a promising way of evaluating the efficacy of MGD treatment. Reduction in acini density and increase in diameter have been reported in IVCM studies [88,162]. In a study of 37 patients, there was a significant decrease in inflammatory cell density in patients receiving anti-inflammatory treatment for MGD over a period of 12 weeks, but this was not seen in the group receiving conventional treatment [88].

Meibomian gland changes related to contact lens wear have been extensively studied; its results, however, have been controversial. While some studies reported increased meibomian gland blockage in contact lens wearers, epidemiological studies have suggested otherwise [7,84,135]. The meibomian gland imaging using IVCM may be the key to resolving this discrepancy. Meibomian gland acini units have already been found to be significantly smaller and higher in density in contact lens–wearing patients, supporting the notion of adverse meibomian gland changes in contact lens wearers. However, it should be noted that the study's sample size was small (a total of 40 patients) and was focused only on soft contact lens wearers with at least 1 year of regular wear [163]. Further longitudinal studies evaluating the chronological changes in meibomian gland morphology in contact lens wearers may be indicated.

The understanding of systemic disorders associated to ocular surface diseases has also improved with the images obtained with IVCM. In Sjögren's syndrome (SS), for instance, meibomian gland involvement was not previously considered to be a major part of the pathology as the condition primarily affects the salivary and tear glands. However, microscopic changes in the meibomian glands have been observed. Acini density seemed to be higher in patients with primary SS than in both MGD patients and normal controls

(138 ± 69 units/mm^2, 57 ± 21 units/mm^2, and 110 ± 31 units/mm^2, respectively), whereas gland orifice was smaller than both MGD patients and controls (27.8 ± 5.9 µm, 50.0 ± 9.1 µm, and 34.7 ± 4.3 µm, respectively) [162]. The use of IVCM in evaluating SS manifestations in the eye will be further discussed in the next section.

Some culprits for MGD are commensals typically found residing in the hair follicles and skin of mammals—*Demodex* mites. Excessive numbers of these parasites around the meibomian orifices and eyelashes can cause inflammation of the eyelids and cornea. These exacerbate meibomian gland blockages leading to dry eye [28]. The excessive presence of *Demodex* mites can be determined by epilating the eyelashes of a patient and counting the number of mites present [73].

However, the *Demodex brevis*, unlike the *Demodex folliculorum*, tends to reside within the meibomian glands and may not be observed after epilation of lashes. As high-powered microscopes are not normally found in eye clinics, the in vitro counting of *D. folliculorum* mites usually only takes place after a certain time period of storage and transportation of the eyelashes. The time lapse between the eyelash epilation and actual counting may alter the number of mites present. IVCM may be a more accurate method of counting *Demodex* mites since no epilation is required and the mites may be viewed in real time. The IVCM images of these mites can be viewed as roundish structures 4–7 µm in diameter within the follicles of the eyelashes [133]. This method has also been employed for other parts of the body, such as the chest, face, and scalp [82].

Sjögren's syndrome: In the autoimmune SS, the body's own immune cells attack exocrine glands and drastically affect their function. It is known to principally affect the salivary and tear glands. Patients with SS therefore suffer from severe dry mouth and dry eye. IVCM may potentially increase the understanding of the cause–effect relationship of the disease. As a systemic condition, SS has substantial manifestations in the eye. When viewed with IVCM, dry eye patients without SS may exhibit an increase in inflammatory cells in the cornea and conjunctiva. The same inflammatory cells have been reported in SS patients but in largely amplified numbers. The higher numbers of inflammatory cells worsen tear stability and damage the ocular surface.

Other conjunctival changes found in SS patients include decreased epithelial cell densities and increased epithelial microcyst densities [165]. The corneal nerve fibers were not spared as its numbers and tortuosity increase [178].

Dry eye: Summary—In the clinical setting, the fundamental clinical examination techniques such as slit-lamp examination usually suffice. However, the information that only IVCM can provide may be important in understanding the microscopic changes in the cellular level. It has also been proven to be useful in evaluating the effectiveness of MGD treatment.

19.3.2.2 Limbal Stem Cell Deficiency

The limbus barricades the conjunctiva from the cornea, preventing conjunctival cells, vessels, and inflammatory cells from invading the cornea. In addition, stem cells involved in corneal wound repair are housed within this structure, specifically in the palisades of Vogt (Figure 19.11) and, as recently discovered with IVCM, the limbal lacuna [26]. LSCD is where the stem cells become unhealthily scarce and the cornea–conjunctiva barrier breaks down. As a result, conjunctival epithelium grows over the cornea (conjunctivalization), often initiating inflammation.

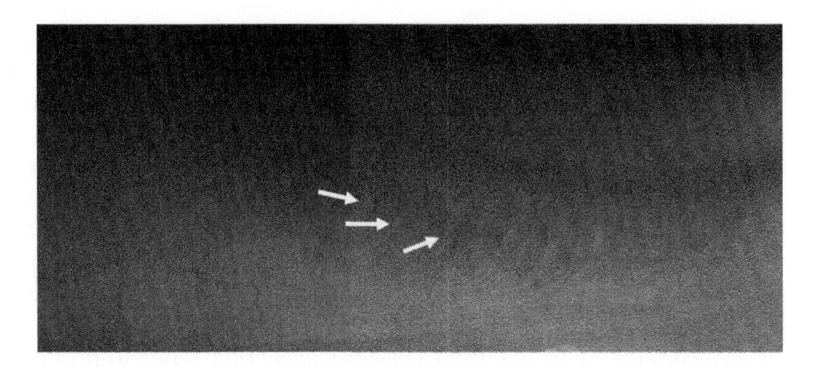

FIGURE 19.11
The palisades of Vogt. A slit-lamp photo of the palisades of Vogt in the inferior limbus of a normal patient (arrows). However, not all patients with healthy eyes will have visible palisades of Vogt, typically being more obvious and pigmented in darker-skinned individuals.

Slit-lamp biomicroscopy signs of LSCD include corneal edema, irregular corneal surface, and extensive corneal fluorescein dye staining (corneal erosions). In the more advanced cases, visible growth of the conjunctival epithelium over the cornea and corneal vascularization may be seen. In LSCD, the cornea varies in transparency, and its irregularity may affect vision drastically. The tendency of the corneal epithelium to break down is the main cause of the symptoms: poor visual quality, sensitivity to light, intermittent pain, and eyelid twitching [34,45].

Impression cytology is currently the main technique to confirm the diagnosis of LSCD when slit-lamp biomicroscopy findings are in doubt. The presence of goblet cells and conjunctival epithelial cells on the cornea in impression cytology confirms the diagnosis of LSCD [33,34].

However, goblet cells may not always be present in the corneas of LSCD. In fact, a previous study noted that only 6 out of 17 conjunctivalized corneas have goblet cells present. However, the authors acknowledged the possibility of not having done a sufficiently thorough scan throughout the affected cornea. In addition, the absence of goblet cells in the cornea in IVCM images may suggest a lower density of goblet cells, possibly because of a massive destruction of these cells, or an accompaniment of another pathology such as aqueous-deficient dry eye [96,121]. Clinical features of LSCD alone currently do not give the clinicians much clue of the etiology, although patient history and presence of other clinical signs may suggest a single cause.

Researchers have reported the appearance of dendritic-like cells in the center of LSCD-affected corneas. In normal corneas, the further one departs from the periphery, the less inflammatory cells one should observe. They postulated that these cells have migrated from the limbus toward the center of the compromised cornea [86,96]. Intraepithelial cysts, 12–52 μm in diameter, were also found within the epithelium of the conjunctivalized cornea. These cysts appeared as dark spaces among the hyperreflective goblet cells [96]. The reason for the presence of these cysts is unknown. Further investigations will be required to determine this.

In the conjunctiva of the LSCD patients, the epithelial basal cells had more prominent hyperreflective nuclei and indistinct edges than the normal conjunctiva. Finally, the effect of LSCD on the corneal nerves is similar to most other ocular surface diseases—a decrease in nerve fiber density. This was more significantly so in the advanced cases of LSCD, where even the Bowman's membrane was undetectable. The inability of IVCM to image the corneal nerves may be due to either an actual damage of the nerves or merely the challenge of focusing beyond the thick conjunctiva tissue in between the objective lens and conjunctivalized cornea.

19.3.2.3 Chemical Burns

Ocular chemical burns are caused by acidic or alkaline agents. These are ocular emergencies and should be managed immediately by thoroughly irrigating the affected eye for more than 30 min with a sterile insipid solution until neutral pH is achieved [99].

Contrary to popular belief, alkaline burns are more threatening to ocular integrity than acidic burns. Exposure to alkaline chemical solution causes saponification of the corneal cell membrane. This enables the insulting agent to penetrate into deeper layers of the cornea and even beyond the ocular surface within minutes of the initial chemical contact [118,175]. On the other hand, acidic chemical solutions cause corneal proteins in the epithelium to coagulate, forming a barrier to prevent further penetration of the chemical into the deeper layers, thus usually causing only superficial damage [175].

In both types of injury, the prognosis of chemical burns depends on the amount and concentration of chemical exposure and promptness and duration of irrigation. Topical pharmaceutical medication is usually sufficient to prevent further long-term adverse effects. Severe ocular damage that requires surgery is rare [99].

Although seldom devastating to the vision, the injurious chemical potentially damages the conjunctival goblet cells and limbal stem cells. The substantially diminished number of goblet cells affects the tear film stability and consequently causes severe dry eye [71,152]. More importantly, the chemical is likely to damage the limbal stem cells, causing LSCD (Section 19.3.2.2) [27].

IVCM and impression cytology are ways that clinicians can utilize to monitor the long-term effects of chemical burns. As mentioned in Section 19.2.2, clinicians' preference is gradually shifting to IVCM. The change in preference is justified by the instant viewing of images: a quicker method of monitoring conjunctival goblet cell and limbal stem cell changes in patients with ocular burns.

19.3.2.4 Keratoconus

Keratoconus, as its name suggests, is the abnormal reshaping of the cornea into a conical shape (Figure 19.12). This degenerative disease causes the cornea to thin and the vision to deteriorate. In the early to moderate stages of the disease, clinical signs such as the small changes in corneal curvature and thickness are extremely subtle and difficult to detect [126]. The cone shape only becomes apparent in the moderate to advanced stages of the disease when the vision has worsened drastically. Keratoconus has been widely accepted as a disease with a genetic association, although other factors such as contact lens wear, excessive eye rubbing, and various systemic diseases also increase the risk of this disease. To this day, its etiology remains unclear [36,126].

On slit-lamp biomicroscopy, prominence of corneal nerves is the earliest sign in keratoconic eyes. Therefore, IVCM findings of corneal nerves are not unexpected. The density of nerve fiber is reduced, while the thickness, prominence, and tortuosity are increased [116,155]. The decrease in density is more substantial in severe cases and in patients on therapeutic contact lens wear. By mapping the corneal nerves with hundreds of IVCM images, Patel and McGhee found that in four patients with keratoconus, the nerve fibers have rearranged to form closed loops at the corneal apex, running parallel to the contour

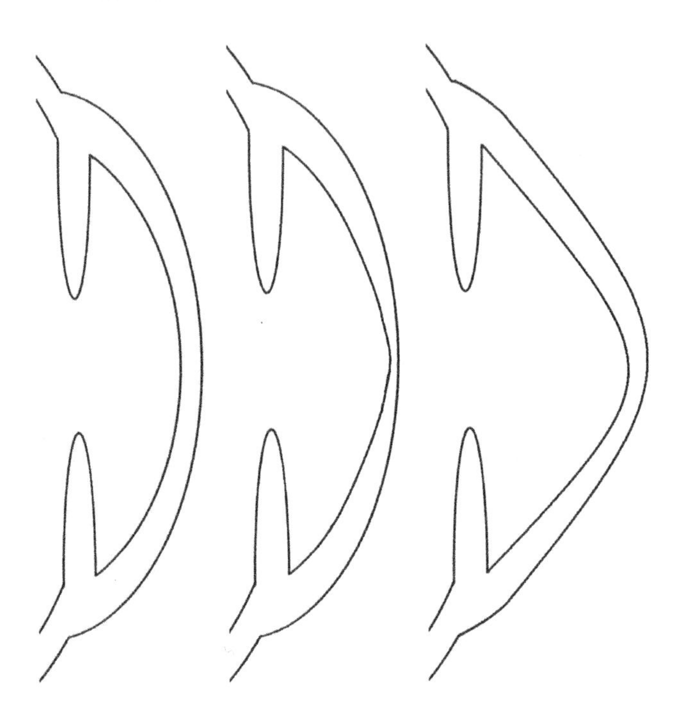

FIGURE 19.12
Progression of keratoconus. The normal cornea (left) starts to thin from the central area of the posterior surface (center) and eventually forms the entire cornea and becomes cone-shaped (right).

of the cornea. This contrasts to the normal whorl pattern of corneal nerve fiber arrangement of normal people [115].

These abnormal IVCM findings of keratoconic corneas are consistent with the reduction in corneal sensitivity as found in previous studies [114]. Whether the changes in corneal nerve fiber precede the clinical manifestations of the disease or are brought about by the change in corneal morphology remains unclear. More longitudinal studies are warranted to determine the sequence of events in nerve fiber changes.

IVCM has revealed that all five corneal layers are affected in keratoconus. Starting from the outermost layer—the epithelium—superficial cells become elongated, the nuclei of the winged-shaped cells are increased, and density of the basal cells decreases while the cells increase in size [47,97,106,155]. The Bowman's membrane is disrupted, possibly explaining the encroachment of epithelial cell processes into the Bowman's membrane [106,138].

In the stromal layer, the keratocytes are activated and disorganized, causing corneal haziness, showing up as increased reflectivity in IVCM images [47,97,106]. Additionally, keratocyte cell density decreases, correlating negatively with severity of disease [47,66,97,106]. Stromal and Descemet's membrane folds, as observed in one study, may further decrease quality of vision [155].

Finally, in the innermost layer—the endothelium—large areas of cell loss, enlargement of cells, and changes in cells shapes and densities have been reported. The magnitude of these changes also seem to correlate with disease severity [47,97,106,155].

Currently, certain kinds of corneal topography imaging are the most utilized imaging technique for the diagnosis and monitoring of keratoconus. Its noncontact method and wider field of view may be reasons for its more widespread use than IVCM. On the other hand, observations of corneal structural changes up to the cellular level can only be made by IVCM. Such details may be vital to the understanding of the pathophysiology and etiology of keratoconus. IVCM may therefore be done in complement to corneal topography in the clinical settings, as well as for research purposes.

19.3.2.5 Pterygium

Pterygium is an abnormal noncancerous growth of the bulbar conjunctiva and forms a wing-shaped raised lesion over the ipsilateral side of the cornea (Figure 19.13). Usually vascularized, it is more frequently formed at the nasal side of the conjunctiva and has a huge link to ultraviolet radiation exposure [110]. Its incidence is therefore greater in individuals who spent a large amount of time outdoors and who live in equatorial regions [90].

Pterygia tissues are usually surgically excised when it grows to the extent of affecting the vision or cosmetically unpleasing. The excised tissues have been used in laboratory histopathological studies to understand this abnormal growth. Tissue studies provide only a glimpse into pterygium pathology (conjunctival stromal and epithelial changes) when it is severe enough to be excised. We are not able to understand the properties and activities of the less advanced pterygium while on the eye [10]. IVCM provides a way for clinicians to observe pterygia in real time at the cellular level, as well as the effects on the neighboring corneal and conjunctival tissues.

In the corneal epithelium adjacent to the pterygium, cell densities decrease while dendritic-like cells increase. In the cornea stroma, the increase in keratocytes activity and density has been observed [111]. Conjunctival goblet cell densities and amount of inflammation on imaging were higher where patients experienced more discomfort linked to pterygium growth [69]. Such information may affect the decision for excision surgery or antigrowth factor intervention [160].

Pterygium growth seems to affect only the superficial surface of the cornea. However, morphological changes in the corneal nerves have been reported. Increased tortuosity, breakages, and localized bulging of subbasal nerve fibers were noticed beneath and around the area of cornea covered by the pterygium [167]. Further studies are warranted

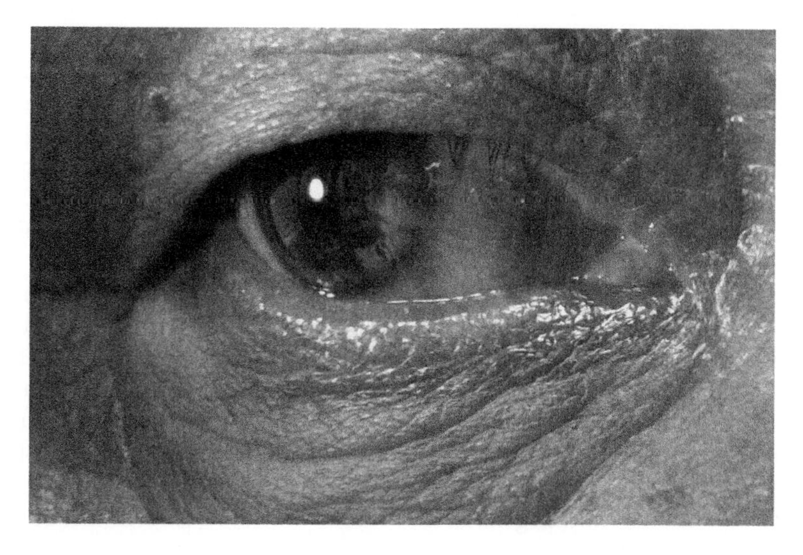

FIGURE 19.13
Pterygium. A fleshy growth over the nasal side of the cornea is presented in this patient.

to determine any effect on corneal sensitivity along with these nerve fibers' morphology in pterygium.

19.3.3 Ocular Surgeries

The two commonly performed corneal surgeries are refractive surgery and corneal grafting. As it is the most densely innervated tissue of the human body, any surgery performed on the cornea would inevitably affect the corneal nerves. Corneal nerve regeneration after surgery involves not only the shifting of its morphology back, or as close as possible, to the presurgical states but also the reconnection of sectioned nerves. Recovery is therefore an extremely long process. Healing of the individual corneal layers is a widely studied topic, with researchers ceaselessly finding ways to speed up the process of wound healing or decrease the extent of the initial wound. IVCM is a useful method to examine both the extent of wound and the recovery of corneal nerves after surgery.

19.3.3.1 Corneal Refractive Surgery

Surgical method for refractive error correction is becoming increasingly common, especially with the development of contemporary *flapless* methods that promises reduced chances of side effects [4]. Refractive surgery alters the refractive status of the cornea by modifying its shape in the epithelial and stromal layers. The current most popular surgical method—LASIK—is gradually giving way to the more contemporary methods of small incision lenticule extraction (SMILE) and refractive lenticule extraction (ReLEx) procedures. The older technique of photorefractive keratectomy (PRK) is much less performed now.

Laser-assisted in situ keratomileusis: Conventional LASIK is performed by making a flap consisting of the epithelium, Bowman's membrane, and the anterior stroma, with the keratome blade, and subsequently applying excimer laser to the stromal bed to make the appropriate ablation according to the desired refractive change (Figure 19.14). Newer techniques (bladeless LASIK) utilize femtosecond lasers to cut the flap instead of a metallic keratome blade.

Flap-related complications, although uncommon, are one of the main concerns of modern-day refractive surgery. Slit-lamp biomicroscopy enables clinicians to examine the flap after surgery in relatively gross detail. However, microscopic changes such as epithelial ingrowth at the edge of the flap are difficult to detect using the slit lamp, especially for less experienced clinicians. Epithelial ingrowth can be easily recognized in IVCM images. Postoperative keratocyte cell count is decreased within the flap and can be monitored with IVCM [119,122].

Corneal flap thickness, as measured by IVCM, was often noticed to be thinner than intended [122]. Furthermore, the high magnification of IVCM gives clinicians a clearer idea of which layer of the cornea is being imaged. The zone in between the flap and the stroma, or the interface zone, can be better visualized with IVCM. Hyperreflective particles were detected in this zone. It is not clear what these particles are, although some researchers believe they are fine metallic debris from the flap-cutting blade. The number of these particles decreases with time [90,119,122]. However, if these particles really are metallic, there is a possibility of oxidation and degradation. This would cause an immune response (diffuse lamellar keratitis) [66].

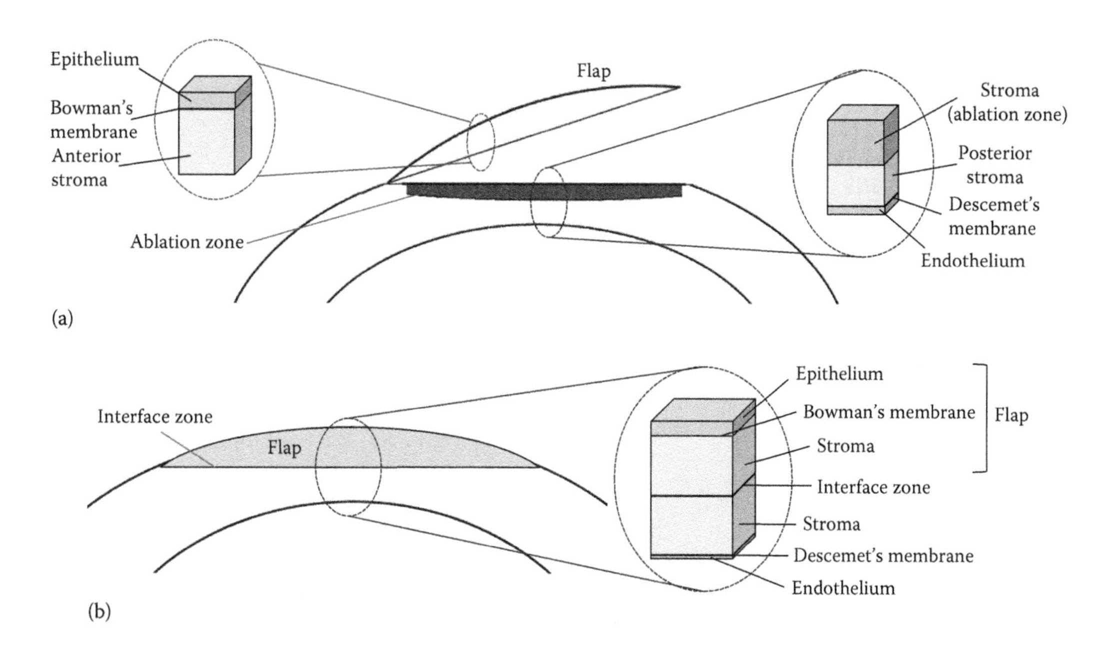

FIGURE 19.14
The corneal layers in LASIK. A schematic illustration of the corneal layers involved in LASIK. The flap consists of the corneal epithelium, Bowman's membrane, and anterior part of the stroma. The exposed area of stroma underneath the flap is modified in shape to correct the refractive error (ablation zone). The posterior part of the stroma, Descemet's membrane, and endothelium are left intact (a). After surgery, the flap is repositioned. The zone between the flap and the stroma bed is the interface zone (b).

Another flap-related complication detectable by IVCM is microfolds at the Bowman's membrane, possibly caused by overstretching of the flap during surgery or an incompatibility between the flap and the reshaped stroma [161]. In IVCM images, their appearance may vary from straight to slightly curved lines and in thickness, length, and orientation. When there is a significant magnitude of microfolds, the quality of vision may be affected [119].

Corneal nerve fiber changes are the main reason for the very common complaint of dry eye after refractive procedures. This is due to the severing of the nerves responsible for stimulating tear secretion during the procedure [1,21]. The decrease in corneal nerve fiber length and density is perhaps the common finding in postoperative refractive surgery patients up to 6 months [30,119]. In fact, a study showed that in the first month post-LASIK, there were close to no nerve fibers in the flap. Nerve fibers in the flap gradually build up in numbers and densities after LASIK but do not return to preoperative values after 3 years [21]. In another study, subbasal nerve fibers demonstrated almost complete restoration to its pre-LASIK numbers after 5 years (Table 19.3) [39].

Corneal lenticular extractions: The newer methods of corneal refractive surgery (SMILE and ReLEx) involve laser-assisted fashioning of a refractive lenticule within the corneal stroma. These procedures still require the creation of a flap with a keratome blade or an external opening to remove the lenticule. This concept allows corneal reshaping, without any ablative loss of corneal stroma. A further possibility is reimplantation of the lenticule at a later stage to address further refractive changes [5].

TABLE 19.3
Summary of IVCM Studies on Post-LASIK Patients

Study	Sample Size	Study Duration	Myopic Correction (Diopters)	Flap Thickness (μm)	Nerve Fiber Findings
Perez-Gomez et al. [119]	12 eyes of 12 patients	6 months	Mean ± SD: −5.0 ± 3.0 Range: −4.5 to −10.0	Intended: 160 Actual: (mean ± SD) 139 ± 10	Unable to image up to a month postoperatively Short, unconnected nerves at 3 months postoperation Anastomosing connections at 6 months postoperation
Darwish et al. [30]	20 eyes of 20 patients	6 months	Mean ± SD: −3.6 ± 1.6 Range: not reported	Intended: 130 Actual: not reported	Decreased in numbers and density in first month by >75% Did not return to preoperative values after 6 months
Calvillo et al. [21]	17 eyes of 11 patients	3 years	Mean: not reported Range: −2.0 to −11.0	Intended: 180 Actual: not reported	Decreased in numbers and density in first month by >90% Returned close to baseline values by 2 years Decreased again in third year to <60% of preoperative numbers
Erie et al. [39]	18 eyes of 12 patients	5 years	Not reported	Intended: 180 Actual: (mean ± SD) 160 ± 28	Decreased in density to 49% of preoperative values 1 year after operation Densities increased to 65% and 66% of preoperative values after 2 and 3 years after operation Returned close to preoperative values after 5 years

Postoperative complications are much less in comparison with LASIK. There are currently no human studies on IVCM's role in monitoring long-term effects of SMILE and ReLEx. However, in animal studies involving white rabbits, keratocytes in the stroma just anterior to the flap were noticeably more reflective than the nonoperated eyes merely 1 day after the ReLEx procedure. The interface zone could be identified in the deeper layer of the cornea by multiple light scattering particles and absence of any cells. The number of these particles was significantly higher in the eyes of LASIK-operated rabbits than in those that underwent the ReLEx procedure, especially with the correction of higher refractive error. Although the authors of that study did not specify the role of these particles, they speculate that the presence of these particles in higher numbers in post-LASIK eyes was due to the damage caused by the excimer laser used in LASIK [128].

Photorefractive keratectomy: In PRK, a flap is not required as the superficial corneal epithelium is directly ablated to reshape the cornea. Due to the level of relative discomfort and longer recovery, PRK is much less commonly performed nowadays. Nevertheless, knowledge of the long-term corneal effects of this procedure is still worth learning as it can correct higher refractive errors that the newer techniques may not account for.

IVCM has revealed changes within the cornea after PRK that conventional clinical techniques would have missed. The Bowman's membrane, for example, which is removed during the procedure, was realized to have not regenerated 5 years after surgery. Anterior stromal keratocytes became unevenly distributed and their nuclei more hyperreflective than those in the normal unoperated eyes [98]. The corneal nerves, however, are less affected by PRK than in LASIK since the former method does not invade the corneal stroma as much as the latter [39].

In modern surgical practices, procedures similar to PRK such as superficial LASIK or laser epithelial keratomileusis (LASEK) have been used [30]. IVCM may have potential to evaluate changes in the cornea after these procedures as well.

Refractive surgery: Summary—The interface zone and flap complications may not be imaged sufficiently with conventional clinical methods for documentation of inflammation and wound healing. IVCM may overcome the barriers of low magnification to enable clinicians to have a better understanding of long-term effects of refractive surgery such as nerve changes. However, clinicians must bear in mind that it may not be wise to perform IVCM in the first few postoperative days due to the risk of flap dislocation.

19.3.3.2 Corneal Grafting

Corneal grafting is the removal of the entire thickness or just the specific layer(s) of the diseased cornea and replacing it with a donor cornea or corneal layer(s). This procedure is indicated when the diseased cornea has reached a stage where it is devastating to the vision and no longer demonstrates the ability to heal. Corneal diseases in which the grafting may be performed include bullous keratopathy, keratoconus, corneal dystrophies, and severe corneal scarring secondary to other causes. Corneal grafting purposes to restore the vision, usually only partially, of patients who suffered from these corneal diseases.

Today, advances in medical technology have enabled surgeons to replace the specific diseased layers of the cornea rather than the entire corneal thickness (penetrating keratoplasty; Figure 19.15). For example, clinicians can choose to just replace the endothelium (endothelial keratoplasty) when the more anterior part of the cornea is not yet affected by Fuch's endothelial dystrophy [101]. In keratoconus where the endothelium is still intact, or other conditions that affect the anterior layers of the cornea, deep anterior lamellar keratoplasty can be performed to specifically replace the stroma and the epithelium [139]. Replacing only certain layers of the cornea may present a smaller risk of graft failure, which is the main complication after corneal grafting [168].

The risk of graft failure/rejection can be as low as 4% in the first year but increasing up to 67% within a decade [142,143,173]. Poor prognostic factors include preexisting ocular conditions (e.g., glaucoma), previous ocular surgery or repeat corneal grafting, and some conditions for which the keratoplasty is performed, for example, fungal keratitis [52,132]. Failed grafts can be recognized on slit-lamp biomicroscopy by signs such as subepithelial infiltrates, corneal haze, and edema [24]. It would be advantageous to detect early signs of graft rejection using more sensitive techniques so that appropriate immunosuppression can begin promptly.

Graft failure in penetrating keratoplasty can be attributed on various causes; one of the most common is endothelial failure. IVCM has allowed researchers to observe the pathology in various layers of the cornea for a more complete assessment.

In the endothelial layer, a dramatic decrease in cell numbers may be observed immediately after surgery, although still remaining at a functional level. However, the numbers continue to fall 20 years after the operation, until the cells reach a critically low level and finally give in to graft failure [13,105]. It is possible that endothelial failure is accompanied by the stromal keratocyte activation. IVCM in the stroma can detect keratocyte activation

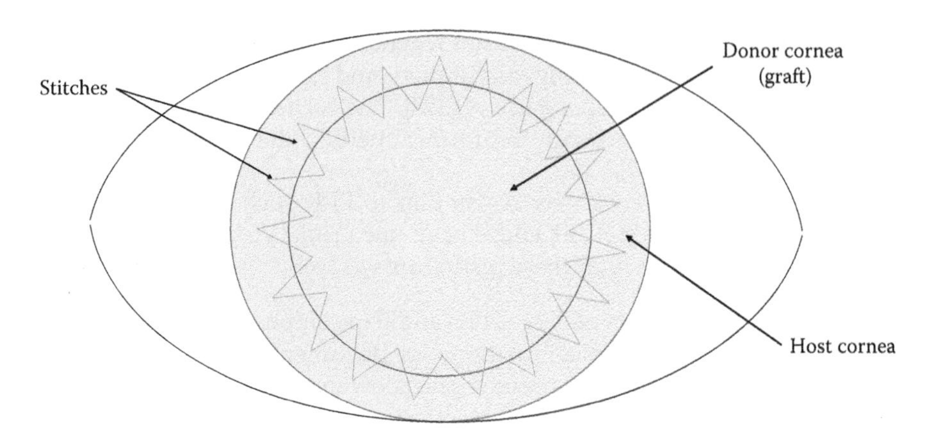

FIGURE 19.15
Penetrating keratoplasty. A schematic illustration of the cornea after penetrating keratoplasty. The full thickness of the center to midperipheral part of the cornea is replaced by a donor cornea, held in place with stitches. These stitches are removed 1–2 years after surgery.

as well as loss of keratocyte within a week after surgery. Keratocyte numbers gradually increase and return to their inactivated states [13,107,147]. Bourne et al. further reported one case of late endothelial failure 4 years after surgery where the keratocytes became activated, likely causing the reduction in corneal transparency.

Most corneal nerve fibers from the donor tissue may not survive the grafting, especially when the entire stroma is replaced. They are significantly decreased after surgery, but their density increases with time [105]. This allows reinnervation of the graft to restore sensation of the cornea [13]. This process is slow. According to a study, corneal sensation is always greater at the periphery than the central as the nerves grow inwards the graft, and the sensation of the cornea is restored at the center after more than 18 months [87].

In the epithelium of the transplanted cornea, the cell areas increase and the cells become irregularly shaped. These cells are quickly disintegrated and replaced by the host's epithelial tissue as the latter grows over the donor cornea. Folds in the stroma and Descemet's membrane after corneal grafting have also been observed with IVCM [147].

IVCM has demonstrated its utility in the monitoring of cellular function of the individual cell types within the donor cornea and has been used in various studies such as the ones described earlier. Such observations have given further insights on the physiological and pathophysiological processes after corneal grafting. This will, in future, allow the development of better techniques. Like LASIK, clinicians have to exercise caution when performing this technique within the first few days after surgery, due to the risk of wound rupture.

19.3.3.3 Glaucoma Surgery

Glaucoma, a major cause of blindness, is a form of optic neuropathy characterized by distinct changes in visual fields and loss of optic nerve fibers, often associated with an inappropriate intraocular pressure (IOP). In chronic glaucoma, patients experience no symptoms until it reaches the moderate to advanced stages, when they notice that their vision is getting poorer and uncorrectable by glasses. Glaucoma is otherwise usually only picked up during routine eye checks and eye screenings. Damage caused by glaucoma cannot be reversed and the treatment is aimed to control its progression [125]. Medications in glaucoma are used to reduce the IOP. Surgical intervention is warranted when medications are unable to control the progression.

Trabeculectomy is the most commonly performed surgery for glaucoma [20]. The procedure involves the creation of a passageway between the anterior chamber and the subconjunctival space. This provides an additional route for the aqueous humor to drain from the eye, significantly reducing the IOP. The drainage of the aqueous results in the elevation of the conjunctiva called the bleb.

Postoperatively, the bleb may stop functioning when it scars and collapses. Outflow of the aqueous is disrupted and the IOP rises again. This risk of bleb failure increases with time. As shown in one study, the incidence of a working bleb may be as low as 42% after 15 years. In cases where the bleb fails, additional surgery may be required; the need for additional surgery increases with time, from 10% at 5 years to 58% at 15 years [172]. Monitoring of the bleb is therefore important to determine if the patient needs further treatment.

Assessment of the bleb is usually done by slit-lamp biomicroscopy [112]. The bleb should appear raised from the surrounding conjunctiva accompanied by a good IOP reading. Such an observation can be extremely vague and may not represent accurately the function of the bleb. For example, a relatively flat bleb may be functioning well as long as there is sufficient cystic space for the aqueous to flow through. It may take an experienced clinician to elicit more subtle features of a functioning bleb. Additional imaging techniques such as optical coherence tomography may provide a better idea of the bleb function [179]. However, for cellular analysis, IVCM remains as the most suitable modality.

The pattern of stromal collagen and the number of microcysts and subepithelial connective tissue density can be observed with IVCM (thickness of the bleb). Generally, the cellular layout in functioning blebs should look spacious in high-magnification scans. The stroma should exhibit a loose meshwork of collagen or the presence of large cystic spaces. A high number of microcysts with loosely arranged subepithelial connective tissue are signs of good bleb function. On the other hand, blebs that have scarred up appear densely packed in the stroma, with a smaller number of microcysts [22,68,91].

Guthoff et al. reported four different types of stromal patterns in IVCM images that were not visible with slit-lamp biomicroscopy—trabecular, reticular, corrugated, and compacted. The trabecular pattern was defined as straight and fine widely spaced fibers. The reticular patterned stroma exhibited straight and crisscrossed fibers with sporadic gaps in between. The corrugated patterned stroma had short, broad, and curved fibers with a disorganized arrangement. The compacted pattern was defined as tightly packed and hyperreflective appearance fibers in parallel arrangement. The trabecular pattern was only seen in blebs with good function, whereas the corrugated and compacted patterns were predominant in failed blebs [41]. These findings may have value in postoperative bleb assessment.

19.3.4 Contact Lens Wear

Contact lens wear is known to most people as an appealing substitute to spectacles. Most clinicians are aware of the risks of microbial keratitis and dry eye that contact lens wear poses [76,159]. Physiological changes such as decreased corneal oxygen intake, deterioration of corneal sensitivity, and infiltration of inflammatory cells may occur [150,181]. Physical alterations to the corneal curvature, thickness, as well as

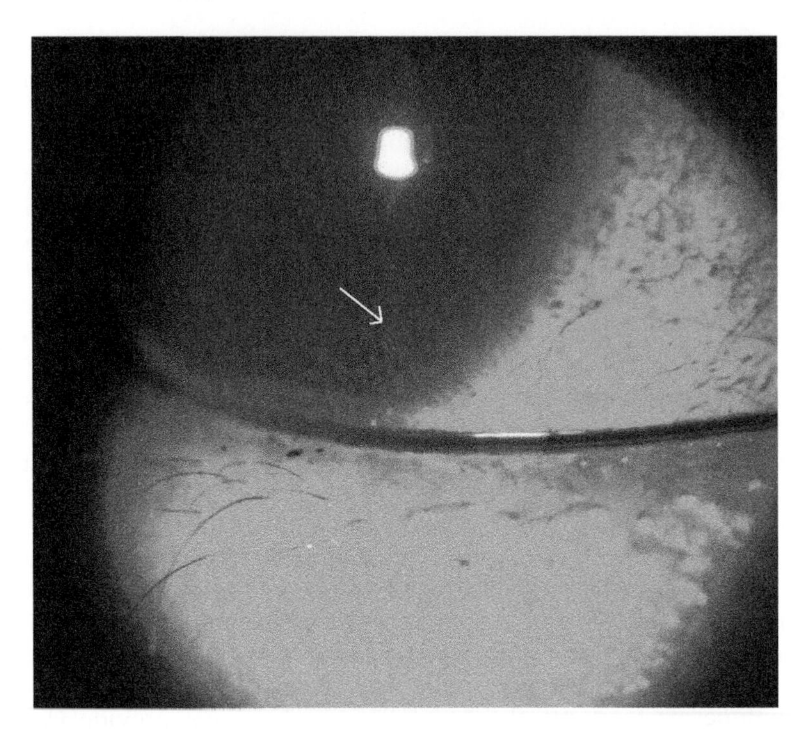

FIGURE 19.16
(See color insert.) Corneal fluorescein dye staining. A slit-lamp photo of corneal fluorescein dye staining that would show up as flourescent green in the cornea (arrow).

regularity can also be induced by contact lens wear [81,92]. With long-term contact lens wear, these changes happen gradually over a course of 5–10 years, depending on the wearing schedule [44,117].

Alterations in the cornea could occur at every layer. On slit-lamp biomicroscopy, changes such as superficial corneal fluorescein staining (Figure 19.16), neovascularization, and endothelial blebs can be spotted if the change is gross enough to be visualized. IVCM has brought the investigation of contact lens-induced changes to the cellular level.

In the epithelium, delayed cell regeneration occurs with contact lens wear. The superficial cells have been observed in IVCM images to increase in size and surface area as quickly as after 4 weeks of extended contact lens wear. Researchers attributed the increase to delayed cell regeneration, as the older cells spread out in area instead of having fresh ones replace them [37].

In the stroma, IVCM has revealed loss of keratocytes, stromal thickening, and edema. Efron et al. postulated that the percentage decrease in keratocytes is approximately equivalent to the percentage increase in corneal thickness. Microdots were first observed with IVCM in the posterior stroma and were suggested to be the magnified version of posterior stromal opacities that were observed with slit-lamp biomicroscope. These microdots were not detected in non–contact lens–wearing controls [12,153].

Endothelial blebs due to contact lens are caused by increased acidity of the cells in the entire corneal tissue. Blebs are reversible, being most apparent within 20 min after soft contact lens insertion, and start to diminish by 30 min [57]. However, with long-term contact lens wear, a longer time may be needed to allow the endothelia to return to its normal state. In addition, the decrease in endothelial cell density and heterogeneity in

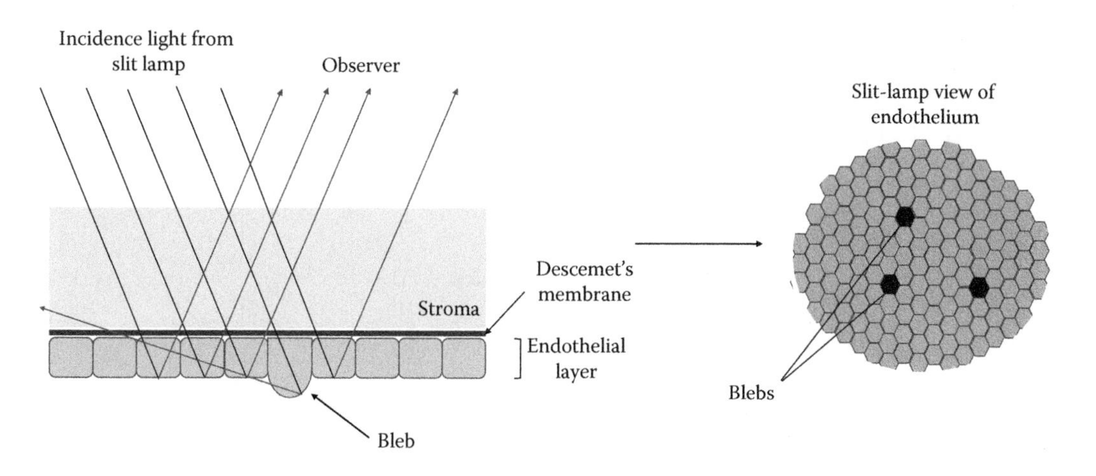

FIGURE 19.17
Endothelial blebs as viewed with slit lamp. A schematic illustration of the slit-lamp optics and view of endothelial blebs. Light incident on the edematous cells is reflected elsewhere, giving the appearance of a missing cell.

the shape of the endothelial cells occurs after long-term contact lens wear. Functional changes such as corneal edema, loss of transparency, and eventually decrease in vision quality follow [25,46].

On slit-lamp biomicroscopy, blebs will appear as *missing* cells among the surrounding intact cells. In actual fact, these cells are merely edematous and interfered with the light reflecting off the cells to the observer's eye, giving the illusion of a *black hole* (Figure 19.17). Large areas of endothelial blebs may therefore sometimes be confused with guttata, which are areas of true endothelial cell loss commonly seen in Fuch's dystrophy. IVCM can be used to distinguish blebs and guttata. The centers of the edematous cells are relatively flatter than the periphery and thus allow light to be reflected back to the observer lens, while the periphery reflects lights elsewhere. Therefore, blebs will not appear as missing cells but as black areas with white centers (Figure 19.18).

Minute inflammatory changes can be observed with IVCM but not slit-lamp biomicroscopy. For example, an increase in Langerhans cell density with number of years of contact lens wear has been reported, even before patients experience any symptoms [181].

The limbus is not spared from contact lens–induced changes. Limbal epithelial cells have been found to be more than 50% larger in contact lens wearers [37]. The white blood cells in the bulbar conjunctival vessels were increased in patients who wore contact lenses with lower oxygen permeability as compared to those who wore lenses with higher oxygen permeability. These changes cannot be detected with slit-lamp biomicroscopy but can be detected with IVCM [102]. Such information may be valuable for the management of contact lens patients and the development for physiologically better contact lenses.

19.3.4.1 Orthokeratology Contact Lens

Orthokeratology contact lenses are rigid gas-permeable contact lenses that are prescribed to be worn overnight. These lenses flatten the cornea while the wearer sleeps and correct for their short-sightedness the following day in a lens- and spectacle-free manner (Figure 19.19).

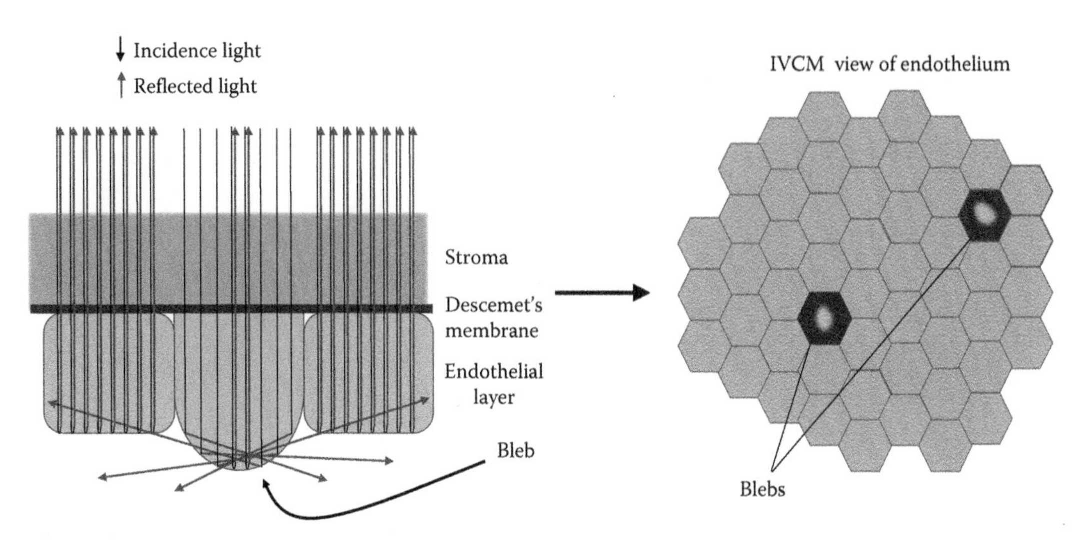

FIGURE 19.18
Endothelial blebs as viewed with IVCM. A schematic illustration of the IVCM optics and view of endothelial blebs. The center of the edematous cells is flatter, thus reflecting incident light straight up to the camera, giving the appearance of a white area in the center of a dark cell.

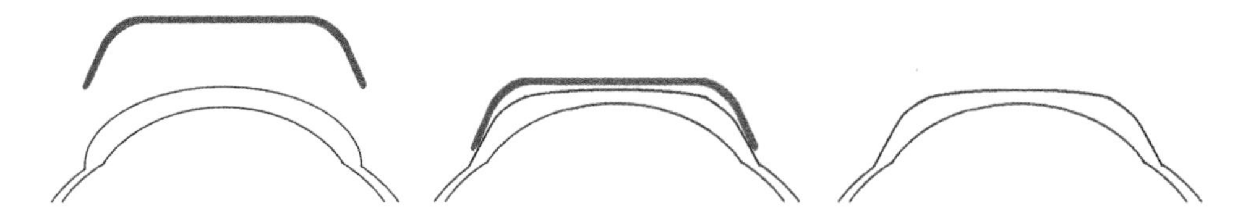

FIGURE 19.19
Orthokeratology contact lens modification of the cornea during sleep. The central cornea is flattened by the lens during sleep and the modified cornea shape is retained for the rest of the day to correct for myopic refractive error.

This method of refractive error correction requires a significant change in the shape of the cornea. Flattening of the cornea is accompanied by transient thinning of the central epithelial layer and thickening of the midperipheral stroma [2]. IVCM has revealed the corresponding changes at the cellular level. Cornea epithelial cells decrease in density, while the superficial epithelial cells increase in size. Apart from the thickened stroma, other layers of the cornea, that is, the Bowman's layer and epithelium, have decreased in thickness. The activation of stromal keratocytes was also noted, although the keratocyte density did not change. All these changes are reversible upon cessation of lens wear [108].

As the corneal stroma and epithelium are altered in thickness, the nerve fiber arrangement in the cornea was also found to change. Lum et al. combined hundreds of IVCM images of corneal nerves through the central and midperipheral cornea to map the nerve pattern. They found that the corneal nerves are distributed peripherally in two orthokeratology contact lens wearers (1 year and 9 years of wear). This pattern of nerve fiber arrangements greatly deviates from the normal pattern, which is a whorl pattern centering slightly inferonasally of the central cornea [83]. It is not known if this arrangement is reversible with the cessation of contact lens wear or the shortest duration of lens wear before this change manifests. Further studies are warranted to resolve these questions, perhaps with IVCM.

19.4 Operational Difficulties

Currently, IVCM is mainly utilized in a research setting more than in the clinic. The inconvenience it poses to the operator and discomfort to the patient may be deterrent factors for its widespread use. Imaging of the eye by IVCM may be challenging for both the operator and the patient. The patient has to remain extremely still during the procedure in order for the operator to locate the area of interest. However, this may be difficult even for the most cooperative patients.

Only a viscous ophthalmic gel lies between the investigative cap and the eye; patients therefore may feel apprehensive about the proximity of an object to the eye and react by constantly moving their eyes. As the field of view of IVCM is only 400 μm at any point of time, even the smallest of eye movements may direct the scan to a completely different region.

Further discomfort may be experienced by the patients when the lens is rotated as the operator changes the depth of scan within the tissue. Even though topical anesthesia is instilled to prevent the sensation of pain, the patient may be aware of the movement of the lens. Patients with very painful eyes (e.g., ulcerative keratitis) may not consent to scanning despite the fact that they may need the scan on an urgent basis. Furthermore, pressure by an examiner in an ulcer with impending perforation is hazardous.

The factors mentioned earlier suggest that a lot of training and a steep learning curve may be required. Localization of the area of interest and identification of visualized structure may be challenging for the amateur operator. Especially in longitudinal research studies and monitoring of patients, relocating the exact regions that were imaged in previous scans may be problematic.

The lack of the universal reference values and cost of the procedure are additional issues to consider. Further studies are warranted to establish normal values and establish the sensitivity and specificity of IVCM compared to other techniques in different conditions.

19.5 Future Directions and Summary

In contrast to conventional light microscopes used for histological analysis of transverse sections, IVCM provides a coronal optical section through the object being examined. This property of IVCM demonstrates its unique ability to provide corneal and conjunctival anatomy at cellular level.

IVCM has now become the early detection and diagnosis technique for various infectious conditions, including amoeba, fungal, and bacterial keratitis. However, it has not yet completely replaced scraping and cultures in the diagnosis of corneal infection. Current clinical applications of IVCM are mostly in the diagnosis of *Acanthamoeba* and fungal keratitis, measuring residual bed thickness after surgical procedures and endothelial cell density.

Technological advancements in the future are expected to improve the confocal microscopy technique leading to 3D image stacks for better understanding of the structure of cornea. Improvements in image resolution, area of scan, depth of field, and even magnification will enhance its use especially in research settings. A flexible confocal system might be able to help visualize areas not accessible otherwise. Noncontact microscope objectives are also being developed and will vastly enhance the utility of IVCM in observations such as tear film and crystalline lens. In addition, quicker scanning times and less operator training may be required should a noncontact method be devised.

The development of various grading and quantifying systems for ocular sign parameters such as cell densities and cell size, as well as the establishment of their normal, is expected in the near future. This will further expand the use of IVCM in both clinical and research environments for better understanding of the anatomy and pathology of the cornea, the conjunctiva, and the ocular surface. IVCM will become a valuable tool for quantitative analysis of the cornea and will enable investigation of corneal wound healing, cellular responses, and nerve regeneration, to name a few. This technology will enable in-depth understanding of ocular surface physiology and pathology.

Acknowledgment

The authors would like to acknowledge Dr. Lawrence Lim from the Singapore National Eye Centre for Figure 19.10 in this chapter.

References

1. Smith, J. A., J. Albeitz et al. (2007). The epidemiology of dry eye disease: Report of the epidemiology subcommittee of the international dry eye workshop. *Ocul Surf* 5(2): 93–107.
2. Alharbi, A. and H. A. Swarbrick (2003). The effects of overnight orthokeratology lens wear on corneal thickness. *Invest Ophthalmol Vis Sci* 44(6): 2518–2523.
3. Amos, W. B. W. and J. G. White (2003). How the confocal laser scanning microscope entered biological research. *Biol Cell* 95: 1058–1063.
4. Ang, M., D. Tan et al. (2012). Small incision lenticule extraction (smile) versus laser in-situ keratomileusis (LASIK): Study protocol for a randomized, non-inferiority trial. *Trials* 13: 75.
5. Angunawela, R. I., A. K. Riau et al. (2012). Refractive lenticule re-implantation after myopic ReLEx: A feasibility study of stromal restoration after refractive surgery in a rabbit model. *Invest Ophthalmol Vis Sci* 53(8): 4975–4985.
6. Arita, R., K. Itoh et al. (2008). Noncontact infrared meibography to document age-related changes of the meibomian glands in a normal population. *Ophthalmology* 115(5): 911–915.
7. Arita, R., K. Itoh et al. (2009). Contact lens wear is associated with decrease of meibomian glands. *Ophthalmology* 116(3): 379–384.
8. Astley, R. A., R. C. Kennedy et al. (2003). Structural and cellular architecture of conjunctival lymphoid follicles in the baboon (*Papio anubis*). *Exp Eye Res* 76(6): 685–694.
9. Babu, K. and K. R. Murthy (2007). Combined fungal and *Acanthamoeba* keratitis: Diagnosis by in vivo confocal microscopy. *Eye (Lond)* 21(2): 271–272.
10. Bal, N., F. Kayaselçuk et al. (2006). Mast cell density in pterygium, and its association with ultraviolet exposure in different climatic conditions: A series of 140 cases. *Turk J Pathol* 22(1): 11–16.
11. Bergmanson, J. P., T. M. Sheldon et al. (1999). Fuchs' endothelial dystrophy: A fresh look at an aging disease. *Ophthalmic Physiol Opt* 19(3): 210–222.
12. Bohnke, M. and B. R. Masters (1997). Long-term contact lens wear induces a corneal degeneration with microdot deposits in the corneal stroma. *Ophthalmology* 104(11): 1887–1896.
13. Bourne, W. M. (2001). Cellular changes in transplanted human corneas. *Cornea* 20(6): 560–569.

14. Bourne, W. M., L. R. Nelson et al. (1997). Central corneal endothelial cell changes over a ten-year period. *Invest Ophthalmol Vis Sci* 38(3): 779–782.
15. Brasnu, E., T. Bourcier et al. (2007). In vivo confocal microscopy in fungal keratitis. *Br J Ophthalmol* 91(5): 588–591.
16. Bron, A. J. (2001). The architecture of the corneal stroma. *Br J Ophthalmol* 85(4): 379–381.
17. Bron, A. J., L. Benjamin et al. (1991). Meibomian gland disease. Classification and grading of lid changes. *Eye (Lond)* 5(pt 4): 395–411.
18. Bron, A. J. and J. M. Tiffany (2004). The contribution of meibomian disease to dry eye. *Ocul Surf* 2(2): 149–165.
19. Bron, A. J., J. M. Tiffany et al. (2004). Functional aspects of the tear film lipid layer. *Exp Eye Res* 78(3): 347–360.
20. Cairns, J. E. (1968). Trabeculectomy. Preliminary report of a new method. *Am J Ophthalmol* 66(4): 673–679.
21. Calvillo, M. P., J. W. Mclaren et al. (2004). Corneal reinnervation after LASIK: Prospective 3-year longitudinal study. *Invest Ophthalmol Vis Sci* 45(11): 3991–3996.
22. Ciancaglini, M., P. Carpineto et al. (2008). Filtering bleb functionality: A clinical, anterior segment optical coherence tomography and in vivo confocal microscopy study. *J Glaucoma* 17(4): 308–317.
23. Clarke, D. W. and J. Y. Niederkorn (2006). The pathophysiology of *Acanthamoeba* keratitis. *Trends Parasitol* 22(4): 175–180.
24. Cohen, R. A., S. J. Chew et al. (1995). Confocal microscopy of corneal graft rejection. *Cornea* 14(5): 467–472.
25. Connor, C. G. and M. E. Zagrod (1986). Contact lens-induced corneal endothelial polymegathism: Functional significance and possible mechanisms. *Am J Optom Physiol Opt* 63(7): 539–544.
26. Cotsarelis, G., S. Z. Cheng et al. (1989). Existence of slow-cycling limbal epithelial basal cells that can be preferentially stimulated to proliferate: Implications on epithelial stem cells. *Cell* 57(2): 201–209.
27. Crawford, A. Z. and C. N. Mcghee (2012). Management of limbal stem cell deficiency in severe ocular chemical burns. *Clin Exp Ophthalmol* 40(3): 227–229.
28. Czepita, D., W. Kuzna-Grygiel et al. (2007). *Demodex folliculorum* and *Demodex brevis* as a cause of chronic marginal blepharitis. *Ann Acad Med Stetin* 53(1): 63–67; discussion 67.
29. Dart, J. K. (1988). Predisposing factors in microbial keratitis: The significance of contact lens wear. *Br J Ophthalmol* 72(12): 926–930.
30. Darwish, T., A. Brahma et al. (2007). Subbasal nerve fiber regeneration after LASIK and LASEK assessed by noncontact esthesiometry and in vivo confocal microscopy: Prospective study. *J Cataract Refract Surg* 33(9): 1515–1521.
31. Davidovits, P. and M. D. Egger (1973). Photomicrography of corneal endothelial cells in vivo. *Nature* 244(5415): 366–367.
32. De Cilla, S., S. Ranno et al. (2009). Corneal subbasal nerves changes in patients with diabetic retinopathy: An in vivo confocal study. *Invest Ophthalmol Vis Sci* 50(11): 5155–5158.
33. Dua, H. S. and A. Azuara-Blanco (1999). Allo-limbal transplantation in patients with limbal stem cell deficiency. *Br J Ophthalmol* 83(4): 414–419.
34. Dua, H. S., J. S. Saini et al. (2000). Limbal stem cell deficiency: Concept, aetiology, clinical presentation, diagnosis and management. *Indian J Ophthalmol* 48(2): 83–92.
35. Duguid, I. G., J. K. Dart et al. (1997). Outcome of *Acanthamoeba* keratitis treated with polyhexamethyl biguanide and propamidine. *Ophthalmology* 104(10): 1587–1592.
36. Edwards, M., C. N. Mcghee et al. (2001). The genetics of keratoconus. *Clin Exp Ophthalmol* 29(6): 345–351.
37. Efron, N. (2007). Contact lens-induced changes in the anterior eye as observed in vivo with the confocal microscope. *Prog Retin Eye Res* 26(4): 398–436.
38. Erdelyi, B., R. Kraak et al. (2007). In vivo confocal laser scanning microscopy of the cornea in dry eye. *Graefes Arch Clin Exp Ophthalmol* 245(1): 39–44.

39. Erie, J. C., J. W. Mclaren et al. (2005). Recovery of corneal subbasal nerve density after PRK and LASIK. *Am J Ophthalmol* 140(6): 1059–1064.
40. Fini, M. E. and B. M. Stramer (2005). How the cornea heals: Cornea-specific repair mechanisms affecting surgical outcomes. *Cornea* 24(8 suppl.): s2–s11.
41. Guthoff, R., T. Klink et al. (2006). In vivo confocal microscopy of failing and functioning filtering blebs: Results and clinical correlations. *J Glaucoma* 15(6): 552–558.
42. Guthoff, R. F., A. Zhivov et al. (2009). In vivo confocal microscopy, an inner vision of the cornea—A major review. *Clin Exp Ophthalmol* 37(1): 100–117.
43. Hillenaar, T., C. Weenen et al. (2009). Endothelial involvement in herpes simplex virus keratitis: An in vivo confocal microscopy study. *Ophthalmology* 116(11): 2077–2086 (e2071–e2072).
44. Holden, B. A., D. F. Sweeney et al. (1985). Effects of long-term extended contact lens wear on the human cornea. *Invest Ophthalmol Vis Sci* 26(11): 1489–1501.
45. Holland, E. J. and G. S. Schwartz (1997). Iatrogenic limbal stem cell deficiency. *Trans Am Ophthalmol Soc* 95: 95–107; discussion: 107–110.
46. Hollingsworth, J. G. and N. Efron (2004). Confocal microscopy of the corneas of long-term rigid contact lens wearers. *Cont Lens Anterior Eye* 27(2): 57–64.
47. Hollingsworth, J. G., N. Efron et al. (2005). In vivo corneal confocal microscopy in keratoconus. *Ophthalmic Physiol Opt* 25(3): 254–260.
48. Houang, E., D. Lam et al. (2001). Microbial keratitis in Hong Kong: Relationship to climate, environment and contact-lens disinfection. *Trans R Soc Trop Med Hyg* 95(4): 361–367.
49. Hu, V. H., P. Massae et al. (2011). In vivo confocal microscopy of trachoma in relation to normal tarsal conjunctiva. *Ophthalmology* 118(4): 747–754.
50. Hu, V. H., H. A. Weiss et al. (2011). In vivo confocal microscopy in scarring trachoma. *Ophthalmology* 118(11): 2138–2146.
51. Ibrahim, O. M., Y. Matsumoto et al. (2010). The efficacy, sensitivity, and specificity of in vivo laser confocal microscopy in the diagnosis of meibomian gland dysfunction. *Ophthalmology* 117(4): 665–672.
52. Ing, J. J., H. H. Ing et al. (1998). Ten-year postoperative results of penetrating keratoplasty. *Ophthalmology* 105(10): 1855–1865.
53. Jalbert, I., F. Stapleton et al. (2003). In vivo confocal microscopy of the human cornea. *Br J Ophthalmol* 87(2): 225–236.
54. Jie, Y., L. Xu et al. (2009). Prevalence of dry eye among adult Chinese in the Beijing eye study. *Eye (Lond)* 23(3): 688–693.
55. Jonuscheit, S., M. J. Doughty et al. (2011). In vivo confocal microscopy of the corneal endothelium: Comparison of three morphometry methods after corneal transplantation. *Eye (Lond)* 25(9): 1130–1137.
56. Kanavi, M. R., M. Javadi et al. (2007). Sensitivity and specificity of confocal scan in the diagnosis of infectious keratitis. *Cornea* 26(7): 782–786.
57. Kaufman, S. C., H. Hamano et al. (1996). Transient corneal stromal and endothelial changes following soft contact lens wear: A study with confocal microscopy. *CLAO J* 22(2): 127–132.
58. Kaye, S. B., C. Lynas et al. (1991). Evidence for herpes simplex viral latency in the human cornea. *Br J Ophthalmol* 75(4): 195–200.
59. Keay, L., K. Edwards et al. (2006). Microbial keratitis predisposing factors and morbidity. *Ophthalmology* 113(1): 109–116.
60. Knop, E. and N. Knop (2005). The role of eye-associated lymphoid tissue in corneal immune protection. *J Anat* 206(3): 271–285.
61. Knop, E., N. Knop et al. (2011). The international workshop on meibomian gland dysfunction: Report of the subcommittee on anatomy, physiology, and pathophysiology of the meibomian gland. *Invest Ophthalmol Vis Sci* 52(4): 1938–1978.
62. Knop, E., N. Knop et al. (2011). The lid wiper and muco-cutaneous junction anatomy of the human eyelid margins: An in vivo confocal and histological study. *J Anat* 218(4): 449–461.
63. Knop, E., D. R. Korb et al. (2012). The lid wiper—A specialized structure at the inner eyelid margin for distribution of the tear film. *Acta Ophthalmol (Copenh)* 90(s249).

64. Kobayashi, A., T. Yoshita et al. (2005). In vivo findings of the bulbar/palpebral conjunctiva and presumed meibomian glands by laser scanning confocal microscopy. *Cornea* 24(8): 985–988.
65. Korb, D. R., J. P. Herman et al. (2010). Prevalence of lid wiper epitheliopathy in subjects with dry eye signs and symptoms. *Cornea* 29(4): 377–383.
66. Ku, J. Y., R. L. Niederer et al. (2008). Laser scanning in vivo confocal analysis of keratocyte density in keratoconus. *Ophthalmology* 115(5): 845–850.
67. Kumar, R. L., A. Cruzat et al. (2010). Current state of in vivo confocal microscopy in management of microbial keratitis. *Semin Ophthalmol* 25(5–6): 166–170.
68. Labbe, A., B. Dupas et al. (2005). In vivo confocal microscopy study of blebs after filtering surgery. *Ophthalmology* 112(11): 1979.
69. Labbe, A., L. Gheck et al. (2010). An in vivo confocal microscopy and impression cytology evaluation of pterygium activity. *Cornea* 29(4): 392–399.
70. Lalive, P. H., A. Truffert et al. (2009). Peripheral autoimmune neuropathy assessed using corneal in vivo confocal microscopy. *Arch Neurol* 66(3): 403–405.
71. Le, Q. H., W. T. Wang et al. (2010). An in vivo confocal microscopy and impression cytology analysis of goblet cells in patients with chemical burns. *Invest Ophthalmol Vis Sci* 51(3): 1397–1400.
72. Ledbetter, E. C., N. L. Irby et al. (2011). In vivo confocal microscopy of equine fungal keratitis. *Vet Ophthalmol* 14(1): 1–9.
73. Lee, S. H., Y. S. Chun et al. (2010). The relationship between *Demodex* and ocular discomfort. *Invest Ophthalmol Vis Sci* 51(6): 2906–2911.
74. Lee, S. Y., A. Petznick et al. (2012). Associations of systemic diseases, smoking and contact lens wear with severity of dry eye. *Ophthalmic Physiol Opt* 32(6): 518–526.
75. Lekhanont, K., D. Rojanaporn et al. (2006). Prevalence of dry eye in Bangkok, Thailand. *Cornea* 25(10): 1162–1167.
76. Lemp, M. A. (1995). Report of the national eye institute/industry workshop on clinical trials in dry eyes. *CLAO J* 21(4): 221–232.
77. Lemp, M. A., P. N. Dilly et al. (1985). Tandem-scanning (confocal) microscopy of the full-thickness cornea. *Cornea* 4(4): 205–209.
78. Liang, H., C. Baudouin et al. (2010). Live conjunctiva-associated lymphoid tissue analysis in rabbit under inflammatory stimuli using in vivo confocal microscopy. *Invest Ophthalmol Vis Sci* 51(2): 1008–1015.
79. Liesegang, T. J. (1997). Contact lens-related microbial keratitis: Part I: Epidemiology. *Cornea* 16(2): 125–131.
80. Lin, P. Y., S. Y. Tsai et al. (2003). Prevalence of dry eye among an elderly Chinese population in Taiwan: The Shihpai Eye Study. *Ophthalmology* 110(6): 1096–1101.
81. Liu, Z. and S. C. Pflugfelder (2000). The effects of long-term contact lens wear on corneal thickness, curvature, and surface regularity. *Ophthalmology* 107(1): 105–111.
82. Longo, C., G. Pellacani et al. (2012). In vivo detection of *Demodex folliculorum* by means of confocal microscopy. *Br J Dermatol* 166(3): 690–692.
83. Lum, E., B. Golebiowski et al. (2012). Mapping the corneal sub-basal nerve plexus in orthokeratology lens wear using in vivo laser scanning confocal microscopy. *Invest Ophthalmol Vis Sci* 53(4): 1803–1809.
84. Marren, S. E. (1994). Contact lens wear, use of eye cosmetics, and meibomian gland dysfunction. *Optom Vis Sci* 71(1): 60–62.
85. Masters, B. R. and A. A. Thaer (1994). Real-time scanning slit confocal microscopy of the in vivo human cornea. *Appl Opt* 33(4): 695–701.
86. Mastropasqua, L., M. Nubile et al. (2006). Epithelial dendritic cell distribution in normal and inflamed human cornea: In vivo confocal microscopy study. *Am J Ophthalmol* 142(5): 736–744.
87. Mathers, W. D., J. V. Jester et al. (1988). Return of human corneal sensitivity after penetrating keratoplasty. *Arch Ophthalmol* 106(2): 210–211.

88. Matsumoto, Y., E. A. Sato et al. (2008). The application of in vivo laser confocal microscopy to the diagnosis and evaluation of meibomian gland dysfunction. *Mol Vis* 14: 1263–1271.
89. Mccarty, C. A., A. K. Bansal et al. (1998). The epidemiology of dry eye in Melbourne, Australia. *Ophthalmology* 105(6): 1114–1119.
90. Mccarty, C. A., C. L. Fu et al. (2000). Epidemiology of pterygium in Victoria, Australia. *Br J Ophthalmol* 84(3): 289–292.
91. Messmer, E. M., M. J. Mackert et al. (2006). In vivo confocal microscopy of normal conjunctiva and conjunctivitis. *Cornea* 25(7): 781–788.
92. Miller, D. (1968). Contact lens-induced corneal curvature and thickness changes. *Arch Ophthalmol* 80(4): 430–432.
93. Millodot, M. (1977). The influence of age on the sensitivity of the cornea. *Invest Ophthalmol Vis Sci* 16(3): 240–242.
94. Millodot, M. (1984). A review of research on the sensitivity of the cornea. *Ophthalmic Physiol Opt* 4(4): 305–318.
95. Minsky, M. (1961). Microscopy apparatus. US 3013467.
96. Miri, A., T. Alomar et al. (2012). In vivo confocal microscopic findings in patients with limbal stem cell deficiency. *Br J Ophthalmol* 96(4): 523–529.
97. Mocan, M. C., P. T. Yilmaz et al. (2008). In vivo confocal microscopy for the evaluation of corneal microstructure in keratoconus. *Curr Eye Res* 33(11): 933–939.
98. Moilanen, J. A., M. H. Vesaluoma et al. (2003). Long-term corneal morphology after PRK by in vivo confocal microscopy. *Invest Ophthalmol Vis Sci* 44(3): 1064–1069.
99. Morgan, S. J. (1987). Chemical burns of the eye: Causes and management. *Br J Ophthalmol* 71(11): 854–857.
100. Mustonen, R. K., M. B. Mcdonald et al. (1998). In vivo confocal microscopy of Fuchs' endothelial dystrophy. *Cornea* 17(5): 493–503.
101. Nanavaty, M. A. and A. J. Shortt (2011). Endothelial keratoplasty versus penetrating keratoplasty for Fuchs endothelial dystrophy. *Cochrane Database Syst Rev* (7): cd008420.
102. Nguyen, T. H., L. T. Dudek et al. (2004). In vivo confocal microscopy: Increased conjunctival or episcleral leukocyte adhesion in patients who wear contact lenses with lower oxygen permeability (Dk) values. *Cornea* 23(7): 695–700.
103. Niederer, R. L. and C. N. Mcghee (2010). Clinical in vivo confocal microscopy of the human cornea in health and disease. *Prog Retin Eye Res* 29(1): 30–58.
104. Niederer, R. L., D. Perumal et al. (2007). Age-related differences in the normal human cornea: A laser scanning in vivo confocal microscopy study. *Br J Ophthalmol* 91(9): 1165–1169.
105. Niederer, R. L., D. Perumal et al. (2007). Corneal innervation and cellular changes after corneal transplantation: An in vivo confocal microscopy study. *Invest Ophthalmol Vis Sci* 48(2): 621–626.
106. Niederer, R. L., D. Perumal et al. (2008). Laser scanning in vivo confocal microscopy reveals reduced innervation and reduction in cell density in all layers of the keratoconic cornea. *Invest Ophthalmol Vis Sci* 49(7): 2964–2970.
107. Niederer, R. L., T. Sherwin et al. (2007). In vivo confocal microscopy of subepithelial infiltrates in human corneal transplant rejection. *Cornea* 26(4): 501–504.
108. Nieto-Bona, A., A. Gonzalez-Mesa et al. (2011). Long-term changes in corneal morphology induced by overnight orthokeratology. *Curr Eye Res* 36(10): 895–904.
109. O'Day, D. M., P. L. Akrabawi et al. (1979). Laboratory isolation techniques in human and experimental fungal infections. *Am J Ophthalmol* 87(5): 688–693.
110. Panchapakesan, J., F. Hourihan et al. (1998). Prevalence of pterygium and pinguecula: The Blue Mountains Eye Study. *Aust NZ J Ophthalmol* 26(suppl. 1): s2–s5.
111. Papadia, M., S. Barabino et al. (2008). In vivo confocal microscopy in a case of pterygium. *Ophthalmic Surg Lasers Imaging* 39(6): 511–513.
112. Park, S. W., H. Heo et al. (2009). Comparison of ultrasound biomicroscopic changes after glaucoma triple procedure and trabeculectomy in eyes with primary angle closure glaucoma. *J Glaucoma* 18(4): 311–315.

113. Parrozzani, R., D. Lazzarini et al. (2011). In vivo confocal microscopy of ocular surface squamous neoplasia. *Eye (Lond)* 25(4): 455–460.
114. Patel, D. V., J. Y. Ku et al. (2009). Laser scanning in vivo confocal microscopy and quantitative aesthesiometry reveal decreased corneal innervation and sensation in keratoconus. *Eye (Lond)* 23(3): 586–592.
115. Patel, D. V. and C. N. Mcghee (2006). Mapping the corneal sub-basal nerve plexus in keratoconus by in vivo laser scanning confocal microscopy. *Invest Ophthalmol Vis Sci* 47(4): 1348–1351.
116. Patel, D. V., T. Sherwin et al. (2006). Laser scanning in vivo confocal microscopy of the normal human corneoscleral limbus. *Invest Ophthalmol Vis Sci* 47(7): 2823–2827.
117. Patel, S. V., J. W. Mclaren et al. (2002). Confocal microscopy in vivo in corneas of long-term contact lens wearers. *Invest Ophthalmol Vis Sci* 43(4): 995–1003.
118. Paterson, C. A., R. R. Pfister et al. (1975). Aqueous humor pH changes after experimental alkali burns. *Am J Ophthalmol* 79(3): 414–419.
119. Perez-Gomez, I. and N. Efron (2003). Change to corneal morphology after refractive surgery (myopic laser in situ keratomileusis) as viewed with a confocal microscope. *Optom Vis Sci* 80(10): 690–697.
120. Petran, M., M. Hadravsky et al. (1968). Tandem scanning reflected light microscope. *J Opt Soc Am* 58: 661–664.
121. Pflugfelder, S. C., S. C. Tseng et al. (1997). Correlation of goblet cell density and mucosal epithelial membrane mucin expression with rose bengal staining in patients with ocular irritation. *Ophthalmology* 104(2): 223–235.
122. Pisella, P. J., O. Auzerie et al. (2001). Evaluation of corneal stromal changes in vivo after laser in situ keratomileusis with confocal microscopy. *Ophthalmology* 108(10): 1744–1750.
123. Pult, H. (2012). Non-contact meibography in diagnosis and treatment of non-obvious meibomian. *J Optom* 5(5): 2–5.
124. Pult, H., B. H. Riede-Pult et al. (2012). Relation between upper and lower lids' meibomian gland morphology, tear film, and dry eye. *Optom Vis Sci* 89(3): e310–315.
125. Quigley, H. A. (1996). Number of people with glaucoma worldwide. *Br J Ophthalmol* 80(5): 389–393.
126. Rabinowitz, Y. S. (1998). Keratoconus. *Surv Ophthalmol* 42(4): 297–319.
127. Radford, C. F., O. J. Lehmann et al. (1998). *Acanthamoeba* keratitis: Multicentre survey in England 1992–1996. National *Acanthamoeba* keratitis study group. *Br J Ophthalmol* 82(12): 1387–1392.
128. Riau, A. K., R. I. Angunawela et al. (2011). Early corneal wound healing and inflammatory responses after refractive lenticule extraction (ReLEx). *Invest Ophthalmol Vis Sci* 52(9): 6213–6221.
129. Rosa, R. H., Jr., D. Miller et al. (1994). The changing spectrum of fungal keratitis in South Florida. *Ophthalmology* 101(6): 1005–1013.
130. Rosenberg, M. E., T. M. Tervo et al. (2002). In vivo confocal microscopy after herpes keratitis. *Cornea* 21(3): 265–269.
131. Roszkowska, A. M., P. Colosi et al. (2004). Age-related modifications of corneal sensitivity. *Ophthalmologica* 218(5): 350–355.
132. Sangwan, V. S., B. Ramamurthy et al. (2005). Outcome of corneal transplant rejection: A 10-year study. *Clin Exp Ophthalmol* 33(6): 623–627.
133. Sattler, E. C., T. Maier et al. (2012). Noninvasive in vivo detection and quantification of Demodex mites by confocal laser scanning microscopy. *Br J Dermatol* 167(5): 1042–1047.
134. Schaefer, F., O. Bruttin et al. (2001). Bacterial keratitis: A prospective clinical and microbiological study. *Br J Ophthalmol* 85(7): 842–847.
135. Schaumberg, D. A., J. J. Nichols et al. (2011). The international workshop on meibomian gland dysfunction: Report of the subcommittee on the epidemiology of, and associated risk factors for, MGD. *Invest Ophthalmol Vis Sci* 52(4): 1994–2005.
136. Sheppard, C. J. and T. Wilson (1979). Effect of spherical aberration on the imaging properties of scanning optical microscopes. *Appl Opt* 18(7): 1058–1063.

137. Sheppard, C. J. R. and A. Choudhury (1977). Image formation in the scanning microscope. *Opt Acta* 24: 1051–1073.
138. Sherwin, T., N. H. Brookes et al. (2002). Cellular incursion into Bowman's membrane in the peripheral cone of the keratoconic cornea. *Exp Eye Res* 74(4): 473–482.
139. Shimmura, S. and K. Tsubota (2006). Deep anterior lamellar keratoplasty. *Curr Opin Ophthalmol* 17(4): 349–355.
140. Shimomura, Y. (2008). Herpes simplex virus latency, reactivation, and a new antiviral therapy for herpetic keratitis. *Nihon Ganka Gakkai Zasshi* 112(3): 247–264; discussion 265.
141. Singh, R., A. Joseph et al. (2005). Impression cytology of the ocular surface. *Br J Ophthalmol* 89(12): 1655–1659.
142. Sit, M., D. J. Weisbrod et al. (2001). Corneal graft outcome study. *Cornea* 20(2): 129–133.
143. Smiddy, W. E., W. J. Stark et al. (1986). Clinical and immunological results of corneal allograft rejection. *Ophthalmic Surg* 17(10): 644–649.
144. Smith, G. T. and H. R. Taylor (1991). Epidemiology of corneal blindness in developing countries. *Refract Corneal Surg* 7(6): 436–439.
145. Snyder, M. C., J. P. Bergmanson et al. (1998). Keratocytes: No more the quiet cells. *J Am Optom Assoc* 69(3): 180–187.
146. Svishchev, G. M. (1969). Microscope for the study of transparent light scattering objects in incident light. *Opt Spectrosc* 30: 188–911.
147. Szaflik, J. P., A. Kaminska et al. (2007). In vivo confocal microscopy of corneal grafts shortly after penetrating keratoplasty. *Eur J Ophthalmol* 17(6): 891–896.
148. Tavakoli, M., P. A. Kallinikos et al. (2007). Corneal sensitivity is reduced and relates to the severity of neuropathy in patients with diabetes. *Diabetes Care* 30(7): 1895–1897.
149. Taylor, K. I. and H. R. Taylor (1999). Distribution of azithromycin for the treatment of trachoma. *Br J Ophthalmol* 83(2): 134–135.
150. Thakur, A. and M. D. Willcox (2000). Contact lens wear alters the production of certain inflammatory mediators in tears. *Exp Eye Res* 70(3): 255–259.
151. Thomas, P. A. (2003). Fungal infections of the cornea. *Eye (Lond)* 17(8): 852–862.
152. Tiffany, J. M. (2003). Tears in health and disease. *Eye (Lond)* 17(8): 923–926.
153. Trittibach, P., R. Cadez et al. (2004). Determination of microdot stromal degenerations within corneas of long-term contact lens wearers by confocal microscopy. *Eye Contact Lens* 30(3): 127–131.
154. Tu, E. Y., C. E. Joslin et al. (2008). The relative value of confocal microscopy and superficial corneal scrapings in the diagnosis of *Acanthamoeba* keratitis. *Cornea* 27(7): 764–772.
155. Ucakhan, O. O., A. Kanpolat et al. (2006). In vivo confocal microscopy findings in keratoconus. *Eye Contact Lens* 32(4): 183–191.
156. Uchino, M., M. Dogru et al. (2006). The features of dry eye disease in a Japanese elderly population. *Optom Vis Sci* 83(11): 797–802.
157. Vaddavalli, P. K., P. Garg et al. (2011). Role of confocal microscopy in the diagnosis of fungal and *Acanthamoeba* keratitis. *Ophthalmology* 118(1): 29–35.
158. Vaddavalli, P. K., P. Garg et al. (2006). Confocal microscopy for Nocardia keratitis. *Ophthalmology* 113(9): 1645–1650.
159. Vajdic, C., B. A. Holden et al. (1999). The frequency of ocular symptoms during spectacle and daily soft and rigid contact lens wear. *Optom Vis Sci* 76(10): 705–711.
160. Van Setten, G., M. Aspiotis et al. (2003). Connective tissue growth factor in pterygium: Simultaneous presence with vascular endothelial growth factor—Possible contributing factor to conjunctival scarring. *Graefes Arch Clin Exp Ophthalmol* 241(2): 135–139.
161. Vesaluoma, M., J. Perez-Santonja et al. (2000). Corneal stromal changes induced by myopic LASIK. *Invest Ophthalmol Vis Sci* 41(2): 369–376.
162. Villani, E., S. Beretta et al. (2011). In vivo confocal microscopy of meibomian glands in Sjögren's syndrome. *Invest Ophthalmol Vis Sci* 52(2): 933–939.
163. Villani, E., G. Ceresara et al. (2011). In vivo confocal microscopy of meibomian glands in contact lens wearers. *Invest Ophthalmol Vis Sci* 52(8): 5215–5219.

164. Wakamatsu, T. H., M. Dogru et al. (2008). Tearful relations: Oxidative stress, inflammation and eye diseases. *Arq Bras Oftalmol* 71(6 suppl.): 72–79.
165. Wakamatsu, T. H., E. A. Sato et al. (2010). Conjunctival in vivo confocal scanning laser microscopy in patients with Sjögren syndrome. *Invest Ophthalmol Vis Sci* 51(1): 144–150.
166. Wang, L., J. Zhang et al. (2008). In vivo confocal microscopic characteristics of fungal keratitis. *Life Sci J* 5(1): 51–54.
167. Wang, Y., F. Zhao et al. (2010). In vivo confocal microscopic evaluation of morphologic changes and dendritic cell distribution in pterygium. *Am J Ophthalmol* 150(5): 650–655 (e651).
168. Watson, S. L., A. Ramsay et al. (2004). Comparison of deep lamellar keratoplasty and penetrating keratoplasty in patients with keratoconus. *Ophthalmology* 111(9): 1676–1682.
169. Webb, R. H., G. W. Hughes et al. (1987). Confocal scanning laser ophthalmoscope. *Appl Opt* 26(8): 1492–1499.
170. West-Mays, J. A. and D. J. Dwivedi (2006). The keratocyte: Corneal stromal cell with variable repair phenotypes. *Int J Biochem Cell Biol* 38(10): 1625–1631.
171. Whitcher, J. P., M. Srinivasan et al. (2001). Corneal blindness: A global perspective. *Bull World Health Organ* 79(3): 214–221.
172. Wilensky, J. T. and T. C. Chen (1996). Long-term results of trabeculectomy in eyes that were initially successful. *Trans Am Ophthalmol Soc* 94: 147–164.
173. Williams, K. A., S. M. Muehlberg et al. (1997). Long-term outcome in corneal allotransplantation. The Australian corneal graft registry. *Transplant Proc* 29(1–2): 983.
174. Wirtschafter, J. D., J. M. Ketcham et al. (1999). Mucocutaneous junction as the major source of replacement palpebral conjunctival epithelial cells. *Invest Ophthalmol Vis Sci* 40(13): 3138–3146.
175. Wright, P. (1982). The chemically injured eye. *Trans Ophthalmol Soc UK* 102(pt 1): 85–87.
176. Yeh, D. L., S. S. Stinnett et al. (2006). Analysis of bacterial cultures in infectious keratitis, 1997 to 2004. *Am J Ophthalmol* 142(6): 1066–1068.
177. Zarei-Ghanavati, S., A. Ramirez-Miranda et al. (2011). Limbal lacuna: A novel limbal structure detected by in vivo laser scanning confocal microscopy. *Ophthalmic Surg Lasers Imaging* 42(online): e129–e131.
178. Zhang, M., J. Chen et al. (2005). Altered corneal nerves in aqueous tear deficiency viewed by in vivo confocal microscopy. *Cornea* 24(7): 818–824.
179. Zhang, Y. Q., Q. Wu et al. (2008). Evaluating subconjunctival bleb function after trabeculectomy using slit-lamp optical coherence tomography and ultrasound biomicroscopy. *Chin Med J* 121(14): 1274–1279.
180. Zhivov, A., O. Stachs et al. (2006). In vivo confocal microscopy of the ocular surface. *Ocul Surf* 4(2): 81–93.
181. Zhivov, A., J. Stave et al. (2007). In vivo confocal microscopic evaluation of Langerhans cell density and distribution in the corneal epithelium of healthy volunteers and contact lens wearers. *Cornea* 26(1): 47–54.

20

Biomechanical Modeling of Blood Vessels for Interpretation of Tortuosity Estimates

Martynas Patašius, Vaidotas Marozas, Darius Jegelevičius, Arūnas Lukoševičius, Irmantas Kupčiūnas, and Audris Kopustinskas

CONTENTS

20.1 Related Work

In general, the ophthalmologists evaluate tortuosity of retinal blood vessels using subjective estimates, for example, optometric scales [1]. But objective estimates also exist.

For such estimates, it is generally assumed that blood vessel is a planar curve that does not intersect itself. It can be defined parametrically. In computer memory, it can be stored discretely (finite number of points). For every point of a continuous curve (and most of the points of discrete curve), it is possible to calculate curvature. The curvature of a parametric curve can be calculated from derivatives of coordinates by the following formula:

$$k = \frac{x'y'' - y'x''}{(x'^2 + y'^2)^{3/2}}. \tag{20.1}$$

One of the most simple methods to estimate the tortuosity of the curve using curvature is the ratio between the integral of module or square of curvature and curve's length L [2]:

$$\tau_1 = \frac{1}{L}\int_{t_1}^{t_2} |k(t)|\,dt. \tag{20.2}$$

A possible modification of this method uses the curvatures of edges of the vessel instead of the center line. That takes into account the fact that tortuosity is calculated not for the idealized lines, but for objects that have width [3]. Later, this modification has been generalized [4]:

$$\tau_{1b} = \frac{1}{L} \int_{t_1}^{t_2} \left(\frac{|k_1(t)|^p + |k_2(t)|^p}{2} \right)^{-p} dt. \tag{20.3}$$

Here
 k_1 and k_2 are the curvatures of edges of blood vessel in specific points
 p is the empirically chosen parameter (authors recommended the value 4) [4]

One more similar estimate has been made using modules of different angles of blood vessel edges instead of curvatures [5].

One more estimate is the integral of square of derivative of curvature divided by the length of the curve [6,7]:

$$\tau_2 = \frac{1}{L} \int_{t_1}^{t_2} (k'(t))^2 dt. \tag{20.4}$$

Such estimate is based on intuition that the curve with constant curvature should not be considered tortuous. In 1993, an analogy supporting this intuition has been used while discussing splines: it is easy to drive a car or a bicycle along the circular road (it is enough to hold the steering wheel strongly), but it is harder to drive where the curvature changes [8]. However, the tortuosity estimate given with this analogy (the integral of square of ratio of curvature's derivative and curvature) [8] is hard to apply when the line can be straight.

Perhaps the most intuitive definition of tortuosity is arc–chord ratio [2]. In this case, if the length of the arc (curve) is L and the distance between ends of curve (chord length) is S, the tortuosity is defined as

$$\tau_3 = \frac{L}{S}. \tag{20.5}$$

However, this estimate is infinite for circles, although it is not considered a tortuous curve [9,10].

Scientists of University of Padua [9] have proposed a modification of arc–chord ratio without this flaw. First, the line is divided into N parts where the sign of curvature is constant (with hysteresis). Then arc–chord ratio is calculated for each part. The tortuosity estimate itself is calculated by the following formula:

$$\tau_4 = \frac{N-1}{L} \cdot \sum_{i=1}^{N} \left(\frac{L_i}{S_i} - 1 \right). \tag{20.6}$$

Later, this method has been modified [11]:

$$\tau_5 = \frac{N-1}{N} \cdot \frac{1}{L} \cdot \sum_{i=1}^{N} \left(\frac{L_i}{S_i} - 1 \right). \tag{20.7}$$

The influence of the quality of blood vessel detection for the estimates can be decreased by using splines or digital low-frequency filters.

20.2 Biomechanical Modeling of Blood Vessel Using the Finite Element Method

As it can be seen, there are many tortuosity estimates. They are supposed to correlate with blood pressure. Thus it seems worth to investigate their behavior in simplified conditions.

Finite elements method was used to model a blood vessel. The wall of the vessel was cylindrical (internal diameter 6 mm and external diameter 8 mm). A small (1.7 mm in diameter) spherical defect was added inside the vessel, thus making it asymmetrical. The defect can be thought as simulating atherosclerosis plaque. The distribution of blood pressure was assumed to be constant inside the vessel. Young's module of the vessel wall (including the defect) was chosen to be 5 MPa [12] while Poisson's ratio was 0.45 [12]. The vessel was modeled as immersed in a box (50 mm × 20 mm × 20 mm) of material with Young's module 1 kPa and Poisson's ratio 0.3 [13]. The surrounding material simulates the tissue of the retina (Figure 20.1) [14].

The static solutions were found for a range of values of blood pressure.

The outer surface of the vessel wall was *cut* into 50 segments lengthwise. Then all the slices were approximated by circles; see Figure 20.2. The tortuosity of projection of

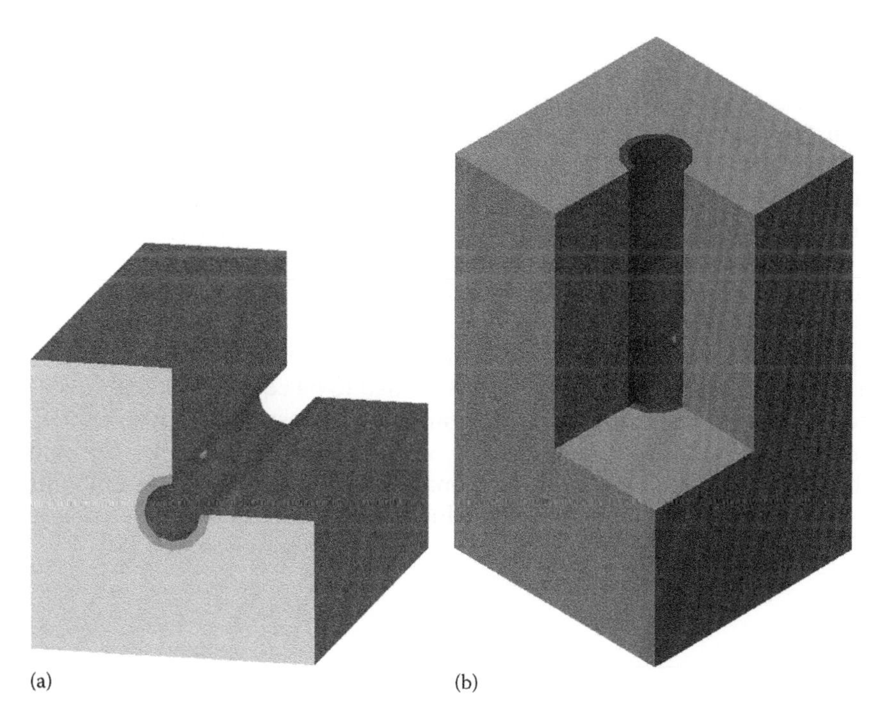

FIGURE 20.1
A blood vessel's model in finite elements: (a) general view with a part being removed and (b) isometric projection with a part being removed [21]. In this model, tetrahedral finite elements were used. (From Patašius, M. et al., Model based investigation of retinal vessel tortuosity as a function of blood pressure: Preliminary results, in *29th Annual International Conference of the IEEE Engineering in Medicine and Biology Society in conjunction with the Biennial Conference of the French Society of Biological and Medical Engineering (SFGBM) (elektroninis išteklius)*, Lyon, France, August 23–26, 2007, IEEE, Piscataway, NJ, 2007, pp. 6459–6462.)

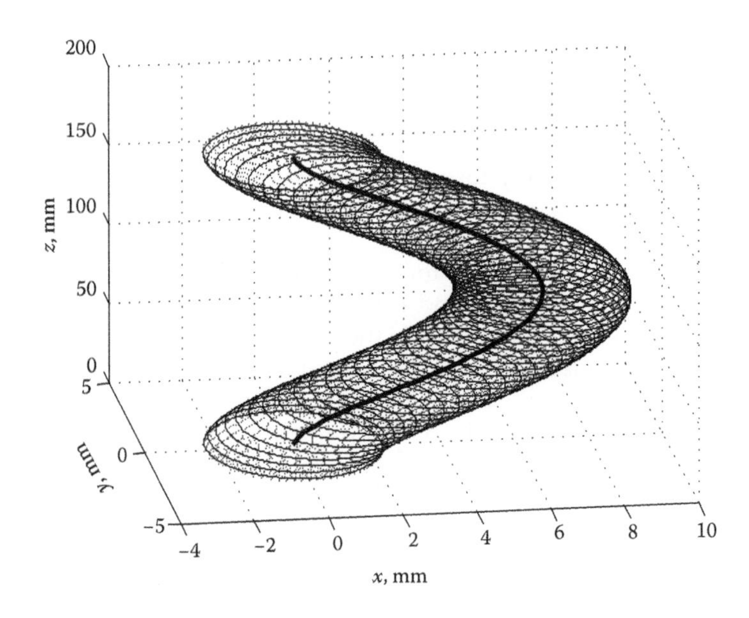

FIGURE 20.2
Approximating the blood vessel's wall segments by circles and making the central line (data used were meant for illustration of the method, not of results).

the curve going through the centers of these circles was estimated using the methods described in the following [14].

Tortuosity indices' dependencies on the pressure are shown in Figure 20.3.

As Figure 20.9 shows, the estimates given by the integral of square of derivative of curvature, arc–length ratio, and method proposed by the scientists of the University of Padova increase quadratically, and the integral of module of curvature increases linearly. In all cases, the dependency is monotonic. Thus, in principle, all those indices can be used to estimate the pressure [14].

The dependency between tortuosity estimates and blood vessel wall's Young's modulus has been found similarly (the pressure was assumed to be equal to 10 kPa).

As it can be seen from Figure 20.4, the values of the estimates given by the integral of derivative of curvature, arc–length ratio, and method proposed by the scientists of University of Padua are inversely proportional to the square of Young's modulus of the blood vessel wall, while the integral of module of curvature is inversely proportional to Young's modulus. Thus all those dependencies are monotonous as well [14].

20.3 Experimental Validation of Blood Vessel Model

The blood vessel model in finite elements has also been validated experimentally.

In the first experiment, a section of silicone tube K70 produced by *Kartell* was used as the phantom of the blood vessel. The inner diameter of the tube was 5 mm, outer diameter—8 mm, and length—about 20 cm. The ends of the tube were fixed. One terminal

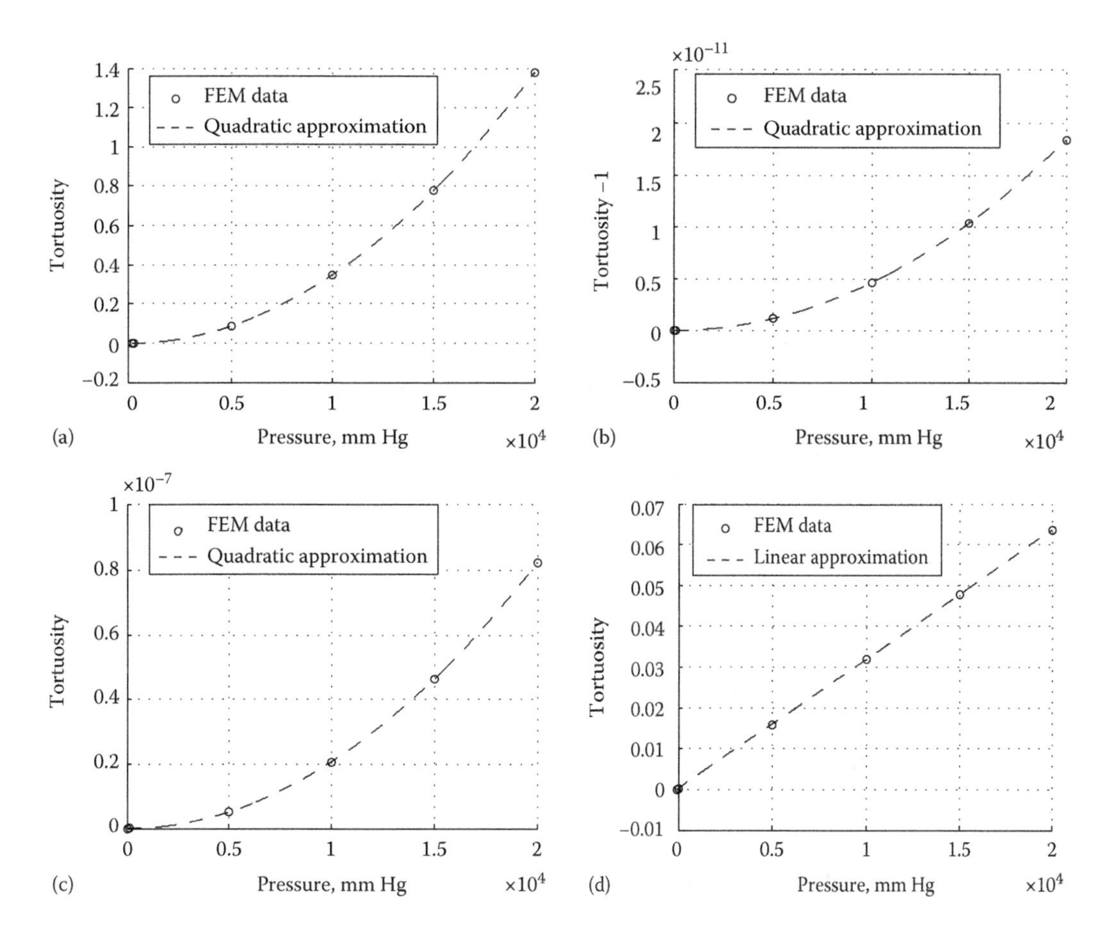

FIGURE 20.3
The estimates of tortuosity as functions of internal pressure: integral of square of derivative of curvature (a), arc–length ratio (b), method proposed by the scientists of University of Padova (c), and integral of module of curvature (d). (From Patašius, M. et al., Model based investigation of retinal vessel tortuosity as a function of blood pressure: Preliminary results, in *29th Annual International Conference of the IEEE Engineering in Medicine and Biology Society in conjunction with the Biennial Conference of the French Society of Biological and Medical Engineering (SFGBM) (elektroninis išteklius)*, Lyon, France, August 23–26, 2007, IEEE, Piscataway, NJ, 2007, pp. 6459–6462.)

end of the tube was connected to a leak-proof camera with a manometer, and another end was closed with a pressure transducer. A hand pump was used to increase the pressure inside the camera and the tube (Figure 20.5) [15].

The goal of the experiment was to estimate the changes of the tube diameter as the function of inner pressure inside the tube. The discrete steps of applied pressure were 100, 140, 200, and 260 mm Hg (13.3, 18.7, 26.7, and 34.7 kPa) [15].

The tube was photographed using a 7 megapixel camera in front of a black background (see Figure 20.6). The size of the resulting images was 3072 × 2304 pixels. The scale of a caliper was kept in the image to enable measurements in absolute units. Then the maximal gradients (limits of the tube) were found in the images, and the diameters along the tube were calculated. Finally, a mean diameter and its 95% confidence interval were calculated for each image of the tube as the pressure was increased [15].

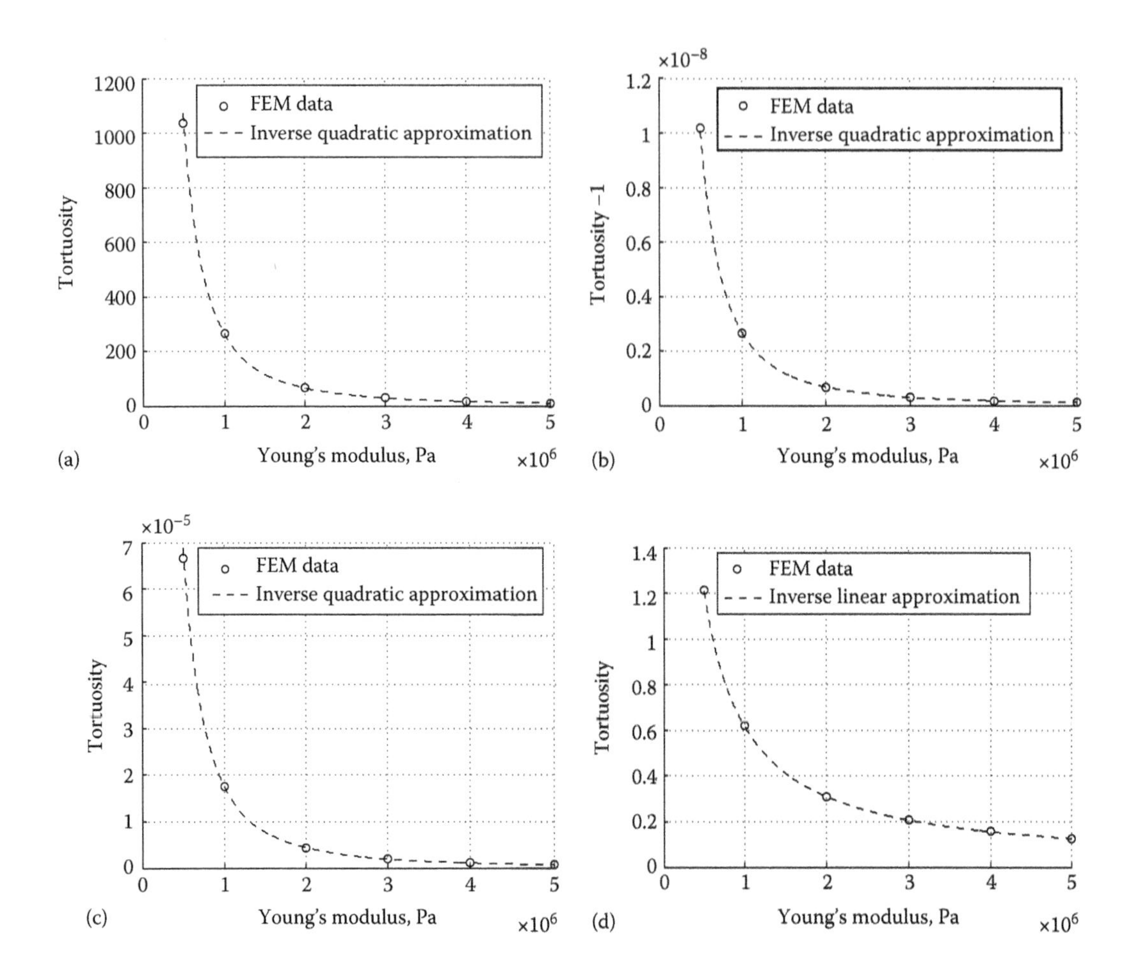

FIGURE 20.4
The estimates of tortuosity as functions of blood vessel wall's Young's modulus: integral of square of derivative of curvature (a), arc–length ratio (b), method proposed by the scientists of University of Padova (c), and integral of module of curvature (d). (From Patašius, M. et al., Model based investigation of retinal vessel tortuosity as a function of blood pressure: Preliminary results, in *29th Annual International Conference of the IEEE Engineering in Medicine and Biology Society in conjunction with the Biennial Conference of the French Society of Biological and Medical Engineering (SFGBM) (elektroninis išteklius)*, Lyon, France, August 23–26, 2007, IEEE, Piscataway, NJ, 2007, pp. 6459–6462.)

A model of such tube was made using Comsol Multiphysics. The tube was modeled by a cylinder of the same size parameters as the real tube. The mechanical properties of silicone, Young's modulus of 1000 psi (6.865 MPa) and Poisson's ratio of 0.48, were found in the literature [16]. The model had 16,428 degrees of freedom.

It has been found that in all four steps of pressure increase, 1 mm of tube was represented by 20 pixels in the image. There were 580–582 crosscuts of the tube where diameters were estimated for each case. As expected, the diameter of the tube was found to increase linearly as the pressure increases (Table 20.1) [15].

The results of modeling using finite elements (Table 20.2) have also shown the linear growth [15].

It should be noted that in both cases, the growth of diameter is linear, but absolute values are not the same. The difference can be explained by the different mechanical

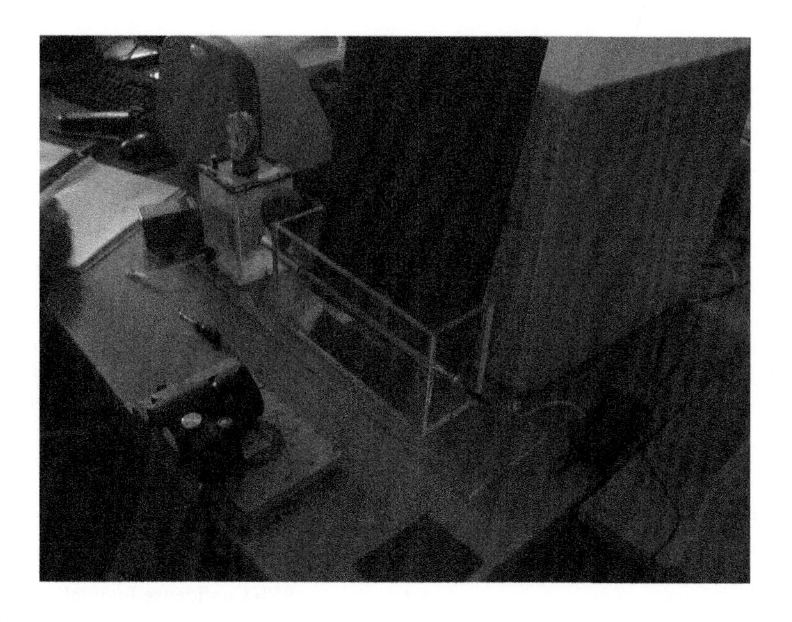

FIGURE 20.5
The experiment with a silicon tube. (From Patašius, M. et al., Comparison of methods of estimation of blood vessel diameter, *Biomedicininė inžinerija = Biomedical Engineering: Tarptautinės konferencijos pranešimų medžiaga, 2007 m. spalio 25-26 d, Kaunas/Kauno technologijos universitetas,* Technologija, Kaunas, Lithuania, 2007, pp. 129–132.)

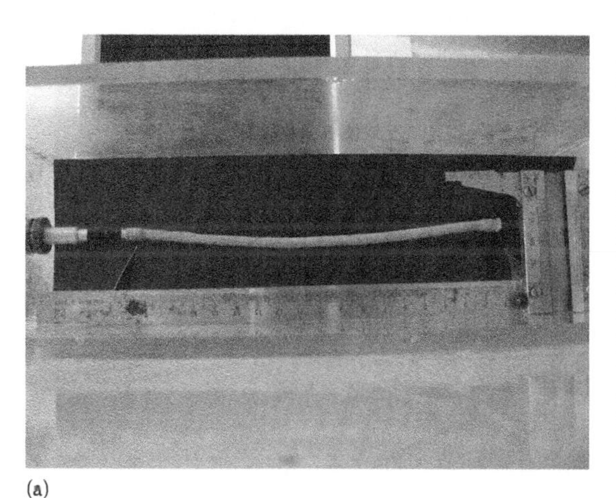

(a)

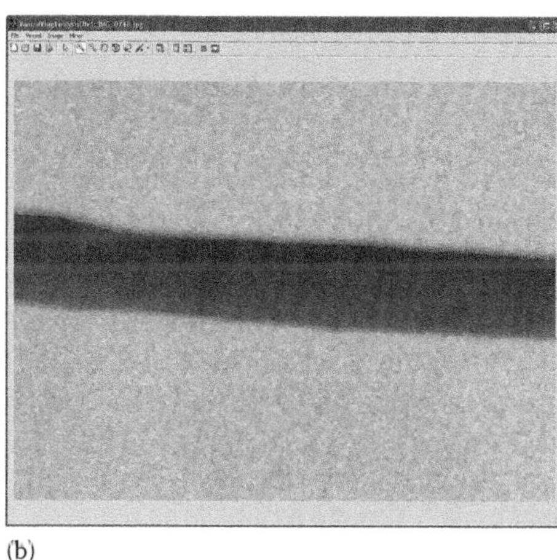

(b)

FIGURE 20.6
(See color insert.) A sample picture of the latex tube (a) and finding the limits of the tube (b). (From Patašius, M. et al., Preliminary validation of FEM based blood vessel model, *Biomedicininė inžinerija = Biomedical engineering: tarptautinės konferencijos pranešimų medžiaga, 2008 m. spalio 23–24 d, Kaunas/Kauno technologijos universitetas,* Technologija, Kaunas, Lithuania, 2008, pp. 70–73.)

properties of silicone and dimensions of the tube and by the error of estimation of representation of 1 mm in the image.

The correspondence of growth trends has let to make a conclusion that the tool is suitable for the detection of deformations. However, the deformations proved to be too small to detect changes of tortuosity. That, in turn, has led to the conclusion that a different, latex, tube should be used, since it would be deformed more easily [15].

TABLE 20.1

Results of the Experiment with Silicone Tube Using Image Analysis

	Average Diameter		95% Confidence Interval	
Pressure, mm Hg	**Pixels**	**mm**	**Lower Limit, Pixels**	**Upper Limit, Pixels**
100	157.163	7.858	156.983	157.344
140	157.393	7.870	157.210	157.576
200	157.663	7.883	157.488	157.838
260	158.022	7.901	157.837	158.208

Source: Patašius, M. et al., Comparison of methods of estimation of blood vessel diameter, *Biomedicininė inžinerija = Biomedical Engineering: Tarptautinės konferencijos pranešimų medžiaga, 2007 m. spalio 25-26 d, Kaunas/Kauno technologijos universitetas*, Technologija, Kaunas, Lithuania, 2007, pp. 129–132.

TABLE 20.2

Dependence between Tube's Diameter and Pressure Using Finite Elements

		95% Confidence Interval	
Pressure, mm Hg	**Average Diameter, mm**	**Lower Limit, mm**	**Upper Limit, mm**
100	8.015	8.0146	8.0155
140	8.021	8.0205	8.0217
200	8.030	8.0293	8.0310
260	8.039	8.0381	8.0403

Source: Patašius, M. et al., Comparison of methods of estimation of blood vessel diameter, *Biomedicininė inžinerija = Biomedical Engineering: Tarptautinės konferencijos pranešimų medžiaga, 2007 m. spalio 25-26 d, Kaunas/Kauno technologijos universitetas*, Technologija, Kaunas, Lithuania, 2007, pp. 129–132.

Thus further experiments were done with a self-made latex tube. Chemask® Peelable latex made by Chemtronics was used [17].

The latex was solved in the water with ammonia. A brush was then used to cover heat shrink tubing RC/PBF1/8 3.2/1.6 (produced by DSG-CANUSA) with the solution. The process was repeated several times. To achieve controlled asymmetry, the latex coating was applied more, twice as many times on one side than on the other. Then hot water was applied to shrink the heat shrink tubing and make the taking off of the latex tube easier [17].

The latex tube was put in the container to hang freely with both ends fixed (Figure 20.6a). The air pressure was increased up to 100 mm Hg (13.3 kPa) and then decreased to 20 mm Hg (2.66 kPa) with steps of 10 mm Hg (1.33 kPa). For each step, two photographs were taken. Violet background has been put behind the tube to increase the contrast [17].

While analyzing the photographs, the edges of the tube were recognized as the local maximums of the color gradient (Figure 20.6b). Using the scale, it has been found that 1 mm corresponds to about 12 pixels in the images [17].

For finite elements model, the tube was assumed to be cylindrical with outer radius equal to 0.25 cm, inner radius—0.175 cm, length—18.5 cm, and the distance between the axes of symmetry of outer and inner cylinders—0.25 mm. Young's modulus of latex rubber has been assumed to be 11.7 dyn/cm^2 (1.17 MPa) [18] and Poisson's ratio—0.5 [19], although it is likely that those estimates describe a different type of latex rubber. The model had 51,346 elements and 286,809 degrees of freedom [17].

Several parameters were used to describe the shape of the tube: the mean diameter of the tube and four tortuosity estimates of the central line—arc–length ratio, integral of squared derivative of curvature, integral of module of curvature, and integral of square of curvature. Because of irregularities of the tube, the tortuosity estimates were calculated not for the raw recognized tube central line, but for B-spline, approximating the central line [17].

Figure 20.7 shows the dependency between the average diameter and internal pressure. It should be noted that while the absolute values of the diameters do differ (indicating errors in mechanical parameter estimation), in both cases, the tendency of linear growth of mean diameter is observed.

Results show that absolute values of the tortuosity estimates do differ (measurements in pixels were used in case of image analysis and measurements in meters—in case of finite element method [FEM] modeling), but their manner of growth is similar [17].

Figure 20.8 shows the dependencies between estimates of the tube's tortuosity and internal pressure. It should be noted that the absolute values are different (partially because in the case of image analysis, pixels were used to measure length, while meters were used in case of finite element modeling). However, in all cases, the growth of tortuosity estimates for image analysis and for finite element modeling is similar [17].

To make the quadratic growth easier to see, Figure 20.9 shows the values of those estimates as functions of squares of internal pressure.

As it can be seen, the dependencies between the square of internal pressure and the aforementioned tortuosity estimates are close to linear, just as the results of modeling would indicate [17].

In general, it can be said that the described finite element models seem to be sufficiently adequate to investigate the relationship between the shape of retinal blood vessels (especially the venules, having no muscular layers) and blood pressure, when other conditions stay constant. That should be true for the period that is sufficiently short to exclude changes related to the growth of blood vessels and similar phenomena of biological nature. This conclusion is supported by the fact that latex tubes have been used to investigate the relationship between tortuosity of blood vessels and blood pressure previously and have been found to be adequate blood vessel models [20,21].

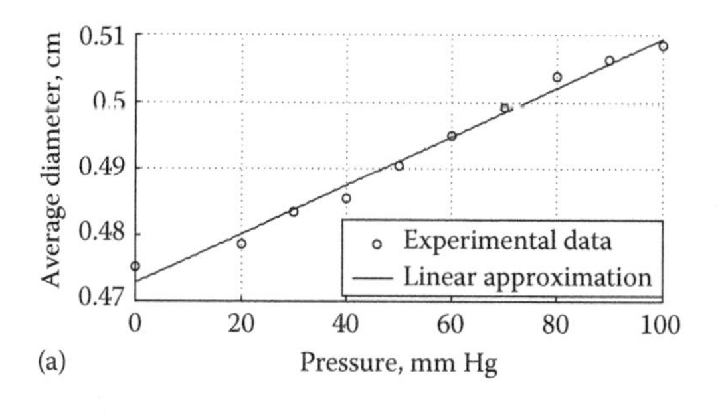

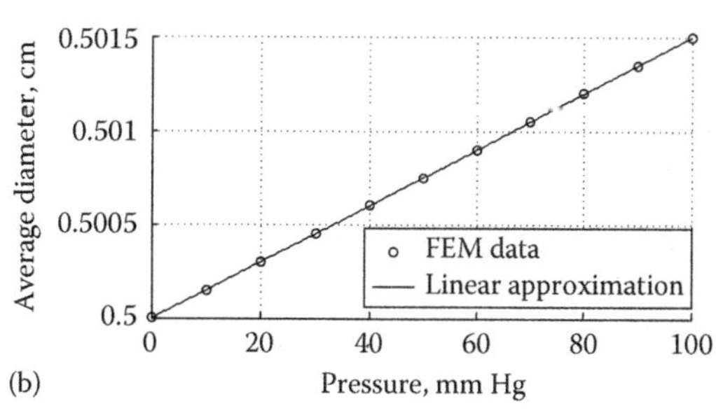

FIGURE 20.7
The average diameter of latex tube as the function of internal pressure—results of the experiment (a) and of finite element modeling (b). (From Patašius, M. et al., Preliminary validation of FEM based blood vessel model, *Biomedicininė inžinerija = Biomedical engineering: tarptautinės konferencijos pranešimų medžiaga, 2008 m. spalio 23–24 d, Kaunas/Kauno technologijos universitetas,* Technologija, Kaunas, Lithuania, 2008, pp. 70–73.)

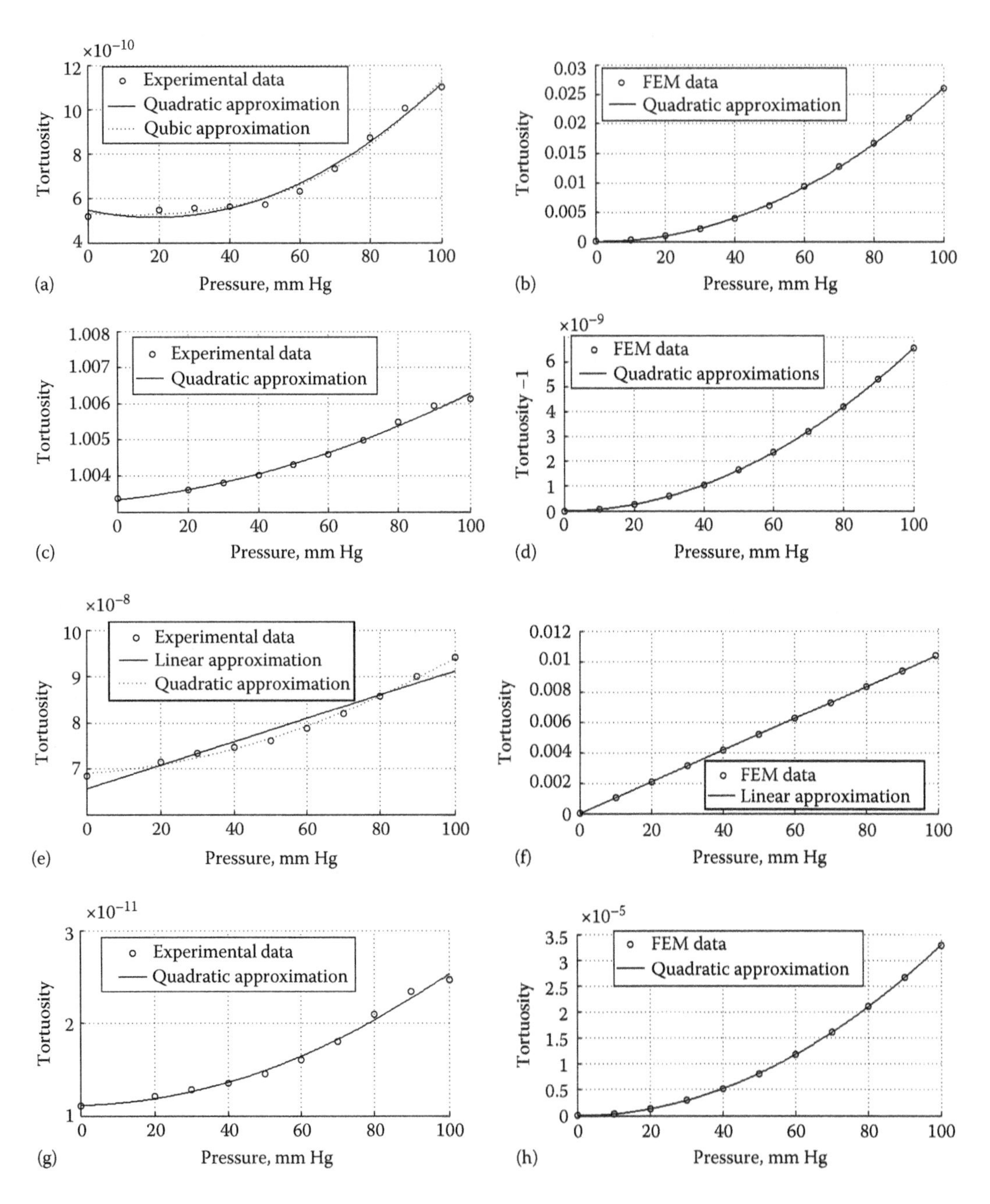

FIGURE 20.8
Tortuosity of the latex tube as a function of internal pressure—results of experiment (a, c, e, and g) and finite element modeling (b, d, f, and h) for different tortuosity estimates: integral of square of derivative of curvature (a and b), arc–length ratio (c and d), integral of module of curvature (e and f), and integral of square of curvature (g and h). (From Patašius, M. et al., Preliminary validation of FEM based blood vessel model, *Biomedicininė inžinerija = Biomedical engineering: tarptautinės konferencijos pranešimų medžiaga, 2008 m. spalio 23–24 d, Kaunas/Kauno technologijos universitetas*, Technologija, Kaunas, Lithuania, 2008, pp. 70–73.)

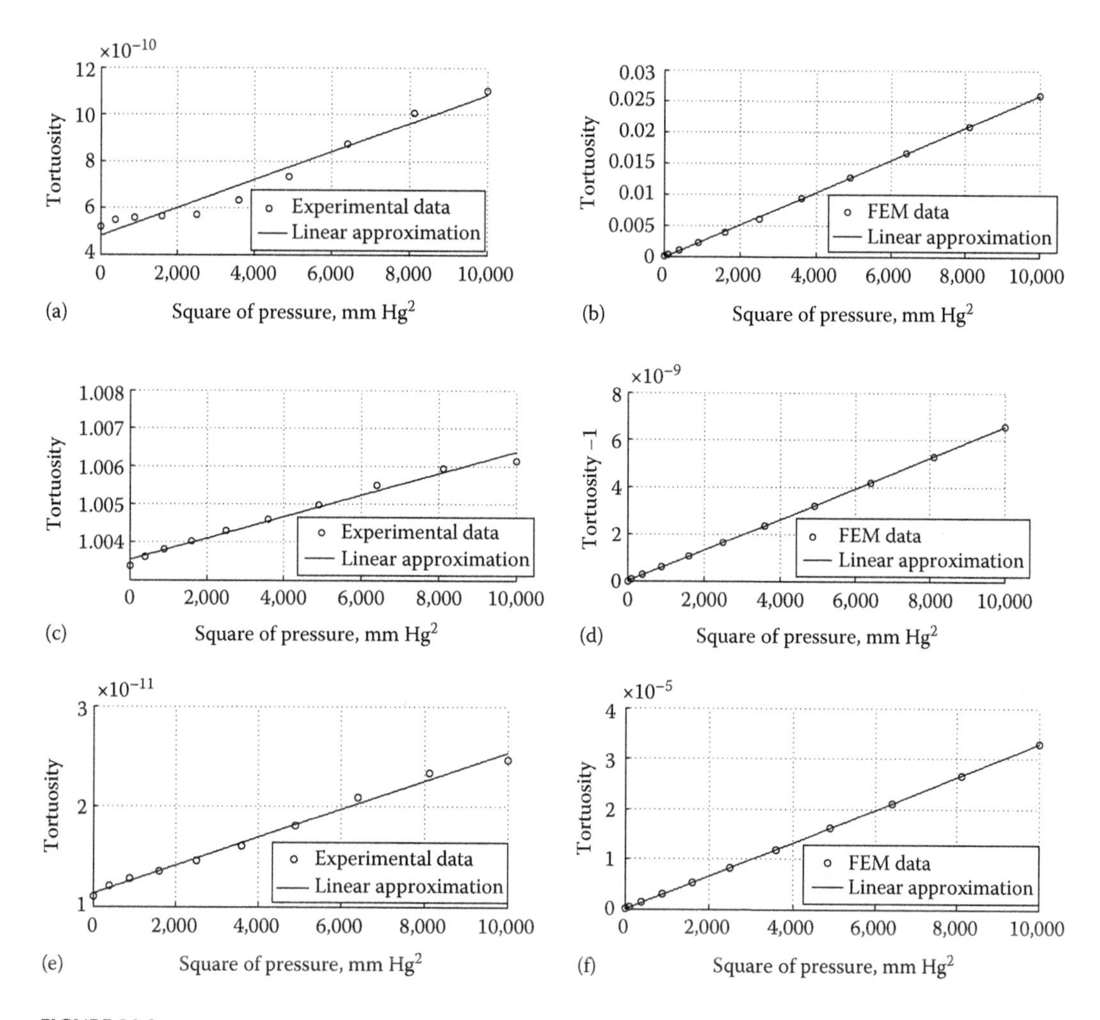

FIGURE 20.9
Tortuosity of the latex tube as a function of square of internal pressure—results of experiment (a, c, and e) and finite element modeling (b, d, and f) for different tortuosity estimates: integral of square of derivative of curvature (a and b), arc–length ratio (c and d), and integral of square of curvature (e and f).

References

1. Pearson, R. M., Optometric grading scales for use in everyday practice, *Optometry Today*, 43(20), 2003, 39–42.
2. Hart, W. E., Goldbaum, M., Cote, B., Kube, P., Nelson, M. R., Automated measurement of retinal vascular tortuosity, *International Journal of Medical Informatics*, 53(2/3), February 1999, 239–252.
3. Azegrouz, H., Trucco, E., Dhillon, B., MacGillivray, T., MacCormick, I. J., Thickness dependent tortuosity estimation for retinal blood vessels, in *28th Annual International Conference of the IEEE Engineering in Medicine and Biology Society (EMBS'06)*, New York, 2006, pp. 4675–4678.
4. Trucco, E., Azegrouz, H., and Dhillon, B. Modeling the tortuosity of retinal vessels: Does caliber play a role? *IEEE Transactions on Biomedical Engineering*, 57(9), 2010, 2239–2247.

5. Bhuiyan, A., Nath, B., Ramamohanarao, K., Kawasaki, R., Wong, T., Automated analysis of retinal vascular tortuosity on color retinal images, *Journal of Medical Systems*, 36(2), 2012, 689–697, doi: 10.1007/s10916-010-9536-6.
6. Patašius, M., Marozas, V., Lukoševičius, A., Jegelevičius, D., Evaluation of tortuosity of eye blood vessels using the integral of square of derivative of curvature, in *Proceedings of the 3rd IFMBE European Medical and Biological Engineering Conference*, Prague, Czech Republic, November 2005, vol. 11, pp. 660–663.
7. Patašius, M., Akies dugno kraujagyslių vingiuotumo įvertinimo metodai, Magistro darbas, Kauno Technologijos Universitetas, Kaunas, Lithuania, 2006.
8. Mächler, M. Very smooth nonparametric curve estimation by penalizing change of curvature. Research Report 71, Seminar für Statistik, Eidgenossische Technische Hochschule, Zürich, CH8092 Zürich, Switzerland, 1993.
9. Grisan, E., Foracchia, M., Ruggeri, A., A novel method for automatic evaluation of retinal vessel tortuosity, in *Proceedings of the 25th Annual International Conference of the IEEE EMBS*, Cancun, Mexico, September 17–21, 2003.
10. Goh, K. G., Hsu, W., Li Lee, M., Wang, H., ADRIS: An automatic diabetic retinal image screening system, in *Medical Data Mining and Knowledge Discovery*, vol. 60, K. J. Cios, Ed., *Studies in Fuzziness and Soft Computing*, Physica-Verlag, New York, pp. 181–210, 2001.
11. Grisan, E. and Ruggeri, A., A markov random field approach to outline lesions in fundus images, in *Proceedings of Fourth European Conference of the International Federation for Medical and Biological Engineering*, vol. 22, J. V. Sloten, P. Verdonck, M. Nyssen, and J. Haueisen, Eds., pp. 472–475. Springer Berlin, Heidelberg, 2008.
12. Finol, E. A., Martino, E. S. D., Vorp, D. A., Amon, C. H., Fluid–structure interaction and structural analyses of an aneurysm model, in *Proceedings of the 2003 Summer Bioengineering Conference*, Key Biscane, FL, June 25–29, 2003, pp. 75–76.
13. Di Puccio, F., Paola, F., Guarneri, G., Finite element modelling of balloon angioplasty, in *IASTED International Conference BIOMECHANICS*, Rhodes, Greece, 2003, pp. 97–102.
14. Patašius, M., Marozas, V., Lukoševičius, A., Jegelevičius, D., Model based investigation of retinal vessel tortuosity as a function of blood pressure: Preliminary results, in *29th Annual International Conference of the IEEE Engineering in Medicine and Biology Society in conjunction with the Biennial Conference of the French Society of Biological and Medical Engineering (SFGBM) (elektroninis išteklius)*, Lyon, France, August 23–26, 2007. IEEE, Piscataway, NJ, 2007, pp. 6459–6462.
15. Patašius, M., Kupčiūnas, I., Marozas, V., Kopustinskas, A., Comparison of methods of estimation of blood vessel diameter, *Biomedicininė inžinerija = Biomedical Engineering: Tarptautinės konferencijos pranešimų medžiaga, 2007 m. spalio 25-26 d, Kaunas/Kauno technologijos universitetas*, Technologija, Kaunas, Lithuania, 2007, pp. 129–132.
16. O'Hara, G. P., Mechanical properties of silicone rubber in closed volume. Technical Report ARLCSB-TR-83045, US Army Armament Research and Development center, Large caliber weapon systems laboratory, Benet weapons laboratory, 1983.
17. Patašius, M., Marozas, V., Kopustinskas, A., Preliminary validation of FEM based blood vessel model, *Biomedicininė inžinerija = Biomedical engineering: tarptautinės konferencijos pranešimų medžiaga, 2008 m. spalio 23–24 d, Kaunas/Kauno technologijos universitetas*, Technologija, Kaunas, Lithuania, 2008, pp. 70–73.
18. Gallerani, M., Ursino, M., Artioli, E., An experimental study of wave propagation in the latex rubber tube [arterial tree model], in *Images of the Twenty-First Century, Proceedings of the Annual International Conference of the IEEE Engineering in Medicine and Biology Society*, Seattle, WA, 1989, vol. 3, pp. 871–872.
19. Binns, R. L., Ku, D. N., Effect of stenosis on wall motion. A possible mechanism of stroke and transient ischemic attack, *Arteriosclerosis, Thrombosis, and Vascular Biology*, 9(6), 1989, 842–847.

20. Kylstra, J. A., Wierzbicki, T., Wolbarsht, M. L., Landers, M. B., Stefansson, E., The relationship between retinal vessel tortuosity, diameter, and transmural pressure, *Graefe's Archive for Clinical and Experimental Ophthalmology*, 224(5), 1986, 477–480.
21. Patašius, M., Akies dugno vaizdų automatinė analizė, Doctoral dissertation, Kaunas University of Technology, Kaunas, Lithuania, 2010.

21

Hybrid Finite Element Simulation for Bioheat Transfer in the Human Eye

Hui Wang, Qing-Hua Qin, and Ming-Yue Han

CONTENTS

21.1 Introduction

Prediction of bioheat performance in biological system is important in many diagnostic and therapeutic applications. Generally, analytical analysis is usually difficult in practice because of geometrically complex biological tissues, typically for the human eye considered in this chapter. For example, the human eyeball consists of several subdomains with different material properties and has complicated geometries for each subdomain. Currently, the application of computational methods in modeling biological eye system has attracted considerable attention of researchers throughout the world.

Among the numerical methods developed so far, finite element and boundary element techniques have been widely used to analyze bioheat transfer phenomena in the human eye. For example, the finite element formulations for 2D human eye structures were, respectively, developed by Scott [24] and Ng and Ooi [11], who used the commercialized software FEMLAB 3.1 as computational tool. By considering the circulation of aqueous humor, Ooi and Ng [15] utilized the finite element technique to conduct heat transfer analysis in the 2D eye model. In addition, the 3D cylindrical computational model of the human eye was established by Brinkmann et al. [3] using the finite element theory.

In the previously mentioned analysis using finite element method (FEM), the entire solution domain is firstly divided into many elements, which can have independent material definitions, and then in each element, the physical fields are approximated by appropriate shape function interpolations. The weak-form integral functional associated with the governing equations and boundary conditions is established to produce the final stiffness equations. However, the time-consuming mesh generation, domain integrals, and discontinuity of heat flux between elements are main disadvantages in the conventional FEM. Besides, other domain-based discretization methods like the finite volume method (FVM) [5,10] and the finite difference method (FDM) [9] were also employed to study transient temperature response caused by laser source in the human eye.

Besides the domain-type methods mentioned previously, the boundary element method (BEM) or dual reciprocity BEM (DRBEM) involving boundary integrals only was also developed for the numerical thermal analysis in the human eye [12–14,17]. Different to the FEM, FVM, and FDM, the time-consuming domain integrals that appeared in the FEM were replaced with dimensional-reduced boundary integrals in the BEM formulation. However, the efficient treatment of singular or near-singular boundary integrals is usually complicated and tedious, and besides the boundary integral equation for boundary nodal physical quantities, extra integral equation is required to evaluate the interior fields inside the domain. Specially, for the multidomain problems, the BEM requires the establishment of independent boundary integral equation for each subdomain, and then the linkage of these equations is accomplished by satisfaction of continuity conditions on the interface of adjacent subdomains. As a result, the coefficient matrix of the resulting equations becomes unsymmetrical and large. More discussion on FEM and BEM can be found in literatures [2,20–22].

In order to alleviate some of these difficulties in the BEM and FEM and simultaneously retain their advantages, a novel hybrid finite element model with the fundamental solution as trial function, named as HFS-FEM, was initially developed by Wang and Qin [27] for simple thermal analysis and now has been extended to solve complicated heat transfer [23,25,31,32] and mechanical problems [4,29,30,32–34]. Besides, they also applied the HFS-FEM to perform heat transfer in the human eyeball with complicated geometry, but the influence of blood perfusion rate was not considered in their study [28]. In the formulation of HFS-FEM, two independent fields (one is defined in the element domain and another on the element boundary) are constructed using the fundamental solution and conventional shape function as used in the BEM and FEM, and then a new hybrid variational functional is constructed to link the two independent fields and to produce the final standard force–displacement equation system. Noting that the intra-element field being approximated with the linear combination of fundamental solutions satisfies analytically the related governing equation, the domain integrals in the hybrid functional can be directly converted into elementary boundary integrals and doesn't cause an appreciable increase in computational effort. It is worthy pointing out that no singular integrals are involved in the HFS-FEM, although the fundamental solutions are employed. It is because the sources used for the evaluation of fundamental solution are placed outside the element of interest, like the known method of fundamental solution (MFS) [6,26]; thus, the source point and field point never overlap during the computation. In addition, different to other hybrid FEMs [18], the basic idea of the proposed hybrid finite element model is the use of the novel interpolation kernels composed of fundamental solutions inside the multiedge element.

In this chapter, the HFS-FEM is extended to predict the steady-state temperature distribution of the 2D human eyeball under the nature convection and tear evaporation conditions.

For this purpose, the established hybrid functional is required to include the convection integral term. To investigate the influence of blood perfusion rate, which appears in the Pennes bioheat governing equation, the eyeball bioheat model is modified by introducing the blood perfusion parameter in the sclera layer and then solved by the use of the present hybrid finite element formulation.

21.2 Mathematical Model for Bioheat Transfer in the Human Eye

21.2.1 Bioheat Governing Partial Differential Equation

A typical 2D model of the human eye as sketched in Figure 21.1 is taken into consideration here. In the figure, only the cornea, iris, aqueous humor, sclera, vitreous, and optic nerve are involved. In fact, between the sclera and the vitreous, one may find two tissue layers known as the retina and the choroid. For simplicity, since these layers are relatively thin, they are modeled together with the sclera and the optic nerve as a single homogeneous region. Moreover, for the sake of simplicity, each of the subdomains is assumed to be thermally isotropic and homogeneous, based on the assumption in some literatures [11–13,24].

For convenience, the cornea and the aqueous humor are denoted by R_1 and R_2, respectively, as shown in Figure 21.2. The other two regions, that is, the lens and the vitreous, are denoted by R_3 and R_4, respectively. Besides, the iris and the sclera having the same thermal conductivities are contiguous, so they can be modeled as a single homogeneous region denoted by R_5 in the practical computation. All regions are assumed to be isotropic and homogeneous.

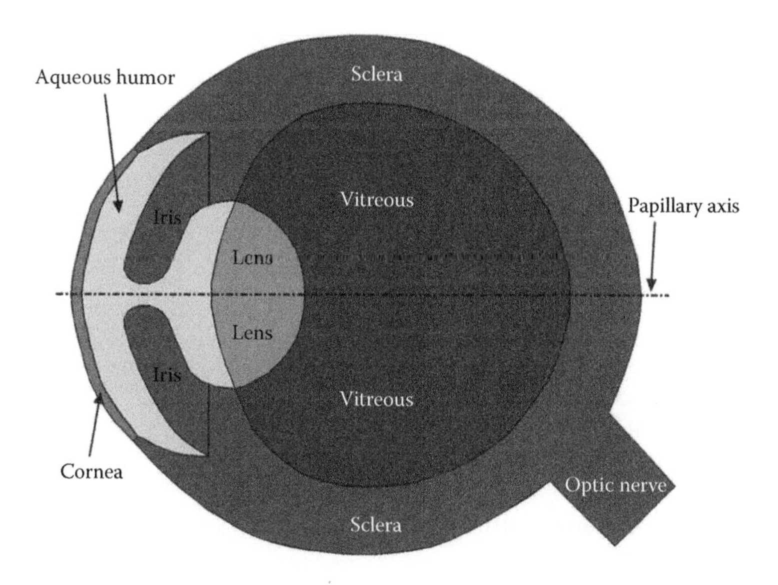

FIGURE 21.1
Sketch diagram of the human eye.

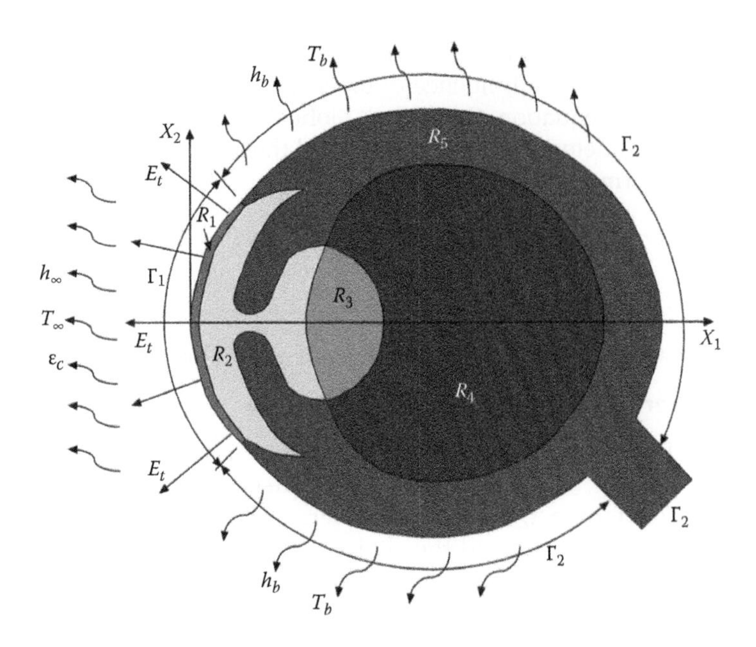

FIGURE 21.2
Illustration of boundary conditions applied on the outer surface of eyeball.

Making use of the rectangular coordinate system (X_1, X_2) with the arrangement of the axis coinciding with the papillary axis, the governing equation representing the bioheat transfer usually is written by the well-known Pennes equation addressing the effect of blood perfusion and metabolic activities in the biological system [16]:

$$k\nabla^2 T + \rho_b c_b w_b (T_b - T) + Q_m + Q_i = \rho c \frac{\partial T}{\partial t}, \tag{21.1}$$

where ∇^2 denotes the Laplace operator, which has the following expression in 2D space:

$$\nabla^2 = \frac{\partial^2}{\partial X_1{}^2} + \frac{\partial^2}{\partial X_2{}^2} \tag{21.2}$$

where
- t is the time variable
- ρ represents the density of the tissue
- c stands for the tissue specific heat
- k is the tissue thermal conductivity
- w_b is the blood flow rate
- ρ_b is the density of blood
- c_b is the blood specific heat
- T is the unknown tissue temperature
- T_b is the blood temperature
- Q_m is the metabolic heat source term
- Q_i is the internal heat source maybe caused by external laser heating, electric disturbance, or radiation of electromagnetic waves

In Equation 21.1, the first term on the left-hand side represents the heat conduction in the tissue caused by the temperature gradient, the second term stands for the heat transport between the tissue and microcirculatory blood perfusion, and the third and last terms are two internal heat generations, respectively, due to tissue metabolism and outer heating sources, while the term on the right-hand side reflects the heat change over time as heat spreads throughout space.

In this work, our interest is to determine the maximum temperature increase in the human eye and then we assume that steady-state temperature is reached. Besides, in the human eye, only small parts of the eyeball such as sclera and optic nerve are perfused and have evident metabolic activities [7], so the blood perfusion and metabolic heat generation can be neglected in most parts of the eyeball [11,12]. In this study, only the blood perfusion behavior in the region R_5 is involved. For this case, the resulting bioheat governing partial differential equation (21.1) is reduced to the following steady-state Helmholtz-type equation

$$k\nabla^2 T(\mathbf{x}) + \rho_b c_b w_b (T_b - T) = 0 \quad \mathbf{x} \in R_5 \tag{21.3}$$

in the region R_5, and Laplace-type equation

$$k\nabla^2 T(\mathbf{x}) = 0 \quad \mathbf{x} \in R_i \ (i = 1,2,3,4) \tag{21.4}$$

in the remaining regions by neglecting the influence of blood perfusion.

21.2.2 Boundary Conditions

In the eyeball model, the following three types of boundary conditions are involved during the bioheat transfer in the biological system:

1. *Convection, radiation, and tear evaporation on the corneal outer surface*
   Since the cornea is the only region in the eye that is exposed to the environment, the heat loss caused through convection and radiation should be considered. Also, the evaporation of tears on the corneal outer surface increases the cooling rate on the corneal surface. Thus, the three forms of cooling mechanism can be put together and the related boundary condition on the surface of cornea is written by

$$q \equiv -k\frac{\partial T}{\partial n} = h_\infty (T - T_\infty) + \varepsilon_c \sigma (T^4 - T_\infty^4) + E_t \quad \text{on } \Gamma_1 \tag{21.5}$$

   or

$$q \equiv -k\frac{\partial T}{\partial n} = [h_\infty + \varepsilon_c \sigma (T + T_\infty)(T^2 + T_\infty^2)](T - T_\infty) + E_t \quad \text{on } \Gamma_1 \tag{21.6}$$

   where
   n is the unit outward normal to the surface
   h_∞ is the heat transfer coefficient between the eye and ambient environment
   T_∞ is the sink temperature of the environmental fluid
   σ is the Stefan–Boltzman constant with value 5.669×10^{-8} W/m^2 K^4
   E_t is the heat loss term due to tear evaporation
   ε_c is the corneal emissivity, which is equal to 0.975

It should be noted that the radiation effect is much smaller than the convection effect in practice, especially for the larger convection coefficient [28]. This can be seen from Equation 21.5, in which the environmental convection coefficient h_∞ is usually much larger than the term

$$\varepsilon_c \sigma (T + T_\infty)(T^2 + T_\infty^2).$$

Thus, in the practical analysis, the radiation effect can be ignored. As a result, the boundary condition applied on the corneal outer surface can be simplified as

$$q \equiv -k \frac{\partial T}{\partial n} = h_\infty (T - T_\infty) + E_t \quad \text{on } \Gamma_1. \tag{21.7}$$

2. *Convection condition on the outer surface of sclera*

   On the outer surface Γ_2 of the sclera, the heat flows run into the eye from the blood acting as heating source in the ophthalmic artery to the sclera. This heating mechanism may be modeled using the following convection boundary condition:

$$q \equiv -k \frac{\partial T}{\partial n} = h_b (T - T_b) \quad \text{on } \Gamma_2, \tag{21.8}$$

   where
   h_b denotes the blood convection coefficient from the sclera to the body core
   T_b is the blood temperature

3. *Continuous conditions between adjacent regions*

   Continuous conditions usually exist on the common interface between two contiguous regions under perfectly bonded assumption. Here, for any two adjacent regions R_i and R_j in the eyeball, the corresponding continuous conditions in terms of temperature T and heat flow gradient $q \equiv -k(\partial T/\partial n)$ can be written as

$$\left.\begin{array}{l} T\big|_{\text{in } R_i} = T\big|_{\text{in } R_j} \\ q\big|_{\text{in } R_i} + q\big|_{\text{in } R_j} = 0 \end{array}\right\} \quad \text{on } R_i \cap R_j. \tag{21.9}$$

21.2.3 Simple Dimensionless Transformation

Due to the significant scale difference of variables in the governing equation, the dimensionless variables defined as follows are introduced:

$$x_1 = \frac{X_1}{L_0}, \quad x_2 = \frac{X_2}{L_0}, \quad \Phi = \frac{(T - T_b)k_0}{Q_0 L_0^2}, \quad K = \frac{k}{k_0}, \tag{21.10}$$

where
L_0 is a reference length of the biological body
k_0, ρ_0, c_0, and Q_0 are, respectively, the reference values of the thermal conductivity, density, specific heat, and heat source term

Thus, we have

$$\frac{\partial T}{\partial X_1} = \frac{Q_0 L_0^2}{k_0} \frac{1}{L_0} \frac{\partial \Phi}{\partial x_1}, \qquad \frac{\partial T}{\partial X_2} = \frac{Q_0 L_0^2}{k_0} \frac{1}{L_0} \frac{\partial \Phi}{\partial x_2}$$
$$\frac{\partial^2 T}{\partial X_1^2} = \frac{Q_0 L_0^2}{k_0} \frac{1}{L_0^2} \frac{\partial^2 \Phi}{\partial x_1^2}, \qquad \frac{\partial^2 T}{\partial X_2^2} = \frac{Q_0 L_0^2}{k_0} \frac{1}{L_0^2} \frac{\partial^2 \Phi}{\partial x_2^2}. \tag{21.11}$$

Through this transformation, the governing equations (21.3) and (21.4) can be rewritten as follows:

$$K\nabla^2 \Phi - S_b \Phi = 0 \quad \left(S_b = \frac{L_0^2 \rho_b c_b \omega_b}{k_0} \right) \tag{21.12}$$

and

$$K\nabla^2 \Phi = 0, \tag{21.13}$$

where the Laplace operator is expressed in terms of dimensionless variables (x_1, x_2)

$$\nabla^2 = \frac{\partial^2}{\partial x_1^2} + \frac{\partial^2}{\partial x_2^2}. \tag{21.14}$$

At the same time, the corresponding boundary conditions reduce to

$$\begin{cases} q = -K\dfrac{\partial \Phi}{\partial n} = H_\infty(\Phi - \Phi_\infty) + \tilde{E}_t & \text{on } \Gamma_1 \\ q = -K\dfrac{\partial \Phi}{\partial n} = H_\infty(\Phi - \Phi_\infty) & \text{on } \Gamma_2, \end{cases} \tag{21.15}$$

where

$$H_\infty = \frac{h_\infty L_0}{k_0}, \qquad \tilde{E}_t = \frac{E_t}{Q_0 L_0}. \tag{21.16}$$

21.3 Hybrid Finite Element Formulation

To perform the finite element analysis, the eyeball domain under consideration is firstly discretized with finite number of connected elements. For each element, two independent temperature fields are introduced, respectively, within the element and on the element boundary, and then hybrid functional is employed to connect them and establish the finite element formulation.

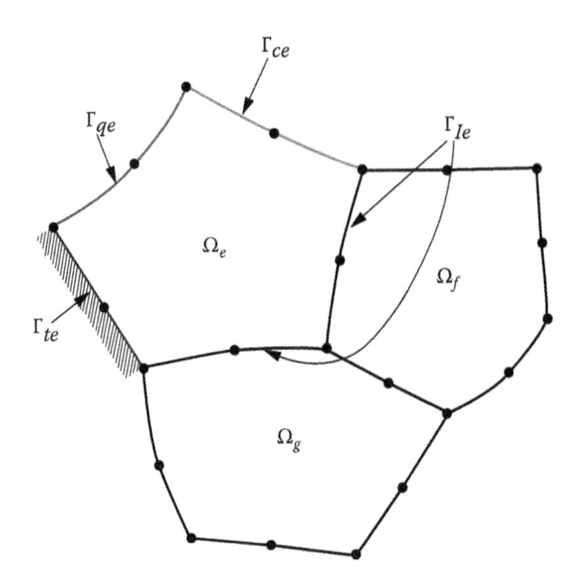

FIGURE 21.3
Illustration of hybrid elements.

21.3.1 Intra-element Fields

In the present hybrid finite element model, the dimensionless temperature field within a particular element Ω_e shown in Figure 21.3 is approximated with the linear combination of fundamental solutions, as was done in the classical meshless MFS [6,8,26,35,36]:

$$\Phi(P) = \sum_{i=1}^{n_s} G^*(P,Q_i)c_{ei} = \{\mathbf{N}\}\{\mathbf{c}_e\} \tag{21.17}$$

in which the vector

$$\{\mathbf{N}\} = \{G^*(P,Q_1) \quad G^*(P,Q_2) \quad \cdots \quad G^*(P,Q_{n_s})\} \tag{21.18}$$

and

$$\{\mathbf{c}\} = \{c_1 \quad c_2 \quad \cdots \quad c_{n_s}\}^{\mathrm{T}}. \tag{21.19}$$

In Equation 21.17, P is the field point that may be located inside the element or on the element boundary, Q_i is the source point arranged outside the element to avoid the singularity of the fundamental solution with unknown source intensity c_j, n_s represents the number of source points, and $G^*(P, Q_i)$ is the so-called fundamental solution, that is, the temperature response at point P due to the point heat source applied at point Q_i.

Further, the derivative of Equation 21.17 in terms of normal vector n yields the following dimensionless heat flux:

$$q \equiv -k\frac{\partial \Phi}{\partial n} = \{n_1 \quad n_2\}\begin{Bmatrix} -k\dfrac{\partial \Phi}{\partial x_1} \\ -k\dfrac{\partial \Phi}{\partial x_2} \end{Bmatrix} = \{n_1 \quad n_2\}\begin{Bmatrix} -k\dfrac{\partial \{\mathbf{N}\}}{\partial x_1} \\ -k\dfrac{\partial \{\mathbf{N}\}}{\partial x_2} \end{Bmatrix}\{\mathbf{c}_e\} = \{\mathbf{Q}\}\{\mathbf{c}_e\}. \tag{21.20}$$

For the governing equation (21.12), the fundamental solution is required to satisfy the following equation:

$$K\nabla^2 G^*(P,Q_i) - S_b G^*(P,Q_i) + \delta(P,Q_i) = 0, \tag{21.21}$$

which has the solution

$$G^*(P,Q_i) = -\frac{1}{2\pi K} K_0\left(\sqrt{\frac{S_b}{K}} r\right). \tag{21.22}$$

For the governing equation (21.13), the fundamental solution is required to satisfy

$$K\nabla^2 G^*(P,Q_i) + \delta(P,Q_i) = 0, \tag{21.23}$$

which gives

$$G^*(P,Q_i) = -\frac{1}{2\pi K} \ln r. \tag{21.24}$$

In Equations 21.21 through 21.24, δ stands for the Dirac delta function, K_0 is the modified Bessel function of the second kind with order 0, and $r = \|P - Q_i\|$ is the distance of the field point P and source point Q_i.

21.3.2 Element Frame Field

In the context of hybrid FEMs [18,19], the independent element frame field is typically introduced to fulfill the requirement of continuous conditions between adjacent elements. In this study, the frame temperature field is defined over the element boundary by

$$\tilde{\Phi}_e(P) = \sum_{i=1}^{n_d} \tilde{N}_i d_i = \{\tilde{\mathbf{N}}\}\{\mathbf{d}_e\}, \tag{21.25}$$

where

- n_d is the number of nodes for the specific element e
- $\tilde{N}_i$ stands for the shape functions as was used in the BEM and FEM [1,2]
- d_i is the unknown nodal temperature at node i

Typically, for the element e occupying the domain Ω_e, as shown in Figure 21.3, there are 5 edges and 10 nodes. For each edge, the employed nonlinear shape functions can be written in terms of the local natural coordinate ξ, that is,

$$\begin{aligned}
\tilde{N}_1(\xi) &= -\frac{\xi(1-\xi)}{2} \\
\tilde{N}_2(\xi) &= 1-\xi^2 \\
\tilde{N}_3(\xi) &= \frac{\xi(1+\xi)}{2}.
\end{aligned} \tag{21.26}$$

21.3.3 Weak-Form Hybrid Functional

To establish the linkage between the two independent fields (21.17) and (21.25) and, at the same time, include the convection boundary condition in this study, a modified element hybrid variational functional constructed based on the author's previous work is written as [27,32]

$$\Pi_{me} = -\frac{1}{2}\int_{\Omega_e}\left\{K\left[\left(\frac{\partial \Phi}{\partial x_1}\right)^2 + \left(\frac{\partial \Phi}{\partial x_2}\right)^2\right] + S_b\Phi^2\right\}d\Omega - \int_{\Gamma_{qe}}\bar{q}\tilde{\Phi}\,d\Gamma + \int_{\Gamma_e} q(\tilde{\Phi}-\Phi)\,d\Gamma$$

$$-\frac{1}{2}\int_{\Gamma_{ce}} H_\infty(\tilde{\Phi}-\Phi_\infty)^2 d\Gamma, \tag{21.27}$$

where

Γ_{qe} and Γ_{ce} are the element boundaries with specified heat flux and convection condition, respectively

Ω_e represents the entire element domain with boundary Γ_e, as shown in Figure 21.3

Besides, in the figure, Γ_{te} and Γ_{Ie}, respectively, stand for the element boundary on which the temperature is prescribed and the common element boundary between adjacent elements.

It is obvious that

$$\Gamma_e = \Gamma_{te} + \Gamma_{qe} + \Gamma_{ce} + \Gamma_{Ie}. \tag{21.28}$$

In the functional (21.27), the last boundary integral represents the convective effect, and $\bar{q}$ represents the specified boundary heat flux.

By invoking the divergence theorem

$$\int_{\Omega}\left(\frac{\partial f}{\partial X_1}\frac{\partial h}{\partial X_1} + \frac{\partial f}{\partial X_2}\frac{\partial h}{\partial X_2}\right)d\Omega = \int_{\Gamma} h\frac{\partial f}{\partial n}d\Gamma - \int_{\Omega} h\nabla^2 f d\Omega \tag{21.29}$$

for any continuous functions f and g in the domain, the first-order variation of the functional (21.27) can be expressed as

$$\delta\Pi_{me} = \int_{\Omega_e}(K\nabla^2\Phi - S_b\Phi)\delta\Phi\,d\Omega + \int_{\Gamma_{te}} q\delta\tilde{\Phi}\,d\Gamma$$

$$+\int_{\Gamma_{qe}}(q-\bar{q})\delta\tilde{\Phi}\,d\Gamma + \int_{\Gamma_{ce}}[q - H_\infty(\tilde{\Phi}-\Phi_\infty)]\delta\tilde{\Phi}\,d\Gamma + \int_{\Gamma_e}\delta q(\tilde{\Phi}-\Phi)d\Gamma \tag{21.30}$$

from which it can be seen that the first, third, and fourth integrals enforce the governing equation, specified heat flux condition, and convection condition, respectively. The second integral will disappear when $\tilde{\Phi}$ is assumed to prior satisfy the specified temperature constraint on the boundary Γ_{te}. The last integral enforces the equality of Φ and $\tilde{\Phi}$ along the element frame Γ_e.

Since the internal field Φ defined in Equation 21.17 analytically satisfies the governing equation of the problem, the domain integral in the functional (21.27) can be straightforwardly converted into boundary integral defined on the element boundary, and we finally have

$$\Pi_{me} = -\frac{1}{2}\int_{\Gamma_e} q\Phi \, d\Gamma + \int_{\Gamma_e} q\tilde{\Phi} \, d\Gamma - \int_{\Gamma_{2e}} \bar{q}\tilde{\Phi} \, d\Gamma - \int_{\Gamma_{3e}} \frac{H_\infty}{2}(\tilde{\Phi} - \Phi_\infty)^2 d\Gamma. \tag{21.31}$$

Substituting Equations 21.17, 21.20, and 21.25 into Equation 21.31 yields

$$\begin{aligned}\Pi_{me} = &-\frac{1}{2}\{\mathbf{c}_e\}^{\mathrm{T}}[\mathbf{H}_e]\{\mathbf{c}_e\} - \{\mathbf{d}_e\}^{\mathrm{T}}\{\mathbf{g}_e\} + \{\mathbf{c}_e\}^{\mathrm{T}}[\mathbf{G}_e]\{\mathbf{d}_e\} \\ &-\frac{1}{2}\{\mathbf{d}_e\}^{\mathrm{T}}[\mathbf{F}_e]\{\mathbf{d}_e\} + \{\mathbf{d}_e\}^{\mathrm{T}}\{\mathbf{f}_e\} - \{\mathbf{a}_e\}.\end{aligned} \tag{21.32}$$

By virtue of the stationary condition

$$\left.\begin{aligned}\frac{\partial \Pi_{me}}{\partial\{\mathbf{c}_e\}^{\mathrm{T}}} = \{0\} \\ \frac{\partial \Pi_{me}}{\partial\{\mathbf{d}_e\}^{\mathrm{T}}} = \{0\}\end{aligned}\right\}, \tag{21.33}$$

we have the following stiffness equations for determining all unknowns:

$$\left.\begin{aligned}[\mathbf{K}_e]\{\mathbf{d}_e\} = \{\mathbf{g}_e\} - \{\mathbf{f}_e\} \\ \{\mathbf{c}_e\} = [\mathbf{H}_e]^{-1}[\mathbf{G}_e]\{\mathbf{d}_e\}\end{aligned}\right\}, \tag{21.34}$$

where

$$\left.\begin{aligned}&[\mathbf{H}_e] = \int_{\Gamma_e} \{\mathbf{Q}\}^{\mathrm{T}}\{\mathbf{N}\} d\Gamma && [\mathbf{G}_e] = \int_{\Gamma_e} \{\mathbf{Q}\}^{\mathrm{T}}\{\tilde{\mathbf{N}}\} d\Gamma \\ &[\mathbf{F}_e] = \int_{\Gamma_{ce}} h\{\tilde{\mathbf{N}}\}^{\mathrm{T}}\{\tilde{\mathbf{N}}\} d\Gamma && \{\mathbf{f}_e\} = \int_{\Gamma_{ce}} H_\infty \Phi_\infty \{\tilde{\mathbf{N}}\}^{\mathrm{T}} d\Gamma \\ &\{\mathbf{g}_e\} = \int_{\Gamma_{eq}} \{\tilde{\mathbf{N}}\}_e^{\mathrm{T}} \bar{q} \, d\Gamma && \{\mathbf{a}_e\} = \int_{\Gamma_{ce}} \frac{H_\infty \Phi_\infty^2}{2} d\Gamma\end{aligned}\right\}. \tag{21.35}$$

21.4 Numerical Examples

To simulate the temperature distribution and investigate the effect of blood perfusion on the temperature variation in the human eye model, the presented approach is applied to a practical example in the following and the obtained results are compared with those from ABAQUS. For reference, the values of some control parameters related to the outer boundary conditions are listed in Table 21.1 [11,12]. Here, the ambient convection coefficient is set

TABLE 21.1
Control Parameters Related to Boundary Conditions

Control Parameters	Value
Blood temperature, T_b	37 (°C)
Blood convection coefficient, h_b	65 (W/m^2 K)
Ambient temperature, T_∞	25 (°C)
Ambient convection coefficient, h_∞	10 (W/m^2 K)
Evaporation rate of tear	40 (W/m^2)

to be 10 W/m^2 K, which corresponds to a natural convection, and the ambient temperature is taken to be 25°C, a general temperature of air at spring and autumn [12]. The evaporation rate of tear is set to be 40 W/m^2, which is in the range [20, 100] W/m^2 and corresponds to tear evaporation in the normal eye [24,28]. Besides, the thermal conductivities of the specified five regions are, respectively, 0.58 W/m K in R_1 and R_2, 0.4 W/m K in R_3, 0.603 W/m K in R_4, and 1.0042 W/m K in R_5 [11–13]. To understand the importance of blood flow in the thermoregulation of the human eye, the density and specific heat of blood are, respectively, taken to be 1050 kg/m^3 and 3600 J/kg/K, and the blood perfusion rate in R_5 is assumed to vary in the range of [0, 0.0005, 0.0010, 0.0015] mL/s/mL.

In addition, it should be mentioned that the geometric dimensions of the computing model employed in this chapter are taken from the literature [12] and regenerated, so the geometric dimension of the computing model here might be different from that in the existing reference [12], and then the results may have some discrepancy with the existing eye model.

To perform the hybrid finite element analysis, the eyeball domain is discretized with 1374 eight-node hybrid elements, and a total of 4243 nodal degrees of freedom are included, as shown in Figure 21.4.

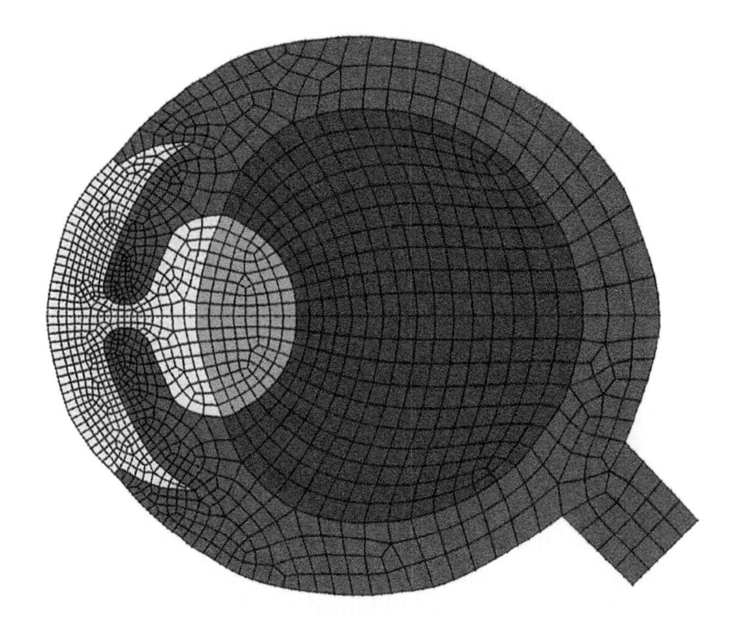

FIGURE 21.4
Finite element mesh for bioheat analysis in the eyeball.

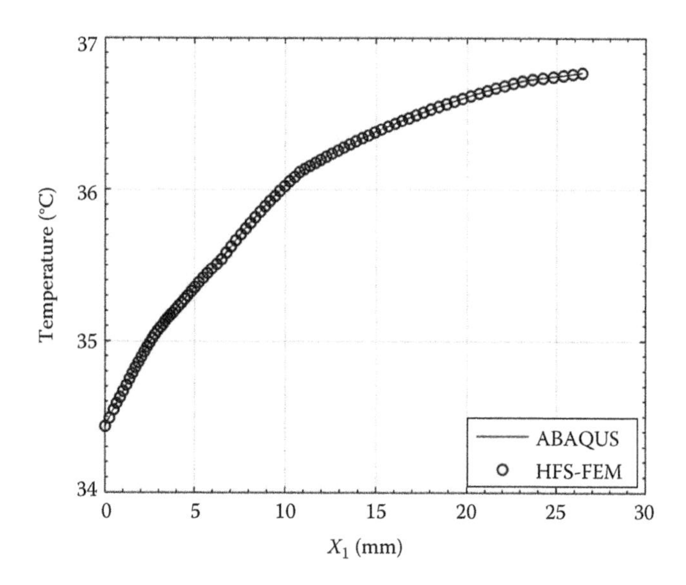

FIGURE 21.5
Temperature distribution along the papillary axis of eyeball.

21.4.1 Validation Study

To verify the proposed hybrid finite element formulation, the case in which the blood perfusion rates in all regions of the eyeball are neglected is firstly considered. The absence of the blood perfusion enables us to seek the solution of bioheat transfer in the system of standard Laplace-type partial differential equation. The distribution of temperature along the papillary axis is plotted in Figure 21.5, in which the results from ABAQUS with the same element mesh as shown in Figure 21.4 are provided for the purpose of comparison. It can be seen that a good agreement between the proposed HFS-FEM and ABAQUS is captured. The temperatures at the center of the corneal surface are, respectively, 34.435°C and 34.436°C from the two methods. The temperature discrepancy between the two methods is only 0.001°C or percentage 0.004% at the center of the corneal surface. Moreover, the temperature isotherms in the entire domain are displayed in Figure 21.6, in which the solid lines represent the results of the proposed HFS-FEM and the dashed lines represent those of ABAQUS. As expected, we observe that there is a good agreement between the results of HFS-FEM and ABAQUS. Thus, the presented hybrid finite element model is verified.

21.4.2 Investigation of Blood Perfusion Rate in the Sclera

To reveal the importance of blood flow in the thermoregulation of the eyeball, we introduce the blood perfusion rate only in the sclera in the study. As a result, the bioheat transfer in the sclera is governed by the Helmholtz-type partial differential equation, while in the remaining regions, the bioheat behavior is governed by the Laplace-type partial differential equation. By the present hybrid finite element formulation, it is easy to treat such mixed problem, and just different fundamental solutions are required to generate the kernel matrix of the element interior temperature field. The structure of the present algorithm keeps unvaried. For different values of blood perfusion rates in the sclera, the induced temperature distribution along the papillary axis of eyeball is displayed in Figure 21.7,

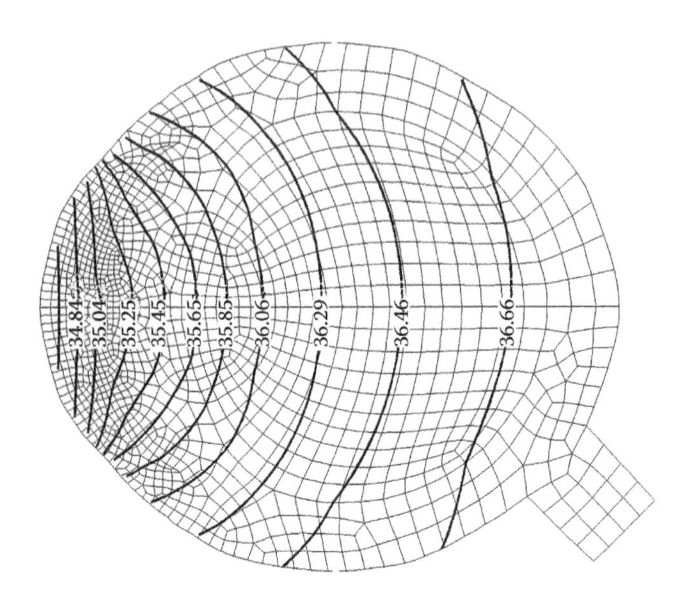

FIGURE 21.6
Isothermal lines in the eyeball domain.

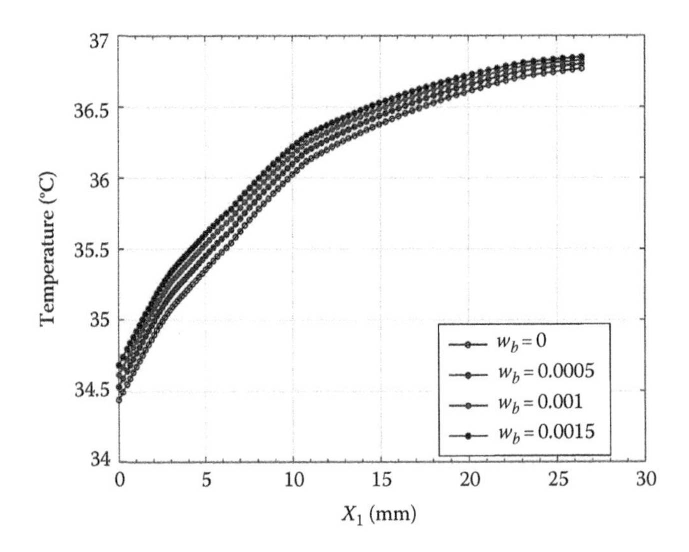

FIGURE 21.7
(See color insert.) Temperature distribution along the papillary axis of eyeball for various blood perfusion rates.

from which it is found that the higher the temperature is, the larger the blood perfusion rate becomes. The main reason is that the presence of blood perfusion activity in the sclera makes the heat energy rapidly flow from the blood vessels in the sclera region into the eyeball, compared to the case without blood perfusion; thus, a heating effect takes place. To see more clearly the influence of blood perfusion, the temperature change at the center of the corneal surface is tabulated in Table 21.2. We can see that there is an approximately steady increase in the value of [0.07, 0.09]°C for the temperature at the center of the corneal surface for every increment in the value of 0.0005 mL/s/mL for blood perfusion rate.

TABLE 21.2

Temperature Change at the Center of the Corneal Surface

Blood Perfusion Rate in the Sclera (mL/s/mL)	Temperature (°C)
$w_b=0$	34.435
$w_b=0.0005$	34.529
$w_b=0.0010$	34.610
$w_b=0.0015$	34.681

21.5 Conclusion

A hybrid finite element model with fundamental solutions as the intra-element trial function was developed to investigate the steady-state bioheat transfer in a normal human eye. By using the fundamental solution in the proposed hybrid finite element formulation, the constructed hybrid variational functional involving the convection effect includes element boundary integrals only. Results from the presented algorithm are firstly compared with those from ABAQUS in the absence of blood perfusion activity within the sclera, and the agreement between them shows the promise of the present hybrid finite element model for heat transfer applications in the human eye. Further, to reveal the influence of blood perfusion in the eye model, a further analysis is performed by adjusting the specified values of blood perfusion rate in the sclera. Numerical results show that the change of blood perfusion rate can significantly affect the temperature distribution in the eyeball by blood heating effect.

Acknowledgments

The research in this chapter is partially supported by the Natural Science Foundation of China under grant no. 11102059 and the Foundation for University Key Teacher by the Henan Province, China, under grant no. 2011 GGJS-083.

References

1. Bathe, K. J. 1996. *Finite Element Procedures*. Englewood Cliffs, NJ: Prentice Hall.
2. Brebbia, C. A., Telles, J. C. F., and Wrobel, L. C. 1984. *Boundary Element Techniques: Theory and Applications in Engineering*. New York: Springer-Verlag.
3. Brinkmann, R., Koop, N., Droege, G., Grotehusmann, U., Huber, A., and Birngruber, R. 1994. Investigations on laser thermokeratoplasty. In *Proceedings of the SPIE*, pp. 120–130, Budapest, Hungary.
4. Cao, L. L., Wang, H., and Qin, Q. H. 2012. Fundamental solution based graded element model for steady-state heat transfer in FGM. *Acta Mechanica Solida Sinica* 25(4): 377–392.

5. Chua, K. J., Ho, J. C., Chou, S. K., and Islam, M. R. 2005. On the study of the temperature distribution within a human eye subjected to a laser source. *International Communications in Heat and Mass Transfer* 32(8): 1057–1065.
6. Fairweather, G. and Karageorghis, A. 1998. The method of fundamental solutions for elliptic boundary value problems. *Advances in Computational Mathematics* 9(1/2): 69–95.
7. Flyckt, V. M. M., Raaymakers, B. W., and Lagendijk, J. J. W. 2006. Modelling the impact of blood flow on the temperature distribution in the human eye and the orbit: Fixed heat transfer coefficients versus the Pennes bioheat model versus discrete blood vessels. *Physics in Medicine and Biology* 51(19): 5007–5021.
8. Mathon, R. and Johnson, R. L. 1977. The approximate solution of elliptic boundary value problems by fundamental solutions. *SIAM Journal on Numerical Analysis* 14: 638–650.
9. Mainster, M. A., White, T. J., and Tips, J. H. 1990. Corneal thermal response to the CO_2 laser. *Applied Optics* 9(3): 665–667.
10. Narasimhan, A., Jha, K. K., and Gopal, L. 2010. Transient simulations of heat transfer in human eye undergoing laser surgery. *International Journal of Heat and Mass Transfer* 53(1): 482–490.
11. Ng, E. Y. K. and Ooi, E. H. 2006. FEM simulation of the eye structure with bioheat analysis. *Computer Methods and Programs in Biomedicine* 82(3): 268–276.
12. Ooi, E. H., Ang, W. T., and Ng, E. Y. K. 2007. Bioheat transfer in the human eye: A boundary element approach. *Engineering Analysis with Boundary Elements* 31(6): 494–500.
13. Ooi, E. H., Ang, W. T., and Ng, E. Y. K. 2008. A boundary element model of the human eye undergoing laser thermokeratoplasty. *Computers in Biology and Medicine* 38(6): 727–737.
14. Ooi, E. H., Ang, W. T., and Ng, E. Y. K. 2009. A boundary element model for investigating the effects of eye tumor on the temperature distribution inside the human eye. *Computers in Biology and Medicine* 39(8): 667–677.
15. Ooi, E. H. and Ng, E. Y. K. 2008. Simulation of aqueous humor hydrodynamics in human eye heat transfer. *Computers in Biology and Medicine* 38(2): 252–262.
16. Pennes, H. H. 1948. Analysis of tissue and arterial blood temperatures in the resting human forearm. *Journal of Applied Physiology* 1(2): 93–102.
17. Peratta, A. 2008. 3D low frequency electromagnetic modelling of the human eye with boundary elements: Application to conductive keratoplasty. *Engineering Analysis with Boundary Elements* 32(9): 726–735.
18. Pian, T. H. H. and Wu, C. C. 2006. *Hybrid and Incompatible Finite Element Methods*. Boca Raton, FL: Chapman & Hall.
19. Qin, Q. H. 2000. *The Trefftz Finite and Boundary Element Method*. Southampton, U.K.: WIT Press.
20. Qin, Q. H. 2005. Trefftz finite element method and its applications. *Applied Mechanics Reviews* 58: 316–337.
21. Qin, Q. H. and Mai, Y. W. 2002. BEM for crack–hole problems in thermopiezoelectric materials. *Engineering Fracture Mechanics* 69(5): 577–588.
22. Qin, Q. H. and Wang, H. 2009. *Matlab and C Programming for Trefftz Finite Element Methods*. Boca Raton, FL: CRC Press.
23. Qin, Q. H. and Wang, H. 2013. Special circular hole elements for thermal analysis in cellular solids with multiple circular holes. *International Journal of Computational Methods* 10(4): 1350008.
24. Scott, J. A. 1988. A finite element model of heat transport in the human eye. *Physics in Medicine and Biology* 33(2): 227–242.
25. Wang, H., Cao, L. L., and Qin, Q. H. 2012. Hybrid graded element model for nonlinear functionally graded materials. *Mechanics of Advanced Materials and Structures* 19(8): 590–602.
26. Wang, H. and Qin, Q. H. 2008. Meshless approach for thermo-mechanical analysis of functionally graded materials. *Engineering Analysis with Boundary Elements* 32(9): 704–712.
27. Wang, H. and Qin, Q. H. 2009. Hybrid FEM with fundamental solutions as trial functions for heat conduction simulation. *Acta Mechanica Solida Sinica* 22(5): 487–498.
28. Wang, H. and Qin, Q. H. 2010. FE approach with Green's function as internal trial function for simulating bioheat transfer in the human eye. *Archives of Mechanics* 62(6): 493–510.

29. Wang, H. and Qin, Q. H. 2010. Fundamental-solution-based finite element model for plane orthotropic elastic bodies. *European Journal of Mechanics-A/Solids* 29(5): 801–809.
30. Wang, H. and Qin, Q. H. 2011. Fundamental-solution-based hybrid FEM for plane elasticity with special elements. *Computational Mechanics* 48(5): 515–528.
31. Wang, H. and Qin, Q. H. 2011. Special fiber elements for thermal analysis of fiber-reinforced composites. *Engineering Computation* 28(8): 1079–1097.
32. Wang, H. and Qin, Q. H. 2012. Boundary integral based graded element for elastic analysis of 2D functionally graded plates. *European Journal of Mechanics-A/Solids* 33: 12–23.
33. Wang, H. and Qin, Q. H. 2012. A fundamental solution-based finite element model for analyzing multi-layer skin burn injury. *Journal of Mechanics in Medicine and Biology* 12(5): 1250027.
34. Wang, H. and Qin, Q. H. 2012. A new special element for stress concentration analysis of a plate with elliptical holes. *Acta Mechanica* 223: 1323–1340.
35. Wang, H., Qin, Q. H., and Kang, Y. L. 2005. A new meshless method for steady-state heat conduction problems in anisotropic and inhomogeneous media. *Archive of Applied Mechanics* 74(8): 563–579.
36. Wang, H., Qin, Q. H., and Kang, Y. L. 2006. A meshless model for transient heat conduction in functionally graded materials. *Computational Mechanics* 38(1): 51–60.

22

Effects of Electromagnetic Fields on Specific Absorption Rate and Heat Transfer in the Human Eye

Teerapot Wessapan and Phadungsak Rattanadecho

CONTENTS

Nomenclature

C	Specific heat capacity (J/(kg K))
E	Electric field intensity (V/m)
e	The tear evaporation heat loss (W/m^2)
f	Frequency of incident wave (Hz)
H	Magnetic field (A/m)
h	Convection coefficient (W/(m^2 K))
j	Current density (A/m^2)
k	Thermal conductivity (W/(m K))
n	Normal vector
p	Pressure (N/m^2)
Q	Heat source (W/m^3)

T	Temperature (K)
u	Velocity (m/s)
t	Time

Greek Letters

β	Volume expansion coefficient (1/K)
μ	Magnetic permeability (H/m)
ε	Permittivity (F/m)
σ	Electric conductivity (S/m)
ω	Angular frequency (rad/s)
ρ	Density (kg/m^3)
ω_b	Blood perfusion rate (1/s)
Γ	External surface area

Subscripts

am	Ambient
b	Blood
ext	External
i	Subdomain
met	Metabolic
r	Relative
ref	Reference
0	Free space, initial condition

22.1 Introduction

The electromagnetic (EM) waves of the different power levels and frequencies penetrate deep into the human body causing health risks. In recent years, there has been some increasing public concern with the interaction between the human body and the EM fields. Since the eye is one of the most sensitive organs to the EM fields, the high-intensity EM fields may lead to a variety of ocular effects. However, the resulting thermophysiologic response of the eye to EM fields is not well understood. Therefore, it is important to investigate the ocular effects occurred during exposure to EM fields. Although the safety standards written in terms of maximum tissue specific absorption rate (SAR) values are regulated, they are not stated in terms of maximum temperature increase in the eye caused by EM energy absorption. The eye temperature increasing gradually can cause serious long-term effects on eyesight and vision. There have been medical case reports of cataract formation in humans via microwave radiation [1]. It is reported that a temperature increase in the eye of 3°C–5°C leads to induce cataract formation [2] and a temperature above 41°C is necessary for production of posterior lens opacities [3]. Therefore, to gain insight into the phenomenon of eye temperature distribution induced by EM fields, it is necessary to have a detailed knowledge of the absorbed power distribution and the temperature distribution.

Previous studies focused on the effects of EM fields on the human eye [4,5]. Nevertheless, their analysis has been conducted based on the maximum SAR values permitted by public safety standards regulation [6,7]. For example, in studies of an interaction between the EM fields and the human eye, most of them have mainly focused on SAR and have not considered the heat transfer. Consequently, it could not be fully understood. In addition, there have been few experimental data on the correlation of SAR levels with the temperature increase in the human tissue. Therefore, a modeling of heat transport is needed to completely explain the actual process of interaction between the EM fields and the human eye.

Thermal modeling of human tissue is important as a tool to explore the effects of external heat sources and investigate abnormalities in the tissue. Recently, the modeling of heat transport in human tissue has been considered by many researchers [8–20]. Most studies of heat transfer analysis in the human eye used heat conduction equation [8–14]. Some studies carried out on natural convection in human eye based on heat conduction model [15,16]. Ooi and Ng [16,17] studied the effect of aqueous humor (AH) hydrodynamics on the heat transfer in the eye based on heat conduction model. Meanwhile, the Pennes' bioheat equation [18,19], based on the heat diffusion equation for a blood-perfused tissue, is used for modeling of heat transfer in the human eye as well [20,21]. Ooi and Ng also developed a 3D model of the human eye [22], extending their 2D model [21]. Recently, researchers have used the porous media models to investigate the transport phenomena in biological media instead of a simplified bioheat model [23–25]. Shafahi and Vafai [26] proposed the porous media along with natural convection model to analyze the eye thermal characteristics during exposure to thermal disturbances. Narasimhan and Vishnampet [27] proposed the porous medium model of the sclera and the choroid to study the effect of choroidal blood flow on transscleral drug delivery to the retina. Many researchers have been tried to conduct the advanced model using the coupled model of heat and laser irradiation in the human eye [28–30]. Results from similar models of Ooi et al. [30] for various applications were also presented in continuation [31–34].

Although the porous media and natural convection models of the human eye have been used in the previous biomedical studies [15–16,26,27], most studies of the human eye exposed to EM fields have not been considering the porous media approach, and natural convection approach is sparse or nonexistent. Wessapan and Rattanadecho [35] investigated the SAR and temperature distributions of EM fields in the eye using porous media theory. There are few studies on an interaction between the temperature and the EM fields in realistic physical model of the human organs especially the eye due to its complexity. Therefore, to provide information on exposure levels and health effects from EM fields, it is necessary to simulate both of the EM fields and the heat transfer, based on porous media theory within an anatomical model particularly the eye.

In this study, a 2D eye model was exploited to simulate the SAR and temperature distributions. EM wave propagation in the eye was investigated by using Maxwell's equations. An analysis of heat transfer in the eye exposed to a transverse magnetic (TM) mode of EM fields was investigated using a developed heat transfer model (included the conduction and natural convection heat transfer mode), which was proposed by Shafahi and Vafai [26]. The SAR and the temperature distribution in various parts of the human eye during exposure to EM fields at 900 MHz, which are obtained by numerical solution of EM wave propagation and heat transfer equation, are presented. This chapter is based on empirical data from the work of Wessapan and Rattanadecho [35], with permission from ASME.

22.2 Problem Formulation

In fact, the human exposures to EM radiation have increased exponentially. The human eye is exposed daily to radiation from sources such as mobile phones, microwave oven,

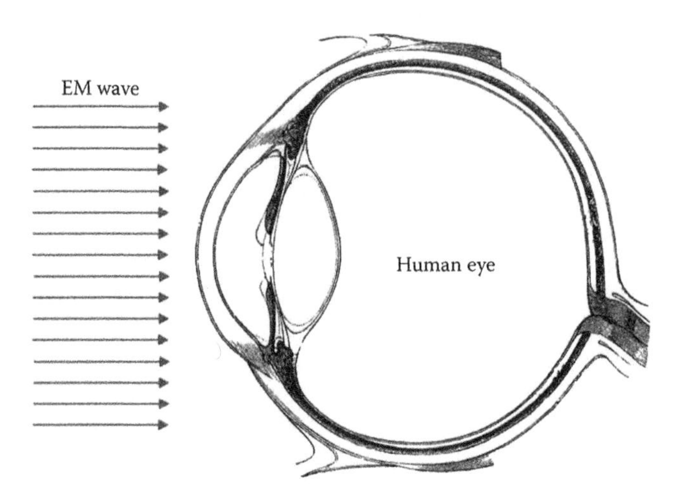

FIGURE 22.1
(See color insert.) EM fields from an EM radiation device.

monitors, and wireless networks and other EM fields commonly found in our daily life. It is known that the human eye is one of the most sensitive organs to EM radiation. This is because the crystalline lens and the cornea are nonvascular tissue with low metabolism and the eye has no thermal sensors and protective reflexes. An investigation of the human eye exposure to EM fields can be done with difficulty due to the eye's complex geometry and its being a heterogeneous tissue. Moreover, this investigation cannot be done by experiments due to the ethical considerations. Exposing a human to EM fields for experimental purposes is still restricted. It is more convenient and ethical to develop a realistic human eye model through numerical simulation. Figure 22.1 shows radiation of EM fields from an EM radiation device to the human body. These EM fields fall on the human eye that causes heating in the deeper tissue, which leads to tissue damage and cataract formation.

Our first step in the evaluation of the effects of a certain exposure to EM fields in the eye is to determine the induced internal EM fields and their spatial distributions. Thereafter, with the EM energy absorption resulting in an increased temperature in the eye, other interactions could be then considered. This study considers the coupling between the EM and heat transfer equations to model the distribution of temperature fields induced by EM radiation in the eye.

In this study, the eye model, which is based on a physical model we developed in the previous research [26], comprises seven types of tissue including posterior chamber, anterior chamber, cornea, iris, sclera, lens, and vitreous. Different types of tissue have different dielectric and thermal properties. In the sclera layer, there are two more layers known as choroid and retina that are relatively thin compared to the size of the sclera itself. To simplify the problem, these layers are assumed to be homogeneous. The iris and the sclera, which have the same properties, are modeled together as one homogenous region [16]. Figure 22.2 shows the 2D eye model used in this study [35]. The dielectric [36,37] and thermal properties [16] of tissue are shown in Tables 22.1 and 22.2, respectively. Each tissue is assumed to be homogeneous and electrically as well as thermally isotropic.

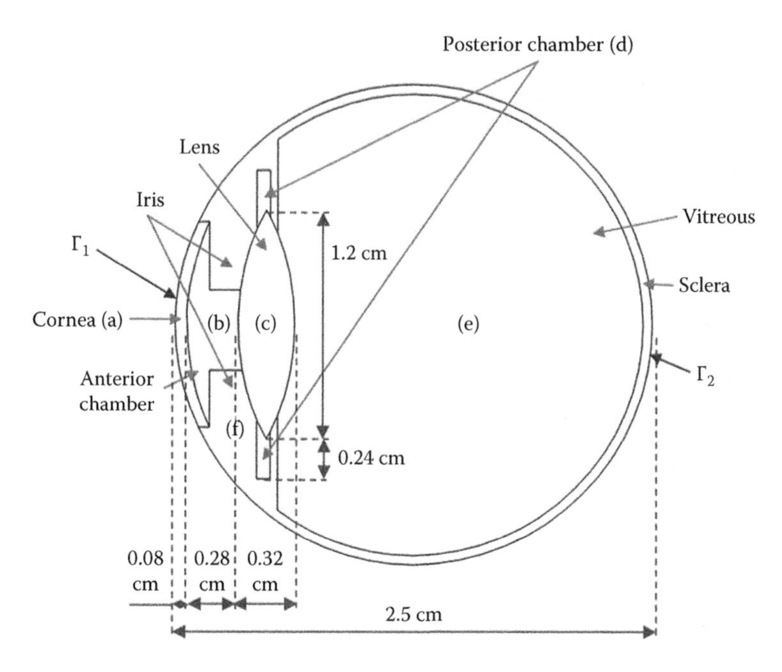

FIGURE 22.2
Human eye vertical cross section. (From Wessapan, T. and Rattanadecho, P., *ASME Trans. J. Heat Transfer*, 134, 091101, 2012. With permission.)

TABLE 22.1
Dielectric Properties of Tissues at 900 MHz

Tissue	ε_r	σ (S/m)
Cornea (a)	52.0	1.85
Anterior chamber (b)	73.0	1.97
Lens (c)	51.3	0.89
Posterior chamber (d)	73.0	1.97
Vitreous (e)	74.3	1.97
Sclera (f)	52.1	1.22
Iris (f)	52.1	1.22

Source: Wessapan, T. and Rattanadecho, P., *ASME Trans. J. Heat Transfer*, 134, 091101, 2012. With permission.

22.3 Mathematical Model Formulation

The intensity of the internal fields in the body depends on various parameters such as an operating frequency, the power intensity, a mode of propagation, the body geometry, the tissue dielectric properties, a distance from EM source, and the presence of other objects in the body vicinity. When the EM waves pass from one medium to another, they can be absorbed, reflected, refracted, or transmitted, depending on the dielectric property of the

TABLE 22.2
Thermal Properties of Human Eyes

Tissue	ρ (kg/m^3)	k (W/m °C)	C_p (J/kg °C)	μ (N s/m^2)	β (1/K)
Cornea (a)	1050	0.58	4178	—	—
Anterior chamber (b)	996	0.58	3997	0.00074	0.000337
Lens (c)	1000	0.4	3000	—	—
Posterior chamber (d)	996	0.58	3997	—	—
Vitreous (e)	1100	0.603	4178	—	—
Sclera (f)	1050	1.0042	3180	—	—
Iris (f)	1050	1.0042	3180	—	—

Source: Wessapan, T. and Rattanadecho, P., *ASME Trans. J. Heat Transfer*, 134, 091101, 2012. With permission.

exposed body and the operating frequency of the EM source. Most of the absorbed EM energies are converted into heat.

22.3.1 Electromagnetic Wave Propagation Equation

EM waves are a phenomenon in the form of self-propagating waves in a free space or in matter. EM waves consist of electric and magnetic fields oscillating in phase perpendicular to each other and to the direction of wave propagation. Maxwell's equations for electric and magnetic fields are used to investigate EM wave propagation in different media and radiation. An EM wave propagating in a linear, isotropic, homogeneous medium can basically be described by Maxwell's equations:

$$\nabla \times \bar{E} = -\frac{\partial \bar{B}}{\partial t} \tag{22.1}$$

$$\nabla \times \bar{B} = \frac{1}{c^2}\frac{\partial \bar{E}}{\partial t} \tag{22.2}$$

$$\nabla \cdot \bar{E} = 0 \tag{22.3}$$

$$\nabla \cdot \bar{B} = 0 \tag{22.4}$$

where
$\bar{E}$ is the electric field intensity (V/m)
$\bar{B}$ is the magnetic flux density (Wb/m^2 or T)
c is the light velocity in the medium (m/s)
$c_0 = 2.99792458 \times 108$ is the speed of light in free space

$$c = \frac{c_0}{n} \tag{22.5}$$

where n is the refractive index of the medium, $n = \sqrt{\varepsilon_r}$ and ε_r is the relative dielectric constant. The other relevant boundary conditions are already given in Figure 23.3.

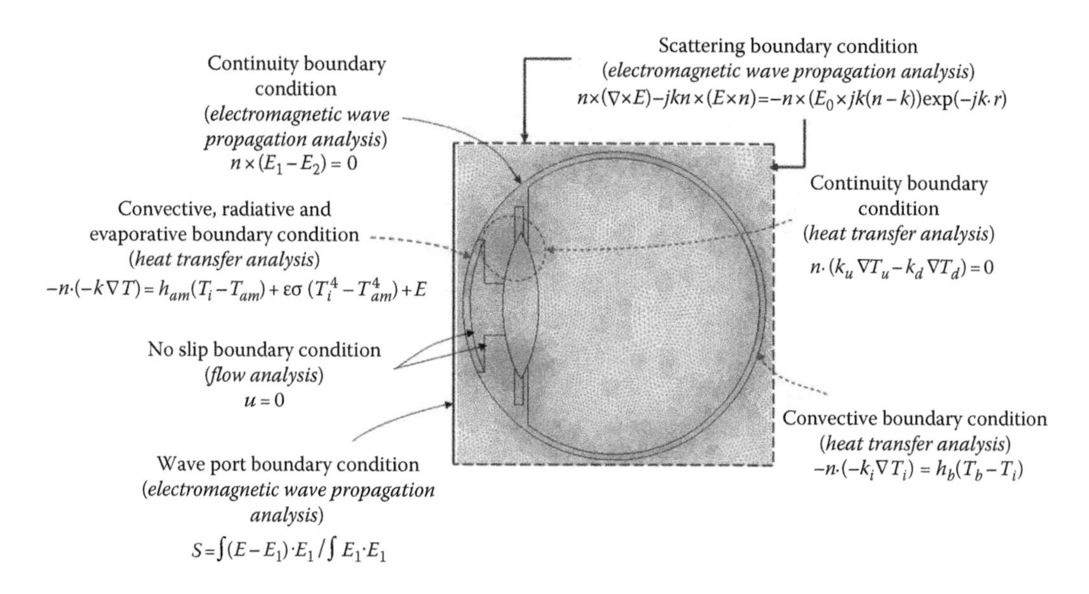

FIGURE 22.3
Boundary condition for the analysis of EM wave propagation and heat transfer. (From Wessapan, T. and Rattanadecho, P., *ASME Trans. J. Heat Transfer*, 134, 091101, 2012. With permission.)

Maxwell's equations for free space are expressed by

$$\nabla \times \bar{E} = j\omega B \tag{22.6}$$

$$\nabla \times \bar{B} = \frac{-1}{c^2} j\omega \vec{E} \tag{22.7}$$

$$\nabla \cdot \bar{E} = 0 \tag{22.8}$$

$$\nabla \cdot \bar{B} = 0 \tag{22.9}$$

where
- ω is the angular frequency (rad/s)
- $j = \sqrt{-1}$

The general form of Maxwell's equations is simplified to demonstrate the EM fields penetrated in the eye as the following equation:

$$\nabla \times \left(\left(\varepsilon_r - \frac{j\sigma}{\omega\varepsilon_0} \right)^{-1} \nabla \times H_z \right) - \mu_r k_0^2 H_z = 0 \tag{22.10}$$

where
- H is the magnetic field (A/m)
- μ_r is the relative magnetic permeability
- ε_r is the relative dielectric constant
- $\varepsilon_0 = 8.8542 \times 10^{-12}$ F/m is the free space permittivity
- k_0 is the free space wave number (1/m)

22.3.1.1 Boundary Condition for Wave Propagation Analysis

This study investigated ocular changes during exposure to EM radiation with a particular power density. A schematic description of a boundary condition is shown in Figure 22.3: the uniform wave flux falls on the left side of the eye. Therefore, for the left boundary, an EM simulator uses a TM wave propagation port with a specified power density:

$$S = \frac{\int \left((E - E_1) \cdot E_1\right) dA_1}{\int \left(E_1 \cdot E_1\right) dA_1} \tag{22.11}$$

where
- E is the electric field intensity (V/m)
- E_1 is fundamental value of electric field for port 1

Boundary conditions along the interfaces between different mediums are considered as continuity boundary conditions:

$$n \times (E_1 - E_2) = 0 \tag{22.12}$$

The outer side of the calculated domain, that is, free space, is considered as a scattering boundary condition:

$$n \times \left(\nabla \times E_z\right) - jkE_z = -jk(1 - k \cdot n)E_{0z} \exp(-jk \cdot r) \tag{22.13}$$

where
- k is the wave number (m^{-1})
- n is the normal vector
- $j = \sqrt{-1}$
- E_0 is the incident plane wave (V/m)
- E_z is the transverse component of the electric field

Microwave EM exposure levels are expressed in terms of power density (in W/m^2 or W/ft^2).

However, for microwave band, both the electric field intensity (in V/m) and the magnetic field intensity (in A/m) are used to represent the fields. According to the International Commission of Non-Ionizing Radiation Protection (ICNIRP) guidelines [6], an average SAR (in W/kg) (or whole-body average SAR) is defined as the ratio of the total absorbed power in the exposed body to its mass where the local SAR refers to the absorbed energy value per unit volume or mass, which can be arbitrarily small. The SAR is defined as

$$\text{SAR} = \frac{\sigma}{2\rho}|E|^2 \tag{22.14}$$

where
- σ is the electric conductivity (S/m)
- ρ is the tissue density (kg/m^3)

The SAR can also be determined from the increase in tissue temperature over a short period of time following the exposure as

$$\frac{\Delta T}{\Delta t} = \frac{\text{SAR}}{C} \tag{22.15}$$

where
- ΔT is the temperature increase
- Δt is the exposure duration
- C is the specific heat

22.3.2 Heat Transfer Equation

From a macroscopic point of view, thermal effects resulting from the EM waves' absorption inside the biological tissue are expressed in terms of the bioheat equation [18,19] based on the heat diffusion equation, which can be written as

$$\rho C \frac{\partial T}{\partial t} = \nabla \cdot (k \nabla T) + \rho_b C_b \omega_b (T_b - T) + Q_{met} + Q_{ext} \tag{22.16}$$

where
- ρ is the tissue density (kg/m^3)
- C is the tissue heat capacity (J/(kg K))
- k is the tissue thermal conductivity (W/(m K))
- T is the tissue temperature (°C)
- T_b is the blood temperature (°C)
- ρ_b is the blood density (kg/m^3)
- C_b is the blood heat capacity
- ω_b is the blood perfusion rate (1/s)
- Q_{met} is the metabolism heat source (W/m^3)
- Q_{ext} is the external heat source (EM heat source density) (W/m^3)

$$Q_{ext} = \frac{\sigma}{2} |E|^2 \tag{22.17}$$

This study utilized two pertinent thermal models to investigate the heat transfer behavior of the eye when exposed to the EM fields.

Model I: Conventional heat transfer model [21]

This model assumes the metabolic heat generation and the blood perfusion in the eye to be zero. The governing equation therefore looked just like the classical heat conduction equation:

$$\rho_i C_i \frac{\partial T_i}{\partial t} = \nabla \cdot (k_i \nabla T_i) + Q_{ext}; \quad i = a, b, c, d, e, f \tag{22.18}$$

where
- i denotes each subdomain in the eye model as shown in Figure 22.2
- ρ is the tissue density (kg/m^3)
- C is the tissue heat capacity (J/(kg K))
- k is the tissue thermal conductivity (W/(m K))
- T is the tissue temperature (K)
- t is the time

Model II: Developed heat transfer model [26]

In this model, the fluid motion is considered only inside the anterior chamber [16]. There is a blood flow in the iris/sclera part, by which the blood flow plays a role to adjust the temperature of the eye [26]. For the rest of the parts, the metabolic heat generation is neglected due to the fact that these parts comprise mainly water [16]. The governing equation for the flow of heat in cornea, posterior chamber, lens, and vitreous is the same as Equation 22.18.

This model accounts for the existence of AH in the anterior chamber. The heat transfer process consists of both conduction and natural convection, which can be expressed as follows:

Continuity equation

$$\nabla \cdot u_i = 0; \quad i = b \tag{22.19}$$

Momentum equation

$$\rho_i \frac{\partial u_i}{\partial t} + \rho_i u_i \nabla \cdot u_i = -\nabla p_i + \nabla \cdot \left[\mu \left(\nabla u_i + \nabla u_i^T \right) \right] + \rho_i g \beta_i \left(T_i - T_{ref} \right); \quad i = b \tag{22.20}$$

where

β is the volume expansion coefficient (1/K)
u is the velocity (m/s)
p is the pressure (N/m^2)
μ is the dynamic viscosity of AH (N s/m^2)
T_{ref} is the reference temperature that we consider here as 37°C

The effects of buoyancy due to the temperature gradient are modeled using the Boussinesq approximation, which states that the density changes to the temperature change and the pressure perturbations are negligible [16].

The energy equation is expressed as follows:

$$\rho_i C_i \frac{\partial T_i}{\partial t} - \nabla \cdot (k_i \nabla T_i) = -\rho C_i u_i \cdot \nabla T_i + Q_{ext} \tag{22.21}$$

The sclera/iris is modeled as a porous medium with blood perfusion, by which the local thermal equilibrium is assumed between the blood and the tissue. A modified Pennes' bioheat equation [26,38] is used to calculate the temperature distribution in the sclera/iris tissue:

$$(1-\varepsilon)\rho_i C_i \frac{\partial T_i}{\partial t} = \nabla \cdot ((1-\varepsilon) k_i \nabla T_i) + \rho_b C_b \omega_b (T_b - T_i) + Q_{ext}; \quad i = f \tag{22.22}$$

where ε is the porosity.

22.3.2.1 Boundary Condition for Heat Transfer Analysis

The heat transfer analysis excluding the surrounding space is considered only in the eye. The cornea surface as shown in Figure 22.3 is considered as the convective, radiative, and evaporative boundary condition for all of the models:

$$-n \cdot (-k\nabla T) = h_{am}(T_i - T_{am}) + \varepsilon\sigma(T_i^4 - T_{am}^4) + e \quad \text{on } \Gamma_1 \; i = a \tag{22.23}$$

where

Γ_i is the external surface area corresponding to section i

e is the tear evaporation heat loss (W/m^2)

T_{am} is the ambient temperature (K)

h_{am} is the convection coefficient (W/(m^2 K))

The blood temperature generally assumed to be the same as the body's core temperature causes heat to be transferred into the eye [16]. The surface of the sclera is assumed to be a convective boundary condition for all of the models:

$$-n \cdot (-k_i\nabla T_i) = h_b(T_b - T_i) \quad \text{on } \Gamma_2 \; i = f \tag{22.24}$$

where

h_b is the convection coefficient of blood

Γ_1 and Γ_2 are the corneal surface and the sclera surface of the eye, respectively

22.3.3 Calculation Procedure

The computational scheme used in this study is applied to assemble a finite element model and compute a local heat generation. The EM calculation is carried out by using tissue properties. To obtain a good approximation, a fine mesh is specified in the sensitive areas, by which a variable mesh method for solving the problem is proposed as in Figure 22.4. The governing equations with initial and boundary conditions are then solved. The 2D model with triangular elements is used to discretize the domain, and the Lagrange quadratic is then used to approximate temperature and SAR variation across each element. To reduce the global mesh size, a mesh convergence test was performed. The mesh with approximately 10,000 elements is obtained.

22.4 Results and Discussion

In this analysis, the effect of power density (5, 10, 50, and 100 mW/cm^2) on distributions of SAR and temperature profiles in the eye is systematically investigated using two models: the conventional heat transfer model and the developed heat transfer model. The models of the EM and thermal fields are solved numerically. The dielectric and thermal properties as in Tables 22.1 and 22.2, respectively, are used for the simulation. In this study, we follow the guidelines of the ICNIRP, the radiated power used at the maximum SAR value of 2 W/kg (general public exposure) and 10 W/kg (occupational exposure) [6].

22.4.1 Verification of the Model

In order to verify the accuracy of the present numerical models, the simulated results from this study are validated against the numerical results obtained by Shafahi and Vafai [26] who studied the same geometric model as this. Moreover, the numerical results are then

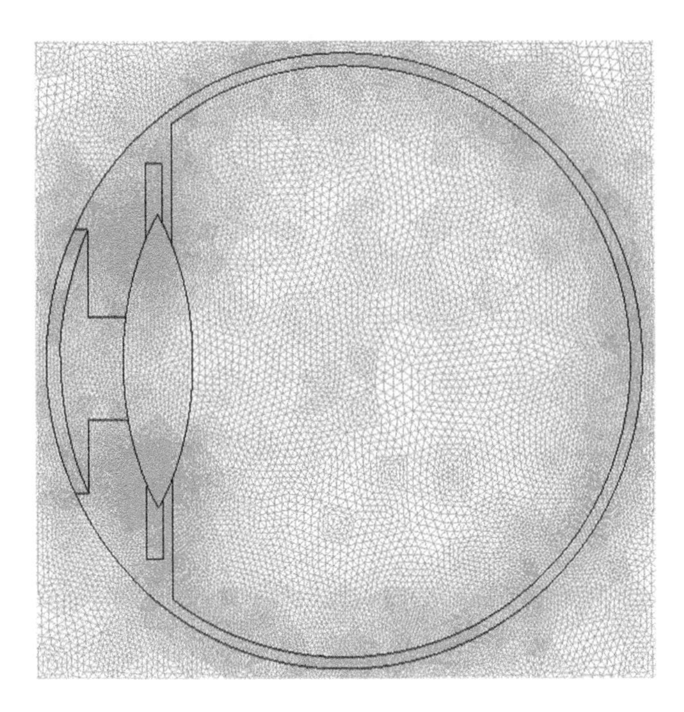

FIGURE 22.4
A 2D finite element mesh of human eye model.

compared to the experimental results of the rabbit obtained from Lagendijk [8]. The validation case assumes that the rabbit body temperature is 38.8°C, the tear evaporation heat loss is 40 W/m^2, the ambient temperature is 25°C, and the convection coefficient of ambient air is 20 W/(m^2 K). The results of the selected test case are presented in Figure 22.5 for the temperature distribution in the eye. Figure 22.5 clearly shows a good agreement of the temperature distribution in the eye between the present solution and that of Shafahi and Vafai [26] and Lagendijk [8]. In the figure, the simulated results of the conventional heat transfer model and the developed heat transfer model provides a good agreement with the simulated results obtained from Shafahi and Vafai [26]. This favorable comparison provides confidence in the results of the present numerical model.

22.4.2 Electric Field Distribution

To illustrate the penetrated electric field distribution inside the eye, the predicted results obtained from our proposed models are required.

22.4.2.1 Effect of Power Density on Electric Field Distribution

Due to the different dielectric characteristics of the various tissue layers, a different fraction of the supplied EM energy will become absorbed in each layer in the eye. Consequently, the reflection and transmission components at each layer contribute to the resonance of standing wave in the eye. Figure 22.6 shows the simulation of an electric field pattern inside the eye exposed to EM field in TM mode operating at the frequency of 900 MHz propagating along the vertical cross section of the eye model, by which the varying power densities are done. As is obvious from Figure 22.6, the higher values of the electric fields in

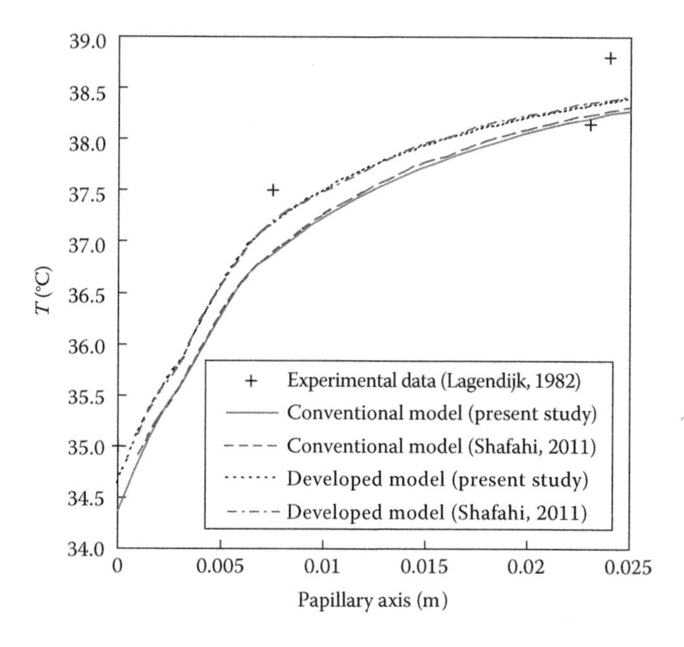

FIGURE 22.5
Comparison of the calculated temperature distribution to the temperature distribution obtained by Shafahi and Vafai and the Lagendijk's experimental data; h_{am} = 20 W/(m² K) and T_{am} = 25°C. (From Wessapan, T. and Rattanadecho, P., *ASME Trans. J. Heat Transfer*, 134, 091101, 2012. With permission.)

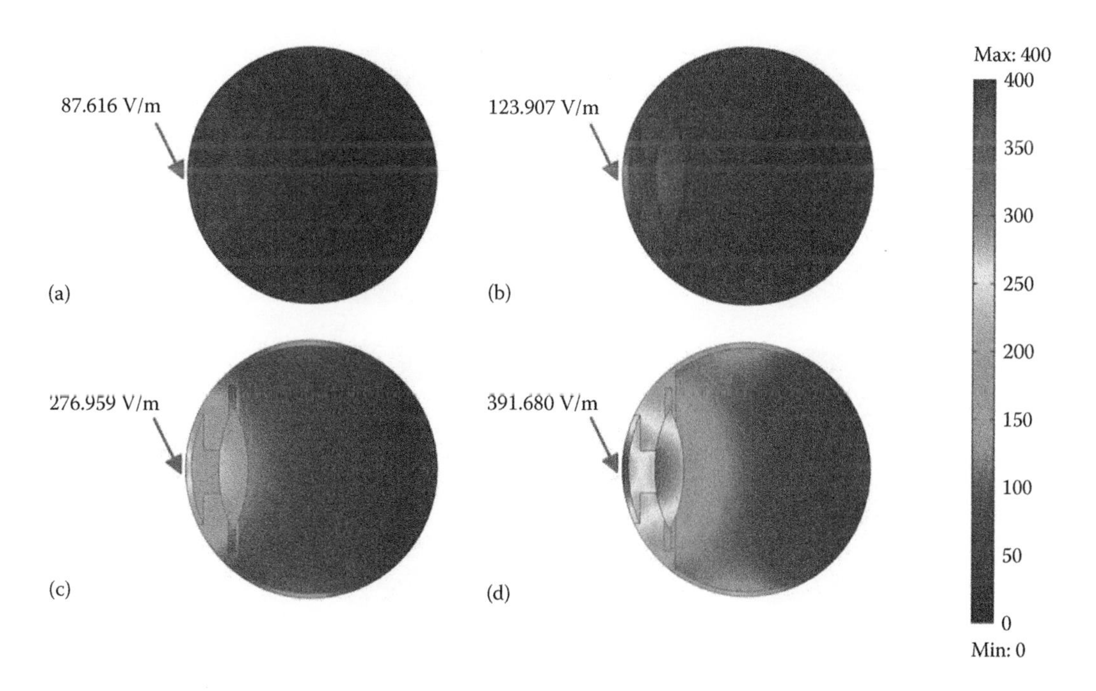

FIGURE 22.6
Electric field distribution (V/m) in human eye exposed to the EM frequency of 900 MHz at the power densities of (a) 5 mW/cm², (b) 10 mW/cm², (c) 50 mW/cm², and (d) 100 mW/cm². (From Wessapan, T. and Rattanadecho, P., *ASME Trans. J. Heat Transfer*, 134, 091101, 2012. With permission.)

all cases occur in the outer part area of the eye, especially in the cornea and lens. The three highest electric field intensity values in the eye at all power densities occur in the cornea, lens, and iris, respectively. This is because the lower value of their dielectric properties (ε_r) shown in Table 22.1 corresponds to Equation 22.10, as well as these tissues are located close to the exposed surface, by which it causes the EM fields to penetrate easily into these tissues. The electric fields deep inside the eye are extinguished where the electric field attenuates due to the absorbed EM energy and the electric fields are then converted to heat. Moreover, the electric field distribution also showed a strong dependence on the dielectric properties of the tissue. Certainly, the maximum electric field intensity at the higher power density is greater than that of the lower power density. The maximum electric field intensities are 391.680, 276.959, 123.907, and 87.616 V/m at the power densities of 100, 50, 10, and 5 mW/cm^2, respectively.

22.4.3 SAR Distribution

22.4.3.1 Effect of Power Density on SAR Distribution

For the SAR distribution in the eye, we found that the amplitude corresponds to the electric fields. Figure 22.7 shows the SAR distribution evaluated on the vertical cross section of the eye exposed to the EM frequency of 900 MHz at various power densities. The results of the SAR values in the eye are evident from Figure 22.7. The SAR values are increased corresponding to the electric field intensities (Figure 22.6). The maximum SAR values are 135.15, 67.575, 13.525, and 6.763 W/kg at the power densities of 100, 50, 10, and 5 mW/cm^2, respectively. Comparing to the maximum SAR value of 2 W/kg (general public exposure)

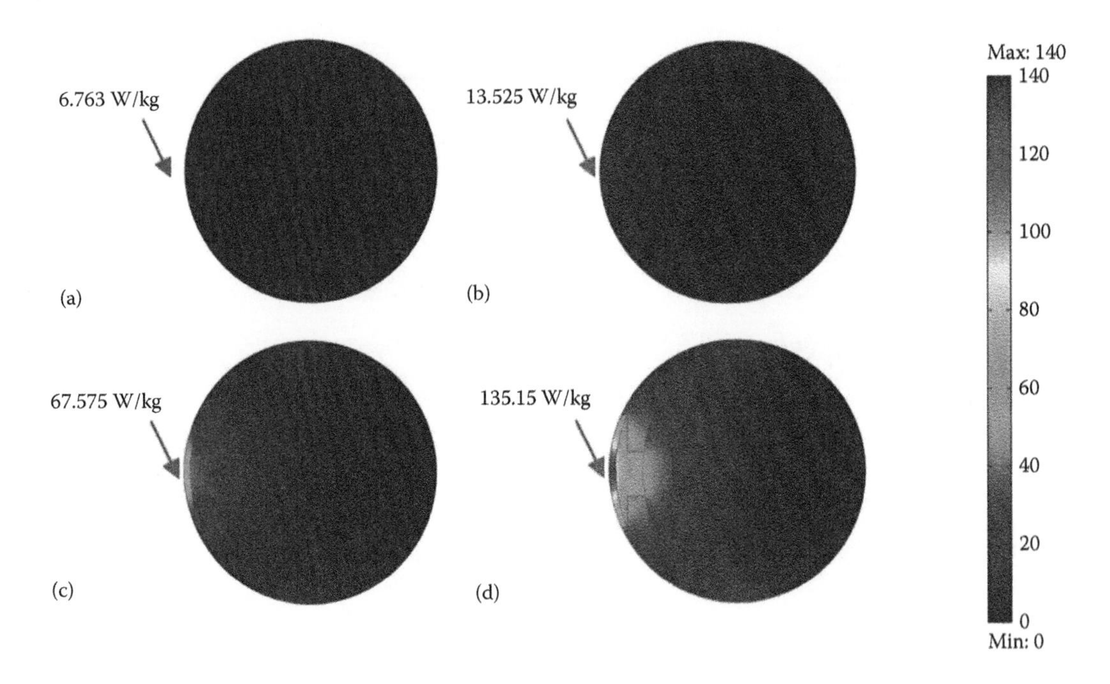

FIGURE 22.7
SAR distribution (W/kg) in human eye exposed to the EM frequency of 900 MHz at the power densities of (a) 5 mW/cm^2, (b) 10 mW/cm^2, (c) 50 mW/cm^2, and (d) 100 mW/cm^2. (From Wessapan, T. and Rattanadecho, P., *ASME Trans. J. Heat Transfer*, 134, 091101, 2012. With permission.)

and 10 W/kg (occupational exposure) [6], the resulting SAR values from this study are higher than the ICNIRP exposure guidelines for occupational exposure in most cases except for the power density of 5 mW/cm^2. Besides the electric field intensity, the magnitude of dielectric and thermal properties in each tissue will directly affect the amount of SAR in the eye. For all power densities, the highest SAR values are obtained only in the region of the cornea, but not in lens and iris as electric field distributions. This is because the cornea has a much higher value of its dielectric properties (σ) than those of the lens and iris, as well as the cornea located close to the exposed surface, at which the electric field intensity is strongest. It is found that the SAR distribution pattern in the eye, which corresponds to Equation 22.14, strongly depends on the effect of the dielectric properties (σ, shown in Table 22.1) and thermal properties (ρ, shown in Table 22.2). With penetration into the eye, the SAR values decrease rapidly along the distance from the EM source.

22.4.4 Temperature Distribution

In order to study the heat transfer in the eye, the coupled effects of the EM wave propagation, the unsteady heat transfer, and the initial and boundary conditions are then investigated. Due to these effects, the electric field distribution (see Figure 22.6) and the SAR distribution (see Figure 22.7) are then converted into heat by absorption of the tissue.

22.4.4.1 Effect of Heat Transfer Model on Temperature Distribution

Since this study has focused on the volumetric heating effect into the multilayer tissues of the eye induced by EM fields, the effect of ambient temperature variation has been neglected in order to gain insight into the interaction between the EM fields and the human tissue as well as the correlation between the SAR and the heat transfer mechanism. For this reason, the ambient temperature has been set to the human body temperature of 37°C, and the tear evaporation has been neglected. Moreover, the effect of thermoregulation mechanisms has also been neglected due to the small temperature increase occurred during exposure process. The convective coefficient due to blood flow inside the sclera is set to 65 W/m^2 K [16].

For the eye exposed to the EM fields for a period of time, the temperature in the eye (Figure 22.8) is increased corresponding to the SAR (Figure 22.7). This is because the electric fields in the eye attenuate owing to the energy absorbed and thereafter the absorbed energy is converted to the thermal energy, which increases the eye temperature. Figure 22.8 shows the temperature distribution in the vertical cross section of the eye at various times exposed to the EM frequency of 900 MHz at the power density of 100 mW/cm^2 calculated using the conventional heat transfer model (Model I) (Figure 22.8a) and developed heat transfer model (Model II) (Figure 22.8b).

It is found that by using the different heat transfer models, the distribution patterns of temperature at a particular time are quite different. The hot spot zone is strongly displayed at 10 min for both heat transfer models at the anterior chamber area, owing to the extensive penetration of EM power of internal regions and higher dielectric properties (ε_r) of the anterior chamber tissue. This higher dielectric property of the anterior chamber represents the stronger absorption ability of EM fields than those of the cornea and lens. The outer corneal surface has a lower temperature than that of the anterior chamber, even if it has higher SAR value (Figure 22.7). This is because heat is dissipated to the ambient via convection and radiation since the main heat transfer mechanism of the conventional heat transfer model is the thermal conduction of the eye, whereas the developed heat transfer

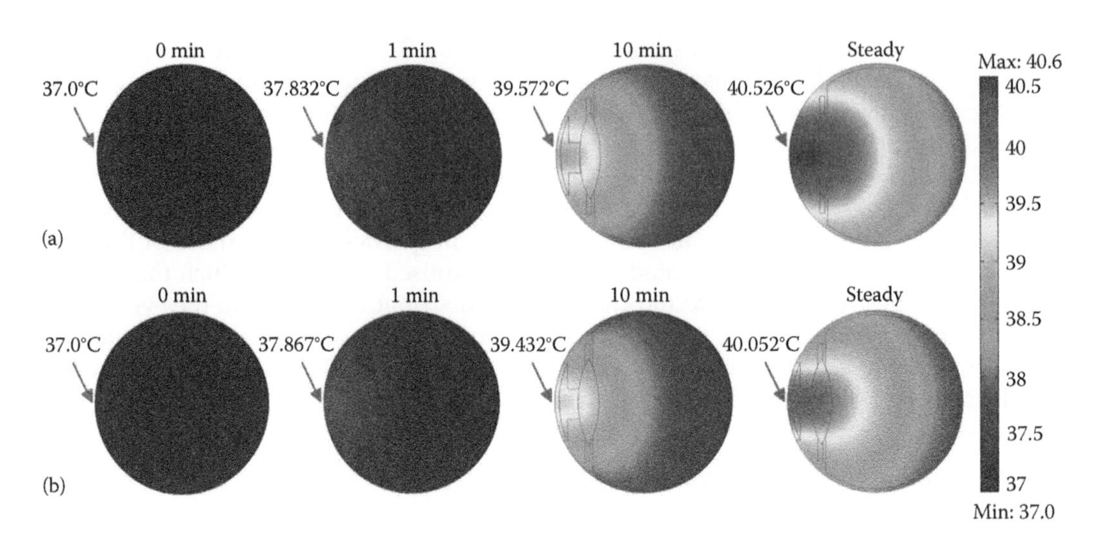

FIGURE 22.8
The temperature distribution in the human eye at various times exposed to the EM frequency of 900 MHz at the power density of 100 mW/cm^2 calculated using (a) the conventional heat transfer model and (b) the developed heat transfer model. (From Wessapan, T. and Rattanadecho, P., *ASME Trans. J. Heat Transfer*, 134, 091101, 2012. With permission.)

model accounts for the natural convection in the anterior chamber as well. Therefore, the developed heat transfer model with higher dissipation rates of heat generated by EM fields can obtain higher cooling effect than that of the conventional heat transfer model.

Consider the temperature increase distribution at the extrusion line (Figure 22.9). Figure 22.10 shows the temperature increase versus papillary axis (along the extrusion line) of the eye exposed to the EM frequency of 900 MHz at various times. In the early stage of

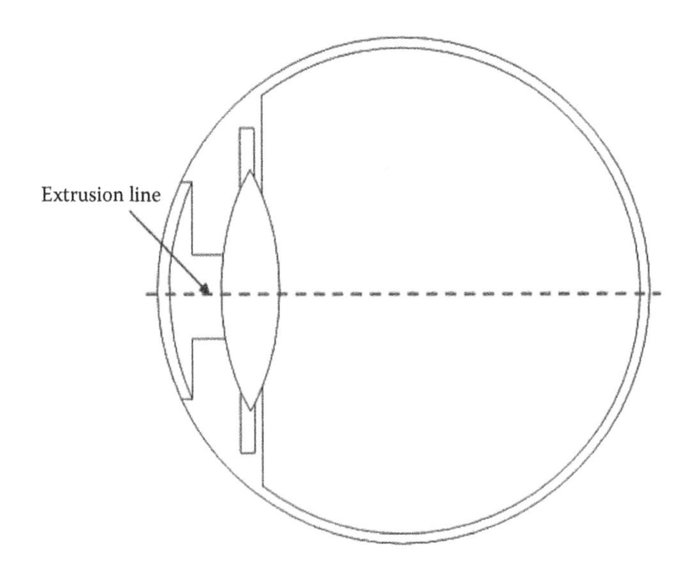

FIGURE 22.9
The extrusion line in the human eye where the temperature distribution is considered. (From Wessapan, T. and Rattanadecho, P., *ASME Trans. J. Heat Transfer*, 134, 091101, 2012. With permission.)

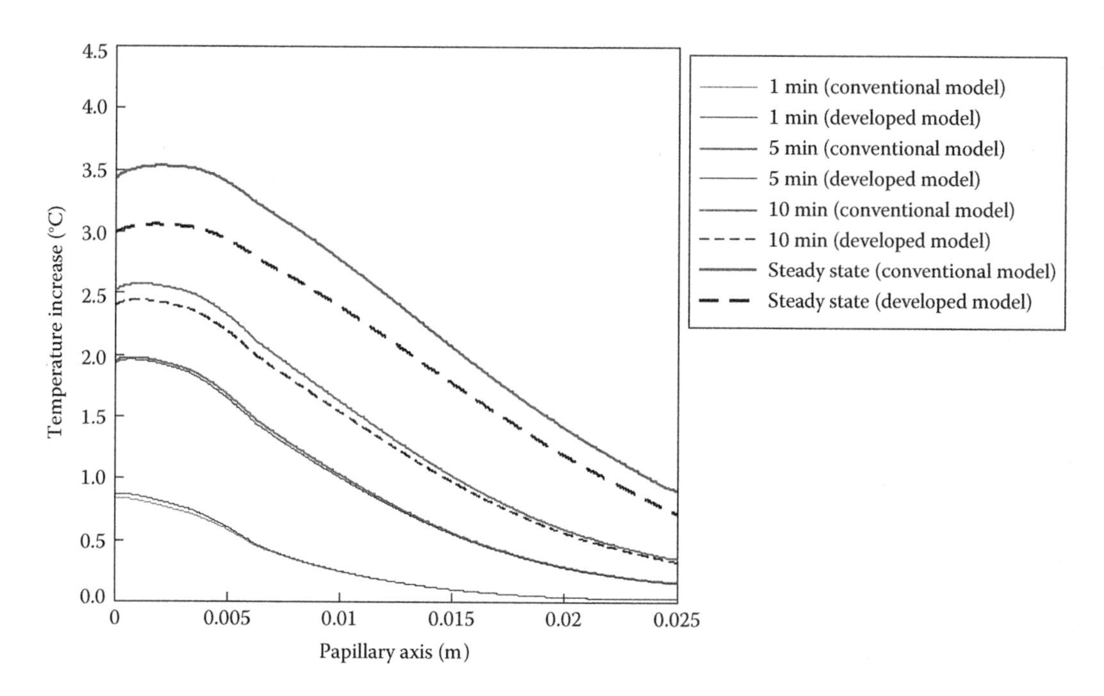

FIGURE 22.10
Temperature increase versus papillary axis of the human eye exposed to the EM frequency of 900 MHz at various times. (From Wessapan, T. and Rattanadecho, P., *ASME Trans. J. Heat Transfer*, 134, 091101, 2012. With permission.)

exposure (1 min), the calculated temperature in the anterior chamber, obtained from the conventional heat transfer model, is little lower than that of developed heat transfer model. This is because natural convection in the developed heat transfer model causes a substantial accumulation of warmer fluid in the upper half of the anterior chamber. Surprisingly, just after 10 min of exposure, the temperature increase of the conventional heat transfer model is higher than that of developed heat transfer model. This is due to the presence of blood perfusion in the iris/sclera tissue, which covers an internal surface area of the eye. This blood perfusion provides buffer characteristic to the eye temperature, which is expected to occur in the realistic physiological conditions. Moreover, the natural convection and formation of two circulatory patterns with opposite direction in the anterior chamber, shown in Figure 22.11, play the important roles on the cooling processes in the eye, especially inner corneal surface, when a large temperature gradient is produced by EM fields after 10 min. The circulation pattern implies that the generated heat in the anterior chamber is convected in two directions: one is to the corneal surface and the other is to the lens surface.

22.4.4.2 Effect of Power Density on Temperature Distribution

In addition, each power density level is applied to investigate the effects of power density (the power irradiated on the eye surface). Figure 22.12 shows the comparison of the temperature distribution in the eye at time approaching to steady-state condition with the frequency of 900 MHz corresponding to the power densities of 5, 10, 50, and 100 mW/cm^2. It is found that the power densities significantly influence the temperature increase in the eye.

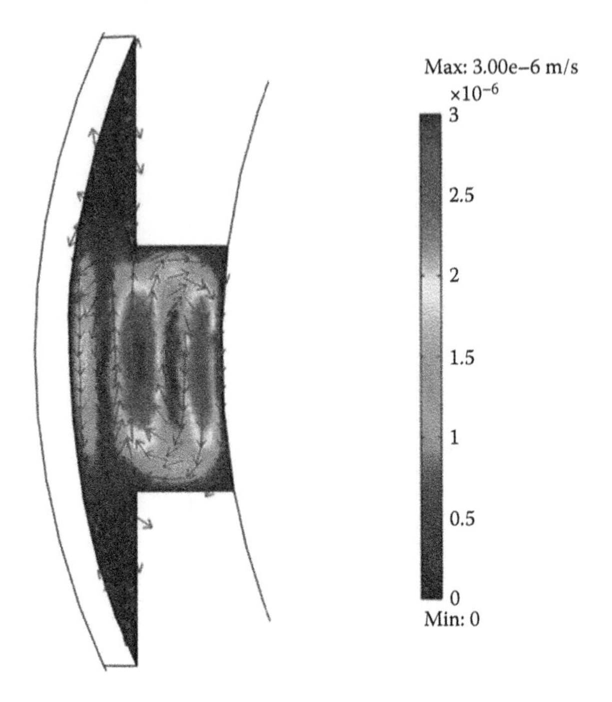

FIGURE 22.11
The velocity distribution inside the anterior chamber in the human eye when exposed to the EM frequency of 900 MHz. (From Wessapan, T. and Rattanadecho, P., *ASME Trans. J. Heat Transfer*, 134, 091101, 2012. With permission.)

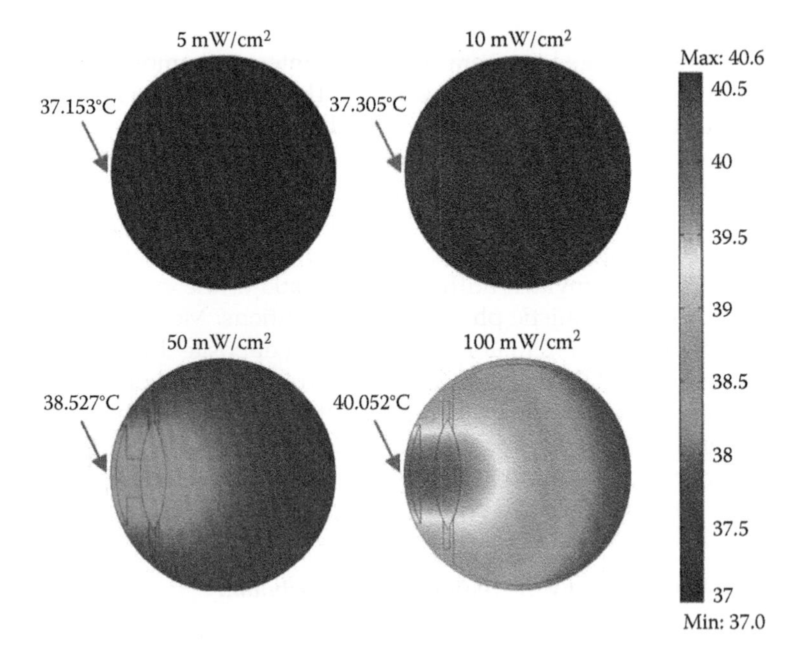

FIGURE 22.12
The temperature distribution in the eye exposed to the EM frequency of 900 MHz at various power densities calculated using (a) the conventional heat transfer model and (b) the developed heat transfer model. (From Wessapan, T. and Rattanadecho, P., *ASME Trans. J. Heat Transfer*, 134, 091101, 2012. With permission.)

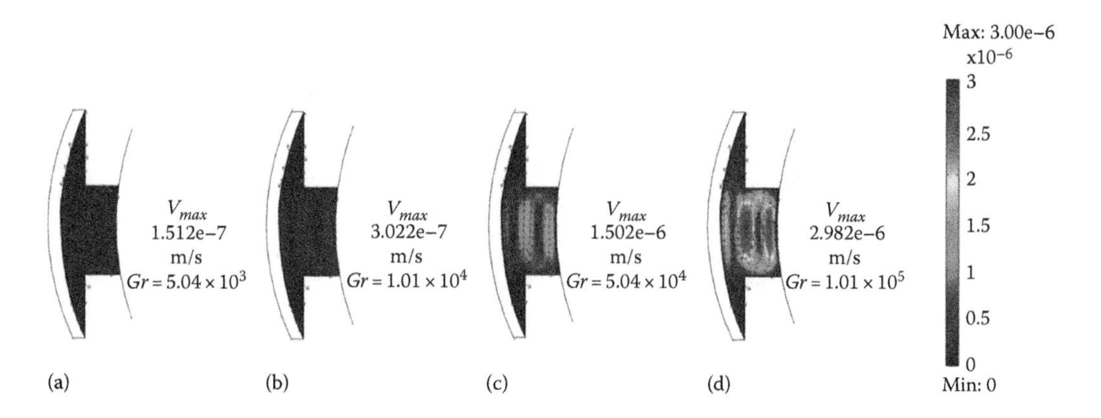

FIGURE 22.13
The velocity distribution inside the anterior chamber in the eye exposed to the EM frequency of 900 MHz at the power densities of (a) 5 mW/cm^2, (b) 10 mW/cm^2, (c) 50 mW/cm^2, and (d) 100 mW/cm^2. (From Wessapan, T. and Rattanadecho, P., *ASME Trans. J. Heat Transfer*, 134, 091101, 2012. With permission.)

Greater power density provides greater heat generation inside the eye, thereby increasing the rate of temperature rise. By using the developed heat transfer model, the maximum temperature increases are 0.153°C, 0.305°C, 1.527°C, and 3.052°C at the power densities of 5, 10, 50, and 100 mW/cm^2, respectively.

Figure 22.13 shows the circulatory patterns in the anterior chamber in the eye exposed to the EM frequency of 900 MHz at various power densities. These circulatory patterns in the anterior chamber vary corresponding to the power densities that produced the temperature gradient in the eye. Therefore, in the case of a lower power density, the circulatory patterns have a lower speed, where a circulatory pattern with a higher power density flows faster. At the lower power density with low flow speed, the heat transfer in the anterior chamber occurs mainly by conduction across the fluid layer. In the case of the higher power density with higher flow speed, different flow regimes are encountered, with a progressively increasing heat transfer. The fluid motion within the anterior chamber is driven by the power density that is associated with the Grashof number Gr. The Grashof number is defined as $Gr = g\beta q D^5/(k\upsilon^2)$, in which D is the eye diameter (m), q is the internal power density (W/m^2), and υ is the kinematic viscosity (m^2/s). The range of Grashof numbers investigated is 5.04×10^3–1.01×10^5 as shown in Figure 22.13.

22.4.5 Concluding Remarks

This study presents the numerical simulation of the SAR and temperature distributions in the eye exposed to TM mode of EM fields. The results of the SAR values in this study are increased corresponding to the electric field intensities. Besides the electric field intensity, the magnitude of dielectric and thermal properties in each tissue will directly affect the amount of SAR in the eye.

In this study, it is found that the highest level of SAR value is the cornea, while the highest temperature is the anterior chamber. In different heat transfer models, the temperature results obtained from a developed heat transfer model, considered natural convection and porous media theory, are compared to the results obtained from a conventional heat transfer model in order to highlight the advantages and the weakness of each model. It is found that by using the different heat transfer models, the distribution patterns of temperature at a particular time are quite different. In all cases, the temperatures obtained from the developed heat transfer model have a lower temperature than that of the conventional heat transfer model. This is due to the presence of blood perfusion that provides buffer characteristic to the eye temperature, as well as the natural convection in the anterior chamber. It is found that greater power density results in a greater heat generation inside the eye, thereby increasing the rate of temperature increase. Moreover, it is found that the temperature distributions in the eye induced by EM fields are not directly related to the SAR distribution due to the effect of dielectric properties, thermal properties, blood perfusion, and penetration depth of the EM power.

The numerical simulations in this study show several important features of the energy absorption in the eye. This information can be used as a guideline for limiting human eye exposure from EM wave radiation.

Acknowledgment

The authors wish to express appreciation to the Thailand Research Fund (TRF) for their support.

References

1. Emery, A. F., Kramar, P., Guy, A. W., and Lin, J. C. 1975. Microwave induced temperature rises in rabbit eyes in cataract research. *J. Heat Transfer—T ASME* 97:123–128.
2. Buccella, C., Santis, V. D., and Feliaiani, M. 2007. Prediction of temperature increase in human eyes due to RF sources. *IEEE Trans. Electromagn. Compat.* 49:825–833.
3. Lin, J. C. 2003. Cataracts and cell-phone radiation. *IEEE Ant. Prop. Magazine* 45:171–174.
4. Fujiwara, O. and Kato, A. 1994. Computation of SAR inside eyeball for 1.5-GHz microwave exposure using finite-difference time domain technique. *IEICE Trans.* E77-B:732–737.
5. Gandhi, O. P., Lazzi, G., and Furse, C. M. 1996. Electromagnetic absorption in the human head and neck for mobile telephones at 835 and 1900 MHz. *IEEE Trans. Microw. Theory Tech.* 44:1884–1897.
6. International Commission on Non-Ionizing Radiation Protection (ICNIRP). 1998. Guidelines for limiting exposure to time-varying electric, magnetic and electromagnetic fields (up to 300 GHz). *Health Phys.* 74:494–522.
7. IEEE. 1999. IEEE standard for safety levels with respect to human exposure to radio frequency electromagnetic fields, 3 kHz to 300 GHz. IEEE Standard C95.1-1999.
8. Lagendijk, J. J. W. 1982. A mathematical model to calculate temperature distribution in human and rabbit eye during hyperthermic treatment. *Phys. Med. Biol.* 27:1301–1311.
9. Scott, J. 1988. A finite element model of heat transport in the human eye. *Phys. Med. Biol.* 33:227–241.
10. Scott, J. 1988. The computation of temperature rises in the human eye induced by infrared radiation. *Phys. Med. Biol.* 33:243–257.
11. Amara, E. H. 1995. Numerical investigations on thermal effects of Laser–Ocular media interaction. *Int. J. Heat Mass Transfer* 38:2479–2488.
12. Hirata, A., Matsuyama, S., and Shiozawa, T. 2000. Temperature rises in the human eye exposed to EM waves in the frequency range 0.6–6 GHz. *IEEE Trans. Electromagn. Compat.* 42:386–393.

13. Chua, K. J., Ho, J. C., Chou, S. K., and Islam, M. R. 2005. On the study of the temperature distribution within a human eye subjected to a laser source. *Int. Commun. Heat Mass Transfer* 32:1057–1065.
14. Limtrakarn, W., Reepolmaha, S., and Dechaumphai, P. 2010. Transient temperature distribution on the corneal endothelium during ophthalmic phacoemulsification: A numerical simulation using the nodeless variable element. *Asian Biomed.* 4:885–892.
15. Kumar, S., Acharya, S., Beuerman, R., and Palkama, A. 2006. Numerical solution of ocular fluid dynamics in a rabbit eye: Parametric effects. *Ann. Biomed. Eng.* 34:530–544.
16. Ooi, E. and Ng, E. Y. K. 2008. Simulation of aqueous humor hydrodynamics in human eye heat transfer. *Comput. Biol. Med.* 38:252–262.
17. Ooi, E. H. and Ng, E. Y. K. 2011. Effects of natural convection inside the anterior chamber. *Int. J. Numer. Methods Biomed. Eng.* 27:408–423.
18. Pennes, H. H. 1948. Analysis of tissue and arterial blood temperatures in the resting human forearm. *J. Appl. Physiol.* 1:93–122.
19. Pennes, H. H. 1998. Analysis of tissue and arterial blood temperatures in the resting human forearm. *J. Appl. Physiol.* 85:5–34.
20. Flyckt, V. M. M., Raaymakers, B. W., and Lagendijk, J. J. W. 2006. Modeling the impact of blood flow on the temperature distribution in the human eye and the orbit: Fixed heat transfer coefficients versus the pennes bioheat model versus discrete blood vessels. *Phys. Med. Biol.* 51:5007–5021.
21. Ng, E. Y. K. and Ooi, E. H. 2006. FEM simulation of the eye structure with bioheat analysis. *Comput. Methods Programs Biomed.* 82:268–276.
22. Ooi, E. H. and Ng, E. Y. K. 2006. Ocular temperature distribution: A mathematical perspective. *J. Mech. Med. Biol.* 9:199–227.
23. Nakayama, A. and Kuwahara, F. 2008. A general bioheat transfer model based on the theory of porous media. *Int. J. Heat Mass Transfer* 51:3190–3199.
24. Mahjoob, S. and Vafai, K. 2009. Analytical characterization of heat transfer through biological media incorporating hyperthermia treatment. *Int. J. Heat Mass Transfer* 52:1608–1618.
25. Khanafer, K. and Vafai, K. 2009. Synthesis of mathematical models representing bioheat transport. In *Advances in Numerical Heat Transfer*, eds. W. J. Minkowycz, E. M. Sparrow, and J. P. Abraham, pp. 1–28. London, U.K.: Taylor & Francis Group.
26. Shafahi, M. and Vafai, K. 2011. Human eye response to thermal disturbances. *J. Heat Transfer—T ASME* 133:011009.
27. Narasimhan, A. and Vishnampet, R. 2012. Effect of choroidal blood flow on transscleral retinal drug delivery using a porous medium model. *Int. J. Heat Mass Transfer* 55:5665–5672.
28. KumarJha, K. and Narasimhan, A. 2011. Three-dimensional bio-heat transfer simulation of sequential and simultaneous retinal laser irradiation. *Int. J. Thermal Sci.* 50:1191–1198.
29. Narasimhan, A. and Sadasivam, S. 2013. Non-Fourier bio heat transfer modelling of thermal damage during retinal laser irradiation. *Int. J. Heat Mass Transfer* 60:591–597.
30. Ooi, E. H., Ang, W. T., and Ng, E. Y. K. 2008. A boundary element model of the human eye undergoing laser thermokeratoplasty. *Comput. Biol. Med.* 28:727–738.
31. Ooi, E. H., Ang, W. T., and Ng, E. Y. K. 2008. A boundary element model for investigating the effects of eye tumor on the temperature distribution inside the human eye. *Comput. Biol. Med.* 39:667–677.
32. Tan, J. H., Ng, E. Y. K., and Acharya, U. R. 2011. Evaluation of topographical variation in ocular surface temperature by functional infrared thermography. *Infrared Phys. Technol.* 54:469–477.
33. Tan, J. H., Ng, E. Y. K., and Acharya, U. R. 2010. Evaluation of tear evaporation from ocular surface by functional infrared thermography. *Med. Phys.* 37:6022–6034.
34. Tan, J. H., Ng, E. Y. K., Acharya, U. R., and Chee, C. Study of normal ocular thermogram using textural parameters. *Infrared Phys. Technol.* 53:120–126.
35. Wessapan, T. and Rattanadecho, P. Specific absorption rate and temperature increase in human eye subjected to electromagnetic fields at 900 MHz. *ASME Trans. J. Heat Transfer* 134:091101.

36. Bernardi, P., Cavagnaro, M., Pisa, S., and Piuzzi, E. 2000. Specific absorption rate and temperature increases in the head of a cellular-phone user. *IEEE Trans. Microw. Theory Tech.* 48:1118–1126.
37. Park, S., Jeong, J., and Lim, Y. 2004. Temperature rise in the human head and brain for portable handsets at 900 and 1800 MHz. *4th International Conference on Microwave and Millimeter Wave Technology, ICMMT 2004*, Beijing, China.
38. Nakayama, A. and Kuwahara, F. 2008. A general bioheat transfer model based on the theory of porous media. *Int. J. Heat Mass Transfer* 51:3190–3199.

23

Dry Eye Characterization by Analyzing Tear Film Images

Beatriz Remeseiro, Manuel G. Penedo, Carlos García-Resúa, Eva Yebra-Pimentel, and Antonio Mosquera

CONTENTS

Dry eye is an increasingly popular syndrome in modern society, which affects a wide sector of the population and worsens with age. Dry eye diagnosis is very difficult to accomplish, specially because of its multifactorial nature. Thus, there are several clinical tests to measure the tear quality and quantity. Some of them assess the tear film by evaluating the interference lipid pattern. This chapter describes an automatic image processing methodology to perform the analysis of the interference lipid pattern using the Tearscope plus and Doane's interferometer as the instruments to acquire tear film images.

23.1 Tear Film

The tear film is a highly specialized structure, which covers the anterior conjunctiva and cornea, being essential to maintain a healthy and functional visual system. It plays important functions such as the following [31]:

Optical function: The tear film fills in the irregularities in the corneal epithelium, thereby providing a perfect, smooth, regular optical surface. So, absence of the tear film provokes blurred vision.

Lubrication function: This allows to minimize the friction between eyelid margins and palpebral conjunctiva during blinking.

Cleaning function: The tear film, together with blinking action, removes debris and desquamated epithelial cells from the epithelium.

Antimicrobial function: The tear film is the first line of defense against ocular surface infection. It contains proteins, such as lysozyme or lactoferrin, that inhibit microbiological contamination.

Nutritional function: Corneal surface must be avascular to guarantee its transparency. So, the nutrition is driven by the tear film. Oxygen from the ambient air dissolves in the tear fluid and is transferred to the corneal epithelium.

The total volume of the tear film is 7.0 ± 2.0 μL with a thickness ranging from 6 to 10 μm. Along the upper and lower lids, it forms a tear meniscus or marginal tear strips. This represents 70% of the total volume of tear fluid within the palpebral aperture [32]. A small proportion lies beneath the eyelids between the palpebral and bulbar conjunctiva, and the remainder covers the cornea and the exposed bulbar conjunctiva [31].

The tear film is a matrix-like structure composed of water, electrolytes, immunoglobulins, antimicrobial molecules, or mucins. The composition of the tear film is distributed specially into three tear film layers: a superficial lipid layer, an intermediate aqueous phase, and an underlying mucous layer (see Figure 23.1).

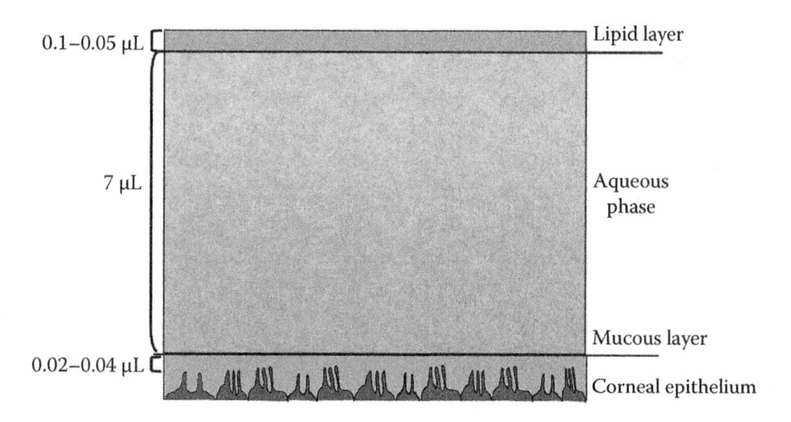

FIGURE 23.1
Structure of the tear film.

23.1.1 Lipid Layer

This is the thinnest layer of the tear film (0.1–0.05 μL) and is comprised by polar and nonpolar lipids. The main function of the lipid layer is the reduction of evaporation from the aqueous phase. Also, it prevents surface contamination of the film with skin lipids and is the focus of various interferential techniques for tear film assessment. This layer is subdivided into two further layers [31]: an anterior lipid layer formed by nonpolar lipids, mainly mixed wax esters and sterol esters, and a posterior lipid layer formed by high-polar lipids, free sterols, free fatty acids, and phospholipids.

23.1.2 Aqueous Phase

This is the thickest layer of the tear film (7 μL) [31,32] and is mainly formed by proteins, such as lysozyme, lactoferrin, or albumin; metabolites; electrolytes; and enzymes. This phase provides the proper functions of the tear film.

23.1.3 Mucous Layer

This layer (0.02–0.04 μL) [31] is mainly formed by glycoproteins to maintain the corneal and conjunctival surfaces hydrated. Furthermore, this allows the lids to slide with minimal friction during the blinking [32].

23.2 Dry Eye Disease

In 2007, the *International Dry Eye Workshop* (DEWS) established the main characteristics of the *dry eye disease* (DED) and published the finest definition of it [34]:

> Dry eye is a multifactorial disease of the tears and ocular surface that results in symptoms of discomfort, visual disturbance and tear film instability with potential damage to the ocular surface. It is accompanied by increased osmolarity of the tear film and inflammation of the ocular surface.

DED is an inflammatory status of the ocular surface driven by increased tear film osmolarity and derived by poor quality/quantity of the tear film. This disease affects quality of life, provokes visual disturbance, and can lead to damage of the ocular surface.

DED has increased its prevalence in the last few years, reaching from 10% to 35% of the general population, and if only contact lens (CL) wearers are considered, this prevalence is even greater [34]. Current style of life, harmful environments such as pollution, tasks that favors increased tear film evaporation, and the aging of population have increased DED prevalence, which is currently considered an endemic condition.

DEWS [34] divided DED into two main categories: *aqueous tear-deficient dry eye* (ADDE) and *evaporative dry eye* (EDE).

23.2.1 Aqueous Tear-Deficient Dry Eye

This type of DED is due to a failure of lachrymal tear secretion and is mainly derived from a Sjogren syndrome. Also, there are other factors that can occasion ADDE, such as lachrymal gland infiltration, sarcoidosis, lymphoma, obstruction of the lachrymal gland ducts, or reflex hyposecretion [34]. This type of DED is age-related and is not the principal focus of this chapter.

23.2.2 EDE

This type of DED refers to a normal lachrymal secretory function, but there is a tear film deficit due to an excessive water loss from the exposed ocular surface. This is the type of dry eye most commonly found in young to middle-aged people and related to ambient conditions, such as air conditioning, and/or CL wear [34]. The etiology of EDE can be divided as intrinsic or extrinsic causes, which are relevant for treatment and therapeutic protocols.

23.2.2.1 Intrinsic EDE

The causes of this type of EDE are derived from intrinsic disease that can affect lid structures. One of these types of EDE is the disorders of lid aperture, where excessive palpebral fissure increases tear film evaporation and is associated with ocular drying and tear hyperosmolarity. This occurs in particular gaze positions that increase palpebral fissure. Poor lid apposition also affects tear film quality due to poor tear film resurfacing. Low blink rate can dry the ocular surface by increasing the period between blinks, so the ocular surface is more exposed to water loss [9]. This leads to a common dry eye derived from computer use, due to the performance of tasks that require concentration [39]. The main cause of EDE is the *meibomian gland dysfunction* (MGD) [13], which is an obstruction of the meibomian glands and is associated to other dermatological conditions, such as acne rosacea or seborrhoeic dermatitis [36]. MGD can be simple, where the gland orifices remain located in the skin of the lid, or cicatricial, where the duct orifices are drawn subsequently onto the lid and tarsal mucous and, hence, are unable to deliver oil to the surface of the tear film [34].

23.2.2.2 Extrinsic EDE

Dry eye is due to some extrinsic exposure, such as ocular surface disorders, where disease of ocular surface may lead to imperfect surface wetting and then dry eye [34]. Topical drugs also can induce toxic response from the ocular surface, mainly due to preservatives, which cause surface epithelial cell damage. This even worsens when frequent instillation is needed [41]. So, in these cases, it should be recommended to change them by nonpreserved drops. Vitamin A deficiency is another cause of EDE [50] because it is essential for the development of goblet cells that are necessary for tear mucin secretion [30]. Allergic conjunctivitis provokes a response at the ocular surface that may lead to loss of surface membrane mucins [34], affecting conjunctival and corneal epithelium. Another extrinsic cause of EDE is CL wear. The CL disrupts normal tear physiology through thinning and breakup of the tear film, rupturing the lipid layer with consequent increases in tear film evaporation [29]. The presence of a CL can produce EDE even in a normal individual. This is an important factor to take into account since CL wear is prevalent in the developing world [38]. The primary reasons for CL intolerance are discomfort and dryness [42], and it was found that 50% of CL wearers report dry eye symptoms [10]. The prelens lipid layer thickness was less in dry eye subjects and correlated well with the prelens tear film thinning time. This, together with poor lens wettability, could be a basis for a higher evaporative loss during lens wear and was attributed to potential changes in tear film lipid composition, rather than to a loss of meibomian gland oil delivery [34].

23.2.3 Evaporation of the Tear Film in EDE

For any type of DED, hyperosmolarity is a precipitating event leading to the pathological changes associated with dry eye. In EDE, the rate of evaporation that results in critical osmolarity will depend on the tear flow rate. Evaporation rate is influenced by six factors, including ambient conditions, hormonal regulation, blink rate, area of palpebral aperture, tear film compartments, and tear film lipid layer [21].

The outermost layer of the tear film, the tear film lipid layer, is a combination of polar and nonpolar lipids that are the secretion of the meibomian glands. As commented earlier, the chief function of the lipid layer is to retard water evaporation from the surface of the open eye [21]. In the normal tear film, much of the lipid layer is a structure that remains stable over a series of blinks, as it approaches the lower lid margin in the down-phase of the blink and unfolding in the up-phase, with little mixing of lipid within the lipid layer or between the lipid layer and the reservoirs [12].

A stable tear film is one in which a minimum amount of tears evaporate. The evaporation rate is determined primarily by the status of the lipid layer, the protein constituents, the aqueous components, and the mucin coating the corneal epithelia [21].

There is some evidence that evaporation is affected by lipid layer thickness, but it is currently not known specifically how lipid composition alters either the stability or thickness of the lipid layer [13]. It has been proposed that the polar lipids act as a surfactant that helps spread the nonpolar lipids over the aqueous component of the tear film, provide a barrier between the two layers, and are also a structure that supports the nonpolar phase, which is responsible for creating a seal that decreases evaporation from the tear film [21].

23.3 Tear Film Assessment

DED is a multifactorial syndrome, so several tests are necessary in order to obtain a clear diagnosis. There are a wide number of tests to evaluate different aspects of the tear film and can be grouped into two main groups, depending on which tear film parameters they measured. On the one hand, quantitative tear film tests are related with the lachrymal gland secretion function and assess tear film tear secretion. On the other hand, qualitative tear film tests reflect the ability of the tear film to remain stable, which is essential to cover the anterior eye and perform its functions. Although there are a broad variety of clinical tests, a deep description of them will be presented since the focus of this chapter is to describe in detail the techniques based on the interferential phenomena. In the next sections, the tests more used in clinical trials are briefly explained.

23.3.1 Quantitative Tear Film Tests

Quantitative tear film tests assess the quantity of tear film and the most common ones are the following:

The Schirmer test. It measures the tear flow reflexively stimulated by insertion of a filter paper into the conjunctival sac [33].

Phenol red thread test. It consists of a thread impregnated with phenol red, which is pH sensitive and changes from yellow to red over the pH range of normal tears [52].

Tear meniscus height. It measures the tear reservoir along the low lid, which is an indicator of tear volume. It is not invasive and only needs the observation of the tear meniscus by a slit lamp [24].

23.3.2 Qualitative Tear Film Tests

Qualitative tear film tests assess the stability of tear film and the most common ones are the following:

Tear breakup time (*BUT*). This is the most commonly used test of tear film stability and consists in measuring the time that the tear film maintains stability after fluorescein instillation [17].

Not invasive tear breakup time (*NIBUT*). This test is similar to BUT, apart from the use of a grid projected onto the precorneal tear film for the observation of distortion and/or abnormality in the image, so fluorescein instillation is avoided [18].

23.4 Assessment of the Tear Film by Interference Phenomena

The tear film is transparent, which makes it difficult for direct observation during clinical assessments. For example, to assess whether tear film is present, BUT test requires staining the preocular tear film, whereas NIBUT test projects a grid on corneal surface. This problem is even greater if we want to directly observe the component structures of the tear film. However, by applying simple optic principles, structure of anterior tear film lipid layer can be appreciated in vivo.

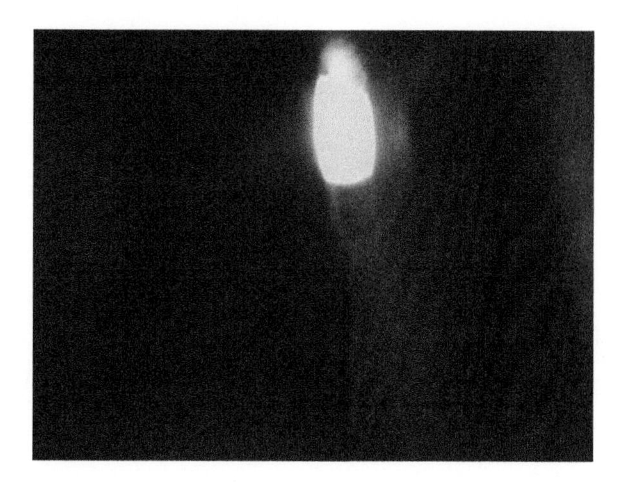

FIGURE 23.2
Appearance of lipid layer by biomicroscope with slit-lamp examination.

23.4.1 Specular Reflection

When a light source incidents on an interface between two refractive index media, a small percentage of the incident light is speculary reflected. Because the refractive index of the lipid layer is higher than that of the aqueous layer, there is a second interface, between the two layers, which can be visible in specular observation. The observation of this specular reflections permits the evaluation of the preocular tear film structure. This has been used to observe the anterior lipid layer with slit-lamp biomicroscopy, but only allows the observation of a 1 mm × 2 mm area, because the light source of the biomicroscope subtends only a small angle (see Figure 23.2). To solve this, McDonald [47] introduced a hemispherical medical lamp to obtain large reflection by the tear film, so larger areas of superficial lipid layer can be evaluated, and posterior devices followed this design (see Figure 23.3).

23.4.2 Interference Phenomena: Interpretation of the Observations

When observing the appearance of the lipid layer by this technique, the presence of interference fringes can be appreciated. These interference fringes result from the wave characteristics of light, and the fact that when coherent rays of light of a given wavelength are combined and brought to a common focus, they will interfere, either constructively or destructively, depending on the degree to which the periodic fluctuations of their electromagnetic fields are in phase. To observe interference phenomena, it is necessary to use coherent light sources, that is, sources whose phase difference remains constant in time. A simple manner in which this can be accomplished is by using a single light source and its optical image.

In the case of the tear film, there are two interfering beams: the beam reflected from the air–lipid interface of the tear film and the beam reflected from the lipid–aqueous interface of the tear film. These two beams originate from the same point of the single light source and, in fact, are two images of it, so the beams satisfy the requirement of coherence. Figure 23.4 shows a schema of this phenomena between

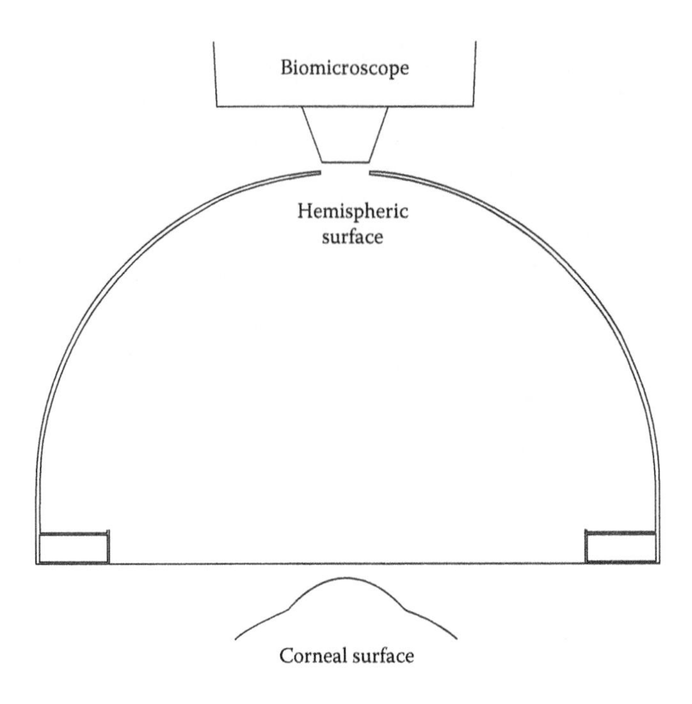

FIGURE 23.3
Hemispherical light source to obtain large reflection by the tear film.

two flat boundaries, air–lipid boundary and lipid–aqueous boundary, which follow the next expression:

$$m(d,\phi',\lambda)=\frac{2n(\lambda)\cos(\phi')}{\lambda} \tag{23.1}$$

where
m is the interferential order
d is the distance between both boundaries, that is, lipid layer thickness
ϕ' is the refracted angle and always is normal or almost normal to the corneal surface
λ is the wavelength of light
$n(\lambda)$ is the refraction index, which depends on wavelength

This interference phenomena can be visible by specular reflection commented earlier, and the observer can appreciate an interference pattern, formed by fringes and/or colors and commonly known as tear film *lipid layer pattern* (LLP). Color fringes are related with lipid layer thickness; so, the determination of lipid layer thickness can be extrapolated. However, the lipidic reflection does not always show a color pattern. The observation of a colorless pattern (gray color) is because its thickness is below the minimal thickness to produce interference fringes. Korb [31] established the lipid layer thickness that corresponded to each color (see Table 23.1), by using a custom-designed hemicylindrical broad-spectrum illumination source and slit-lamp biomicroscope.

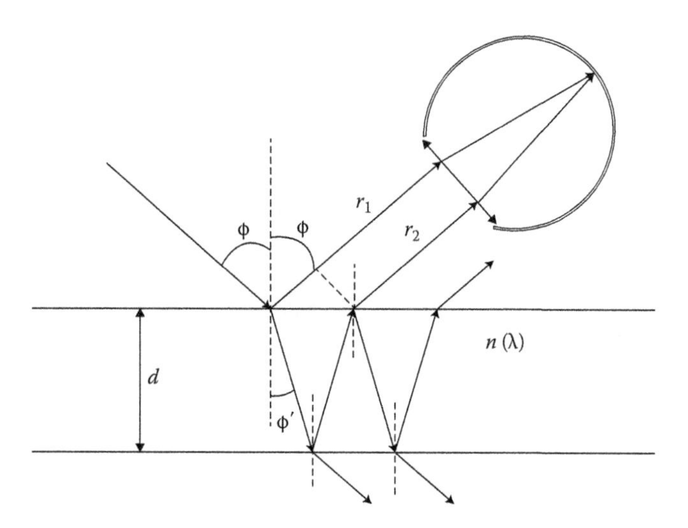

FIGURE 23.4
Optical diagram, which shows the interference. Both light beams r_1 and r_2 originate from the same source: r_1 is the light beam reflected from the air–lipid interface of the tear film and r_2 is the light beam reflected from the lipid–aqueous interface of the tear film. The thickness d generates an optical path difference between them and will produce interference fringes after recombination. ϕ is the incidence angle, equal to the reflected angles; ϕ' is the refracted angle and $n(\lambda)$ is the refraction index.

TABLE 23.1
Correspondence of the Color Interference Pattern with Lipid Layer Thickness

Color	Lipid Layer Thickness (nm)
Gray to white	30–60
Gray/yellow	75
Yellow	90
Yellow/brown	105
Brown/yellow	120
Brown	135
Brown/blue	150
Blue/brown	165
Blue	180

Subsequently, many devices, based on optical principles described here, have been designed to assess the LLP. This chapter is focused on two relevant methods: the Tearscope plus and the Doane's interferometer.

23.4.3 Tearscope Plus

The Tearscope plus [6] is a handheld instrument designed by Guillon that can be used alone or in conjunction with the biomicroscope [26] (see Figure 23.5). The first way makes faster the LLP evaluation, although is recommended to use with the biomicroscope to obtain images with high magnification. The observation of the LLP is usually made at

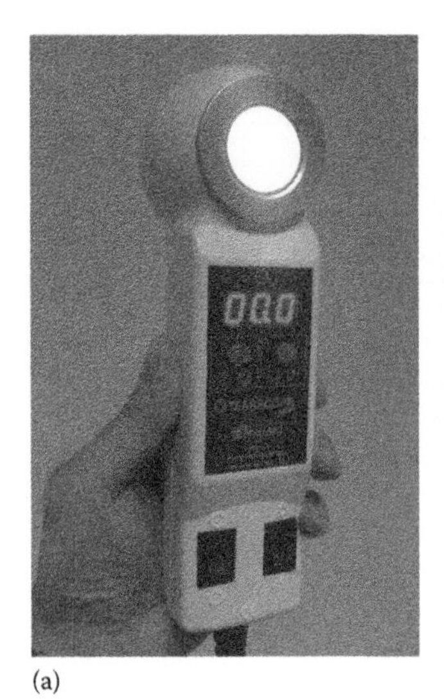

(a)

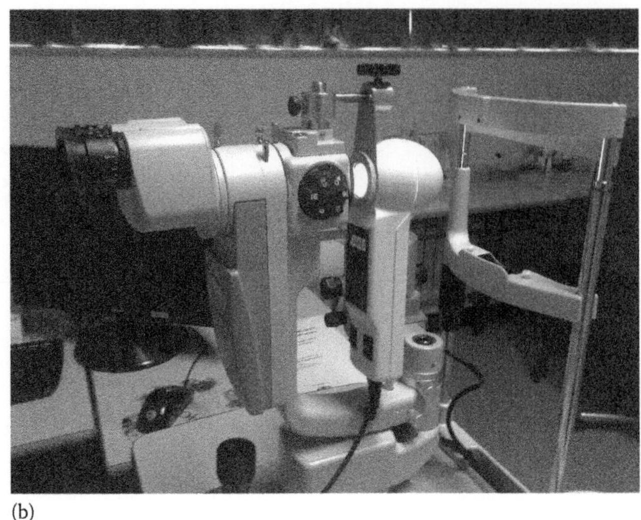

(b)

FIGURE 23.5
Tearscope plus. This device enables specular reflection over the entire cornea through a cylindrical source of white fluorescent light onto the lipid layer. (a) Tearscope plus handheld instrument. (b) Tearscope plus attached to a slit lamp, which enables high magnification.

16–40 × objective magnification. The Tearscope plus acts as the light source, and it projects a cylindrical source of cool white fluorescent light onto the lipid layer. Thus, any observed phenomena are unique to the specific light source of this device. The Tearscope plus lighting system is a diffuse hemispherical light source with a central hole to allow observation [26].

Guillon proposed five main grades of lipid layer thickness interference patterns for observations made using the Tearscope plus [26]. These patterns are based on the morphology and the color (see Figure 23.6):

Open meshwork (13–50 nm). It represents a very thin, poor, and minimal lipid layer stretched over the ocular surface. Its appearance is gray, marble-like pattern that indicates a poor tear film prone to EDE.

Closed meshwork (13–50 nm). It indicates more lipid than open meshwork, less stretching of the lipid film. It is a gray, marble-like pattern, but with closed meshwork and tight pattern.

Wave (50–70 nm). It is thicker than meshwork with wavy, gray streak effect. This represents average tear film stability.

Amorphous (80–90 nm). It is associated with a thick, white, yellowish even, and well-mixed lipid layer that may show colors during the blink. Ideal candidate for CL fitting.

Color fringe (brown 90–140 nm, blue 180 nm). It represents a thicker lipid layer with a mix of brown and blue color fringes well spread out over the surface. Good candidate for CL wear with possible tendency for greasing problems or lipid deposits if a CL is fitted.

Although this method offers a useful technique to evaluate the quality and structure of the tear film, it is affected by the subjective interpretation of the observer. Thicker lipid

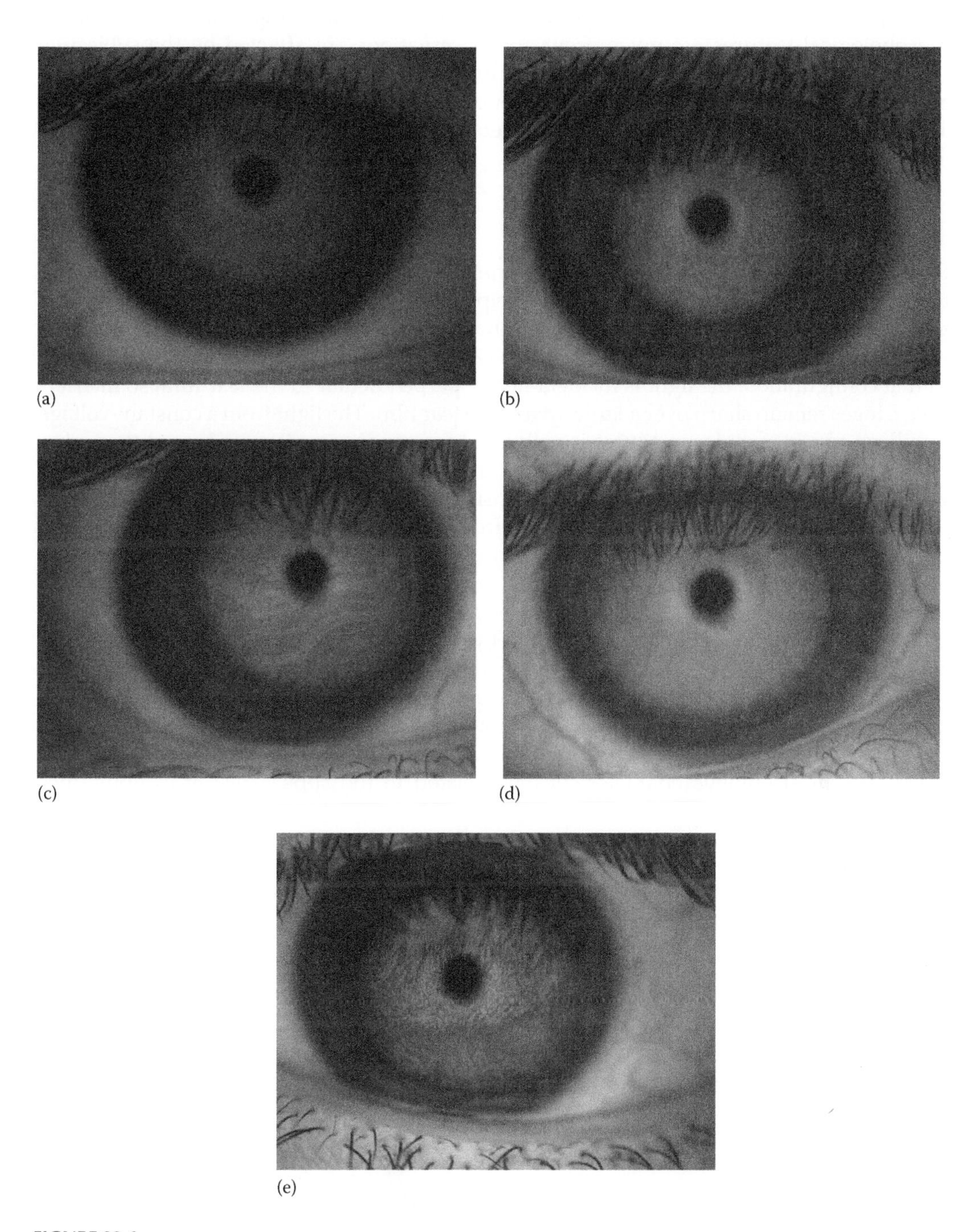

FIGURE 23.6
Lipid layer interference patterns observed with the Tearscope plus. (a) Open meshwork, (b) closed meshwork, (c) wave, (d) amorphous, and (e) color fringe.

layers (≥90 nm) are readily observed since they produce color and wave patterns. However, thin lipid layers (≤60 nm) are difficult to visualize, since color fringes and other distinct morphological features are not present and observations are affected by the subjective interpretation of the observer [31]. Training also affects the interpretation of the LLP. Thus, a learning curve for Tearscope tear interference pattern grading was established [40]. The Tearscope plus can be also used with a camera attached to a slit lamp [23], so LLP videos can be stored for further analysis.

23.4.4 Doane's Interferometer

Doane [20] designed and constructed an instrument that allows measurement of the in vivo tear film through an application of the principle of thin film interferometry. Basically, the tear film interferometer consists of a light source and an observation system and captures images using a video-based system. Figure 23.7 shows a scheme of this interferometer [23]. In that configuration, the light is incident nearly perpendicular to the tear film, so interference fringes remain sharp over a large area of the tear film. The light from a constant-voltage stabilized tungsten–halogen source is collected by a condensing lens, is passed through a narrowband interference filter, has a half maximum bandwidth <8 nm, is centered at 546 nm wavelength, and is used to illuminate a translucent screen S. This screen then acts as an extended source, and light from it is reflected from the front-surface diagonal mirror M. This mirror and a large condensing lens, both having central apertures, form a cone of light that is incident upon the surface of the tear film. After reflection from the two surfaces of the tear film, the specularly reflected light passes through the apertures in the center of the condensing lens and diagonal mirror and is collected by a focusing lens L, which forms an image of the surface of the tear film on a photographic film plane or video camera sensor [20].

Initially, the method of categorizing the images followed that of Thai et al. [51]. However, the change to a digital camera made this unworkable, due to the level of detail seen in the digital images. In order to rework the categories, large selections of images were analyzed. The most obvious characteristics are related to the appearance of contour lines

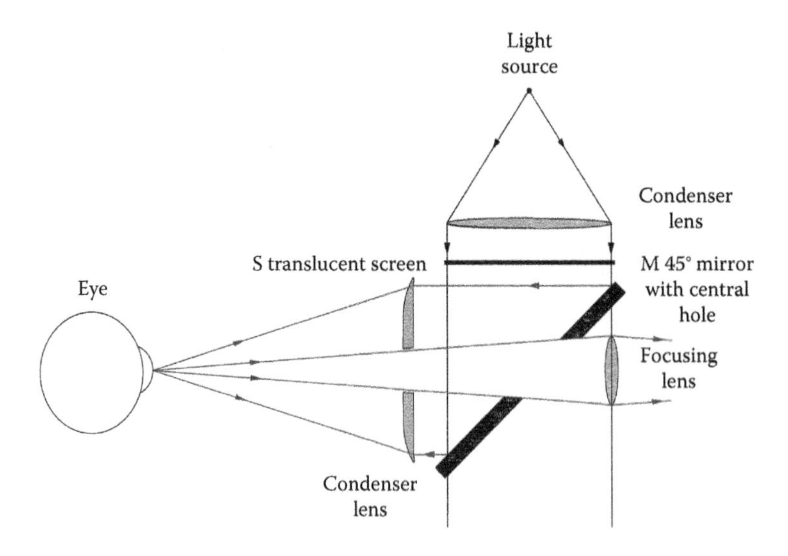

FIGURE 23.7
Schematic illustration of the Doane's interferometer.

suggesting variations in the lipid layer thickness. These were either gray or made up of colored fringes. The presence or absence of disturbances in the tear film was also noted. These features suggested groups described in terms of *strong* fringes, with either a regular pattern or a broken pattern; *fine* fringes, with very little color differentiation; and *debris*, indicating small to medium disturbances within the underlying pattern.

An overall observation of the tear film with white light allows classification into five distinct patterns with the following appearances (see Figure 23.8):

Strong fringes. It contains obvious color fringes with an appearance of spreading across the cornea.

Coalescing strong fringes. It is defined by obvious color fringes, but coalescing into islands of color.

Fine fringes. It has gray fringes spreading across the cornea.

Coalescing fine fringes. It is composed of gray fringes, but coalescing into islands of gray.

Debris. It includes obvious disturbances in the tear film, likely to be of varying origin.

Once again, this useful technique is difficult to carry out due to the inconsistency in analyzing the images. Significant changes can occur in relatively short time intervals, resulting in successive images that can be dramatically different from each other.

23.5 Automatic Classification of Tear Film Images

Experts carry out tear film assessment by means of the evaluation of the lipid layer through a manual process, which consists in classifying images obtained with the Tearscope plus or the Doane's interferometer into one of their corresponding categories. This clinical task is not only difficult and time-consuming, but also affected by the subjective interpretation of the observers.

It was demonstrated that the evaluation of the interference lipid pattern using Tearscope images can be automated with the benefits of being faster and unaffected by subjective factors [43,23]. The key of these researches lies in characterizing the interference phenomena as a color texture pattern through image processing techniques. Color is one of the discriminant features of the Guillon's categories because some patterns show distinctive color characteristics, and texture is used to characterize the interference patterns of the Guillon's categories, since thick lipid layers show clear patterns while thinner ones are more homogeneous. In a similar way, a representative set of texture extraction methods and three color spaces were proposed in [45] to characterize the Guillon's patterns. Regarding machine learning algorithms, the behavior of five popular classifiers was analyzed in [44], and a statistical comparison between them was proposed.

On the other hand, the evaluation of the interference lipid pattern using Doane images can be also automated according to [46]. In this research, a comparative study was performed by analyzing the results obtained with five texture extraction techniques and three color spaces. The general methodology proposed for both Tearscope and Doane images is common, with slight differences in some of its stages. Figure 23.9 depicts this research methodology for automatic tear film classification.

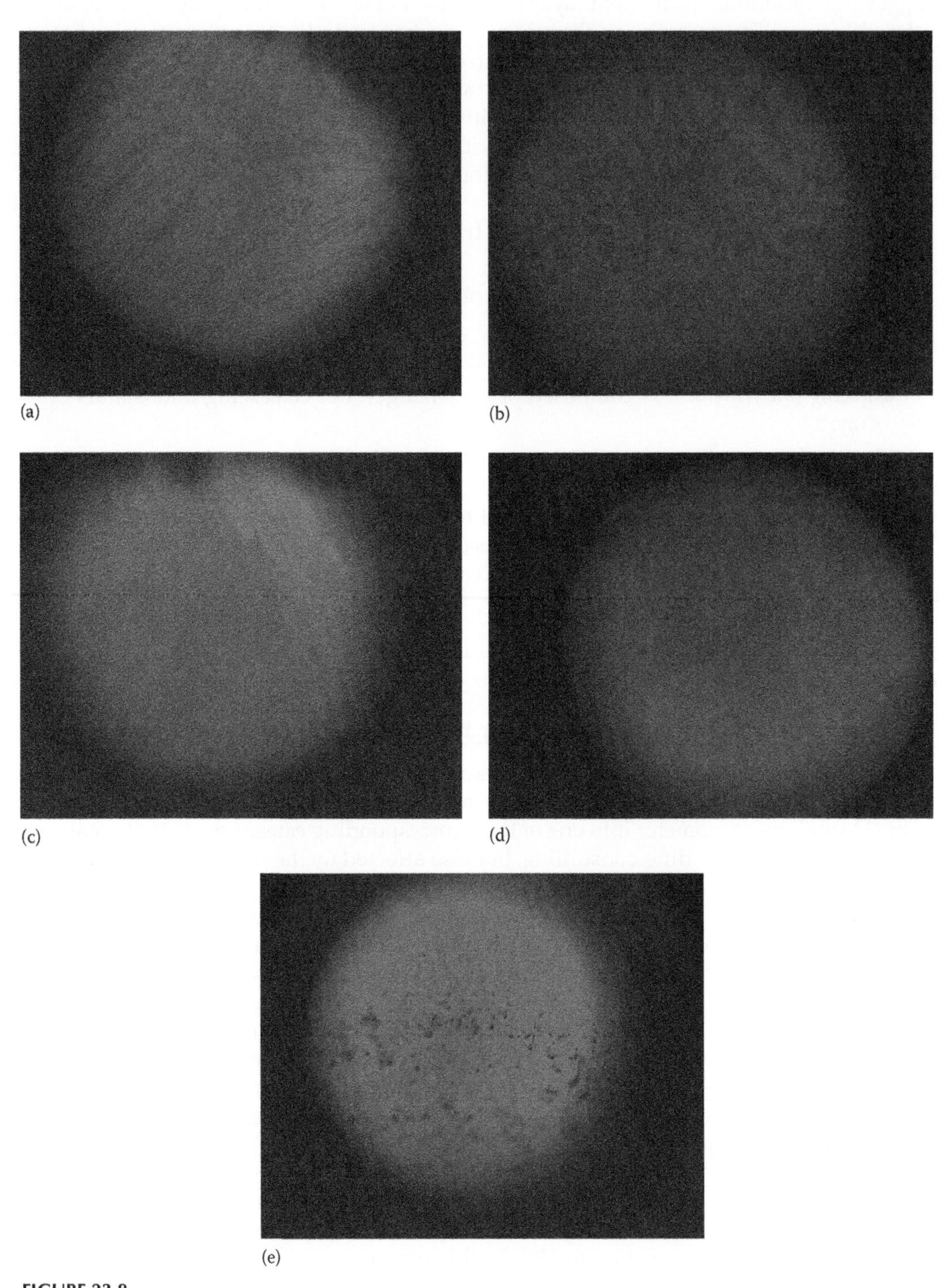

(a) (b) (c) (d) (e)

FIGURE 23.8
(See color insert.) Lipid layer interference patterns observed with the Doane's interferometer. (a) Strong fringes, (b) coalescing strong fringes, (c) fine fringes, (d) coalescing fine fringes, and (e) debris.

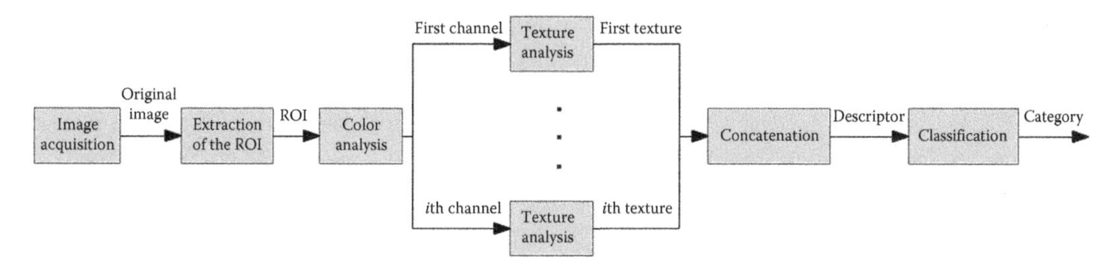

FIGURE 23.9
Steps of the general methodology.

Firstly, the input image is acquired using the Tearscope plus or the Doane's interferometer. Secondly, the region of interest (ROI) of the input image in RGB is extracted. After that, this extracted region in RGB is converted into different channels, which depend on the color analysis technique considered. Next, the texture features of each channel are extracted, and their individual descriptors are generated. Then, the individual descriptors are concatenated in order to generate the final descriptor of the input image, which contains its color and texture features. Finally, the descriptor is classified into one of the corresponding categories using a machine learning algorithm. Following, every stage will be explained in detail apart from the concatenation step due to its simplicity.

23.5.1 Image Acquisition

The input image acquisition is carried out according to two different procedures, one per each instrument considered. Next, both procedures are explained in depth.

23.5.1.1 Tearscope Images

The image acquisition is carried out with the Tearscope plus [6] attached to a Topcon SL-D4 slit lamp [5]. The interference patterns are observed through a slit-lamp microscope, with magnification set at 200×. Since the lipid tear film is not static between blinks, a video is recorded and analyzed by an optometrist in order to select the best image for processing. The interference phenomena is recorded using a Topcon DV-3 digital video camera [3] and stored via the Topcon IMAGEnet i-base [4] at a spatial resolution of 1024×768 pixels per frame and in the RGB color space. Then, an image is selected to go through the next step only when the lipid tear film is completely expanded after the eye blink.

23.5.1.2 Doane Images

In this case, the image acquisition is carried out with the Doane's interferometer [20] and a digital PC-attached CMEX-1301 camera [1]. The program ImageFocus [2] is used for image capture, and images are stored at a spatial resolution of 1280×1024 in the RGB color space. A video of approximately 4 fps is recorded for up to 1 min, and then an optometrist analyzes it in order to select the best image to be processed in the next step.

23.5.2 Extraction of the ROI

Before analyzing the color and the texture corresponding to the interference phenomena, it is necessary to extract the region where they appear. Both kinds of images contain several parts of the eye that lack information for the automatic classification, such as eyelashes (see Figures 23.6 and 23.8). Experts usually analyze the central part of the images, ignoring these irrelevant areas and focusing on the area in which the predominant pattern is clear. This leads to the second step, which consists in preprocessing the images in order to extract the ROI [45,46], where the automatic classification will take place. This stage of the methodology is different for each type of image, so both options are subsequently described.

23.5.2.1 Tearscope Images

The bottom part of the iris is where the tear has higher contrast, and so it is the area analyzed by optometrists to assess the tear film by interference phenomena. This region corresponds to the most illuminated area of the image because of the acquisition procedure. Thus, the input image in RGB is transformed to the $L \times {}^*a \times {}^*b$ (Lab) color space, and only its component of luminance L is selected to this stage. Next, a set of previously ring-shaped templates, that cover the different shapes the ROI can have, is considered. The ROI is located using the *normalized cross-correlation technique* [48] between the L channel and the set of templates. Thus, the ROI is selected as the area with maximum normalized cross-correlation value. As a result, a subtemplate is produced and the ROI is located as a rectangle inside it. Figure 23.10 depicts the stages for extracting the ROI when the Tearscope plus is used to acquire the images.

23.5.2.2 Doane Images

The central part of the image is where its predominant pattern appears and so it is the area analyzed by practitioners in order to evaluate the tear film. This region corresponds to the surface of the cornea, characterized by green or yellow tonalities. Thus, only the green channel of the input image in RGB is considered in this stage. Next, the pixels whose gray level is less than a threshold are considered as the background, and the rest

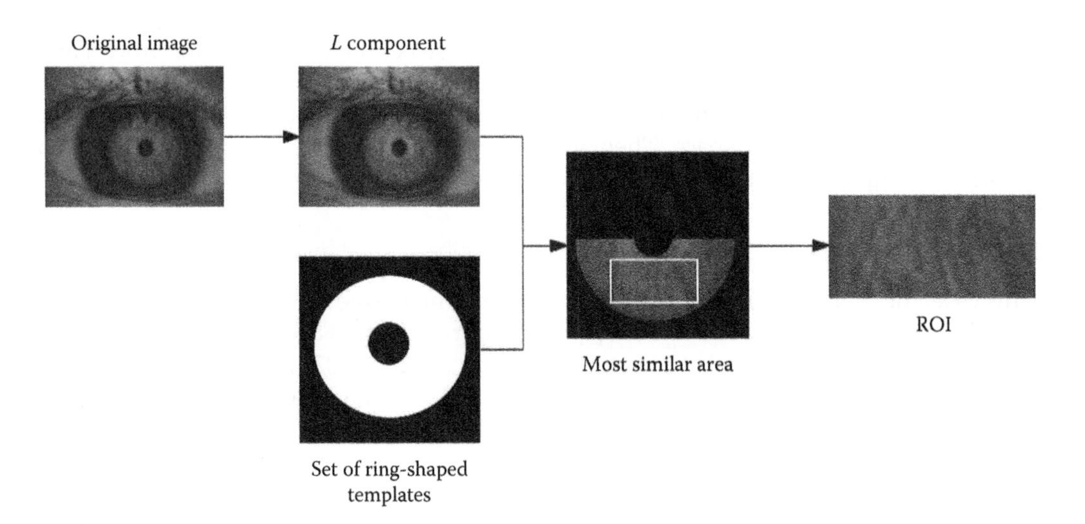

FIGURE 23.10
Extraction of the ROI from images acquired with the Tearscope plus.

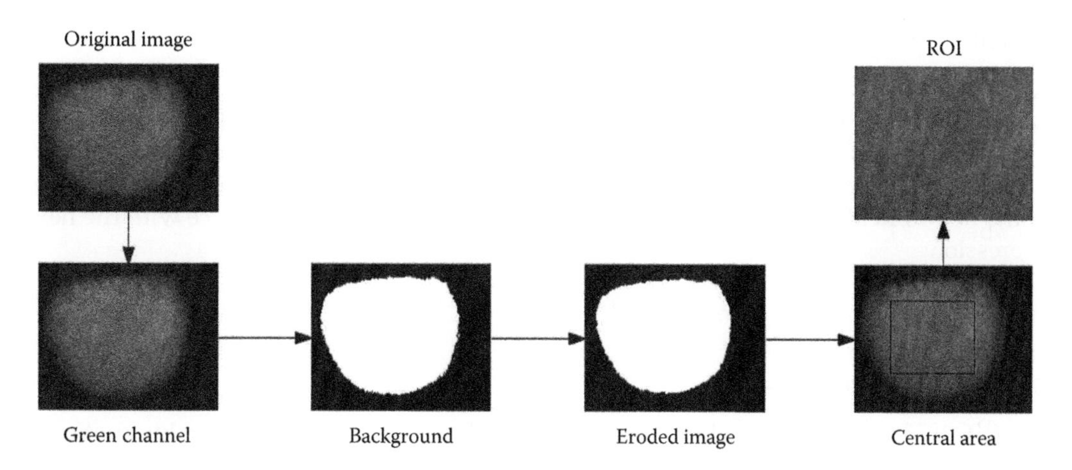

FIGURE 23.11
Extraction of the ROI from images acquired with the Doane's interferometer.

of them represent the surface of the cornea. Then, the morphological operator of erosion is applied to shrink the area of the cornea and eliminate some irrelevant parts that can appear around it. After that, the rectangle defined by the background is considered and its size is reduced to an established percentage, and so the ROI is delimited. Figure 23.11 shows the extraction of the ROI, step by step, when Doane's interferometer is used to acquire the tear film images.

23.5.3 Color Analysis

Color is one of the discriminant features of the images acquired with the Tearscope plus and the Doane's interferometer, since some categories show distinctive color characteristics. For this reason, the stage of color analysis is proposed in the methodologies presented in [45,46]. Thus, besides grayscale images, which do not analyze color information, the use of Lab and RGB images is also considered in both researches. Figure 23.12 shows the different channels that the color analysis produces as the inputs to the texture analysis step. Next, these three options for color analysis are explained.

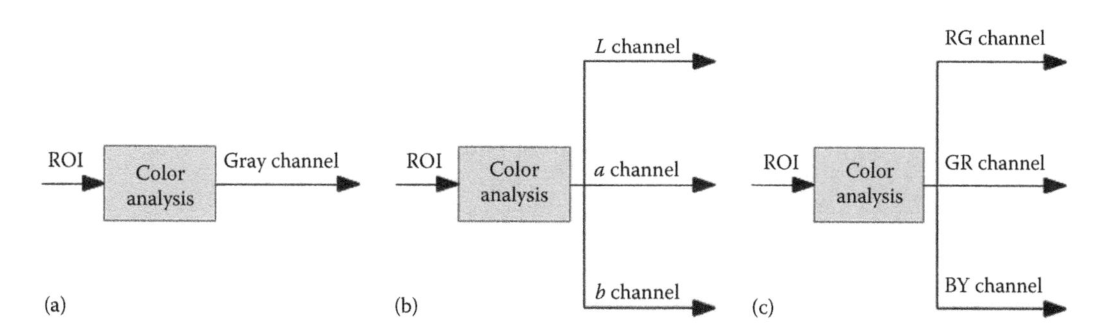

FIGURE 23.12
Color analysis using (a) grayscale images, (b) Lab color space, and (c) opponent colors.

23.5.3.1 Grayscale

A grayscale image is one in which the only color are shades of gray varying from black to white. It is only necessary to specify a single intensity value for each pixel, so less information needs to be provided.

Using grayscale images to analyze the texture entails transforming the three channels of the ROI in RGB (*R*, *G*, and *B*) to only one gray channel (*Gr*) in accordance with the next expression:

$$Gr = 0.299 \cdot R + 0.587 \cdot G + 0.114 \cdot B \tag{23.2}$$

23.5.3.2 Lab Color Space

The CIE 1976 Lab color space [37] is a chromatic color space, specified by the International Commission on Illumination, which describes all the colors visible to the human eye. Lab is a 3D model where its three coordinates represent (1) the luminance of the color *L*, (2) its position between magenta and green *a*, and (3) its position between yellow and blue *b*. Its use is recommended by CIE in images with natural illumination, and its colorimetric components, which are differences of colors, make this color space appropriate for texture analysis.

Using the Lab color space to analyze texture involves converting the three channels of the ROI in RGB to the three channels of Lab (*L*, *a*, and *b*). This transformation has to be done by calculating first *X*, *Y*, and *Z* as intermediate channels:

$$\begin{bmatrix} X \\ Y \\ Z \end{bmatrix} = \begin{bmatrix} 0.4124563 & 0.357580 & 0.180423 \\ 0.212671 & 0.715160 & 0.072169 \\ 0.019334 & 0.119193 & 0.950227 \end{bmatrix} \cdot \begin{bmatrix} R \\ G \\ B \end{bmatrix} \tag{23.3}$$

$$\begin{aligned} X &= \frac{X}{0.950456} \\ Z &= \frac{Z}{1.088754} \end{aligned} \tag{23.4}$$

Next, the Lab channels are calculated according to

$$L = \begin{cases} 116 \cdot Y^{1/3} - 16 & \text{for } Y > 0.008856 \\ 903.3 \cdot Y & \text{for } Y \le 0.008856 \end{cases} \tag{23.5}$$

$$\begin{aligned} a &= 500(f(X) - f(Y)) + 128 \\ b &= 200(f(Y) - f(Z)) + 128 \end{aligned} \tag{23.6}$$

where

$$f(t) = \begin{cases} t^{1/3} & \text{for } t > 0.008856 \\ 7.787t + 16/116 & \text{for } t \le 0.008856 \end{cases} \tag{23.7}$$

23.5.3.3 RGB Color Space: Opponent Colors

The RGB color space [49] is an additive color space defined by three chromaticities: (1) the channel red R, (2) the channel green G, and (3) the channel blue B. Despite being one of the most frequently used color spaces for image processing, it is not perceptually uniform. For this reason, the opponent process theory of human color vision, proposed by Hering [28] in the 1800s, is used instead of using directly the RGB color space. This theory states that the human visual system interprets information about color by processing three opponent channels: red versus green (R_G), green versus red (G_R), and blue versus yellow (B_Y).

Using opponent colors to analyze the texture makes it necessary to calculate the three opponent colors from the ROI in RGB, which are defined as

$$\begin{aligned} R_G &= R - p * G \\ G_R &= G - p * R \\ B_Y &= B - p * (R + G) \end{aligned} \tag{23.8}$$

where p is a low-pass filter.

23.5.4 Texture Analysis

Texture analysis is an important and useful area of study in machine vision. Most natural surfaces exhibit texture, and a successful vision system must be able to deal with the textured world surrounding it. Regarding tear film classification, previous works [45,46] have demonstrated the utility of making use of texture to characterize the interference patterns, one of the discriminant features of the lipid layer categories.

In order to deal with this step, five popular texture analysis methods [16] were proposed in the two aforementioned researches: *Butterworth filters*, *Gabor filters*, and *the discrete wavelet transform*, as signal processing methods; *Markov random fields* (MRFs) as a model-based method; and *co-occurrence features* as a statistical method. These methods are subsequently described.

23.5.4.1 Butterworth Filters

Butterworth band-pass filters [25] are frequency domain filters that have a flat response in the band-pass frequency, which gradually decays in the stopband. A Butterworth band-pass filter can be represented in 1D as

$$f(\omega) = \frac{1}{1 + ((\omega - \omega_c)/\omega_0)^{2n}} \tag{23.9}$$

where

- n is the order of the filter
- ω is the angular frequency
- ω_0 is the cutoff frequency
- ω_c is the center frequency

The order n of the filter defines the slope of the decay; the higher the order, the faster the decay.

A bank of nine second-order filters is used, so that the whole frequency spectrum is covered by the band-pass frequencies considered. By that means, the filter bank maps each input image into nine filtered images, one per frequency band. Next, the quantitative vector to each image has to be created. Therefore, each frequency band results have to be normalized and the histograms of their output images have to be computed. Uniform histograms with nonequidistant bins are used instead of the traditional ones. In order to obtain uniform histograms, the next process is followed: given all the filtered images in a frequency band, their pixels are sorted and the limits of the histogram are defined so that each bin contains a maximum of N/N_{bins} pixels, where N is the number of pixels in the corresponding frequency and N_{bins} the number of histogram bins.

Using 16-bin histograms, the descriptor of an input image has 16 components per frequency band. Thus, the nine individual descriptors can be combined by just concatenating them.

23.5.4.2 Gabor Filters

Gabor filters [22] are complex exponential signal modulated by Gaussians widely used in texture analysis. A 2D Gabor filter [19], using Cartesian coordinates in the spatial domain and polar coordinates in the frequency domain, can be defined as

$$g_{x_0,y_0,f_0,\theta_0} = exp\{i[2\pi f_0(x\cos\theta_0 + y\sin\theta_0) + \phi]\}gauss(x,y) \quad (23.10)$$

where

$$gauss(x,y) = a \cdot exp\{-\pi[a^2(x\cos\theta_0 + y\sin\theta_0)^2 + b^2(x\sin\theta_0 - y\cos\theta_0)^2]\} \quad (23.11)$$

a and b model the shape of the filter, while x_0, y_0, f_0, and θ_0 represent the location in the spatial and frequency domains, respectively.

A bank of filters is created with 16 Gabor filters centered at 4 frequencies and 4 orientations. Thus, the filter bank maps each input image to 16 filtered images, one per frequency–orientation pair. Using the same idea as in Butterworth filters, the feature vector is created by generating the uniform histogram with nonequidistant bins. The individual descriptors associated to each filter are combined by means of their concatenation, and different numbers of bins can be considered.

23.5.4.3 Discrete Wavelet Transform

The discrete wavelet transform [35] generates a set of wavelets by scaling and translating a *mother wavelet*, which is a function defined both in the spatial and frequency domains, that can be represented in 2D as

$$\phi^{a,b}(x,y) = \frac{1}{\sqrt{a_x a_y}}\phi\left(\frac{x-b_x}{a_x}, \frac{y-b_y}{a_y}\right) \quad (23.12)$$

where

$a = (a_x, a_y)$ governs the scale

$b = (b_x, b_y)$ the translation of the function

The values of *a* and *b* control the band-pass of the filter in order to generate high-pass (H) or low-pass (L) filters.

The wavelet decomposition of an image consists in applying wavelets horizontally and vertically in order to generate four subimages at each scale (LL, LH, HL, and HH), which are then subsampled by a factor of 2. It is an iterative method, which consists in repeating the process over the LL subimage and results in the standard pyramidal wavelet decomposition.

Some statistical measures are used to create the descriptor from an input image: mean, absolute average deviation, and energy. These measures are, respectively, defined as

$$\mu = \frac{1}{N}\sum_{i=1}^{N} p(i) \tag{23.13}$$

$$aad = \frac{1}{N}\sum_{i=1}^{N} |p(i) - \mu| \tag{23.14}$$

$$e = \frac{1}{N^2}\sum_{i=1}^{N} p(i)^2 \tag{23.15}$$

Thus, the feature descriptor of an input image is constructed from the μ and the *aad* of the input and LL images and from the *e* of the LH, HL, and HH images.

Different mother wavelets can be considered, such as Haar or Daubechies. Haar is the simplest nontrivial wavelet and Daubechies is one representative type of basis for wavelets. Daub*i* represents the Daubechies orthonormal wavelet, where the number of vanishing moments is equal to half the coefficient *i*. Notice that the Haar wavelet is equivalent to Daub2. Regarding the scales, different numbers of scales can also be considered depending on the size of the input image.

23.5.4.4 Markov Random Fields

MRFs [11] are model-based texture analysis methods that construct an image model whose parameters capture the essential perceived qualities of the texture. An MRF model is based upon the assumption that a pixel intensity distribution is conditionally dependent upon only its local neighborhood and independent of the rest of the image. Thus, MRFs generate a texture model by expressing the gray values of each pixel in an image as a function of the gray values in its neighborhood.

The concept of neighborhood is defined as the set of pixels within a distance *d*, using the Chebyshev distance. The Markov process for textures is modeled using a *Gaussian Markov random field* (GMRF) defined as [53]

$$X(c) = \sum \beta_{c,m}[X(c,m) + X(c-m)] + e_c \tag{23.16}$$

where

e_c is the zero mean Gaussian distributed noise
m is an offset from the center cell c
$\beta_{c,m}$ are the parameters that weigh a pair of symmetric neighbors to the center cell

The β coefficients describe the Markovian properties of the texture and the spatial interactions among pixels. Equation 23.16 can be represented in matrix notation as

$$X(c) = \beta^T Q_c + e_c \tag{23.17}$$

Consequently, the β coefficients can be estimated through least squares fitting:

$$\beta = \left[\sum_{c \in I} Q_c Q_c^T\right]^{-1} \left[\sum_{c \in I} Q_c X(c)\right] \tag{23.18}$$

The texture descriptor of an input image is obtained by calculating the directional variances proposed by Cesmeli and Wang [15], which are defined as

$$f_i = \frac{1}{N \times M} \sum_{c \in I} [X(c) - \beta_i Q_{ci}]^2 \tag{23.19}$$

For a distance d, the descriptor comprises $4d$ features. Different distances can be considered and their descriptors can be combined by means of their concatenation.

23.5.4.5 Co-Occurrence Features

Haralick et al. introduced co-occurrence features [27], a popular and effective texture descriptor based on the computation of the conditional joint probabilities of all pairwise combinations of gray levels, given an interpixel distance d and an orientation θ. The method generates a set of *gray level co-occurrence matrices* (GLCM) and extracts several statistical measures from their elements.

As in the aforementioned method, the *Chebyshev* distance is considered. Therefore, for a distance $d=1$, four orientations are considered (0°, 45°, 90°, and 135°) and four GLCM are generated. In general, the number of orientations and, accordingly, the number of matrices for a distance d is $4d$.

From each GLCM, a set of 14 statistics proposed by Haralick et al. [27] are computed. For explanatory purposes, the definition of 3 of these 14 statistical measures is shown:

$$f_1 = \sum_{i=1}^{N} \sum_{j=1}^{N} \left(\frac{P_{\theta,d}(i,j)}{R} \right)^2 \tag{23.20}$$

$$f_2 = \sum_{n=0}^{N-1} n^2 \left\{ \sum_{|i-j|=n} \left(\frac{P_{\theta,d}(i,j)}{R} \right) \right\} \tag{23.21}$$

$$f_3 = \frac{\sum_{i=1}^{N} \sum_{j=1}^{N} [i, jP_{\theta,d}(i,j)/R] - \mu_x \mu_y}{\sigma_x \sigma_y} \tag{23.22}$$

where

$P_{\theta,d}(i,j)$ are the elements of the matrix
N is the number of distinct gray levels
R is a normalizing constant
μ_x, μ_y, σ_x, and σ_y are the means and standard deviations of the marginal distributions associated with $P_{\theta,d}(i,j)$
The angular second-moment feature f_1 is a measure of homogeneity of the image
The contrast feature f_2 is a measure of the amount of local variations present in the image
The correlation feature f_3 is a measure of gray-tone linear dependencies in the image

The mean and the range of these 14 statistics are calculated across matrices, and a set of 28 features composes the texture descriptor for a distance *d*. Different distances can be considered and combined in different ways by only concatenating their individual descriptors.

23.5.5 Classification

After performing the previous steps, an input image leads to a quantitative vector containing color and texture features. These features should be distinctive in order to classify the vector into one of the corresponding categories. In this sense, machine learning supplies algorithms that improve automatically through experience based on data, in a process also known as training. Data can be seen as examples that illustrate relations between features and classes. In the problem at hand, the images are the examples with their quantitative vectors as features, while the categories correspond to the classes.

In [43,44], several machine learning algorithms applied to Tearscope images were statistically analyzed in terms of accuracy. The same general conclusion was reached in both researches: the *support vector machine* (SVM) was selected as the most competitive method. On the other hand, the experiments performed over Doane images presented in [46] also used the SVM as machine learning algorithm.

SVM is a supervised learning algorithm based on the statistical learning theory. It revolves around the notion of a *margin*, either side of a hyperplane that separates two classes [14]. This algorithm necessarily reaches a global minimum and avoids ending in a local minimum. Also, SVM avoids problems of overfitting, and with an appropriate kernel, it can work well even if the data are not linearly separable. However, SVM methods are binary; so, multiclass problems, as tear film classification, have to be transformed to a set of multiple binary problems.

23.5.6 Results

Several experiments were performed in [45] using the five different texture extraction methods in the three color spaces previously presented. A similar kind of experiment was performed in [46]. All the experimental results presented in both of them were obtained using two different datasets annotated by optometrists, which are the following:

Tearscope images. This dataset [8] is composed of 105 images acquired with the Tearscope plus from healthy subjects with ages ranging from 19 to 33 years old. It includes 29 open meshwork, 29 closed meshwork, 25 wave, and 25 color fringe images.

Doane images. This dataset [7] is composed of 106 images acquired with the Doane's interferometer from patients between 39 and 71 years old. It includes 11 strong fringes, 25 coalescing strong fringes, 30 fine fringes, 26 coalescing fine fringes, and 14 debris images.

Regarding the texture extraction methods, the different experiments performed are summarized in Table 23.2. Each of these experiments was performed in grayscale, Lab, and opponent colors. Tables 23.3 and 23.4 show the best result for each texture–color pair, where the best result per color space is highlighted. These results are presented in terms of percentage accuracy, a measure which represents the rate percent of the images that are correctly classified according to their category. Also, the parameter configuration of each pair is specified in brackets.

Table 23.3 shows a remarkable improvement in accuracy due to the use of color information. This improvement is because color is one of the discriminant features of the Guillon's categories. Regarding texture extraction methods, co-occurrence features produce best results closely followed by Gabor filters, both of them providing classification results with maximum accuracy over 95%, when they are combined with the Lab color space. On the other hand, results in Table 23.4 show that, in general, the use of color information slightly improves the accuracy obtained in grayscale, and the Lab color space outperforms the

TABLE 23.2

Experiments Performed over Tearscope and Doane Images with Each Texture Extraction Method

	Tearscope Images	Doane Images
Butterworth filters	Using the 9 frequency band filters and 16-bins histograms, each frequency band was analyzed separately. Additionally, the adjacent frequency bands were combined by means of the concatenation of their individual descriptors.	
Gabor filters	3-bin, 5-bin, 7-bin, and 9-bin histograms were analyzed using the bank of 16 Gabor filters.	From 3- to 19-bin histograms, 2 × 2 were analyzed using the bank of 16 Gabor filters.
Discrete wavelet transform	Each feature was analyzed individually to determine its relevance, using the Haar algorithm as the mother wavelet and two scales. Then, two alternative descriptors were created according to the statistical measures presented above (see Section 23.5.4.3): one composed of the features obtained from the mean, the absolute average deviation, and the energy (12 features) and other composed of the features obtained from only the mean and the absolute average deviation (6 features).	Scales from 1 to 8 were analyzed using all the statistical measures presented above (see Section 23.5.4.3). The mother wavelets considered were Haar and Daubechies (Daub4, Daub6, and Daub8).
MRFs	Each distance from 1 to 10 was analyzed individually in order to compare different neighborhoods.	Each distance from 1 to 10 was analyzed individually, as well as the combination of the adjacent distances by means of the concatenation of their descriptors.
Co-occurrence features	Each distance from 1 to 7 was analyzed individually, as well as the combination of the adjacent distances through the concatenation of their descriptors.	Each distance from 1 to 17 was analyzed individually, as well as the combination of the adjacent distances through the concatenation of their descriptors.

TABLE 23.3

Comparison of Different Feature Extraction Methods Using Tearscope Images: Best SVM Categorization Accuracy (%) and Parameter Configuration in the Three Color Spaces

	Grayscale	Lab	Opp. Colors
Butterworth filters	83.81 (freqs. 1–9)	93.33 (freqs. 5–7)	90.48 (freqs. 2–4)
Gabor filters	88.57 (3 bins)	95.24 (7 bins)	88.57 (5 bins)
Discrete wavelet transform	85.72 (12 feats.)	89.52 (6 feats.)	85.71 (6 feats.)
MRFs	83.81 (dist. 4)	83.81 (dist. 3)	84.76 (dist. 1)
Co-occurrence features	**92.38** (dist. 7)	**96.19** (dist. 6)	**92.38** (dist. 3–4)

Note: The best result for each color space is given in bold.

TABLE 23.4

Comparison of Different Feature Extraction Methods Using Doane Images: Best SVM Categorization Accuracy (%) and Parameter Configuration in the Three Color Spaces

	Grayscale	Lab	Opp. Colors
Butterworth filters	86.79 (freqs. 3–5)	86.79 (freqs. 2–3)	88.68 (freqs. 1–4)
Gabor filters	85.85 (13 bins)	91.51 (17 bins)	83.96 (3 bins)
Discrete wavelet transform	86.79 (Haar 4 sc.)	89.62 (Daub4 7 sc.)	88.68 (Haar 4 sc.)
MRFs	83.96 (dist. 1–5)	91.51 (dist. 1–9)	83.96 (dist. 3–6)
Co-occurrence features	**92.45** (dist. 12)	**93.40** (dist. 2–10)	**89.62** (dist. 9)

Note: The best result for each color space is given in bold.

other two options for color analysis. This improvement is due to the presence of color features in Doane images, which are representative of each category. Respecting texture information, co-occurrence features produce best results, independently of the color space, with maximum accuracy over 90%.

These results, with maximum accuracies over 95% and 90% regarding images acquired with the Tearscope plus and the Doane's interferometer, respectively, demonstrated that it is possible to precisely evaluate the interferometry patterns through a completely automatic procedure. The clinical significance of these results should be highlighted, since the systematic and objective computerized method for analysis and classification is highly desirable, allowing for homogeneous diagnosis and relieving the experts from this tedious time-consuming task.

References

1. CMEX-1300x camera. Euromex Microscopen BV, Arnhem, the Netherlands.
2. ImageFocus Capture and Analysis Software. Euromex Microscopen BV, Arnhem, the Netherlands.
3. Topcon DV-3 digital video camera. Topcon Medical Systems, Oakland, NJ.
4. Topcon IMAGEnet i-base. Topcon Medical Systems, Oakland, NJ.

5. Topcon SL-D4 slit lamp. Topcon Medical Systems, Oakland, NJ.
6. *Tearscope Plus Clinical Hand Book and Tearscope Plus Instructions.* Keeler Ltd., Windsor, U.K./Broomall, PA, 1997.
7. VOPTICAL DO. VARPA optical dataset annotated by optometrists from the Department of Life Sciences, Glasgow Caledonian University, Glasgow, U.K., 2012.
8. VOPTICAL I1. VARPA optical dataset annotated by optometrists from the Faculty of Optics and Optometry, University of Santiago de Compostela, Santiago de Compostela, Spain, 2012. http://www.varpa.es/voptical I1.html, last accessed: March 2013.
9. M. B. Abelson, G. W. Ousler 3rd, L. A. Nally, D. Welch, and K. Krenzer. Alternative reference values for tear film break up time in normal and dry eye populations. *Adv Exp Med Biol*, 506(Pt B):1121–1125, 2002.
10. C. G. Begley, R. L. Chalmers, G. L. Mitchell, K. K. Nichols, B. Cafery, T. Simpson, R. DuToit, J. Portello, and L. Davis. Characterization of ocular surface symptoms from optometric practices in North America. *Cornea*, 20(6):610–618, 2001.
11. J. Besag. Spatial interaction and the statistical analysis of lattice systems. *J R Stat Soc B*, 36:192–236, 1974.
12. A. J. Bron, J. M. Tifany, S. M. Gouveia, N. Yokoi, and L. W. Voon. Functional aspects of the tear film lipid layer. *Exp Eye Res*, 78(3):347–360, 2004.
13. A. J. Bron and J. M. Tifany. The contribution of meibomian disease to dry eye. *Ocul Surf*, 2(2):149–165, 2004.
14. C. Burges. A tutorial on support vector machines for pattern recognition. *Data Min Knowl Dis*, 2(2):1–47, 1998.
15. E. Cesmeli and D. Wang. Texture segmentation using, Gaussian–Markov random fields and neural oscillator networks. *IEEE Trans Neural Netw*, 12, 2001.
16. C. H. Chen, L. F. Pau, and P. S. P. Wangs. *The Handbook of Pattern Recognition and Computer Vision* (2nd edn.). World Scientific Publishing Co., Inc., River Edge, NJ, 1998.
17. P. Cho and B. Brown. Review of the tear break-up time and a closer look at the tear break-up time of Hong Kong Chinese. *Optom Vis Sci*, 70(1):30–38, 1993.
18. P. Cho and W. Douthwaite. The relation between invasive and noninvasive tear break-up time. *Optom Vis Sci*, 72(1):17–22, 1995.
19. J. G. Daugman. Uncertainty relation for resolution in space, spatial frequency, and orientation optimized by two-dimensional visual cortical filters. *J Opt Soc Am A*, 2(7):1160–1169, 1985.
20. M. G. Doane. An instrument for in vivo tear film interferometry. *Opt Vis Sci*, 66(6):383–388, 1989.
21. G. N. Foulks. The correlation between the tear film lipid layer and dry eye disease. *Surv Ophthalmol*, 52(4):369–374, 2007.
22. D. Gabor. Theory of communication. *J Inst Electr Eng*, 93:429–457, 1946.
23. C. García-Resúa, M. J. Giráldez-Fernández, M. G. Penedo, D. Calvo, M. Penas, and E. Yebra-Pimentel. New software application for clarifying tear film lipid layer patterns. *Cornea*, 32(4):538–546, 2012.
24. C. García-Resúa, J. Santodomingo-Rubido, M. Lira, M. J. Giráldez, and E. Y. Vilar. Clinical assessment of the lower tear meniscus height. *Ophthalmic Physiol Opt*, 29(5):487–496, 2009.
25. R. Gonzalez and R. Woods. *Digital Image Processing*. Pearson/Prentice Hall, Upper Saddle River, NJ, 2008.
26. J. P. Guillon. Non-invasive Tearscope plus routine for contact lens fitting. *Cont Lens Anterior Eye*, 21(Suppl. 1):31–40, 1998.
27. R. M. Haralick, K. Shanmugam, and I. Dinstein. Texture features for image classification. *IEEE Trans Syst Man Cybern Syst Man Cybern*, 3:610–621, 1973.
28. E. Hering. *Outlines of a Theory of the Light Sense*. Harvard University Press, Cambridge, MA, 1964.
29. F. J. Holly. Tear film physiology and contact lens wear. II. Contact lens-tear film interaction. *Am J Optom Physiol Opt*, 58(4):331–341, 1981.

30. Y. Hori, S. Spurr-Michaud, C. L. Russo, P. Argueso, and I. K. Gipson. Differential regulation of membrane-associated mucins in the human ocular surface epithelium. *Invest Ophthalmol Vis Sci*, 45(1):114–122, 2004.
31. D. R. Korb. *The Tear Film: Structure, Function and Clinical Examination*. Butterworth-Heinemann, London, U.K., 2002.
32. J. R. Larke. *The Eye in Contact Lens Wear*. Butterworth-Heinemann, Oxford, U.K., 1997.
33. J. H. Lee and P. M. Hyun. The reproducibility of the Schirmer test. *Korean J Ophthalmol*, 2(1):5–8, 1988.
34. M. A. Lemp, C. Baudouin, J. Baum, M. Dogru, G. N. Foulks, S. Kinoshita, P. Laibson et al. The definition and classification of dry eye disease: Report of the definition and classification subcommittee of the international dry eye workshop (2007). *Ocul Surf*, 5(2):75–92, 2007.
35. S. G. Mallat. A theory for multiresolution signal decomposition: The wavelet representation. *IEEE Trans Pattern Anal Mach Intell*, 11:674–693, 1989.
36. J. P. McCulley and J. M. Dougherty. Blepharitis associated with acne rosacea and seborrheic dermatitis. *Int Ophthalmol Clin*, 25(1):159–172, 1895.
37. K. McLaren. The development of the CIE 1976 (L*a*b) uniform colour-space and colour-difference formula. *J Soc Dyers Colourists*, 92(9):338–341, 1976.
38. T. T. McMahon and K. Zadnik. Twenty-five years of contact lenses: The impact on the cornea and ophthalmic practice. *Cornea*, 19(5):730–740, 2000.
39. K. Nakamori, M. Odawara, T. Nakajima, T. Mizutani, and K. Tsubota. Blinking is controlled primarily by ocular surface conditions. *Am J Ophthalmol*, 124(1):24–30, 1997.
40. J. J. Nichols, K. K. Nichols, B. Puent, M. Saracino, and G. L. Mitchell. Evaluation of tear film interference patterns and measures of tear breakup time. *Optom Vis Sci*, 79(6):363–369, 2002.
41. P. J. Pisella, P. Pouliquen, and C. Baudouin. Prevalence of ocular symptoms and signs with preserved and preservative free glaucoma medication. *Br J Ophthalmol*, 86(4):418–423, 2002.
42. N. Pritchard and D. Fonn. Dehydration, lens movement and dryness ratings of hydrogel contact lenses. *Ophthalmic Physiol Opt*, 15(4):281–286, 1995.
43. L. Ramos, M. Penas, B. Remeseiro, A. Mosquera, N. Barreira, and E. Yebra-Pimentel. Texture and color analysis for the automatic classification of the eye lipid layer. In *LNCS: Advances in Computational Intelligence, International Work Conference on Artificial Neural Networks—IWANN 2011*, vol. 6692, pp. 66–73, Torremolinos-Málaga, Spain, 2011.
44. B. Remeseiro, M. Penas, A. Mosquera, J. Novo, M. G. Penedo, and E. Yebra-Pimentel. Statistical comparison of classifiers applied to the interferential tear film lipid layer automatic classification. *Comput Math Methods Med*, 2012:207315, 2012.
45. B. Remeseiro, L. Ramos, M. Penas, E. Martínez, M. G. Penedo, and A. Mosquera. Colour texture analysis for classifying the tear film lipid layer: A comparative study. In *International Conference on Digital Image Computing: Techniques and Applications (DICTA)*, pp. 268–273, Noosa, Queensland, Australia, December 2011.
46. B. Remeseiro, A. Tomlinson, K. Oliver, E. Martin, N. Barreira, and A. Mosquera. Automatic grading system for human tear films (unpublished yet).
47. J. E. McDonald. Surface phenomena of the tear film. *Am J Ophthalmol*, 67(1): 56–64, 1969.
48. J. C. Russ. *The Image Processing Handbook* (3rd edn.). CRC Press Inc., Boca Raton, FL, 1999.
49. S. J. Sangwine and R. E. N. Horne. *The Colour Image Processing Handbook*. Chapman & Hall, London, U.K., 1998.
50. A. Sommer and N. Emran. Tear production in vitamin A—Responsive xerophthalmia. *Am J Ophthalmol*, 93(1):84–87, 1982.
51. L. C. Thai, A. Tomlinson, and M. G. Doane. Effect of contact lens materials on tear physiology. *Optom Vis Sci*, 81(3):194–204, 2004.
52. A. Tomlinson, K. J. Blades, and E. I. Pearce. What does the phenol red thread test actually measure? *Optom Vis Sci*, 78(3):142–146, 2001.
53. J. W. Woods. Two-dimensional discrete Markovian fields. *IEEE Trans Inf Theory*, 18(2):232–240, 1972.

24

Thermography and the Eye: A Look at Ocular Surface Temperature

Dawn K.A. Lim, Caroline Ka Lin Chee, and Thet Naing

CONTENTS

24.1 Background

The role of temperature measurement in the human body has been described since 400 BC by the Greek physician Hippocrates. Heat emission, as a by-product of tissue metabolism, is transferred to the body surface by conduction, convection, through the human vascular system [1]. The measurement of ocular surface temperature (OST) to aid the understanding of ocular physiology has been widely reported in the literature since the 1960s [2–8].

Interest in eye temperature spans over decades, since the time of Dohnberg, who attempted to measure the eye temperature with a mercury thermometer, as far back as 1876 [9]. Contact methods have been criticized for inducing tearing that destroys thermal equilibrium [3]; thus, temperature measurement of the eye has been superseded by technologic innovations in noncontact methods such as infrared thermography.

This chapter describes the application of infrared images in ophthalmology.

24.2 Infrared Imaging of the Eye

The source of infrared radiation is heat or thermal radiation from the human body. This lies within the electromagnetic spectrum, which is invisible to the naked eye. Over the

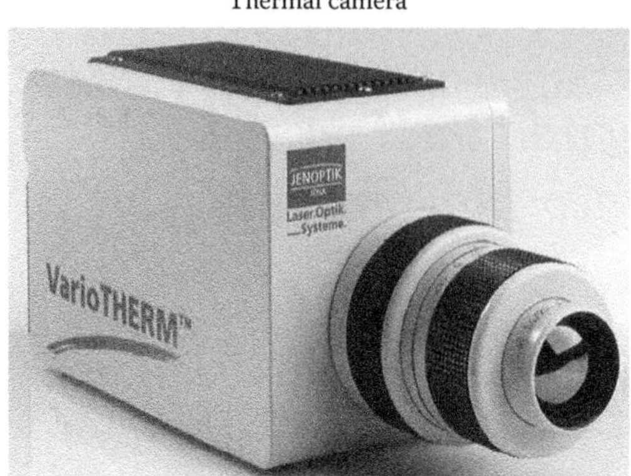

FIGURE 24.1
An example of an infrared camera, VarioTHERM® head II, by Jenoptik, Germany.

years, technologic adaptations from military prototypes have been applied to the development of infrared cameras for medical use, with increasing sensitivity and reliability, results of which can be appreciated in a color-coded display.

Mapstone was amongst the first to describe observations from the use of infrared camera on the eye [2–8]. He proposed that the surface temperature of the eye can be determined by measuring the quantity of radiation emitted. Mapstone then variously described thermography recordings in various conditions such as anterior uveitis, internal carotid stenosis, and ischemic anterior segments using the Bofors infrared system.

The current generation of infrared cameras is more portable, with faster frame speeds, reproducibility, and sensitivity. These use imaging systems of focal plane array, which image a desired field of view without scanning, analogous to a typical camera, through which the film captures the 2-D image directly projected by the lens at an image plane.

An example of specifications seen in an infrared camera (Figure 24.1: VarioTHERM® II, Jenoptik, Germany) include the following:

- Focal plane array detector with 256 × 256 pixel resolution
- Bandwidth of 3.4–5.0 μm
- Thermal resolution of 0.1°C
- Accuracy of ±2%
- Frame speeds of 50 Hz
- Range of lenses to choose from, based on the desired field of view

24.3 Thermal Profile of the Ocular Surface

Normal ocular thermograms have been described [3,5,10], with central or averaged OST ranging from 32.9°C to 36°C, with a normal temperature difference between the limbus and central cornea to be 0.37°C ± 0.21°C (mean ± SD). On a color-coded display, red

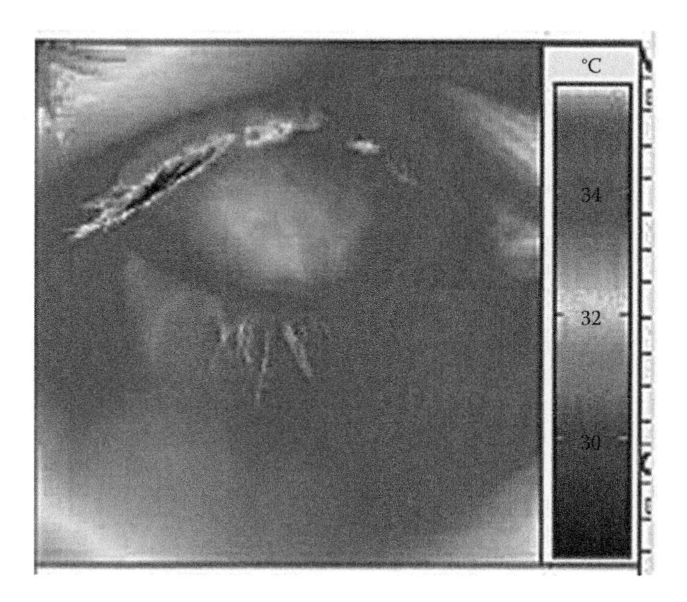

FIGURE 24.2
(See color insert.) A normal ocular thermogram in color-coded display.

represents warmer areas of the ocular surface, whereas blue represents the cooler zones or isotherms.

Typical descriptions of cool areas and warmer areas of the ocular surface are as follows (Figure 24.2):

Cooler isotherms:

- Center of cornea

Warmer isotherms:

- Medial and lateral canthi and palpebral skin.

Mapstone [3] proposed that thermal patterns in and around the eye can be explained away by how surface heat is conducted over a concave or convex surface, with differential warming of the overlying tear film. A convex surface (such as the cornea) tends to demonstrate a greater net loss of heat compared to a concave surface like the canthi. This is because convected loss depends on a free passage of air over a surface. Hence, there will be no obstruction to flow over a convex surface, whereas a concave surface (canthi) contains isolated pockets of skin that will retain some heat within the walls of the concavity, hence resulting in the observed warmer isotherms.

Factors that account for the cooler isotherm over the center of the cornea include the following:

- Its avascularity.
- It is the area most distal from the limbal vasculature.
- The anterior chamber in a normal eye is deeper centrally compared to the periphery, hence a higher rate of conductive loss, perhaps due to the greater temperature gradient from the iris to the central corneal surface.

It has also been observed that steeper corneas exhibit a significantly steeper gradient [9], perhaps because of a greater rate of evaporative loss from an increased surface area.

24.4 OST and Ocular Factors

24.4.1 Blinking

Blinking facilitates the spread of warm tears over the cornea and conjunctiva, as the tear film thins after each blink, the surface will appear to cool. Hence, the more rapid cooling of the ocular surface in dry eye conditions appears to be related to reduced tear film stability and the increased rate of evaporation [9,10].

24.5 OST and Extraocular Factors

No effect of gender or race on OST has been observed in previous studies [9–11]. The effect of age on OST remains controversial, with some conflicting evidence that may suggest a negative correlation between age and OST [11], possibly due to changes in tear production and stability of the tear film.

Factors that have been proposed to influence OST include the following:

- Diurnal variation in body temperature
- Room temperature

A positive correlation between body temperature and room temperature has been reported [12,13].

24.6 OST and Ocular Pathology

24.6.1 Anterior Segment Pathology

Observational studies have been carried out variously to investigate the use of thermography in various ocular pathologies.

Increased blood flow from inflammatory conditions of the ocular surface, namely, the cornea and the conjunctiva, may result in detectable changes of the OST, such as scleritis, keratitis, and other forms of anterior segment inflammation such as acute anterior uveitis [4,9].

The role of ocular thermography in establishing the stability of the tear film layer and its relationship to dry eyes have been investigated [14,15]. A steeper thermal gradient from the corneal center to the limbus and a faster rate of cooling after each blink have been observed in dry eyes [9].

A study of OST and postoperative glaucoma eyes that have undergone trabeculectomy [16] suggests that thermography may have a role in evaluating bleb function. It was noted that functional blebs have lower temperatures than nonfunctional blebs. It is likely that the lower OST is due to the conductive loss of heat from the flow of aqueous humor, out of the scleral flap to perfuse the underlying subconjunctival space in a well-functioning bleb.

In refractive surgery, authors have proposed the use of thermography to measure the extent of thermal loading and to predict the likelihood of postoperative haze [17,18] following refractive procedures such as photorefractive keratectomy.

24.6.2 Posterior Segment Pathology

The potential of thermography in investigating posterior segment disorders remains limited. Negative correlation between OST and reduced blood flow to the eye in cases of carotid artery stenosis has been described [8,19]. Previous studies have also attempted to establish trends of OST in nonproliferative diabetic retinopathy and central vein occlusion [20,21] disorders of the eye. However, doubts remain as to how OST may predict posterior segment pathologies accurately even in cases of posterior segment inflammation, as it has been proposed that any heat produced by posterior segment inflammation will be dissipated by the highly vascularized retina, so any thermal gradient will be minimal and unlikely to influence OST [9].

24.7 Limitations and the Future of Ocular Thermography

To date, there is still insufficient knowledge of the normal thermogram, and without this, it is difficult to classify abnormalities [22,23].

Unanswered questions that remain and acceptable normal limits of OST awaiting to be established include its variability with age, axial length, and anterior chamber depth amongst others. The difficulty in interpreting current published data lies with the use of various camera systems that may produce variability in terms of measurement techniques and would require validation in terms of data procurement and applicability to the clinical setting; the small sample sizes through which these studies, largely of an observational nature, have been conducted; and the diurnal, intra- and interindividual variability in OST measurement that may confound studies of these nature. More work needs to be done to build systems of greater sensitivity that can detect temperature differences down to 0.01°C, especially for use in an organ as small and delicate as the eye. Efficiency in current systems are also limited by its convenience and speed at which the results are made available as data obtained via infrared cameras have to be separately analyzed via customized software programs that further limit its utility in a busy clinical setting. Till then, this method of assessing the OST is at best experimental, and there are certainly frontiers to be further explored and improved upon in ocular thermography.

References

1. Purslow C, Wolffsohn JS. Ocular surface temperature: A review. *Eye Contact Lens* 2005 May;31(3):117–123.
2. Mapstone R. Measurement of corneal temperature. *Exp Eye Res* 1968;7:237–243.

3. Mapstone R. Ocular thermography. *Br J Ophthalmol* 1970;54:751–754.
4. Mapstone R. Corneal thermal patterns in anterior uveitis. *Br J Ophthalmol* 1968;52:917–921.
5. Mapstone R. Normal thermal patterns in cornea and periorbital skin. *Br J Ophthalmol* 1968; 52:818–827.
6. Mapstone R. Thermometry and the eye. *Trans Ophthalmol Soc UK* 1969;88:693–699.
7. Mapstone R. Determinants of ocular temperature. *Br J Ophthalmol* 1968;52:729–741.
8. Mapstone R. Anterior segment hyperaemia and ischaemia. *Trans Ophthalmol Soc UK* 1970;90:329–335.
9. Morgan PB, Soh MP, Efron N, Tullo AB. Potential applications of ocular thermography. *Optom Vis Sci* 1993 July;70(7):568–576.
10. Efron N, Young G, Brennan NA. Ocular surface temperature. *Curr Eye Res* 1989;8:901–906.
11. Alio J, Padron M. Influence of age on the temperature of the anterior segment of the eye. *Ophthalmic Res* 1982;14:153–159.
12. Schwartz B. Environmental temperature and the ocular temperature gradient. *Arch Ophthalmol* 1965;74:237–243.
13. Freeman RD, Fatt I. Environmental influences on ocular temperature. *Invest Ophthalmol* 1973; 12:596–602.
14. Kamao T, Yamaguchi M, Kawasaki S, Mizoue S, Shiraishi A, Ohashi Y. Screening for dry eye with newly developed ocular surface thermographer. *Am J Ophthalmol* 2011 May;151(5):782–791.
15. Craig JP, Singh I, Tomlinson A, Morgan PB, Efron N. The role of tear physiology in ocular surface temperature. *Eye (Lond)* 2000 August;14(Pt 4):635–641.
16. Kawasaki S, Mizoue S, Yamaguchi M, Shiraishi A, Zheng X, Hayashi Y, Ohashi Y. Evaluation of filtering bleb function by thermography. *Br J Ophthalmol* 2009 October;93(10):1331–1336.
17. Betney S, Morgan PB, Doyle SJ et al. Corneal temperature changes during photorefractive keratectomy. *Cornea* 1997;16:158–161.
18. Maldonado-Codina C, Morgan PB, Efron N. Thermal consequences of photorefractive keratectomy. *Cornea* 2001;20:509–515.
19. Morgan PB, Smyth JV, Tullo AB, Efron N. Ocular temperature in carotid artery stenosis. *Optom Vis Sci* 1999 December;76(12):850–854.
20. Sodi A, Giambene B, Miranda P, Falaschi G, Corvi A, Menchini U. Ocular surface temperature in diabetic retinopathy: A pilot study by infrared thermography. *Eur J Ophthalmol* 2009 November–December;19(6):1004–1008.
21. Sodi A, Giambene B, Falaschi G, Caputo R, Innocenti B, Corvi A, Menchini U. Ocular surface temperature in central retinal vein occlusion: Preliminary data. *Eur J Ophthalmol* 2007 September–October;17(5):755–759.
22. Tan JH, Ng EYK, Rajendra Acharya U, Chee C. Study of normal ocular thermogram using textural parameters. *Infrared Phys Technol* 2010;53(2):120–126.
23. Tan JH, Ng EYK, Rajendra Acharya U, Chee C. Infrared thermography on ocular surface temperature: A review. *Infrared Phys Technol* 2009;52(4):97–108.

Index

D

K

L

M

N

O

P

Q

R

S

T

For Product Safety Concerns and Information please contact our EU representative GPSR@taylorandfrancis.com Taylor & Francis Verlag GmbH, Kaufingerstraße 24, 80331 München, Germany

Printed and bound by CPI Group (UK) Ltd, Croydon, CR0 4YY
01/05/2025
01858336-0001